Cross-Cultural Research in Health, Illness and Well-Being

Series editor

Pranee Liamputtong, School of Science and Health, Western Sydney University, Penrith, NSW, Australia

This new series examines determinants of health from a cross-cultural perspective. The focus of this perspective is on factors which could influence and determine the health and well-being of people. These factors include biological and genetic factors; health behaviors; socio-cultural and socio-economic factors and environment factors. This series fills a gap by including books which are research-based and contain diverse issues relevant to determinants of health including emerging health issues, such as HIV/AIDS and other infectious and non-infectious diseases/illnesses from a cross-cultural perspective. Volumes in the series will be a valuable resource for researchers and students in sociology, quality of life studies, anthropology, medicine, public health, social work and medicine.

More information about this series at http://www.springer.com/series/13178

Pranee Liamputtong
Editor

Children and Young People Living with HIV/AIDS

A Cross-Cultural Perspective

Springer

Editor
Pranee Liamputtong
School of Science and Health
Western Sydney University
Penrith, NSW, Australia

ISSN 2366-6056 ISSN 2366-6064 (electronic)
Cross-Cultural Research in Health, Illness and Well-Being
ISBN 978-3-319-29934-1 ISBN 978-3-319-29936-5 (eBook)
DOI 10.1007/978-3-319-29936-5

Library of Congress Control Number: 2016942861

Printed on acid-free paper

This Springer imprint is published by Springer Nature
The registered company is Springer International Publishing AG Switzerland

This book is dedicated to:

My late father, Saeng Liamputtong, who passed away in March 2014
My mother, Yindee Liamputtong, who brought up eight children amidst poverty
and
My two children: Zoe Sanipreeya Rice and Emma Inturatana Rice

Preface

Children and young people are at the center of HIV/AIDS epidemic. In 2014, UNAIDS reported that some 36.9 million (34.3–41.4 million) people were living with HIV. Every day, around 7000 persons become infected with HIV and 5000 persons die from AIDS, due mostly to lack of access to HIV prevention, care, and treatment services. Globally, AIDS-related illnesses remain a leading cause of death. The epidemic has spared no country in the world, although in some countries prevalence rates are still low.

HIV/AIDS have caused a "social assault" on the lives of children and young people in the world. Chapters in this volume attest to this. Many have been orphaned by the death of their HIV-positive parents. Young people, according to the United Nations, are "at the center of the HIV/AIDS epidemic." Many young people also bear the burden of caring for family members living with HIV/AIDS. Marginalized young people such as refugees, migrants, street children, and those who have been seen to have transgressed their gender norms (e.g., MSA, lesbians, bisexual, gays and transgender individuals) are most at risk due to the use of illicit drugs, their exposure to unprotected sex (in exchange for food, money and protection), and stigma associated with their marginalized lives. Worldwide, we have witnessed the impact that HIV/AIDS has on the opportunities for these young people to be able to lead healthy adult lives. It is crucial that the voices of these children and young people are heard, and their lived experiences and needs are better understood by health and social care providers, as well as researchers in the field so that culturally sensitive health and social care can be implemented for them.

The focus of this book is on the issues that these children and young people face and their lived experiences associated with HIV/AIDS (both directly and indirectly) throughout different parts of the globe. Chapters in this volume indeed affirm the need for us (health-care providers, researchers, and policymakers) to understand and better respond to the social conditions that dictate the health and well-being of children and young people living with HIV/AIDS.

Up until now, many articles have been written to portray children and young people living with HIV/AIDS in different parts of the world. But to my knowledge, there has not been any a single and recent book which attempts to put together results from empirical research that relates to children and young people who are living with HIV/AIDS. This book is written with the intention to fill this gap. The book comprises mainly chapters written by researchers who carry out their projects in different parts of the world. Each chapter contains theoretical and/or empirical information which is based on real-life situations. The volume also includes some chapters which are based on systematic review of literature. I contend that these chapters can be used as evidence for health-care providers to implement socially and culturally appropriate services to assist individuals and groups of children and young people who are living with HIV/AIDS in many societies.

I hope that the book will be of value to health-care providers who have their interests in working with children and young people living with HIV/AIDS from a cross-cultural perspective. The volume will be useful for students and lecturers in courses like anthropology, sociology, social work, nursing, public health, and medicine. In particular, it will assist health workers in community health centers and hospitals in understanding issues related to HIV/AIDS among children and young people and hence provide culturally sensitive health care to these individuals from different social and cultural backgrounds. The book will also be useful for anyone who is interested in children and young people living with HIV/AIDS in diverse social and cultural settings.

In bringing this book to life, I owe my gratitude to many people. First, I would like to thank all contributors who helped make this book possible. Second, I thank Esther Otten and Hendrikje Tuerlings of Springer who worked with me to bring this book to the final form. Last, Rosemary Oakes has helped edit some of the chapters for me.

This book is dedicated to my parents who brought their children up amidst poverty in Thailand. They believed that only education would improve the lives of their children and hence worked hard to send us to school. I have made my career thus far because of their beliefs and the opportunity that they both have provided for me. I thank them profoundly. I also dedicate this book to my two daughters who have been part of my life and for understanding the ongoing busy life of their mother.

Penrith, Australia
November 2015

Pranee Liamputtong

Contents

Contributors

Jamie Albright is a clinical psychology doctoral student at the University of Virginia. She received her BA in Public Health from Elon University in 2013 and her MA in Psychology from the University of Virginia in 2016. Her research is aimed at identifying ways to support marginalized adolescents' psychosocial well-being using a resilience framework.

Corry Azzopardi received her PhD and MSW from the University of Toronto's Factor-Inwentash Faculty of Social Work. She has been a social worker with the Hospital for Sick Children in Toronto since 2002. Her clinical practice, teaching, and research concentrate in the areas of child maltreatment and pediatric healthcare.

Gonzalo Bacigalupe is professor and director of Family Therapy and Counseling Psychology Programs at the University of Massachusetts Boston and is Ikerbasque Research Professor at the University of Deusto Bilbao. Bacigalupe is coprincipal investigator of a Patient-Centered Outcomes Research Institute Pilot research project. He is research faculty in the Health Equity Scholars Program (HESP) of the UMass Center for Health Equity Intervention Research (CHEIR). His research focuses on the impact of media on family health. He is president of the American Family Therapy Academy, fellow of the American Psychology Association, and member of several peer review journal editorial boards.

Peri J. Ballantyne a health sociologist, is an associate professor in the Department of Sociology, Trent University, Peterborough, Canada, and is affiliated with the Leslie Dan Faculty of Pharmacy, University of Toronto. Her research interests include the social determinants of health across the life course, professional-lay interactions in health care and lay interpretations of health and illness, and the sociology of pharmaceuticals. In qualitative research, she uses in-depth interviewing and focus group methods to understand the impact of social context on the meaning of human phenomenon such as health, illness, dis-/ability, and work/non-work.

Deevia Bhana is a professor in the School of Education, University of KwaZuluNatal, South Africa. Her research includes a focus on childhood sexualities, gender, schooling, and inequalities. She is a coauthor of *Towards Equality? Gender in South African Schools During the HIV/AIDS Pandemic* (2009, UKZN Press) and a coeditor of the book *Babies and/or Books: Pregnancy and Young Parents at School* (HSRC, 2012).

Olenka Bilash is professor of second language and intercultural education in the Department of Secondary Education, Faculty of Education, University of Alberta, Canada. She teaches and publishes in the areas of action research, qualitative research methodology, professional development, transformative practice, and intercultural communication and has worked on projects in Cameroon and South Africa.

Ari Bitnun is an associate professor of Pediatrics, University of Toronto, and a staff physician in the Division of Infectious Diseases, Department of Pediatrics, the Hospital for Sick Children. Ari received his MD from the University of British Columbia and completed his pediatric residency training in Israel and subsequently clinical and research infectious diseases fellowships at the Hospital for Sick Children. He has been involved in pediatric HIV clinical research since 1999 and has been a member of the Family-Centered HIV Clinic at the Hospital for Sick Children since 2004.

Jason Brophy is a pediatric infectious diseases physician and researcher at the Children's Hospital of Eastern Ontario and an assistant professor of pediatrics at the University of Ottawa. He completed his clinical and research fellowships in pediatric infectious diseases fellowship and HIV at the Hospital for Sick Children, University of Toronto. He has a Masters of Health Research Methodology from McMaster University. He is the current chair of the Canadian Pediatric/Perinatal AIDS Research Group. He has also worked as a pediatric HIV clinical advisor with the Clinton Health Access Initiative in Vietnam.

Catherine Campbell is professor and head of social psychology at the London School of Economics, where she directs the Health, Community, and Development Group. She has a particular interest in health inequalities and the role of small-scale collective action in supporting the well-being of marginalized groups, with particular reference to HIV/AIDS, mental health, and the health of women and children. She has published over 150 peer-reviewed papers on these topics.

Tomás Campbell is a clinical psychologist and neuropsychologist and has worked in the HIV field since 1990. Tomás spent 2 years working in an HIV NGO in Zambia in 1993-1994 and realized that psychological interventions with people with HIV had to be intensely practical in order to assist people with HIV to face the everyday challenges of living with the disease. This principle has guided his clinical work and his research interests. His research interests include the identification and mitigation of the neuropsychological impact of HIV in the developing brain, the impact of HIV-related stigma on the mental health of people with HIV and the development of psychological resilience in young people to and their families to face the challenges of life as a positive person. Tomás is a committee member of the British Psychological Society's Faculty for HIV & Sexual Health and a past chair. He is also the former president of the Royal Society of Medicine's Black Ethnic Minority Health Section (2013). He is a trustee of the UK-based Children's HIV Association (CHIVA) and chair of the trustees of AfricAid which supports the Whizzkids Academies in South Africa and Ghana.

Kathryn Cantrell is a doctoral student at University of Massachusetts Boston where she conducts research related to e-health interventions for individuals with chronic illnesses. Kathryn is a certified child life specialist with Developmental Therapeutic Source, LLC, where she provides psychosocial care to children with chronic illnesses. Prior to Kathryn's current positions, she worked at St. Jude Children's Research Hospital as a child life specialist for youth with HIV. Kathryn received her master of arts in child development from Tufts University where she currently lectures courses in pediatric psychology. Kathryn's research interests include supporting coping in youth with chronic illnesses and designing virtual interventions for coping.

Rachel Chickerella was born in Columbus, Ohio, and lives in Boston, Massachusetts. She completed her undergraduate degree at Xavier University majoring in psychology with a double minor in criminal justice in philosophy. While completing her degree, she worked as a research assistant in the Epilepsy Adherence Lab at Cincinnati Children's Hospital, was a peer mediator in a girls' after-school club, and participated in the Inside-Out Prison Exchange Program. Rachel is currently working on her masters in mental health counseling at the University of Massachusetts, Boston. She works as a research assistant for Dr. Bacigalupe looking at the efficacy of online support communities. She also researches trauma informed practice in early childhood education.

Magda Conway has worked with children and HIV for 11 years, being the UK policy lead at the National Children's Bureau and then as a freelance consultant, supporting (among others) the Children's HIV Association and UNICEF. Magda has set up peer support groups, developed numerous participation and peer support projects, delivered training, and written extensively about this group.

Marguerite Daniel is currently an associate professor of development-related health promotion at the HEMIL Centre, University of Bergen. Her research interests include children affected and infected by HIV, the impact on social cohesion of international aid targeting children, and local and global perspectives on child protection, in southern and eastern Africa, in particular Botswana and Tanzania. Her theoretical stance is salutogenic and is concerned with how children thrive in adversity.

Michelle Di Risio is a flex-time PhD student in the Department of Pharmaceutical Sciences, University of Toronto, Toronto, Canada. She is also employed at Hoffmann La Roche in the Medical Affairs Department. Her academic interests are in applying sociological approaches to examine the broader social, political, cultural, and historical organization of various medical concepts such as the meanings of illness and the dying process.

Mangi J. Ezekiel is an employee of Muhimbili University of Health and Allied Science as Lecturer in the Behavioural Sciences department. His background is in medical sociology and anthropology. Prior to joining MUHAS, he worked briefly as a community development worker at Plan International. He is an excellent team worker with interpersonal communication and social skills. After completing his undergraduate and postgraduate studies in Tanzania, he conducted extensive research with young people that culminated into a PhD (medical anthropology) at the University of Oslo in Norway.

Cynthia D. Fair is a professor of human service studies and coordinator of public health studies at Elon University. Her clinical and research interests include HIV-infected and affected youth and women as well as HIV-related stigma and discrimination. Her most recent research is focused on the transition of youth with HIV from pediatric to adult infectious disease care, as well as the reproductive decisions of youth with perinatally acquired HIV infection.

Bonnie Fournier is a PhD candidate and lecturer at the University of Alberta, Faculty of Nursing. Her recent research projects have focused on the role of Ugandan nurses caring for individuals with HIV and AIDS and the experience of Ugandan children who are orphaned and HIV seropositive. Her qualitative research expertise is in participatory action research, photovoice, and other arts-based methods. She has many years of international experience in Zambia working for MSF (Medecins Sans Frontieres), in Uganda, working with children affected by war, in Zimbabwe working as an HIV and AIDS research consultant, and in Qatar teaching nursing.

Simon Gregson trained as demographer at the London School of Economics and Political Science in the late 1980s before completing a DPhil at the Centre for Epidemiology of Infectious Disease at the University of Oxford. He was appointed to the academic staff in the Department of Infectious Disease Epidemiology at Imperial College London in 2001 and was awarded a chair in Demography and Behavioural Science in 2008. Simon set up and directs the Manicaland Project, a longitudinal study using quantitative, qualitative, and mathematical modeling methods to describe and interpret trends in the spread and control of HIV in eastern Zimbabwe.

Jayne Griffiths is a London-based clinical psychologist who has been centrally involved in designing and delivering clinical psychology interventions to HIV-positive people since 2008. She is a member of the Looking Forward Day project group that runs a long-term group based program for young people over the age of 12 years who are aware of their diagnosis. She has also run parenting courses for HIV-positive parents. She is interested in systemic approaches to her family-based clinical work and has also led the Looking Forward group in the development and application of the Tree of Life approach. Jayne has contributed to the development of UK standards about HIV disclosure to HIV-positive young people and has undertaken teaching, advice, and support to primary health-care clinicians working with HIV-positive adolescents in South Africa.

Eleanor Holroyd is a Professor of Nursing, School of Clinical Sciences, Auckland University of Technology, Auckland, New Zealand. She is a senior medical anthropologist working on researches of sex workers, HIV/AID, sex education and barriers for condom use.

Md Shahidul Islam completed his PhD at the School of Health, University of New England, Armidale, Australia. He completed MSc in International Health from Royal Tropical Institute, Amsterdam, the Netherlands; Queen Margaret University, Edinburgh, UK; and Karolinska Institutet, Stockholm, Sweden. He received his bachelor (Hon's) and master degrees in sociology from the University of Dhaka, Bangladesh. Currently, he is teaching at the School of Health, University of New England, Armidale, Australia. He is also an associate professor of sociology discipline at Khulna University, Bangladesh. His teaching and research interests include the sociology of health and medicine, HIV/AIDS, gender, and sexuality.

Larissa Kojoué has a PhD in political sciences. She is a research associate at Les Afriques dans le Monde (LAM, Bordeaux) and African Studies Centre (ASC, Leiden). Her areas of interest include HIV/AIDS, global health, public policies, children, social movements, and human rights in Cameroon.

Joseph T.F. Lau is a Professor and Head of the Division of Health Improvement and the Director of the Centre of Health Behaviors Research of the School of Public Health and Primary Care, the Chinese University of Hong Kong. He is a senior public health scholar working on interdisciplinary evidence-based and theory-based research on HIV prevention and care in China.

Haochu (Howard) Li is an Early Career Researcher in the UNC Project-China, Institute for Global Health and Infectious Diseases, University of North Carolina at Chapel Hill, NC, United States, and a postdoctoral fellow in the School of Public Health, Shandong University, Jinan, China. He is a medical anthropologist trained in multiple disciplines, obtaining a master degree in anthropology, a master degree in health social sciences, and a PhD in public health. His research topics included sexual identity, sexual health, sexual culture, sexual risk behavior, mental health, and health service seeking among men who have sex with men in China. Some of his researches have been published in peer-review journals or presented in international conferences.

Xiaoming Li is a Professor and SmartState Chair for Clinical Translational Research, Department of Health Promotion, Education, and Behavior, Arnold School of Public Health, Columbia, SC, United States. He is a senior psychologist working on interdisciplinary HIV/AIDS studies among migrants, sex workers, and family affected by HIV/AIDS.

Catherine MacPhail has worked in HIV prevention in South Africa for the past 15 years, specifically focusing on adolescents. She is currently working on examining the role of cash transfers and community norms for preventing HIV infection in young South African women, investigating the issues associated with aging, HIV, and sexual health in South Africa and Australia and sexual health of Australian adolescents. She holds a postdoctoral fellowship at the Collaborative Research Network at the University of New England and an honorary appointment at the Wits Reproductive Health and HIV Institute, University of the Witwatersrand.

Vivian Midtbø is currently employed as a researcher at the National Centre for Emergency Primary Health Care, Uni Research, Bergen. She is previously trained as a nurse, and she completed her master of philosophy of health promotion at the University of Bergen in spring 2012. Her research interests include children and adolescents living with HIV, health promotion, primary health care, and clinical development for nurses in the primary health-care sector.

Angela Miller was a senior social worker at the Paediatric HIV Service at Sydney Children's Hospital for 10 years where she provided psychosocial support and counseling to children, families, and pregnant women with HIV. In addition, she coordinated Camp Goodtime and the Positive Kids camps. Angela recently took up a new position as senior social worker/counselor at the Short Street Sexual Health Centre in Sydney.

Paul Miller is a director in the Institute for Educational Administration & Leadership-Jamaica (IEAL-J) and a former professor of Educational Leadership & Management in the School of Graduate Studies, Research & Entrepreneurship, University of Technology, Jamaica. He is currently a reader in education at Brunel University London, where he is also a program leader for the MA education. He has a master of laws degree specializing in minorities (children) rights and the law.

Victor Minichiello is emeritus professor at the University of New England; adjunct professor at The Australian Research Centre in Sex, Health & Society, La Trobe University; and section editor of *BMC Public Health*. He has published extensively on topics related to sexual health, sexualities, and ageism. His recent research projects focus on the sexual and intimacy experiences of older women, male sex work and society, and the use of e-technology to facilitate positive health outcomes.

Pattaraporn Moolchaem is a PhD candidate in the School of Public Health and Human Biosciences, La Trobe University. Her PhD thesis is focusing on the lived experiences, health, and well-being among male-to-female transgendered individuals in Thailand. Pattaraporn has experience working in behavioral and medical research on HIV/AIDS and other sexually transmitted infections among males who have sex with males and transgender people. She has also held a position of lecturer at the Faculty of Nursing, Ratchathani University, Thailand, and associated researcher in gender identity and transgenderism at Transgender ASIA Research Centre based in Hong Kong. Pattaraporn identifies herself as a transsexual woman.

Ami Moore is a social demographer at the University of North Texas, Denton. Her research interests are in health-related studies as well as gender and place of birth factors in the economic assimilation of immigrants in the USA. She has conducted HIV and AIDS research on different population groups in Ghana and Togo. She uses both qualitative and quantitative methodologies in her research. She teaches graduate and undergraduate courses in demography and sociology. She was a Fulbright Scholar twice.

Zivai Mupambireyi is a Zimbabwe-based qualitative social scientist with 13 years of research experience in the field of HIV/AIDS. She obtained a Wellcome Trust Masters fellowship in 2008 and undertook an MSc in health, community, and development at the London School of Economics and Political Science (LSE; www.lse.ac.uk), with a focus on health services research. She is currently enrolled as a PhD student at the University College London (UCL; www.ucl.ac.uk). Her research interests lie in adolescent health, HIV/AIDS, Children and Antiretroviral Therapy with the aim of making recommendations on the best methods of service delivery/implementation.

Christy E. Newman is a senior research fellow at the Centre for Social Research in Health (formerly the National Centre in HIV Social Research) at UNSW. She is a qualitative researcher interested in the social aspects of engaging different populations and professional groups with contemporary health imperatives and health services, particularly in relation to HIV and sexual health care.

Sylvia Niele is currently a registered psychologist working in private practice in Melbourne, Australia. She has also worked in various public mental health settings and been involved in longitudinal research on healthy ageing. Sylvia's interest in HIV/AIDS was sparked while doing volunteer work among street youth in Durban, South Africa, witnessing the devastating impact of the pandemic first hand. This posed the question, "Why is HIV/AIDS continuing to spread in this developing country?" and inspired a return trip to Durban to collect data exploring the role of culture, attitudes, beliefs, and stigma toward HIV/AIDS among this disenfranchised and vulnerable group.

Constance Nyamukapa is currently employed by Imperial College London as Research Associate. Her first degree was in social work (University of Zimbabwe-1996). In 1998 she joined the Manicaland HIV/STD Prevention Project and has been with the project since. In 2000–2001 she was awarded Wellcome Trust fellowship to do an MSc in population and development at London School of Economics and Political Science, UK. In 2003–2007 Constance was awarded scholarship to do PhD at Imperial College London, and her thesis focused on psychosocial well-being of HIV-affected orphans in eastern Zimbabwe. Areas of interest center around HIV impact on OVC (psychosocial well-being and educational outcomes) and general population.

Georgina Yaa Oduro is a lecturer at the Department of Sociology and Anthropology, University of Cape Coast, Ghana. She holds a PhD from the University of Cambridge, UK, and an MA in Human Resource Management from the University of Westminster, London. She completed her PhD in 2010 having researched the topic "Gender relations, sexuality and HIV/AIDS education within the context of Ghanaian youth cultures". She has an interdisciplinary background in sociology, education and management. She is a qualitative researcher with expertise in creative data collection methods such as drawings, stories, essays, body mapping, etc. Her research interests include gender relations, youth cultures, sexuality, sexual health, social contexts of HIV/AIDS and other medical practice in Africa. She has been involved in both local and international research projects and has some publications to her credit. She has also won a number of scholarships and awards.

Adobea Owusu holds a PhD and MA from the University of North Texas (UNT), Denton, Texas, and an MPH from the UNT School of Biomedical Sciences at Forth Worth, Texas, USA. She also holds graduate diploma and bachelor of science (Hons.) from the University of Ghana, Legon. She has a faculty position at the University of Ghana, Legon. Adobea is currently the head of the Social Division of the Institute of Statistical, Social and Economic Research at the University of Ghana, where she teaches graduate courses. Her current research focuses on sexuality, access to health care, and HIV/AIDS.

Asha Persson is a social anthropologist by training and a research fellow at the Centre for Social Research in Health (formerly the National Centre in HIV Social Research) at the University of New South Wales where she does sociologically informed qualitative research on various cultural and lived aspects of HIV, with particular focus on the experiences and needs of previously hidden or under-researched populations within the Australian epidemic, including heterosexuals, children, and couples with mixed HIV status.

Audrey Pettifor is an associate professor in the Department of Epidemiology at the University of North Carolina at Chapel Hill and a faculty fellow at the Carolina Population Center. Her research focuses on determinants of HIV/STI in sub-Saharan Africa with the goal of identifying modifiable risk factors and developing novel interventions to prevent new HIV infections—particularly in young women. Audrey has conducted HIV research in South Africa for over 15 years and also has worked in Malawi, Zimbabwe, Kenya, the Democratic Republic of Congo, and Madagascar.

She has experience in conducting structural interventions including the role of incentives for HIV prevention, community mobilization to change negative gender norms, and interventions to promote linkages to care. She received her PhD in epidemiology and MPH in maternal and child health from the University of California, Berkeley.

Saumya RamaRao is a senior associate with the Population Council's Reproductive Health program. She oversees major product introduction research, generates evidence about health systems and the people who use them, and provides technical assistance for program design and implementation. Her areas of research interest include safe abortion, safe motherhood, and family planning. She conducts on-the-ground research to identify specific reproductive health needs, works closely with Ministry of Health officials and service-delivery organizations to expand their range and quality of services, and provides technical assistance and support to program monitoring and evaluation. She is also a member of the Council's Institutional Review Board providing ethical oversight to institutionally developed projects.

Stanley Read is professor emeritus of Pediatrics at the University of Toronto. He is a consultant in Pediatric Infectious Diseases at the Hospital for Sick Children. He has been director of the HIV/AIDS Family-Centered Care Program since its inception in 1988. He chairs the Scientific Advisory Committee of the Canadian Foundation for AIDS Research and is consultant to the Ministry of Health of the Bahamas. His major research interests include exploring determinates of a functional cure, HIV transmission in babies of HIV-infected women, neurocognitive development in children exposed to antiretrovirals, and gene therapy in HIV infection.

Laura Robertson worked as a social epidemiologist in the Department of Infectious Disease Epidemiology, Imperial College London from 2006 to 2013. While studying for her PhD, she researched orphanhood and its impact on children and young adolescents in the context of the HIV/AIDS epidemic in sub-Saharan Africa, particularly in Zimbabwe. She later evaluated a cash transfer program for orphaned and other vulnerable children, in Manicaland, Zimbabwe. She is currently training to be a mental health nurse at Middlesex University.

Robyn Salter has a master's degree in social work from Carleton University, Ottawa, Ontario, Canada. She is a social worker of the Infectious Diseases Program at Sick Kids in Toronto and has been a social worker in the HIV program since it started in 1988. Her clinical practice and research have focused on psychosocial issues for children, teenagers, and families with HIV including parenting children with HIV, stigma and disclosure of HIV status to children, teens transitioning to adult health care, and issues for parents going through treatment to prevent transmission during pregnancy and early infancy.

Stephanie Savage holds a master's degree in social work from the University of Toronto. She also completed a Universities Without Walls HIV research fellowship. She is currently working with children and families affected by HIV. In her clinical practice, she specializes in health and mental health. Her research has focused on issues for people living with HIV and practice considerations for support providers working with them including HIV nondisclosure criminalization, peer support, and mental health.

Katie D. Schenk is a research assistant professor in the Department of Global and Community Health at George Mason University, Virginia, USA. She is the principal investigator of an NIH-funded research study exploring HIV status disclosure among children and caregivers in Zimbabwe. She teaches courses on global health and research methodology to graduate students. She has extensive research experience focused on mitigating the impacts of HIV on children and families in sub-Saharan Africa. She has conducted fieldwork at diverse research sites, including in Kenya, South Africa, Tanzania, Uganda, Zambia, and Zimbabwe. From 2002 to 2014, she led a portfolio of applied social and behavioral research studies in HIV and sexual and reproductive health at the Population Council, where she now serves on the Institutional Review Board.

John Scott is a professor at the University of New England Australia. He has published approximately 80 books, articles, and book chapters on a broad range of issues associated with the sociology of health and illness and sociology of gender and sexuality. A common theme in his research has been a concern with marginalized social populations and the development of critical and interpretive perspectives to understand the experiences of and social reactions to such populations. His most recent book (edited with Minichiello) is *Male Sex work and Society* (Harrington Park Press).

Morten Skovdal is an associate professor of Global Health at the University of Copenhagen. Morten trained as a community health psychologist at the London School of Economics and Political Science and received his PhD in 2009. Before taking up his academic post, Morten worked as a senior advisor on impact and evidence with Save the Children. Much of his research is focused on children's experiences of the HIV epidemic in sub-Saharan Africa, inspired by the need to appropriate and align HIV technologies and development interventions with local realities.

Stephen Wallder is lecturer in business and management in the Faculty of Educational Studies at the University of Technology, Jamaica. He has over 25 years teaching and industry experience. He has led workplace education programs and advised companies on workplace policies in relation to HIV/AIDS. He was the both chair and vice-chair for the Jamaica Business Council on HIV/AIDS (the Business response umbrella organization to HIV/AIDS in Jamaica).

Nataly Woollett is currently a technical team head at Wits Reproductive Health and HIV Institute (WRHI) where the focus is to integrate psychosocial aspects of health and HIV into public health systems. Nataly, in collaboration with WHO, is also the principal investigator of an RCT intervention study conducted in antenatal clinics for pregnant women experiencing intimate partner violence. Nataly has particular expertise in areas of mental health and HIV, gender-based violence and HIV, trauma and traumatic bereavement, and the special needs of OVC and child/adolescent witnesses of violence. Nataly has trained in the fields of psychology, art therapy, and play therapy. She is currently completing her PhD at Wits University School of Clinical Medicine on the mental health outcomes of HIV-positive adolescents.

About the Editor

Pranee Liamputtong is a medical anthropologist and professor of Public Health at the School of Science and Health, Western Sydney University, Sydney, Australia. Until early 2016, Pranee held a personal chair in Public Health at the Department of Public Health, School of Psychology and Public Health, College of Science, Health and Engineering, La Trobe University, Melbourne, Australia. Pranee has also previously taught in the School of Sociology and Anthropology and worked as a public health research fellow at the Centre for the Study of Mothers' and Children's Health, La Trobe University. Pranee has a particular interest in issues related to cultural and social influences on childbearing, childrearing, women's reproductive and sexual health, and the health of children. She has published several books and a large number of papers in these areas.

Some of her recent books in the health and social sciences include: *The Journey of Becoming a Mother Amongst Women in Northern Thailand* (Lexington Books, 2007); *Community, Health and Population* (Oxford University Press, 2009); *Infant Feeding Practices: A Cross-Cultural Perspective* (Springer 2011); *Motherhood and Postnatal Depression: Narratives of Women and Their Partners* (Springer, 2011); *Health, Illness and Well-Being: Perspectives and Social Determinants* (Oxford University Press, 2012); *Women, Motherhood and HIV/AIDS: A Cross-Cultural Perspective* (Springer, 2013); *Stigma, Discrimination and HIV/AIDS: A Cross-Cultural Perspective* (Springer, 2013); and *Contemporary Socio-Cultural and Political Perspectives in Thailand* (Springer, 2014). Her new book on *Public Health: Local and Global Perspective* has recently been published by Cambridge University Press in early 2016.

Pranee is a qualitative researcher and has also published several method books. Her most recent method books include: *Researching the Vulnerable: A Guide to Sensitive Research Methods* (Sage, 2007); *Performing Qualitative Cross-Cultural Research* (Cambridge University Press, 2010); *Focus Group Methodology: Principles and Practice* (Sage, 2011); *Qualitative Research Methods, 4th Edition*

(Oxford University Press, 2013); *Research Methods in Health: Foundations for Evidence-Based Practice, 2nd Edition* (Oxford University Press, 2013); and *Participatory Qualitative Research Methodologies in Health* (Sage, 2015). She is currently working on a series of books on research methods in the health social sciences for Springer and the third edition of *Research Methods in Health* book for Oxford University Press (due in early 2017).

Chapter 1
Children, Young People and HIV/AIDS: A Cross-Cultural Perspective

Pranee Liamputtong

Contents

1.1 Children, Young People and HIV/AIDS

In 2013, UNAIDS reported some 35.3 million (32.2–38.8 million) people were living with HIV. UNAIDS also suggests that every day, around 7000 persons become infected with HIV and 5000 persons die from AIDS, due mostly to lack of access to HIV prevention, care and treatment services. Globally, AIDS-related illnesses remain a leading cause of death (UNAIDS 2013). The epidemic has spared no country in the world, although in some countries prevalence rates are still low. However, it should be noted that low prevalence rates at national level may mask pockets within a country where the rate is high.

Children and young people, according to the United Nations (2013), are "at the center of the HIV/AIDS epidemic" (Lowenthal et al. 2014a: 143). Currently, about 5.4 million people aged 10–24 are living with HIV/AIDS. Many of these young people acquired HIV perinatally but about 780,000 young people aged 15–24 are newly infected (UNAIDS 2013). Approximately 97 % of the new infections take

P. Liamputtong (✉)
School of Science and Health, Western Sydney University, Penrith 2751, NSW, Australia
e-mail: p.liamputtong@westernsydney.edu.au

P. Liamputtong (ed.), *Children and Young People Living with HIV/AIDS*, Cross-Cultural Research in Health, Illness and Well-Being,
DOI 10.1007/978-3-319-29936-5_1

place in low- and middle-income nations (UNAIDS 2013), and about 90 % of these young people live in resource-poor settings in sub-Saharan Africa (UNAIDS 2012; Lowenthal et al. 2014a, b).

Children and young people who are living with HIV/AIDS are from the most marginalized and vulnerable groups in the world (Orban et al. 2010; Kumar 2012; UNAIDS 2013; Bell and Aggleton 2014). For most young people living with HIV/AIDS, they have to deal with multiple issues including stigma, fears about illness and contamination, concerns about their life expectancy, clinic appointments and medication regimens, as well as a desire to be a 'normal' person, engaging in intimate relationships, and concerns about reproductive health needs (Brown et al. 2000; Jaspan et al. 2009; King et al. 2009; Fair and Albright 2012; Snyder et al. 2014; see also Chaps. 4, 6, 10, 18, 19, 20, and 21 in this volume). Natalie Woollett contends in Chap. 4 that HIV-positive young people are affected by the HIV epidemic in various ways. Not only that they have to deal with their own illnesses and uncertain futures, they also "suffer trauma and grief as they watch their parents and family members die, many lose siblings and their home at the event of a parents' passing as siblings are displaced to various family members and areas in the country". Similarly, Shahidul Islam, John Scott and Victor Minichiello (Chap. 3) write that existing research has pointed to many risks and pressures on the lives of children living with HIV/AIDS. These include withdrawal from school, increased household activity burdens, lack of access to health care, malnutrition, emotional stress, social stigma and discrimination, as well as increased risks of HIV infection, abuse, and exploitation (see also Beard et al. 2010; Leeper et al. 2010; Chi and Li 2013).

Many children have been made orphan by the death of their HIV-positive parents (Watts et al. 2005; Kang et al. 2008; Kumar 2012; Nyberg et al. 2012; Campbell et al. 2014; see Chaps. 2, 3, 4, 9, 16, 20, and 24 in this volume). Often, death of parents leads to the loss of family income and property and this has a detrimental impact on the lives of young people in the family. Many children and young people are forced to withdraw from school and work in order to pay for the medical and household expenses of the family (Harms et al. 2010; Kumar 2012; Chi and Li 2013). Islam and colleagues (Chap. 3) contend that "the passing of one or both parents ultimately results in single parenthood or being orphaned, and possibly placement with alternate caregivers and unstable living arrangements. These experiences can trigger intense grief, feelings of abandonment, and disruptions in attachment security". For young people living in a household infected with HIV/AIDS, they bear the burden of caring for their parents and other family members who are no longer able to take care of themselves (Cluver and Gardner 2007; Evans and Becker 2009; Skovdal et al. 2009; Kumar 2012; Skovdal and Campbell 2013; Pearlstein et al. 2014; see also Chaps. 2, 3, and 16 in this volume). This has great impact on their health and well-being.

There are particular groups of children and young people who seem to be affected more by HIV/AIDS. Young people who have a marginalized gender norm such as men having sex with men (MSM) are at great risk for HIV/AIDS and mental health burdens (Courtenay-Quirk et al. 2006; Beyrer et al. 2010; Geibel et al. 2010;

Dahoma et al. 2011; Kemeny 2011; Semple et al. 2011; Okonofua 2012; Zanoni and Mayer 2014; see also Chaps. 11, 12, 13, and 18 in this volume). Other marginalized young people such as refugees, migrants, ethnic minority groups, and street children are most at risk due to the use of illicit drugs, their exposure to unprotected sex (in exchange for food, money and protection), and stigma associated with their marginalized lives (Orban et al. 2010; MacDonell et al. 2013; see also Chaps. 9, 13, 18, 20, 21, 22, and 24 in this volume). Children and young people from migrant and refugee backgrounds face additional marginalization and challenges resulting from the burdens of trying to adapt into a new living situation, losses and traumas in their country of origin, social isolation, barriers to employment, and poverty (see also Chaps. 9 and 20).

Perinatally-infected children and young people are often referred to as a "hidden population". They are "a forgotten part of the AIDS epidemic" (Dorrell and Katz 2014: 454). Little research has paid attention to the social and psychological impact of living with HIV among this group of young people (Bell et al. 2003; Green and Smith 2004; Fielden et al. 2006; Mellins et al. 2009; CHIPS 2012; Dorrell and Katz 2013, 2014; see also Chaps. 5, 6, 18, 19, 20 and 21 in this volume). Nevertheless, Michelle DiRisio and Peri Ballantyne (Chap. 5) and Asha Persson, Christy Newman and Angela Miller (Chap. 6) have suggested that these young people do have positive experiences if there are sensitive interventions or programs that cater for their needs and concerns.

Girls and young women are affected by HIV/AIDS much more than boys and young men. Similar to gender inequalities among women in general, gender play a significant role in the health and well-being of HIV-positive children and young people (Gupta et al. 2011; Ramjee and Wand 2014; see also Chaps. 3, 4, 7, and 15 in this volume). It has been recognized globally that gender inequalities render girls and young women vulnerable to HIV/AIDS (UNAIDS 2013). Deevia Bhana argues in Chap. 7 that "gender inequalities and harmful gender norms create a burden on women and girls reducing their ability to negotiate safe sex… Unequal gender power relations play a significant role in HIV settings and drives young women's vulnerability to disease" (see also Gupta et al. 2011; Jewkes and Morrell 2010, 2012; Liamputtong 2013a; Fleming et al. 2014; Chap. 15 in this volume).

1.2 Living with HIV/AIDS and Mental Health Issues

Globally, HIV/AIDS and depression are the main causes of the burden of disease for young people (UNICEF 2011; Betancourt et al. 2013; United Nations 2014). Depending on the research methodology and samples of the study, it has been shown that major depression is highly prevalent among HIV-positive individuals, ranging between 18 % and 81 % (Arseniou et al. 2013). In poor nations in particular, mental health problems are at the foreground of disease burden in young people (United Nations 2014). Research has pointed to the increased risk for poor mental health outcomes among young people living with HIV/AIDS (see also Chaps. 3, 4, 9, 12,

18, 20, and 21 in this volume). Often, this is the result of stigma and discrimination towards them. Children whose parents are HIV-positive may also see themselves as "tainted" or "contaminated" due to the HIV status of their parents (Harms et al. 2010; Chi and Li 2013). Islam et al. show this in their chapter (Chap. 3) that, "children were rejected and discriminated against directly and indirectly by peers and community members because of their parents' HIV-positive status". Other researchers have also revealed similar findings (see Mahati et al. 2006; Surkan et al. 2010). Thus, children of HIV-positive parents tend to suffer from emotional distress and depression.

Many of these young people also reside in poor families with high level of food insecurity (Cluver et al. 2011; Boudreau and Fisher 2012; Betancourt et al. 2013; Mellins and Malee 2013; Bernays et al. 2014; Lowenthal et al. 2014a, b; see also Chaps. 3, 4, 9, and 15 in this volume). Other social contexts of HIV including poverty, familial disruption, and orphanhood, may play a significant role in the higher rate of mental health problems among these young people (Domek 2009; Williams et al. 2007; Thom 2012; Lowenthal et al. 2014a, b).

1.3 HIV/AIDS, Stigma and Discrimination

As discussed in the above section, HIV-positive children and young people suffer from psycho-social disadvantages as a consequence of HIV/AIDS-related stigma, directly and indirectly. Literature concerning HIV/AIDS and children and young people reveals the high prevalence of stigma that these vulnerable people encounter in their everyday life (Messer et al. 2010; Chi and Li 2013; Liamputtong 2013b). Almost all chapters in this volume will also attest to this.

Stigma, according to Goffman (1963: 3) is a "process of devaluation" associated with stereotyping and prejudice. It is employed by individuals to define certain attributes of others as "discreditable or unworthy, resulting in the person stigmatized becoming "discounted" or "tainted"" (Thomas 2006: 3175). Stigma has also been referred to as "a reaction to fear or perceived threat" (Sivaram et al. 2009: 234). Parker and Birdsall (2005: 5) contend that stigma is part of prejudiced 'identity', and sets apart "individuals or groups through the attachment of heightened negative perceptions and values" (see also Chaps. 3, 4, 6, 8, 9, 12, 14,17, 18, 19, 20, 21, 22, and 24 in this volume).

Although stigma is a socially constructed concept, it has a negative impact on the life as well as the health and well-being of the individuals who are so labeled (Liamputtong and Kitisriworapan 2012; Liamputtong 2013b). Sontag (1991) contends that HIV/AIDS symbolizes 'sinful' and 'evil'. Hence, people living with HIV/AIDS are perceived as discredited individuals who have "[im]moral characters". As a consequence, they are socially conditioned as "others" (Mason et al. 2001). Often, this leads to discrimination against the discredited persons.

From the onset of the epidemic, HIV/AIDS has been seen not only as a medical condition, but also as a stigmatized illness (Herek and Glunt 1993; Scambler 2003;

Letteney and LaPorte 2004). Since the recognition of HIV/AIDS in 1981, it has provoked forceful reactions from others (Scambler 2003). HIV/AIDS uniquely combined "sex, drugs, death and contagion" (Scambler 2003: 199). This unique combination made HIV/AIDS a powerfully stigmatizing disease. It is also prevalent among those who are already members of stigmatized groups, initially gay men, later injecting drug users (Scambler 2003; Parker and Aggleton 2003). Globally, in countries where HIV/AIDS is predominantly heterosexually transmitted, stigmatization and discrimination are also pervasive. The stigmatization and discrimination of these people have violated human rights of human beings. Clearly, as Mann and Tarantola (1998: 4–5) put it, "those who – before the arrival of HIV/AIDS – were socially marginalized, stigmatized or discriminated against, were found gradually and increasingly to bear the brunt of the HIV/AIDS epidemic. Human rights violations are now recognized to be primordial root causes of vulnerability to the epidemic" (see also Chap. 14 in this volume).

In their chapter with HIV-positive youth in Australia (Chap. 6), Asha Persson, Christie Newman and Angela Miller write that "the social stigma related to having HIV is a fundamental aspect of their disease that sets these young people apart from their peers and profoundly shapes their life experience and sense of self". Many studies have also revealed that stigma associated with HIV/AIDS is a "destructive influence" on the well-being and quality of life of HIV-positive young people (Fair et al. 2011; Martinez et al. 2012; Dorrell and Katz 2013; Mellins and Malee 2013; Rydström et al. 2013).

1.4 HIV/AIDS, Secrecy and Disclosure

Closely related to stigma and discrimination is the notion of secrecy and disclosure (Fielden et al. 2006; Abramowitz et al. 2009; Vijayan et al. 2009; Dorrell and Katz 2013; Rydström et al. 2013; see Chaps. 5, 6, 7, 17, 18, 19, 20, 21, and 22). Secrecy (non-disclosure) is a means that individuals who experience stigma use to hide their "discredited identity" (Goffman 1974). Disclosure has received much attention in literature concerning HIV/AIDS. HIV disclosure or nondisclosure is a complex phenomenon. There are various issues influencing the decision-making and process of disclosure. The experiences of a person living with HIV/AIDS who decides to disclose or not disclose is also diverse. The choice of disclosure or non-disclosure is a reflection of how each HIV-positive person experiences and deals with HIV/AIDS in their everyday life (Bailey and Darak 2013; Dorrell and Katz 2013; Greeff 2013; Sauceda et al. 2013; Chew et al. 2014; Liamputtong and Haritavorn 2015). Disclosure can have both positive and negative consequences (Greeff 2013). It can lead to more social support from family members and others (Ross et al. 2007; Liamputtong and Haritavorn 2015). However, disclosure is intrinsically linked with stigma and discrimination (Scambler 2009; Liamputtong et al. 2012; Liamputtong and Haritavorn 2015). A disclosure of HIV status can also be problematic for many

HIV-positive people. It creates anxiety because these individuals cannot foretell the feelings and reactions of others by their disclosure.

In their research with HIV-positive young people in Australian, Persson et al. tell us that due to fears of being rejected or ostracized, most of them did not disclose their HIV status to their friends and peer network. They did so to protect themselves from stigma and discrimination. For these young people, secrecy, Persson et al. suggest, is "a sensible tactic to avoid social disapproval of an aspect of their life that they consider as marginal in their 'psychic economies' " (Seidman et al. 1999: 18). Within a household, parents may keep the HIV status of their children secret. Often, they are concerned about emotional impact on their children and fear of stigmatization (Nöstlinger et al. 2006; Wiener et al. 2007; Zhang et al. 2013). Due to secrecy in families, young people growing up with HIV have been portrayed as "an isolated and hidden population" (Fielden et al. 2006; Fair and Albright 2012). This might also contribute to the risk of emotional and behavioral problems among these young people (Rydström et al. 2013; see Chap. 6).

Nevertheless, Persson et al. (Chap. 6) also suggest that disclosure can be a "therapeutic emancipation" for young people living with HIV/AIDS. Vivian Midtbo and Marguerite Daniel also illustrate in their chapter (Chap. 17) that disclosure acts as a positive resource for HIV-positive young people in Botswana. Battles and Wiener (2002: 309) point out that disclosure is a "positive factor in long term survival and decreased problem behavior" in young people. Disclosure is also "positively associated with social support and self confidence" (see also Ferris et al. 2007; Lam et al. 2007; Liamputtong and Haritavorn 2015). Positive outcomes of disclosure include: the "promotion of trust, improved adherence, open family communication, and better long-term health and emotional well-being in children" (Wiener et al. 2007, p. 156; Dorrell and Katz 2014: 454).

With the complexity of antiretroviral therapy and its associated need for high adherence in order to enhance the efficacy of HIV drugs and reduce the development of drug resistance, disclosure is essentially important for HIV-positive individuals including children and young people (Brown et al. 2000; Chesney 2003; Giacomet et al. 2003; Naar-King et al. 2006; WHO 2011; Dorrell and Katz 2013; see also Chaps. 5, 12, 17, 18, 20, 21, and 22 in this volume). It is also argued that children and young people would benefit physically and emotionally from taking part in decisions about their care and treatment (Naar-King et al. 2006; Krauss et al. 2013; Dorrell and Katz 2014; Lowenthal et al. 2014a, b).

1.5 Resilience and HIV-Positive Young People

Despite some grim issues presented above, we have also witnessed children and young people who are able to deal with their HIV in a more positive ways. Despite adversarial circumstances, being resilient enables individuals to achieve positive societal functioning (Masten and Obradovic 2006). Resilience recognizes that individuals have internal characteristics and external means that help them to deal with challenges and reach personal ability and well-being (Greene et al. 2004). Although illness and other adversities in life can be challenges, Saleebey (2005) suggests that they may also be 'sources of opportunity' for many people.

Several chapters in this volume illustrate that children and young people living with HIV/AIDS are not totally the victim of their illnesses (see Chaps. 5, 6, 19, and 20). They acted on their own agencies in order to deal with their illnesses. In their research with young HIV-positive people in Canada (Chap. 5), Michelle DiRisio and Peri Ballantyne tell us that, "positive chronic illness identities emerged from the successful management of 'healthy' chronically infected bodies". These young people are portrayed as "pharmaceutical persons". They actively negotiate their health and well-being through an on-going use of medications, and "continual medical monitoring of their selves, by themselves, their families, and their health care professionals". Their chapter illustrates "a positive narrative regarding the potential opportunities of life with HIV that all nations grappling with growing youth prevalence rates might aim to achieve".

Similarly, Asha Persson, Christy Newman and Angela Miller (Chap. 6) tell us that Australian HIV-positive young people in their study did not see HIV as an illness and living with HIV is a 'normal' part of their lives. HIV is "something that can be integrated into life rather than pose an obstacle". Persson et al. contend that "conventional theories of stigma do not readily fit with these stories. Not one of these young people articulated a 'spoiled identity', the hallmark of internalized stigma", as theorized by Goffman (1974). Their data did not point to the sense of self of the young people that "was marked by shame or reduced to their HIV status, even when HIV was seen as central and seminal to their lives". Perceptions of 'normality' among HIV-positive young people have also been discussed by several researchers (see Flicker et al. 2005; Fielden et al. 2006; Dorrell and Katz 2013; Rydström et al. 2013).

1.6 Social Support, Interventions and Health Promotion Programs

Children and young people living with HIV/AIDS need distinctive physical and psychological care in order to assist them to cope with not only their developmental challenges but also other HIV-related issues including stigma, discrimination and the maintenance of health and well-being (Snyder et al. 2014). It can be burdensome for children and young people to take responsibility for their own health care needs. Snyder et al. (2014: 115) contend that young people are "typically unequipped with the skills to navigate health systems and to manage what is a chronic, communicable, and potentially life-threatening disease". Adherence to antiretroviral medication among children and young people is a good example here. Their adherence is much lower than other groups of HIV-positive people (Williams et al. 2007; Nachega et al. 2009; see also Chaps. 4, 5, 6, 18, 19, 20, 21, and 22 in this volume).

Social support, either informal networks or formal structures, play a crucial role in the HIV response for children and young people (Gregson et al. 2013; Skovdal et al. 2013). Generally, social support acts as a "buffer" to diminish distress and strengthen resilience for individuals who experience stressful life events (Richmond and Ross 2008; Drageset et al. 2012; Hoban and Liamputtong 2013; Dumrongthanapakorn and Liamputtong 2015; Walker et al. 2015; Suwankhong and Liamputtong 2016). Social support is linked with better health and quality of life in people who are experiencing adversities in life. It helps to decrease stress associated with the diagnosis of illnesses, improve their emotional well-being, and produces positive changes in their lives. Additionally, social support enhances self-esteem, and provide a sense of belonging and security (Richmond and Ross 2008; Walker et al. 2015; Suwankhong and Liamputtong 2016). There has also been evidence that giving and receiving social support can be a health-promoting behavior (Kawachi and Berkman 2001; Uchino 2004; Umberson et al. 2010; Thoits 2011; Dumrongthanapakorn and Liamputtong 2015; Walker et al. 2015). Social support functions both at the individual and societal levels (Thoits 1995, 2011; Richmond and Ross 2008; Walker et al. 2015; Suwankhong and Liamputtong 2016).

Within the HIV/AIDs general discourse, support groups are widely accepted as valuable means for alleviating the psycho-social impacts of HIV/AIDS (Liamputtong et al. 2009, 2012; UNAIDS 2011; Mburu et al. 2014). I contend that this has also been recognized as a vehicle to help young people to deal with their HIV-positive status (Mupambireyi et al. 2014; see also Chaps. 6, 17, 18, 19, and 20 in this volume). Snyder et al. (2014: 115) suggest that social support provides "the health-enabling 'safe spaces' which help to create important networks and social bonds" among young people living with HIV/AIDS (see also Campbell et al. 2013). In their study in Zimbabwe, Mupambireyi et al. (2014) showed that the children saw support groups as "safe social spaces". They also perceived support groups as "spaces to identify role models and to restore confidence, both in themselves and in their future" (Skovdal and Belton 2014: 5). Research in the US and South Africa have also revealed that support groups helped to improve the psycho-social sequels of newly-diagnosed HIV-positive individuals (Futterman et al. 2010; Hosek et al. 2011; Snyder et al. 2014: 119). Support groups have also been recommended by UNAIDS (2011) as a feasible means for meeting the psycho-social needs of HIV-positive young people in Africa.

Existing research has also suggested that structured support groups have helped to encourage HIV-positive young people to seek care and maintain their care (Horstmann et al. 2010). Snyder et al. (2014: 114) point to the "Hlanganani Program" that was developed to engage HIV-positive young people in care. The program uses "a dynamic, three-session cognitive behavioral support group facilitated by laypersons". Young people, who were diagnosed within the previous 12 months, were invited to attend three sessions in either a clinic or other community space. The program included three issues: Coping and support; HIV health; and HIV prevention. The findings of this pilot study provided an assurance that a structured support group for newly diagnosed HIV-positive young people could be an efficient means for young people to enter and continue long-term HIV care (Snyder et al. 2014).

There are other social support structures and interventions that have been created to assist young people living with HIV/AIDS. These include group homes (Fournier et al. 2014), peer support (Mburu et al. 2014), drop in-style youth centers (Black et al. 2014), dance4life (d4l) social youth movement (Schouten et al. 2014), and community-based organizations (Skeen et al. 2014). In Chap. 15, Catherine MacPhail and Audrey Pettifor provide a number of intervention programs that were implemented to assist young people living with HIV/AIDS.

In this volume, there are a number of chapters that discuss some support networks and innovative health interventions for children and young people living with HIV/AIDS (see Chaps. 6, 15, 16, 17, 18, 19, 20, 21, and 22). I will discuss several interventions in the section below.

Social network technologies provide access to social support for individual living with HIV/AIDS (Fox and Purcell 2010; Kahana et al. 2013). For HIV-positive young people, online patient communities (OPCs) offer a means for them to seek social and emotional support for coping with their illness, diagnosis and its treatment. OPCs are not restricted by geographical locations; individuals can connect with others who are in the same situation (Bacigalupe 2011). Existing research has suggested that participation in OPCs improves young people's empowerment, and this has been found to enhance their adherence to treatment and care (Van Uden-Kraan et al. 2009; Bartlett and Coulson 2011; Mo and Coulson 2012; Bacigalupe 2013).

In Chap. 18, Gonzalo Bacigalupe, Kathryn Cantrell and Rachel Chickerella tell us about the power of online patient communities for HIV-positive young people in their study. They write: "For many YHIV, stigma inhibits the formation of social connections and peer support. But with the growth of online patient communities (OPCs), YHIV are more connected than ever as they provide one another with health information, emotional guidance, and a sense of community that spans geographical barriers". Gonzalo et al. contend that "the social power of OPCs can aid in community support and provide opportunities for story telling and meaning-making that social stigmatization obstructs".

Magda Conway (see Chap. 19) presents an excellent psycho-social peer support called 'Freedom To Be' (F2B), which is "a therapeutic residential intervention for 100 ALHIV that provides psycho-social support, peer support and youth-friendly information/workshops on issues relating to growing up with HIV". The success of F2Bs lies in "the core set of values and ethos" of the program. These values include "respect, non-judgment, equity and acceptance". Conway contends that "for any individual that has faced adversity and difficult experiences, being in an environment where they are respected, listened to, encouraged to express himself or herself in a way that … emotionally safe can be extremely powerful". Conway concludes that "bringing the peer group together to share their experiences, explore challenges and develop personal support networks that will survive into adulthood, goes someway to 'normalizing' HIV for this group".

Tomas Campbell and Jayne Griffiths (Chap. 21) created a program that they referred to as the 'Looking Forward Day' (LfD) as a means to involve HIV-positive young people in their study. The LfD provided these young people the opportunity to discuss their diagnosis, medication, treatment and related difficulties with other HIV-positive youth and professionals. They employed "psychodrama approaches" to explore these young people's emotions and practice skills. Campbell et al. tell us: "By recreating real-life situations or problems, and acting them out in the present, the young people have an opportunity to evaluate their behavior, practice new roles safely and to develop and rehearse new skills". Their philosophical framework was to adopt a "playful approach to serious problems" to "constantly update and modify how issues are covered in order to facilitate ongoing attendance and engagement".

1.7 Researching with Children and Young People Living with HIV/AIDS

Researching children and young people may require different approaches from those used in normal circumstances and often, researchers have to be innovative. Our choice of innovative methods primarily depends on the age, experience, preference and social status of the research participants (Liamputtong and Fernandez 2015). The cultural environment and the physical setting of the research, the questions we pose, and our competence as a researcher, also determine the methods we select. However, regardless of the innovative methods we may choose, showing respect to individuals and taking into account the group differences such as class, age, gender, ethnicity and culture are important fundamental aspects of research that involves children and young people.

Ethical issues are extremely important when our research involves children and young people and particularly when these young people are living with HIV/AIDS (Liamputtong 2007). As discussed in Chap. 23, Katie Schenk and Saumya Ramarao "the design and conduct of research fieldwork frequently gives rise to difficult ethical dilemmas. Children and families affected by HIV may be vulnerable to harmful outcomes including stigma, discrimination, abuse and exploitation; and may have impaired access to power and resources". Also argue that the vulnerable circumstances of children and families "demand that a researcher seeking their participation in a data collection activity must exercise special care and take extra precautions to ensure their protection". Basing on their experience of conducting ethical review, Schenk and Ramarao provide some valuable advice for the design and process of research aimed at enhancing the ethical conduct of research among children and families affected by HIV. In their chapter, Schenk and Ramarao conclude that "it *is* feasible to conduct ethically sound and high quality research among children and families affected by HIV, and that these values extend far beyond our field of HIV research to researchers in other fields working among vulnerable children and families, including malaria and child survival".

Collecting information from children may pose some difficulties as children may not be able to articulate health issues as well as adults (Fleer 2014). It is essential to adopt a sensitive and an innovative way that would allow children to be able to talk about their understanding of the issues under investigation (Jorgenson and Sullivan

2009; Wright 2012a; MacDonald 2013; Agbenyega 2014; Gill and Liamputtong 2014; Liamputong and Fernandez 2015). According to McArdle (2012), and Gill and Liamputtong (2014), most children are familiar with drawing activities. Drawings allow young children's ideas to be visible (Agbenyega 2014) because through drawing activities, children are able to articulate their ideas about things in detail (McArdle 2012; Liamputong and Fernandez 2015). Importantly, through drawing activities, children are able to express things which can be difficult to do through other vocal and literal expressions (Wright 2012a; Agbenyega 2014; Gill and Liamputtong 2014; Liamputong and Fernandez 2015). See Chaps. 2 and 8 in this volume for the adoption of drawing methods in research with children/young people living with HIV/AIDS.

The method of photovoice has emerged as an innovative means of working with marginalised people and in cross-cultural research. The photovoice method rejects traditional paradigms of power and the production of knowledge within the research relationship (Liamputtong 2010). The researchers are more concerned about developing critical consciousness and empowerment amongst their research participants (Castleden et al. 2008; Rhodes et al. 2008). According to Rhodes and associates (2008: 168), photovoice is not simply just "a basic research method". To them, photovoice is "an intervention strategy that facilitates participant empowerment by creating a space for participation and control over the process and builds the capacity of participants to mobilize to explore, describe, and analyze challenges and assets and problem solve". Bonnie Fournier and Olenka Bilash provide an excellent discussion regarding the use of the photovoice method with HIV-positive children in Uganda (see Chap. 24 in this volume).

1.8 About the Book

The book comprises 24 chapters and are separated into four parts. In Part 1, chapters focus on the lived experiences of living with HIV/AIDS among children and young people. Chapters in Part 2 discuss gender and identity issues relating to risk of and living with HIV/AIDS. In Part 3, chapters are focused on health care, human right issues and interventions that allow children and young people to live better lives with their HIV/AIDS. The last part of the volume includes chapters on ethical issues and research methods when research involves children and young people living with HIV/AIDS.

1.9 Conclusion

HIV/AIDS have caused a "social assault" on the lives of children and young people in the world. As readers will see throughout this volume, we have witnessed the impact that HIV/AIDS has on the health, well-being as well as life opportunities for young people to be able to lead healthy adult lives in many parts of the world (Lowenthal et al. 2014a, b). Although HIV-positive children and young people tend to experience adversities in life, there are those who attempt to make their illnesses most positive, particularly if they receive sufficient and effective social support. I contend that children and young people are not passive victims of HIV/AIDS, but that they act in their own agencies to counteract any negativity they might encounter. It is crucial that the voices of these children and young people are heard and their lived experiences and needs are better understood by health and social care providers so that culturally and sensitive health care can be implemented.

References

Abramowitz, S., Koenig, L., Chandwani, S., Orban, L., Stein, R., LaGrange, R., & Barnes, W. (2009). Characterizing social support: Global and specific social support experiences of HIV-infected youth. *AIDS Patient Care and STDs, 23*(5), 323–330.

Agbenyega, J. S. (2014). Beyond alienation: Unpacking the methodological issues in visual research with children. In M. Fleer & A. Ridgeway (Eds.), *Visual methodologies and digital tools for researching with children* (pp. 89–110). Cham: Springer.

Arseniou, S., Arvaniti, A., & Samakouri, M. (2013). HIV infection and depression. *Psychiatry and Clinical Neuroscience, 68*(2), 1–14.

Bacigalupe, G. (2011). Is there a role for social technologies in collaborative healthcare? *Families, Systems & Health, 29*(1), 1–14.

Bacigalupe, G. (2013). *Chronic patients and social networking: Research lessons from a virtual community in the basque country.* Paper presented at the 141st APHA Annual Meeting (November 2–November 6, 2013).

Bailey, A., & Darak, S. (2013). Spaces of disclosure and discrimination: Case studies from India. In P. Liamputtong (Ed.), *Stigma, discrimination and living with HIV/AIDS: A cross-cultural perspective* (pp. 229–245). Dordrecht: Springer.

Bartlett, Y. K., & Coulson, N. S. (2011). An investigation into the empowerment effects of using online support groups and how this affects health professional/patient communication. *Patient Education and Counseling, 83*(1), 113–119.

Battles, H. B., & Wiener, L. S. (2002). From adolescents through young adulthood: Psychosocial adjustment associated with long-term survival of HIV. *Journal of Adolescent Health, 30*(3), 161–168.

Beard, J., Biemba, G., Brooks, M. I., Costello, J., Ommerborn, M., & Bresnahan, M., et al. (2010). Children of female sex workers and drug users: A review of vulnerability, resilience and family-centred models of care. *Journal of the International AIDS Society, 13*(Suppl 2) (S6), 1–8. doi:10.1186/1758-2652-13-S2-S6. Retrieved June 11, 2015, from http://www.biomedcentral.com/content/pdf/1758-2652-13-S2-S6.pdf

Bell, S. A., & Aggleton, P. (2014). Economic vulnerability and young people's sexual relationships in rural Uganda. *Journal of Youth Studies, 17*(6), 814–828.

Bell, D. N., Martinez, J., Botwinick, G., Shaw, K., Walker, L. E., Dodds, S., Sell, R. L., Johnson, R. L., Friedman, L. B., Sotheran, J. L., & Siciliano, C. (2003). Case finding for HIV-positive youth: A special type of hidden population. *Journal of Adolescent Health, 33*(2), 10–22.

Bernays, S., Jarrett, P., Kranzer, K., & Ferrand, R. A. (2014). Children growing up with HIV infection: The responsibility of success. *Lancet, 383*, 1355–1357.

Betancourt, T. S., Meyers-Ohki, S. E., Charrow, A., & Hansen, N. (2013). Annual research review: Mental health and resilience in HIV/AIDS-affected children—a review of the literature and recommendations for future research. *Journal of Child Psychology and Psychiatry, and Allied Disciplines, 54*(4), 423–444.

Beyrer, C., Baral, S. D., Walker, D., Wirtz, A. L., Johns, B., & Sifakis, F. (2010). The expanding epidemics of HIV type 1 among men who have sex with men in low and middle-income countries: Diversity and consistency. *Epidemiology Reviews, 32*(1), 137–151.

Black, S., Wallace, M., Middelkoop, K., Robbertze, D., Bennie, T., Wood, R., & Bekker, L.-G. (2014). Improving HIV testing amongst adolescents through an integrated Youth Centre rewards program: Insights from South Africa. *Children and Youth Services Review, 45*, 98–105.

Boudreau, M. E., & Fisher, C. M. (2012). Providing effective medical and case management services to HIV-infected youth preparing to transition to adult care. *Journal of the Association of Nurses in AIDS Care, 23*, 318–328.

Brown, L. K., Lourie, K. J., & Pao, M. (2000). Children and adolescents living with HIV and AIDS: A review. *Journal of Child Psychology and Psychiatry, 41*(1), 81–96.

Campbell, C., Scott, K., Nhamo, M., Nyamukapa, C., Madanhire, C., Skovdal, M., et al. (2013). Social capital and HIV competent communities: The role of community groups in managing HIV/AIDS in rural Zimbabwe. *AIDS Care, 25*(S1), 114–122.

Campbell, T., Griffiths, J., Beer, H., Legemah, P., & Saine, M. (2014). HIV+ children and their families in the UK: Results from a family-clinic based 'look-back' exercise in London. *Perspectives in Public Health, 134*(1), 31–37.

Castleden, H., Garvin, T., & Huu-ay-aht First Nation. (2008). Modifying photovoice for community-based participatory indigenous research. *Social Science & Medicine, 66*(6), 1393–1405.

Chesney, M. (2003). Adherence to HAART regimens. *AIDS Patient Care and STDs, 17*, 169–177.

Chew, J., Beng, A. L., & Mun, S. (2014). Parental concerns about disclosure of a child's HIV/AIDS status in Singapore. *Social Work in Health Care, 51*, 5–21.

Chi, P., & Li, X. (2013). Impact of parental HIV/AIDS on children's psychological well-being: A systematic review of global literature. *AIDS and Behavior, 17*, 2554–2574.

Cluver, L., & Gardner, F. (2007). Risk and protective factors for psychological well-being of children orphaned by AIDS in Cape Town: A qualitative study of children and caregivers' perspectives. *AIDS Care, 19*(3), 318–325.

Cluver, L., Orkin, M., Gardner, F., & Boyes, M. E. (2011). Persisting mental health problems among AIDS orphaned children in South Africa. *Journal of Child Psychology and Psychiatry, 53*(4), 363–370.

Collaborative HIV Paediatric Study (CHIPS). (2012). Annual report. London. Retrieved from www.chipscohort.ac.uk/summary_data.asp

Courtenay-Quirk, C., Wolitski, R. G., Parsons, J. T., & Gomez, C. A. (2006). Is HIV/AIDS stigma dividing the gay community? Perceptions of HIV-positive men who have sex with men. *AIDS Education and Prevention, 18*(1), 56–67.

Dahoma, M., Johnston, L. G., Holman, A., Miller, L. A., Mussa, M., Othman, A., et al. (2011). HIV and related risk behavior among men who have sex with men in Zanzibar, Tanzania: Results of a behavioral surveillance survey. *AIDS and Behavior, 15*(1), 186–192.

Domek, G. J. (2009). Facing adolescence and adulthood: The importance of mental health care in the global pediatric AIDS epidemic. *Journal of Developmental and Behavioural Pediatrics, 30*, 147–150.

Dorrell, J., & Katz, J. (2013). "I knew I had something bad because no one spoke about it" – disclosure discovery: Experiences of young people with perinatally acquired HIV in the UK. *Vulnerable Children and Youth Studies, 8*(4), 353–361.

Dorrell, J., & Katz, J. (2014). 'You're HIV positive': Perinatally infected young people's accounts of the critical moment of finding out their diagnosis. *AIDS Care, 26*(4), 454–458.

Drageset, S., Lindstrøm, T. C., Giske, T., & Underlid, K. (2012). "The support I need": Women's experiences of social support after having received breast cancer diagnosis and awaiting surgery. *Cancer Nursing, 35*(6), E39–E47.

Dumrongthanapakorn, P., & Liamputtong, P. (2015) Social support coping means: The lived experiences of Northeastern Thai women with breast cancer. *Health Promotion International*. doi:10.1093/heapro/dav023.

Evans, R., & Becker, S. (2009). *Children caring for parents with HIV and AIDS*. Bristol: The Policy Press.
Fair, C., & Albright, J. (2012). "Don't tell him you have HIV unless he's 'The One'": Romantic relationships among adolescents and young adults with perinatal HIV infection. *AIDS Patient Care and STDs, 26*(12), 746–754.
Fair, C., Sullivan, K., & Gatto, A. (2011). Indicators of transition success for youth living with HIV: Perspectives of pediatric and adult infectious disease care providers. *AIDS Care, 23*(8), 965–970.
Ferris, M., Burau, K., Schweitzer, A. M., Mihale, S., Murray, N., Preda, M., … Kline, M. (2007). The influence of disclosure of HIV diagnosis on time to disease progression in a cohort of Romanian children and teens. *AIDS Care, 19*, 1088–1094.
Fielden, S., Scheckter, L., Chapman, G., Alimenti, A., Forbes, J., Sheps, S., Cadell, S., & Frankish, J. (2006). Growing up: Perspectives of children, families and service providers regarding the needs of older children with perinatally acquired HIV. *AIDS Care, 18*, 1050–1053.
Fleer, M. (2014). A digital turn: Post-developmental methodologies for researching with young children. In M. Fleer & A. Ridgeway (Eds.), *Visual methodologies and digital tools for researching with children* (pp. 3–10). Cham: Springer.
Fleming, P. J., Lee, G. J. L., & Dworkin, S. L. (2014). "Real men don't": Constructions of masculinity and inadvertent harm in public health interventions. *American Journal of Public Health, 6*, 1029–1035.
Flicker, S., Skinner, H., Read, S., Veinot, T., McClelland, A., Saulnier, P., & Goldberg, E. (2005). Falling through the cracks of the big cities: Who is meeting the needs of HIV-positive youth? *Canadian Journal of Public Health, 96*(4), 308–312.
Fournier, B., Bridge, A., Pritchard Kennedy, A., Alibhai, A., & Konde-Lule, J. (2014). Hear our voices: A Photovoice project with children who are orphaned and living with HIV in a Ugandan group home. *Children and Youth Services Review, 45*, 55–63.
Fox, S., & Purcell, K. (2010). *Chronic disease and the internet*. Washington, DC: Pew Internet & American Life Project.
Futterman, D., Shea, J., Besser, M., Stafford, S., Desmond, K., Comulada, W. S., et al. (2010). Mamekhaya: A pilot study combining a cognitive-behavioral intervention and mentor mothers with PMTCT services in South Africa. *AIDS Care, 22*(9), 1093–1100.
Geibel, S., Tun, W., Tapsoba, P., & Kellerman, S. (2010). HIV vulnerability of men who have sex with men in developing countries: Horizons studies, 2001–2008. *Public Health Report, 125*, 316–324.
Giacomet, V., Albano, F., Starace, F., Franciscis, A., Giaquinto, C., Gattinara, G. C., Bruzzese, E., Gabiano, C., Galli, L., Viganò, A., Caselli, D., & Guarino, A. (2003). Adherence to antiretroviral therapy and its determinants in children with human immunodeficiency virus infection: A multicentre, national study. *Acta Paediatrica, 92*(12), 1398–1402.
Gill, J., & Liamputtong, P. (2014). The drawing method: Researching young people with a disability. In SAGE cases in methodology (SCiM) (an online resource for students and researchers). Sage: London. doi:http://dx.doi.org/10.4135/978144627305013512929.
Goffman, E. (1963). *Stigma: Notes on the management of spoiled identity*. New York: Simon and Schuster.
Goffman, E. (1974). *Stigma: Notes on the management of spoiled identity*. Harmondsworth: Penguin Books.
Greeff, M. (2013). Disclosure and stigma: A cultural perspective. In P. Liamputtong (Ed.), *Stigma, discrimination and living with HIV/AIDS: A cross-cultural perspective* (pp. 71–95). Dordrecht: Springer.
Green, G., & Smith, R. (2004). The psychosocial and health needs of HIV-positive people in the United Kingdom: A review. *HIV Medicine, 5*(1), 5–46.
Greene, R. R., Galambos, C., & Lee, Y. (2004). Resilience theory. *Journal of Human Behavior in the Social Environment, 8*(4), 75–91.
Gregson, S., Nyamukapa, C., Schumacher, C., Magutshwa-Zitha, S., Skovdal, M., Yekeye, R., et al. (2013). Evidence for a contribution of the community response to HIV decline in eastern Zimbabwe. *AIDS Care, 25*(S 1), 88–96.

Gupta, G. R., Ogen, J., & Warner, A. (2011). Moving forward on women's gender-related HIV vulnerability: The good news, the bad news and what to do about it. *Global Public Health: An International Journal of Research, Policy and Practice, 6*(3), 370–382.

Harms, S., Jack, S., Ssebunnya, J., & Kizza, R. (2010). The orphaning experience: Descriptions from Ugandan youth who have lost parents to HIV/AIDS. *Child and Adolescent Psychiatry and Mental Health, 4*(6), 1–10.

Herek, G. M., & Glunt, E. K. (1993). Public reactions to AIDS in the United States: A second decade of stigma. *American Journal of Public Health, 83*(4), 573–577.

Hoban, E., & Liamputtong, P. (2013). Cambodian migrant women's postpartum experiences in Victoria, Australia. *Midwifery, 29*, 772–778.

Horstmann, E., Brown, J., Islam, F., Buck, J., & Agins, B. D. (2010). Retaining HIV-infected patients in care: Where are we? Where do we go from here? *Clinical Infectious Diseases, 50*(5), 752–761.

Hosek, S., Lemos, D., Harper, G., & Telander, K. (2011). Evaluating the acceptability and feasibility of project ACCEPT: An intervention for youth newly diagnosed with HIV. *AIDS Education and Prevention, 23*(2), 128–144.

Jaspan, H. B., Li, R., Johnson, L., & Bekker, L. G. (2009). The emerging need for adolescent focused HIV care in South Africa. *South African Journal of HIV Medicine, 10*(4), 9–11.

Jewkes, R., & Morrell, R. (2010). Gender and sexuality: Emerging perspectives from the heterosexual epidemic in South Africa and implications for HIV risk and prevention. *Journal of the International AIDS Society, 13*(1), 6.

Jewkes, R., & Morrell, R. (2012). Sexuality and the limits of agency among South African teenage women: Theorising femininities and their connections to HIV risk practices. *Social Science & Medicine, 74*(11), 1729–1737.

Jorgenson, J., & Sullivan, T. (2009). Accessing children's perspectives through participatory photo interviews. *Forum: Qualitative Social Research, 11*(1). Art 8. http://nbn-resolving.de/urn:nbn:de:0114-fqs100189

Kahana, S. Y., Rohan, J., Allison, S., Frazier, T. W., & Drotar, D. (2013). A meta-analysis of adherence to antiretroviral therapy and virologic responses in HIV-infected children, adolescents, and young adults. *AIDS and Behavior, 17*(1), 41–60.

Kang, M., Dunbar, M., Laver, S., & Padian, N. (2008). Maternal versus paternal orphans and HIV/STI risk among adolescent girls in Zimbabwe. *AIDS Care, 20*(2), 214–217.

Kawachi, I., & Berkman, L. F. (2001). Social ties and mental health. *Journal of Urban Health, 78*(3), 458–467.

Kemeny, M. E. (2011). Psychoneuroimmunology. In H. Freidman (Ed.), *The Oxford handbook of health psychology* (pp. 138–161). New York: Oxford University Press. Oxford Handbook Online.

King, E., De Silva, M., Stein, A., & Patel, V. (2009). Interventions for improving the psychosocial well-being of children affected by HIV and AIDS. *Cochrane Database of Systematic Reviews*, 2, CD006733.

Krauss, B. J., Letteney, S., De Baets, A. J., Baggaley, R., & Okero, F. A. (2013). Disclsoure of HIV status to HI-positive children 12 and under: A systematic cross national review of implications for health and well-being. *Vulnerable Children and Youth Studies, 8*(2), 99–119.

Kumar, A. (2012). AIDS orphans and vulnerable children in India: Problems, prospects, and concerns. *Social Work in Public Health, 27*(3), 205–212.

Lam, P. K., Naar-King, S., & Wright, K. (2007). Social support and disclosure as predictors of mental health in HIV positive youth. *AIDS Patient Care and STDs, 21*(1), 20–29.

Leeper, S. C., Montague, B. T., Friedman, J. F., & Flanigan, T. P. (2010). Lessons learned from family-centred models of treatment for children living with HIV: Current approaches and future directions. *Journal of the International AIDS Society, 13*(Suppl. 2), S3. doi:10.1186/1758-2652-13-S2-S3.

Letteney, S., & LaPorte, H. H. (2004). Deconstructing stigma: Perceptions of HIV-seropositive mothers and their disclosure to children. *Social Work in Health Care, 38*, 105–123.

Liamputtong, P. (2007). *Researching the vulnerable: A guide to sensitive research methods*. London: Sage.

Liamputtong, P. (2010). *Performing qualitative cross-cultural research*. Cambridge: Cambridge University Press.

Liamputtong, P. (2013a). Stigma, discrimination, and HIV/AIDS: An introduction. In P. Liamputtong (Ed.), *Stigma, discrimination and living with HIV/AIDS* (pp. 1–19). Dordrecht: Springer.

Liamputtong, P. (2013b). *Qualitative research methods* (4th ed.). Melbourne: Oxford University Press.

Liamputtong, P., & Fernandez, S. (2015). The drawing method and Burmese refugee children's perceptions of health and illness. *Australasian Journal of Early Childhood, 40*(1), 23–32.

Liamputtong, P., & Haritavorn, N. (2015). To tell or not to tell: Disclosure and women living with HIV/AIDS in Thailand. *Health Promotion International, 31*, 23. doi:10.1093/heapro/dau057.

Liamputtong, P., & Kitisriworapan, S. (2012). Deviance, difference and stigma as social determinants of health. In P. Liamputtong, R. Fanany, & G. Verrinder (Eds.), *Health, illness and well-being: Perspectives and social determinants* (pp. 242–256). Melbourne: Oxford University Press.

Liamputtong, P., Haritavorn, N., & Kiatying-Angsulee, N. (2009). HIV and AIDS, stigma and AIDS support groups: Perspectives from women living with HIV and AIDS in central Thailand. *Social Science & Medicine, 69*(6), 862–868.

Liamputtong, P., Haritavorn, N., & Kiatying-Angsulee, N. (2012). Living positively: The experiences of Thai women in central Thailand. *Qualitative Health Research, 22*(4), 441–451.

Lowenthal, E. D., Jibril, H. B., Sechele, M. L., Mathuba, K., Tshume, O., & Anabwani, G. M. (2014a). Disclosure of HIV status to HIV-infected children in a large African treatment center: Lessons learned in Botswana. *Children and Youth Services Review, 45*, 143–149.

Lowenthal, E. D., Bakeera-Kitaka, S., Marukutira, T., Chapman, J., Goldrath, K., & Ferrand, R. A. (2014b). Perinatally acquired HIV infection in adolescents from sub-Saharan Africa: A review of emerging challenges. *Lancet, 383*, 1–14.

MacDonald, A. (2013). Using children's representations to investigate meaning-making in mathematics. *Australasian Journal of Early Childhood, 38*(2), 65–73.

MacDonell, K., Naar-King, S., Huszti, H., & Belzer, M. (2013). Barriers to medication adherence in behaviorally and perinatally infected youth living with HIV. *AIDS and Behavior, 17*(1), 86–93.

Mahati, S. T., Munyati, S., Chitiyo, G., Mashange, W., Chibatamoto, P., & Mupambireyi, P. F. (2006). *A qualitative assessment of orphans and vulnerable children in two Zimbabwean districts*. Cape Town: HSRC Press.

Mann, J., & Tarantola, D. (1998). Responding to HIV/AIDS: A historical perspective. *Health and Human Rights: An International Journal, 2*(4), 5–8.

Martinez, J., Harper, G., Carleton, R. A., Hosek, S., Bojan, K., Glum, G., & The Adolescent Medicine Trials Network, J. (2012). The impact of stigma on medication adherence among HIV-positive adolescent and young adult females and the moderating effects of coping and satisfaction with health care. *AIDS Patient Care and STDs, 26*(2), 108–115.

Mason, T., Carlisle, C., Watkins, C., & Whitehead, E. (2001). Introduction. In T. Mason, C. Carlisle, C. Watkins, & E. Whitehead (Eds.), *Stigma and social exclusion in health care* (pp. 1–13). London: Routledge.

Masten, A. S., & Obradovic, J. (2006). Competence and resilience in development. *Annals of the New York Academy of Sciences, 1094*(1), 13–27.

Mburu, G., Ram, M., Oxenham, D., Haamujompa, C., Iorpenda, K., & Ferguson, L. (2014). Responding to adolescents living with HIV in Zambia: A social–ecological approach. *Children and Youth Services Review, 45*, 9–17.

McArdle, F. (2012). The visual arts: Ways of seeing. In S. Wright (Ed.), *Children, meaning-making and the arts* (2nd ed., pp. 30–56). Frenchs Forest: Pearson Australia.

Mellins, C., & Malee, K. (2013). Understanding the mental health of youth living with perinatal HIV infection: Lessons learnt and current challenges. *Journal of the International AIDS Society, 16*(1), 1–19. http://dx.doi.org/10.7448/IAS.16.1.18593.

Mellins, C. A., Brackis-Cott, E., Leu, C., Elkington, K., Dolezal, C., Wiznia, A., Bamji, M., McKay, M., & Abrams, E. J. (2009). Rates and types of psychiatric disorders in perinatally human immunodeficiency virus-infected youth and seroreverters. *Journal of Child Psychology and Psychiatry, 50*, 1131–1138.

Messer, L. C., Pence, B. W., Whetten, K., Whetten, R., Thielman, N., O'Donnell, K., et al. (2010). Prevalence and predictors of HIV-related stigma among institutional- and community-based caregivers of orphans and vulnerable children living in five less-wealthy countries. *BMC Public Health, 10*(504), 1–7.

Mo, P. K., & Coulson, N. (2012). Developing a model for online support group use, empowering processes and psychosocial outcomes for individuals living with HIV/AIDS. *Psychology & Health, 27*(4), 445–459.

Mupambireyi, Z., Bernays, S., Bwakura-Dangarembizi, M., & Cowan, F. M. (2014). "I don't feel shy because I will be among others who are just like me…": The role of support groups for children perinatally infected with HIV in Zimbabwe. *Children and Youth Services Review, 45*, 106–113.

Naar-King, S., Templin, T., Wright, K., Frey, M., Parsons, J. T., & Lam, P. (2006). Psychosocial factors and medication in HIV-positive youth. *AIDS Patient Care and STDs, 20*(1), 44–47.

Nachega, J. B., Hislop, M., Nguyen, H., Dowdy, D. W., Chaisson, R. E., Regensberg, L., et al. (2009). Antiretroviral therapy adherence, virologic and immunologic outcomes in adolescents compared with adults in Southern Africa. *Journal of Acquired Immune Deficiency Syndrome, 51*, 65–71.

Nöstlinger, C., Bartoli, G., Gordillo, V., Roberfroid, D., & Colebunders, R. (2006). Children and adolescents living with HIV positive parents: Emotional and behavioural problems. *Vulnerable Children and Youth Studies, 1*(1), 29–43.

Nyberg, B. J., Yates, D. D., Lovich, R., Coulibaly-Traore, D., Sherr, L., Thurman, T. R., et al. (2012). Saving lives for a lifetime: Supporting orphans and vulnerable children impacted by HIV/AIDS. *JAIDS Journal of Acquired Immune Deficiency Syndromes, 60*, S127–S135.

Okonofua, F. (2012). Same sex relationships and HIV/AIDS in Africa: Need for research and programmatic focus. *African Journal of Reproductive Health, 16*(4), 9–12.

Orban, L. A., Stein, R., Koenig, L. J., Conner, L. C., Rexhouse, E. L., Lewis, J. V., & LaGrange, R. (2010). Coping strategies of adolescents living with HIV: Disease specific stressors and responses. *AIDS Care, 22*(4), 420–430.

Parker, R., & Aggleton, P. (2003). HIV/AIDS-related stigma and discrimination: A conceptual framework and implications for action. *Social Science & Medicine, 57*, 13–24.

Parker, W., & Birdsall, K. (2005). *HIV/AIDS, stigma and faith-based organizations: A review. Centre for AIDS development, research and evaluation (CADRE) on behalf of Futures Group*. Johannesburg: CADRE.

Pearlstein, S. L., Mellins, C. A., Dolezal, C., Elkington, K. S., Santamaria, E. K., Leu, C. S., & Abrams, E. J. (2014). Youth in transition: Life skills among perinatally HIV-infected and HIV-exposed adolescents. *Journal of Pediatric Psychology, 39*(3), 294–305.

Ramjee, G., & Wand, H. (2014). Geographical clustering of high risk sexual behaviors in "Hot-spots" for HIV and sexually transmitted infections in Kwazulu-Natal, South Africa. *AIDS and Behavior, 18*(2), 317–322.

Rhodes, S. D., Hergenrather, K. C., Wilkin, A. M., & Jolly, C. (2008). Visions and voices: Indigent persons living with HIV in the southern United States use photovoice to create knowledge, develop partnerships, and take action. *Health Promotion Practice, 9*(2), 159–169.

Richmond, C. A. M., & Ross, N. A. (2008). Social support, material circumstance and health behavior: Influences on health in First Nation and Inuit communities of Canada. *Social Science & Medicine, 67*, 1423–1433.

Ross, R., Sawatphanit, W., & Suwansujarid, T. (2007). Finding peace (kwam sa-ngob jai): A Buddhist way to live with HIV. *Journal of Holistic Nursing, 25*(4), 228–235.

Rydström, L.-L., Ygge, B.-M., Tingberg, B., Navèr, L., & Eriksson, L. (2013). Experiences of young adults growing up with innate or early acquired HIV infection: A qualitative study. *Journal of Advanced Nursing, 69*(6), 1357–1365.

Saleebey, D. (2005). The philosophy, principles, and language of the strengths perspective. In D. Saleebey (Ed.), *The strengths perspective in social work practice (Chapter 1)*. New York: Longman.

Sauceda, J. A., Wiebe, J. S., Rao, D., Pearson, C. R., & Simoni, J. M. (2013). HIV-related stigma and HIV disclosure among Latinos on the US-Mexico border. In P. Liamputtong (Ed.), *Stigma, discrimination and living with HIV/AIDS: A cross-cultural perspective* (pp. 187–203). Dordrecht: Springer.

Scambler, G. (2003). Deviance, sick role and stigma. In G. Scambler (Ed.), *Sociology as applied to medicine* (pp. 192–202). Edinburgh: Saunders.

Scambler, G. (2009). Health-related stigma. *Sociology of Health & Illness, 31*(3), 441–455.

Schouten, B., Vlug-Mahabali, M., Hermanns, S., Spijker, E., & van Weert, J. (2014). To be involved or not to be involved? Using entertainment-education in an HIV-prevention program for youngsters. *Health Communication, 29*, 762–772.

Seidman, S., Meeks, C., & Traschen, F. (1999). Beyond the closet? The changing social meaning of homosexuality in the United States. *Sexualities, 2*, 9–34.

Semple, S. J., Strathdee, S. A., Zians, J., McQuaid, J., & Patterson, T. L. (2011). Psychosocial and behavioral correlates of anxiety symptoms in a sample of HIV-positive, methamphetamine-using men who have sex with men. *AIDS Care, 23*(5), 628–637.

Sivaram, S., Zelaya, C., Srikrishnan, A. K., Latkin, C., Go, V. F., Solomon, S., & Celentano, C. (2009). Associations between social capital and HIV stigma in Chennai, India: Considerations for prevention intervention design. *AIDS Education and Prevention, 21*(3), 233–250.

Skeen, S., Tomlinson, M., Macedo, A., Miltz, A., Croome, N., & Sherr, L. (2014). Child development in HIV-positive and HIV-affected children in South Africa and Malawi—What role for community organisations? *Children and Youth Services Review, 45*, 90–97.

Skovdal, M., & Belton, S. (2014). The social determinants of health as they relate to children and youth growing up with HIV infection in sub-Saharan Africa. *Children and Youth Services Review, 45*, 1–8.

Skovdal, M., & Campbell, C. (2013). Public engagement and policymaking for caregiving children of the HIV epidemic in Sub-Saharan Africa. In R. A. Smith (Ed.), *Global HIV/AIDS politics, policy, and activism: Persistent challenges and emerging issues* (Policy and policymaking, Vol. 2, pp. 107–130). Santa Barbara: Praeger.

Skovdal, M., Ogutu, V., Aoro, C., & Campbell, C. (2009). Young carers as social actors: Coping strategies of children caring for ailing or ageing guardians in Western Kenya. *Social Science and Medicine, 69*(4), 587–595.

Skovdal, M., Campbell, C., & Onyango, V. (2013). Supporting 'young carers' in Kenya: From policy paralysis to action. *Child Care in Practice, 19*(4), 318–339.

Snyder, K., Wallace, M., Duby, Z., Aquino, L. D. H., Stafford, S., Hosek, S., Futterman, D., & Bekker, L.-G. (2014). Preliminary results from Hlanganani (Coming Together): A structured support group for HIV-infected adolescents piloted in Cape Town, South Africa. *Children and Youth Services Review, 45*, 114–121.

Sontag, S. (1991). *Illness as metaphor: AIDS and its metaphors*. London: Penguin Books.

Surkan, P. J., Mukherjee, J. S., Williams, D. R., Eustache, E., Louis, E., Jean-Paul, T., et al. (2010). Perceived discrimination and stigma toward children affected by HIV/AIDS and their HIV-positive caregivers in central Haiti. *AIDS Care, 22*(7), 803–815.

Suwankhong, D., & Liamputtong, P. (2016) Social support among women with breast cancer in southern Thailand. *Journal of Nursing Scholarship, 48*(1), 39–47. doi: 10.1111/jnu.12179.

Thoits, P. A. (1995). Stress, coping and social support processes: Where are we? What next? *Journal of Health and Social Behavior, 35*, 53–79.

Thoits, P. A. (2011). Mechanisms linking social ties and support to physical and mental health. *Journal of Health and Social Behavior, 52*(2), 145–161.

Thom, R. (2012). *HAART and mind: Common mental disorders in people living with HIV/AIDS*. South Africa: The Access Series, Reach Publishers.

Thomas, F. (2006). Stigma, fatigue and social breakdown: Exploring the impacts of HIV/AIDS on patient and carer well-being in the Caprivi Region, Namibia. *Social Science & Medicine, 63*, 3174–3187.

Uchino, B. N. (2004). *Social support and physical health: Understanding the health consequences of our relationships*. New Haven: Yale University Press.

Umberson, D., Crosnoe, R., & Reczak, C. (2010). Social relationships and health behavior across the life course. *Annual Review of Sociology, 36*, 139e157.

UNAIDS. (2010). *Global report: UNAIDS report on the global AIDS epidemic*. Geneva: UNAIDS. Available at http://www.unaids.org/sites/default/files/media_asset/20101123_globalreport_en_1.pdf

UNAIDS. (2011). *HIV and AIDS estimates 2011*. Retrieved March 12, 2013, from UNAIDS website. http://www.unaids.org/en/regionscountries/countries/southafrica/

UNAIDS. (2012). *AIDS info – Thailand*. Retrieved from http://www.unaids.org/en/regionscountries/countries/thailand/

UNAIDS. (2013). *Global report. UNADIS report on the global AIDS epidemic 2013*. Available at: http://www.unaids.org/en/media/unaids/contentassets/documents/epidemiology/2013/gr2013/unaids_global_report_2013_en.pdf. Accessed 15 Aug 2014.

UNICEF. (2011). *Adolescent mental health: An urgent challenge for investigation and investment*. Retrieved June 12, 2015, from http://www.unicef.org/sowc2011/pdfs/Adolescent-mental-health.pdf

United Nation (2013). Fact sheet: Adolescents, young people and HIV. Retrieved 9 Apr 2016 from www.unaids.org.

United Nations. (2014). *Mental health matters: Social inclusion of youth with mental health conditions*. New York: United Nations. Retrieved June 12, 2015, from http://www.un.org/esa/socdev/documents/youth/youth-mental-health.pdf.

Van Uden-Kraan, C. F., Drossaert, C. H., Taal, E., Seydel, E. R., & van de Laar, M. A. (2009). Participation in online patient support groups endorses patients' empowerment. *Patient Education and Counseling, 74*(1), 61–69.

Vijayan, T., Benin, A., Wagner, K., Romano, S., & Andiman, W. (2009). We never thought this would happen: Transitioning care of adolescents with perinatally acquired HIV infection from pediatrics to internal medicine. *AIDS Care, 21*, 1222–1229.

Walker, R., Koh, L., Wollersheim, D., & Liamputtong, P. (2015). Peer support training and mobile phones: Enhancing social connectedness of refugee women and implications for health promotion. *Health and Social Care in the Community, 23*(3), 325–336.

Watts, H., Lopman, B., Nyamukapa, C., & Gregson, S. (2005). Rising incidence and prevalence of orphanhood in Manicaland, Zimbabwe, 1998 to 2003. *AIDS, 19*(7), 717–725.

Wiener, L. S., Mellins, C. A., Marhefka, S., & Battles, H. B. (2007). Disclosure of an HIV diagnosis to children: History, current research, and future directions. *Journal of Developmental and Behavioral Pediatrics, 28*, 155–166.

Williams, S. L., Williams, D. R., Stein, D. J., Seedat, S., Jackson, P. B., & Moomal, H. (2007). Multiple traumatic events and psychological distress: The South African Stress and Health Study. *Journal of Traumatic Stress, 20*(5), 845–855.

World Health Organization. (2011). *Guideline on HIV disclosure counselling for children up to 12 years of age*. Geneva: WHO.

Wright, S. (2012). Arts education as a collective experience. In S. Wright (Ed.), *Children, meaning-making and the arts* (2nd ed., pp. 194–225). Frenchs Forest: Pearson Australia.

Zanoni, B. C., & Mayer, K. H. (2014). The adolescent and young adult HIV cascade of care in the United States: Exaggerated health disparities. *AIDS Patient Care and STDs, 28*(3), 128–135.

Zhang, L., Li, X., Zhao, J., Zhao, G., Kaljee, L., & Stanton, B. (2013). Disclosure of parental HIV infection to children and psychosocial impact on children in China: A qualitative study. *Asia Pacific Journal of Counselling and Psychotherapy, 4*(2), 163–174.

Part I
Children, Young People and Living with HIV/AIDS

Chapter 2
Unpacking 'OVC': Locally Perceived Differences Between Orphaned, HIV-Positive and AIDS-Affected Children in Zimbabwe

Morten Skovdal, Catherine Campbell, Zivai Mupambireyi, Laura Robertson, Constance Nyamukapa, and Simon Gregson

Contents

M. Skovdal (✉)
Department of Public Health, University of Copenhagen, Øster Farimagsgade 5, 1014 Copenhagen, Denmark
e-mail: m.skovdal@gmail.com

C. Campbell
Department of Social Psychology, London School of Economics and Political Science, Houghton Street, WC2A 2AE London, UK

Z. Mupambireyi
Centre for Sexual Health and HIV/AIDS Research Zimbabwe (CeSHHAR), 9 Monmouth Road, Avondale West, Harare, Zimbabwe

L. Robertson
School of Public Health, Imperial College London, Norfolk Place, London W2 1PG, UK

C. Nyamukapa • S. Gregson
School of Public Health, Imperial College London, Norfolk Place, London W2 1PG, UK

Biomedical Research and Training Institute, No. 10 Seagrave road, Avondale, Harare, Zimbabwe

P. Liamputtong (ed.), *Children and Young People Living with HIV/AIDS*, Cross-Cultural Research in Health, Illness and Well-Being, DOI 10.1007/978-3-319-29936-5_2

2.1 Introduction

'Orphaned and vulnerable children' (OVC) is an encompassing term used to describe children who are experiencing the effects of living in low resource and high HIV prevalence communities. However, within this social welfare category, there are different layers of vulnerability, raising questions about the capacity of generalized OVC responses to respond to the specific needs of groups of children falling within the OVC umbrella. This chapter examines children's social representations of their HIV-positive, AIDS-affected (living with HIV-positive parents) or orphaned peers – unpacking similarities and differences in layers of vulnerability of children falling within the orphaned and vulnerable children (OVC) category.

Despite progress in the availability of treatment for people living with the human immunodeficiency virus (HIV) and the acquired immune deficiency syndrome (AIDS), the cumulative impact of HIV on households continues to have a devastating effect on the lives of children throughout sub-Saharan Africa (UNAIDS 2013). Researchers and practitioners alike are investing significant resources in mapping out and responding to the needs and circumstances of children living in communities affected by HIV (PEPFAR 2012). However, a gap seems to be emerging between researchers and practitioners. Researchers, alongside an increasingly sophisticated body of HIV literature, identify new labels and classifications to describe and explain patterned needs and circumstances of children. For example, researchers have noted differences between maternal, paternal and double orphaned children (Watts et al. 2005; Kang et al. 2008) – warranting a distinction between type of orphanhood. Whilst many researchers, in the quest for knowledge, map out the unique circumstances and intersecting vulnerabilities of particular groups of children, and in the process make recommendations for policy and practice that are specific to a group of children, leading practitioners and policymakers seem to favor more general responses (e.g., UNICEF 2004; World Bank 2005; PEPFAR 2012; Nyberg et al. 2012).

This can be illustrated by the 2012 OVC programming guidelines developed by the President's Emergency Plan for AIDS Relief (PEPFAR) – the world's leading supporter of OVCs (Nyberg et al. 2012; PEPFAR 2012). The guidelines suggest a focus on strengthening government and civil society services so that they are organised and resourced to respond to the general needs (education, health and well-being, nutrition, social- and child protection) of children in HIV-affected households (Nyberg et al. 2012). A clear benefit of supporting and strengthening the systems that offer more generalised care to OVC, is that it helps circumvent the stigmatisation of particular groups of children (UNICEF et al. 2004; Nyberg et al. 2012). There are examples in the literature where programs targeting particular groups of children (e.g., 'AIDS orphans', 'AIDS-affected children' and 'orphans') may unintentionally resonate with negative community perceptions of, and responses to, the labeled children (Meintjes and Giese 2006; Skovdal 2012).

While systems strengthening is key to taking OVC care and support to scale, and in building supportive and enabling environments for orphaned and vulnerable children (Skovdal and Daniel 2012), questions remain about the capacity of OVC programming, with a systems strengthening focus, to respond to the specific needs of groups of children falling within the OVC umbrella. Is there a danger that OVC programs could be so generalized that they fail to meet the distinctive needs of particular groups of children (e.g. children with disabilities or children caring for sick AIDS-infected adults)? At a time when health and welfare funding is leveling off (Kirigia et al. 2011; Leach-Kemon et al. 2012), might a drive for a generalised OVC response impact more specialized children's services?

The vagueness of the term 'vulnerable children', coupled with the sheer scale of 'AIDS orphanhood' and limited resources, could prevent some service providers from broadening their scope beyond, for example, 'AIDS orphans' and be inclusive of children who may not be orphaned, but equally and in some cases more vulnerable. This has been observed in the cash transfer program for OVC in Kenya, where vulnerable children with caregiving responsibilities did not get enrolled onto the program because both of their parents were alive (Skovdal and Campbell 2013). Similarly, PEPFAR has observed that "some partners singled out "AIDS orphans" for "services", at the expense of supporting children facing other related hardships, which "contributed to unintentional stigmatization, resentment, and psychosocial distress among beneficiaries" (Nyberg et al. 2012:129).

These challenges raise important questions, both pertaining to the capacity of general OVC programs to cater for the different layers of vulnerability that fall within the OVC umbrella, and to the role of social welfare categories in framing support. Contributing to this debate, this chapter examines children's own social representations of their HIV-positive, AIDS-affected or orphaned peers, unpacking perceived similarities and differences in the layers of vulnerability that exist within these three sub-categories that often fall within the OVC welfare category. This chapter contributes to a better understanding of vulnerability of children living in low resource and high HIV prevalence communities and highlights the need for both more general and specific responses (see also Chap. 16 in this volume).

2.2 Theoretical Framework

Why examine children's social representations of their HIV-positive, AIDS-affected and orphaned peers? Social representations refer to the values, ideas and practices that characterize a social context (Moscovici 1973). Social representations enable people to orientate themselves in their material and social world and provide a platform for communication to take place among members of a community – providing people with a code for social exchange and for classifying, naming and shaming various aspects of community life (Moscovici 1973). Children thus draw on social representations to make sense of their social world, co-construct meanings and, in the process, create social identities and representational boundaries between themselves and others (Duveen 2001; Duveen et al. 2004). Labels and welfare categories play an important role in manifesting and cementing these representational boundaries. Social representations theory can therefore be used to get an insight into local understandings of what life is like for particular groups of children, such as those who are HIV-positive, AIDS-affected or orphaned, as well as to highlight differences and similarities between them. These locally perceived differences and similarities provide a useful springboard for further debate and clarity to some of the more dominant social welfare categories in the literature.

2.3 The Study

This study forms part of a larger research project on behavioral, community and STD control interventions in the HIV response. In the course of a study of children's representations of their HIV-affected peers with particular interest in stigma (Campbell et al. 2010, 2012), it became clear that children often had quite different representations of children either HIV-affected, HIV-infected or orphaned in ways which we thought might throw interesting light on the fraught debate about what terms to use to describe children experiencing hardship in the context of HIV – a debate that has often been dominated by adult assessments of children's struggles – giving rise to this sub-study. The project was granted ethical approval by the Medical Research Council of Zimbabwe (MRCZ/A/681) and a research committee at the London School of Economics and Political Science. UNICEF (2002) guidelines for undertaking research with children were followed and written consent was obtained from all participating children and their parents/guardians with the agreement that anonymity was upheld.

The study took place in the Manicaland province of eastern Zimbabwe. Manicaland reached very high levels of HIV prevalence, particularly in the small towns, but fell, in part, due to reductions in sexual risk behavior, from 24 % between 1998 and 2000 to 15 % between 2009 and 2011 (Gregson et al. 2006). Despite the decline, Manicaland has one of the highest HIV prevalence rates in sub-Saharan Africa, leaving many children vulnerable to poor mental health (Nyamukapa et al. 2010). Data were collected from 63 children in both rural and urban sites. Participants were selected through convenience and snowball sampling by local community guides (Flick 2002) and we made efforts to stratify the data by including a mix of female and male, and urban and rural, participants (Bauer and Gaskell 2000). Three of the 63 children participating in the study were not literate and verbally dictated their story to the researcher, who then transcribed it.

Traditional research involving children has been done *on* them, not *with* them, and there is need to ensure that children are active participants in research, rather than mere objects of study (Skovdal and Abebe 2012). Not only do we have a moral obligation to facilitate children's right to participate in research, it is a pragmatic strategy to ensure policies and service delivery resonate with the lived realities of children. The draw-and-write technique has been identified as a way to engage children in age-appropriate qualitative research (Backett-Milburn and McKie 1999; Horstman et al. 2008; Knighting et al. 2011) and has previously been used to explore children's social representations (Campbell et al. 2010, 2012).

The children participating in this study were between the ages 10 and 12 and each created a draw-and-write dataset. A table of participant demographic information follows in Table 2.1. The children were given one of three open-ended prompts: (1) draw a picture and write a story about a child who is themself infected by HIV; (2) draw a picture and write a story about a child who lives in a household where a family member is affected by AIDS; or (3) draw a picture and write a story about a child who is orphaned. Field assistants took care to explain the difference between 'HIV-infected' and 'AIDS-affected' and remained present during the time of the

Table 2.1 Characterization of children who participated in the research

Prompt	# Data sets	Sex	Age	Location
AIDS-affected	26	11 girls, 15 boys	6 10 years, 8 11 years, 12 12 years	19 urban, 7 rural
HIV-positive	16	10 girls, 6 boys	5 10 years, 6 11 years, 5 12 years	7 urban, 9 rural
Orphaned	21	11 girls, 10 boys	4 10 years, 10 11 years, 7 12 years	13 urban, 8 rural
Total	**63**	**32 girls, 31 boys**	**15 10 years, 24 11 years, 24 12 years**	**39 urban, 24 rural**

exercise should the child have any questions. It is possible that this explanation may have affected the story-telling by the children. The exercises were conducted either in home settings or in local community centres. They were free to create stories based on personal experience or that were purely imaginary. We did not ask or attempt to distinguish which or how children themselves might have been affected by HIV.

Draw-and-write data sets were analyzed together and treated as a single unit. If, for example, a child both drew and spoke of a crying child, the code (basic theme) 'crying' would be applied only once to the child's draw-and-write data set. This was done to aid a tally of code occurrences in relation to the number of informants. Using thematic network analysis (Attride-Stirling 2001), emerging themes were identified by 48 codes, or basic themes. They were further condensed into 18 organizing themes and ultimately into three global themes. A frequency count of the basic themes was done. The frequencies listed in Table 2.2 refer to the number of children presenting a particular theme in their drawings and/or stories. As such, for the theme 'crying', 14 out of 21 children drew and/or wrote about a crying orphan. Additionally, the differences in code frequency between the three groups were compared using the Fisher's Exact Test. The full coding framework and a table of theme frequency and calculated p-values are illustrated in Table 2.2. Although the small, non-random sample of children limits the ability to draw strong conclusions from statistical tests, it is helpful to use the statistical analysis to supplement the core qualitative analysis to better understand the similarities and differences among the three subgroups.

2.4 Differences and Similarities Between Orphaned, HIV-Positive and AIDS-Affected Children

Reflecting the global themes of Table 2.2, it is evident that the three groups of children were perceived to experience a host of challenges and difficulties, albeit to varying degrees. They were, however, also believed to have access to, and make use of, a variety of assets, resources and solidarity. We will now draw on Table 2.2 to highlight differences and similarities in the perceived life circumstances of three groups of children affected by the HIV epidemic.

Table 2.2 Basic theme frequency, with calculated p-values for statistical differences between the three groups of OVC

Global themes	Organizing themes	Basic themes	AIDS-affected (N=26) count (%)	HIV-positive (N=16) count (%)	Orphaned (N=21) count (%)	p-values
Challenges and difficulties	Poor health	Child sick	1 (4 %)	16 (100 %)	0 (0 %)	<0.001
		Visibly unwell	3 (12 %)	8 (50 %)	2 (10 %)	0.007
	Barriers to education	No money for school expenses	0 (0 %)	0 (0 %)	9 (43 %)	<0.001
		No time to attend school	5 (19 %)	1 (8 %)	14 (67 %)	<0.001
		Poor academic performances	2 (8 %)	2 (13 %)	0 (0 %)	0.284
	Difficult living situation	Cruel guardian	0 (0 %)	6 (38 %)	8 (38 %)	<0.001
		No food	4 (15 %)	6 (38 %)	16 (76 %)	<0.001
		Parent/guardian sick	22 (85 %)	3 (19 %)	3 (14 %)	<0.001
		Ragged clothing/no shoes	2 (8 %)	1 (8 %)	19 (90 %)	<0.001
	Maltreatment and sigma	Avoided by other children	9 (35 %)	4 (25 %)	4 (19 %)	0.517
		Fear of contracting AIDS	4 (15 %)	2 (13 %)	0 (0 %)	0.154
		Physical abuse	1 (4 %)	5 (31 %)	12 (57 %)	<0.001
		Teased	3 (12 %)	1 (8 %)	9 (43 %)	0.012
		Sexual abuse	1 (4 %)	3 (19 %)	0 (0 %)	0.057
	Psychological challenges	Crying	5 (19 %)	4 (25 %)	14 (67 %)	0.003
		Lonely	4 (15 %)	0 (0 %)	1 (5 %)	0.293
		Unhappy	7 (27 %)	3 (19 %)	10 (48 %)	0.170
Assets and resources	Esteem	Admiration	6 (23 %)	0 (0 %)	7 (33 %)	0.025
		Emotional strength	6 (23 %)	0 (0 %)	3 (14 %)	0.153
		Resilience	7 (27 %)	4 (25 %)	4 (19 %)	0.869
		Perseverance	8 (31 %)	5 (31 %)	8 (38 %)	0.890
	Social actors	Assumes household duties	17 (65 %)	0 (0 %)	4 (19 %)	<0.001
		Dedicated to education	7 (27 %)	1 (8 %)	5 (24 %)	0.282
		Hard working	19 (73 %)	4 (25 %)	16 (76 %)	0.002
		Making life changing decisions	0 (0 %)	3 (19 %)	6 (29 %)	0.006

(continued)

Table 2.2 (continued)

Global themes	Organizing themes	Basic themes	AIDS-affected (N=26) count (%)	HIV-positive (N=16) count (%)	Orphaned (N=21) count (%)	p-values
	Knowledge and skills	Accurate knowledge of AIDS	10 (38 %)	8 (50 %)	0 (0 %)	<0.001
		Caregiving activities	19 (73 %)	1 (8 %)	2 (10 %)	<0.001
		Knows quality patient care	8 (31 %)	0 (0 %)	0 (0 %)	0.001
		Time management	10 (38 %)	0 (0 %)	4 (19 %)	0.010
	Community-level resources	Agricultural (animals, gardens)	15 (58 %)	3 (19 %)	10 (48 %)	0.038
		Community support	6 (23 %)	1 (8 %)	5 (24 %)	0.310
		Healthcare facilities	5 (19 %)	6 (38 %)	2 (10 %)	0.115
		Income generation	5 (19 %)	0 (0 %)	5 (24 %)	0.086
		Medical practitioners helpful	4 (15 %)	1 (8 %)	0 (0 %)	0.160
		Medicine available	5 (19 %)	2 (13 %)	0 (0 %)	0.080
		Schools	7 (27 %)	2 (13 %)	13 (62 %)	0.004
Solidarity	Community-level support	Neighbors helpful	9 (35 %)	3 (19 %)	3 (14 %)	0.249
		NGOs/charities supportive	4 (15 %)	0 (0 %)	3 (14 %)	0.308
		Peer support	4 (15 %)	1 (8 %)	2 (10 %)	0.688
		Police intervene	1 (4 %)	2 (13 %)	3 (14 %)	0.479
	Need for kind treatment	Deserve a better life	6 (23 %)	2 (13 %)	5 (24 %)	0.786
		Children not culpable	3 (12 %)	2 (13 %)	3 (14 %)	0.999
		Call to be nice to children	2 (8 %)	4 (25 %)	6 (29 %)	0.148

2.4.1 Challenges and Difficulties

Across all three groups, stories and drawings contained more reference to challenges and struggles facing children than to sources of community support. In addition to pervasive stigma, all three groups of children were depicted as having to deal with the physical ramifications of HIV/AIDS and other illnesses – afflicting themselves or loved ones, difficult living situations, educational challenges, maltreatment, poverty, and psychosocial difficulties. While all three groups of children were quick to identify the physical manifestations of poverty and disease, they also identified less tangible hardships, such as shame and loneliness. The most frequently identified challenges are outlined below.

2.4.1.1 Poor Health

Although a few children represented AIDS-affected and orphaned children as visibly unwell (12 % and 10 %, respectively), HIV-positive children were, unsurprisingly, significantly more likely to be represented as physically ill compared to their AIDS-affected and orphaned peers (50 %, $p = 0.007$).

> He [an HIV-positive boy] is very thin and looked like a two year old boy. His hair slips back and when he touches it. His leg is like a stick of matches. His hand is like a skeleton's. (Akudzwe, girl, aged 11)

One boy, Adashe (aged 10), drew the picture of an HIV-positive girl as presented below:

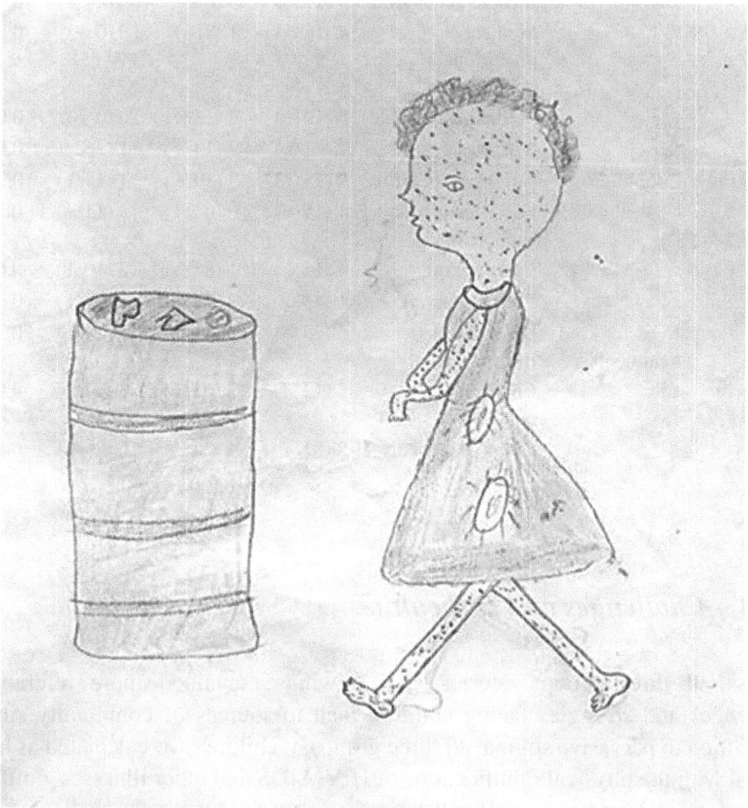

An HIV-positive girl

2.4.1.2 Barriers to Education

Orphaned children were more likely than the other two groups to be represented as facing barriers to education (basic themes "no money for school expenses" – $p<0.001$ and "no time to attend school" – $p<0.001$). Compared to their peers they were also more likely to be described as being bright (to stress the unfairness of their limited access to education) and to live in a context characterized by poverty and neglect, often with elderly guardians who are struggling to pay for school fees, or with extended family members who take little interest in the orphaned child (see also '*Difficult Living Situation*'):

> He [an orphan] is an intelligent boy but there is no money for him [to attend school]. (Anotendwa, girl, aged 10)

In contrast, HIV-positive children were not represented as having any difficulties attending school. Instead, 13 % of the children drawing and writing about HIV-positive children depicted them as performing poorly in school, primarily because of poor health compared to others.

2.4.1.3 Difficult Living Situation

Orphaned and HIV-positive children were more likely than their AIDS-affected counterparts to be represented as living with a cruel guardian ($p<0.001$) and be subject to neglect (basic theme "ragged clothing/no shoes" – $p<0.001$).

> He [an orphan] lives with his aunt. She is very cruel to him. His aunt's children tell him to do all the household work. They do not do anything but wash and eat. He is not going to school. She told him I do not have any money to waste on you. (Anotida, girl, aged 10)

Cruel guardians were often described by the children to fail to provide adequate food or clothing for their charges.

> His [HIV-positive boy] stepmother is very cruel to him . . . everyday he is late for school. If he fails at the end of term, his mother bites him. Sometimes he is not given food to eat. (Cebile, girl, aged 10)

AIDS-affected children, on the other hand, were significantly more likely to be represented as living with sick parents who are unable to sustain the household than their HIV-positive and orphaned peers ($p<0.001$).

2.4.1.4 Maltreatment and Stigma

There were numerous depictions of AIDS-affected, HIV-positive and orphaned children being subject to stigma, discrimination and maltreatment. As illustrated in Table 2.2, all three groups of children were represented as being avoided by their non-affected peers.

> No children will play with her [AIDS-affected girl]. This is because of stigmatization. (Chadamwari, girl, aged 10)
>
> No one likes to visit them [an AIDS-affected family] because they fear to catch the disease. (Chenai, girl, aged 11)

There were, however, differences in the kind of maltreatment and stigma that each of the three groups of children experienced. Orphaned children, for example, compared to their AIDS-affected peers, were significantly more likely to be represented as subject to physical abuse ($p<0.001$), echoing the neglect described earlier, and marginally more likely to be represented as subject to teasing and bullying compared to their HIV-positive and AIDS-affected peers ($p=0.012$).

> Her [an HIV-positive girl] classmates laugh at her, teased her, cartoon her. She feels unwanted. (Chiedza, girl, aged 11)

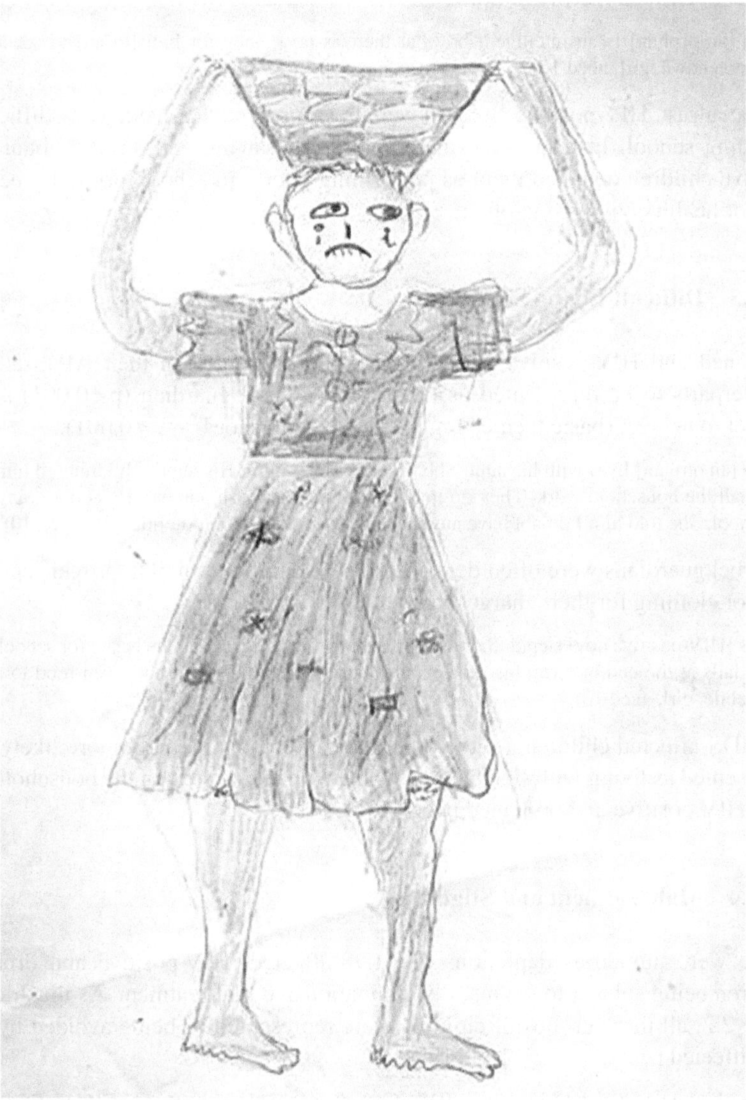

An orphaned girl. (Chiratidzo, girl, aged 11)

2.4.1.5 Psychosocial Challenges

Orphaned children were represented as facing more psychosocial challenges than their counterparts. While all three groups were said to face substantial emotional challenges, these children were significantly more likely to be depicted as crying than either AIDS-affected children or HIV-positive children ($p=0.003$).

This section has highlighted that orphaned, HIV-positive and AIDS-affected children are represented by their non-affected peers to face numerous challenges. Although most of the challenges cut across the three categories of children, highlighting similarities in their struggles, some of the representations suggest a pattern of differences in the hardship they experience. This includes dominant representations of orphaned children as neglected by non-caring guardians, subject to physical abuse, and generally upset by their situation. HIV-positive children, compared to their peers, were represented as experiencing poor health and struggling to concentrate in class because of feeling unwell. Like their AIDS-affected peers, they were represented to experience HIV-related stigma, above and beyond what orphaned children experience. What distinguished AIDS-affected children from their HIV-positive and orphaned peers was their representation of living with AIDS-sick parents.

2.4.2 Assets and Resources

The children identified a variety of community resources and assets, including direct material help, charitable gestures and recognition of children as social actors that benefit 'OVC'. They were said to utilize community support networks that enable them to be more independent. Additionally, the children were represented to draw upon personal traits and strengths to survive and engage in community life.

2.4.2.1 Esteem

AIDS-affected and orphaned children were perceived to receive higher levels of esteem than their HIV-positive counterparts. AIDS-affected and orphaned children were significantly more likely to be described with admiration compared to their HIV-positive peers ($p=0.025$). This admiration emerged as a representation both through how the participating children themselves described the AIDS-affected or orphaned children or how they portrayed them as being recognized by local community members:

> Her [AIDS-affected child] sick mother thanks her every time she cares for her, she will be giving some blessings from God. (Chirango, boy, aged 12)

By implication, the lack of recognition of HIV-positive children's strengths, and the fact that none of the children spoke of them with admiration, suggests that

HIV-positive children are seen as victims and in need of support. No difference was observed in relation to their resilience and perseverance. A quarter of the children portrayed their grouping of children as emotionally resilient and a third of them spoke of them as having perseverance.

2.4.2.2 Social Actors

Reflecting earlier themes that represent HIV-positive children as weak and with more physical challenges, no HIV-infected children were portrayed as contributors to household livelihoods. In contrast, orphaned and AIDS-affected children, in particular, were significantly more likely to be represented as engaging in positive behaviours, such as actively taking on head-of-household responsibilities ($p < 0.001$):

> He [an AIDS-affected boy] is now the breadwinner everyday. He goes to sell tomatoes for them to survive. His two younger sisters clean, wash, and cook. (Andokuhle, boy, aged 11)

Ashirai, a boy aged 12, told us that:

> I take care of my father because I love my father. In my spare time I go and do the selling my cabbages and maize and beans and milk and the money I make goes to buying my father some fruits like avocados.

He also drew a picture of taking care of his father below:

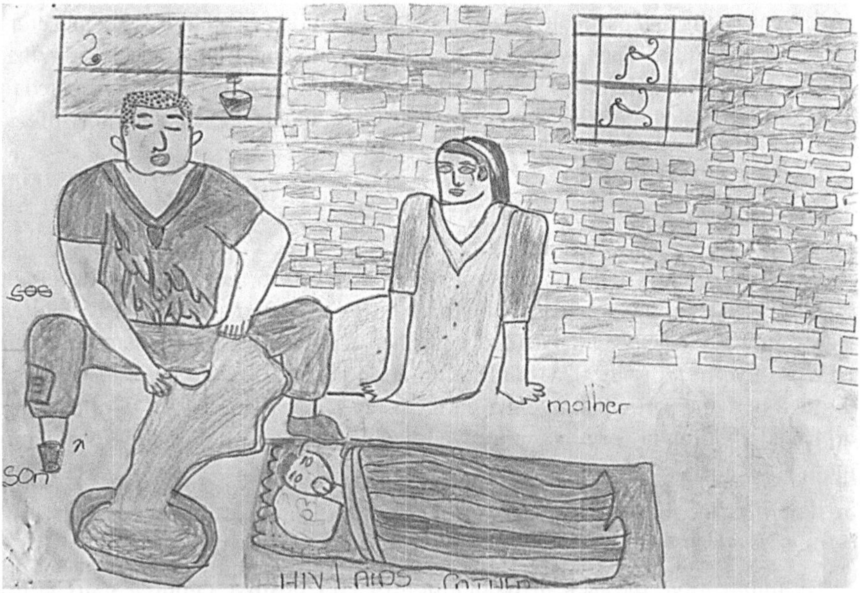

A boy caring for his HIV-positive father

Relatedly, both AIDS-affected and orphaned children were significantly more likely to be represented as hard working compared to HIV-positive children ($p = 0.002$)) – earning them greater recognition as active agents – although all three groups are at least minimally represented as engaging in routine work.

> She [an AIDS-affected girl] has to go early in the morning to the garden to grow some vegetables . . .after work she will go and play with her friends. (Bakhile, boy, aged 12)

This idea was also expressed in the drawing drawn by Zvikomborero, a girl aged 12.

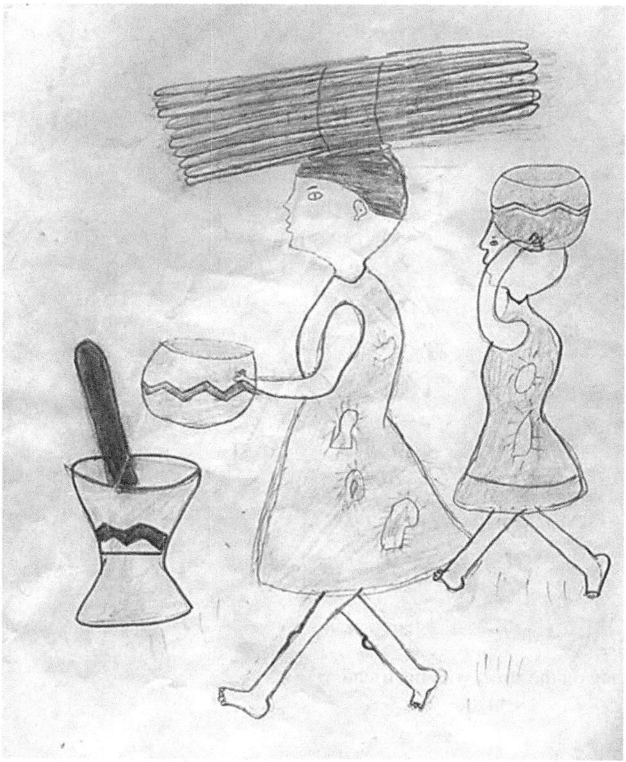

Two orphaned siblings completing chores

In addition, orphaned children, echoing the dominant representation of them being neglected, were illustrated as capable social actors, capable of making critical and complex decisions such as deciding to run away from an abusive family.

> She decided to run away from her [abusive] aunt, so that she can live a good life. She decided to live in the streets. (Washe, girl, aged 11)

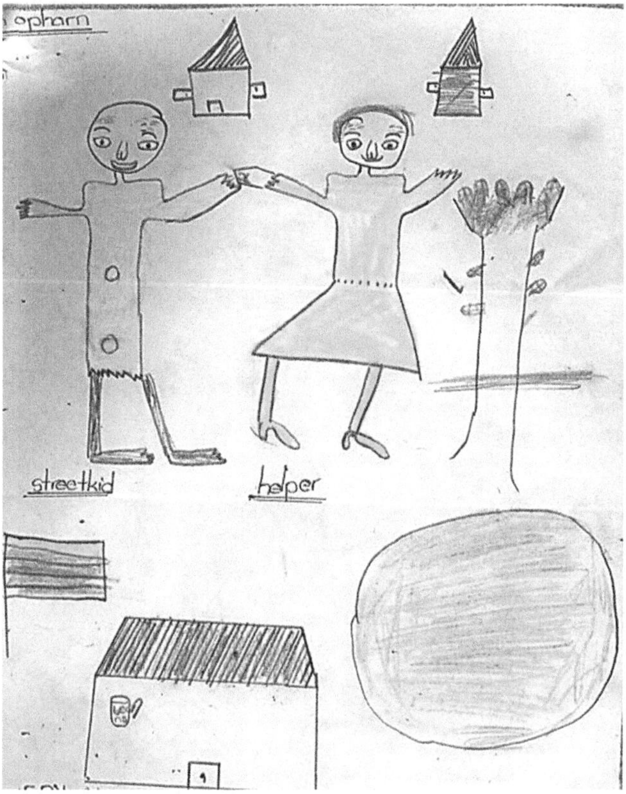

An orphan living on the street with his friend

2.4.2.3 Knowledge and Skills

The three groups of children were portrayed to have significantly different levels of knowledge and skills. Reflecting their representation of AIDS-affected children as social actors, this group of children was portrayed as having substantial know-how of how to care for sick parents, compared to both their HIV-positive and orphaned peers ($p=0.001$). 73 % of the drawings and stories of AIDS-affected children depicted them, one way or the other, as having the knowledge and skills to take good care of sick and immune-compromised relatives. This is what one girl, Wedzerai (aged 11) wrote about an AIDS-affected girl in her story.

> She [AIDS-affected child] always buys fruits for her parents for instance apples, bananas, oranges and pineapple. They always eat few fruits but she encourages them to take a lot because they are good for their health.

They were also depicted as having good time management skills – an outcome of juggling multiple responsibilities simultaneously. There were also significant differences in how the children were perceived to have accurate knowledge about HIV and AIDS. At no point were orphaned children said to have good and accurate knowledge about HIV. HIV-positive children and AIDS-affected children on the other hand, arguably because of their close proximity to HIV, were believed to have good knowledge about HIV ($p<0.001$).

2.4.2.4 Community Resources

AIDS-affected and orphaned children, in particular, were depicted as drawing on a variety of material resources to enable them to cope with their misfortunes and better their situation. They were portrayed as working in the fields or tending a garden as an income-generating activity (no HIV-positive child was portrayed as engaging in income generating work). Both HIV-positive and AIDS-affected children were represented as more likely than orphaned children to know, and make use of, local health facilities.

This section on assets and resources has also highlighted significant differences between the social representations of HIV-positive, AIDS-affected and orphaned children. HIV-positive children were depicted as having good HIV knowledge, but were also described as weak, earning them no esteem or admiration. AIDS-affected and orphaned children on the other hand were more likely to be represented as social actors, taking active roles in sustaining their household. This was particularly the case for AIDS-affected children who were depicted as young carers and admired for their support and commitment to their sick parents.

2.4.3 Solidarity

Many of the drawings and essays gave detail to community-level solidarity, both through the children's representations of the sort of peer, family and community support that is available to AIDS-affected, HIV-positive and orphaned children, but also by indicating their own recognition of the children's strengths and by making calls for treating these three groups of children better.

2.4.3.1 Community Support

As highlighted by Table 2.2, only a minority of the drawings depicted the children as benefitting from communities, local organizations, neighbors, and extended family members. The drawings or stories that did include community support, gave detail to both informal assistance, such as helping with chores or caregiving, or more formally through the support of local community groups or non-governmental organizations.

> Rudo understands the situation at Pamela's [an AIDS-affected child] house so if they are back she helps Pamela doing all the housework . . . Rudo helps her friend Pamela all the time. (Vhukile, boy, aged 12)
>
> He [an orphan] was registered by the Red Cross which paid for fees and books and food, now he goes to school with everything. Every day, he thinks of his parents. And he thanks his grandmother and his uncle and the Red Cross. (Tongoona, boy, aged 11)

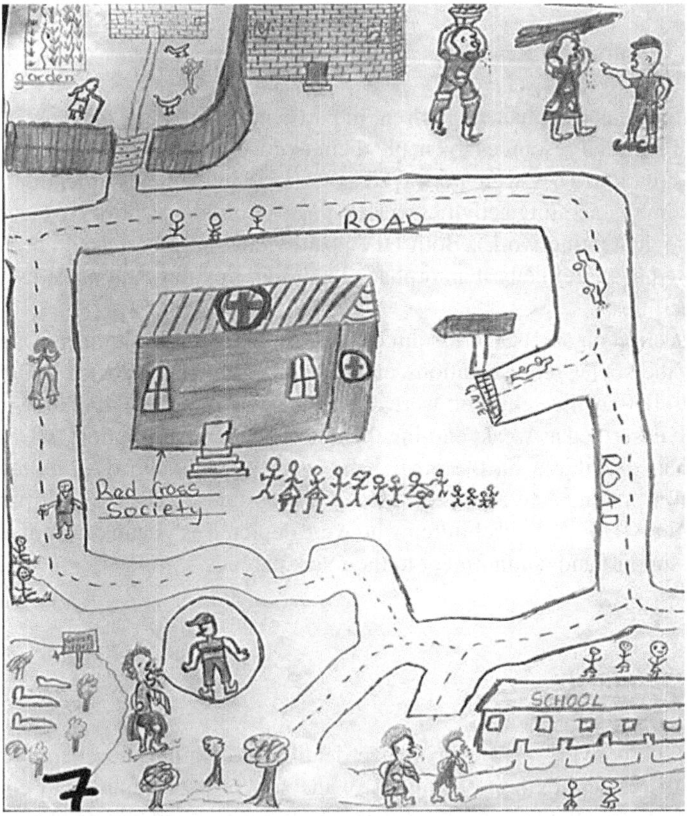

A queue to visit the Red Cross. (Tivongeshe, boy, aged 10)

There were no significant differences in their representation of community support available to the three groups of children.

2.4.3.2 Need for Kind Treatment

A number of the children's written stories concluded with some recommendations that the children, regardless of their life circumstances, need to be treated in a kind and respectful manner. The children acknowledged that each of the three groups of children were undeserving of the scorn and malice that is shown toward them and deserve a better life.

> My advice to them [other children] is that people must show love, support and care to them [HIV positive children]. They must know that they mustn't ruin other children's lives. (Tinaishe, girl, aged 12)

Our child informants recognized that the situation that children falling under the OVC category find themselves in is unjust and undeserved. These stories indicate that children have a visceral understanding that all children deserve kindness and an awareness that they should reach out to children falling under the OVC category.

2.5 Conclusion

To contribute to debates on whether service delivery for children of the HIV epidemic should be targeted to address the unique needs of certain groups of children or remain comprehensive in general areas such as psychosocial support, education, social protection and health, this paper examined similarities and differences in Zimbabwean children's social representations of their HIV-positive, AIDS-affected or orphaned peers.

It is clear from our findings that children, whether they are HIV-positive, AIDS-affected or orphaned, were seen to face many similar struggles and to draw on similar assets or resources to cope with hardship. This highlights the importance of pursuing a more generalized response, for all children falling under the OVC category and that caution should be exercised when defining child vulnerability in terms of orphanhood or household illness (Akwara et al. 2010). However, the social representations analysis presented in this paper suggests that there are also some significant differences between HIV-positive, AIDS-affected and orphaned children, which can be used to inform service delivery. For example, both AIDS-affected and orphaned children were depicted as social actors and were held in high esteem for their efforts to sustain household livelihoods. Their good social behavior was admired by the children participating in the study. Caregiving children in Kenya have been observed to draw on this social recognition of their agency to develop positive social identities that help them cope with adversity (Skovdal et al. 2009; Skovdal and Andreouli 2011). HIV-positive children, in contrast, were not admired in any way. They were portrayed as having poor health, weak and faced with stigma. Orphaned children, more than both HIV-positive and AIDS-affected children were depicted as sad and neglected by non-caring and abusive guardians. This picture could be elaborated through further research into community members' and family members' social representations of HIV-positive, AIDS-affected and orphaned children (Skovdal et al. 2013).

A limitation of the paper is that it does not seek to establish any kind of straightforward relationship between the perceptions that arise from the stories and the daily 'realities' of orphaned and vulnerable children. In fact, some perceptions may reflect stereotypes, and do little to unpack the fact that some children may be both orphaned, HIV-positive, and care for an elderly caregiver. The most we are able to claim is that the representations we have identified above constitute powerful symbolic resources which are likely to play a key role in shaping children's understandings, interactions with peers and responses to personal hardship. It would, therefore, be useful to explore these issues further, both by triangulating the study with adult perceptions, and by interviewing children who self-identify as orphaned, HIV-positive or AIDS-affected about their lived experiences.

Although this paper does not offer much of a solution to how we should define the vulnerability of HIV-positive, AIDS-affected and orphaned children, it does offer a local insight to some of the perceived differences between these three groups of children as well as implications for care and support. Furthermore, social representations, like the ones presented in this paper, typify representational boundaries that are created by children to either create distance or bring themselves closer to the 'other' (e.g., HIV-positive, AIDS-affected or orphaned children). These in and out group boundaries are reflective of children's own fears and anxieties and create a sense of comfort, safety and psychological distancing. Whilst such processes help children, irrespective of their life and living situation, to give meaning to hardship, they can also be used to explain stigmatizing (e.g., children teasing peers living with HIV) or sympathizing (e.g., children respecting AIDS-affected children because of their caregiving) attitudes and behaviors (Jodelet 1991) and highlight avenues for stigma reduction programming (Campbell et al. 2010).

Based on our findings, we conclude that children living in low resource and high HIV prevalence communities can benefit from both a more generalized OVC response and a continued need to unpack differences with the aim of (i) addressing the unique needs of certain sub-groups of children and (ii) to make optimal use of the distinct resources and forms of solidarity that are available to them. Practitioners need to combine the strengths of both approaches and to promote a mix of targeted and generalized systems strengthening responses. How to do so cost-effectively and without increasing stigma are important challenges still to be addressed.

Acknowledgements The Wellcome Trust (award number 084401/Z/07/Z) supported this research. We would like to thank the children participating in this study for their valuable input.

References

Akwara, P. A., Noubary, B., Lim Ah Ken, P., Johnson, K., Yates, R., Winfrey, W., et al. (2010). Who is the vulnerable child? Using survey data to identify children at risk in the era of HIV and AIDS. *AIDS Care, 22*(9), 1066–1085.

Attride-Stirling, J. (2001). Thematic networks: An analytic tool for qualitative research. *Qualitative Research, 1*(3), 385–405.

Backett-Milburn, K., & McKie, L. (1999). A critical appraisal of the draw and write technique. *Health Education Research, 14*, 387–398.

Bauer, M., & Gaskell, G. (2000). *Qualitative researching with text, image and sound: A practical handbook for social research*. London: Sage.

Campbell, C., Skovdal, M., Mupambireyi, Z., & Gregson, S. (2010). Exploring children's stigmatisation of AIDS-affected children in Zimbabwe through drawings and stories. *Social Science & Medicine, 71*(5), 975–985.

Campbell, C., Skovdal, M., Mupambireyi, Z., Madanhire, C., Robertson, L., Nyamukapa, C. A., et al. (2012). Can AIDS stigma be reduced to poverty stigma? Exploring Zimbabwean children's representations of poverty and AIDS. *Child: Care, Health and Development, 38*(5), 732–742.

Duveen, G. (2001). Representations, identities, resistance. In K. Deaux & G. Philogène (Eds.), *Representations of the social* (pp. 254–270). Oxford: Blackwell.

Duveen, G., Lloyd, B. B., & British Psychological Society Conference. (2004). *Social representations and the development of knowledge*. Cambridge: Cambridge University Press.

Flick, U. (2002). *An introduction to qualitative research* (2nd ed.). London: Sage.

Gregson, S., Garnett, G., Nyamukapa, C., Hallett, T., Lewis, J., Mason, P., et al. (2006). HIV decline associated with behavior change in eastern Zimbabwe. *Science, 311*, 664–666.

Horstman, M., Aldiss, S., Richardson, A., & Gibson, F. (2008). Methodological issues when using the draw and write technique with children aged 6 to 12 years. *Qualitative Health Research, 18*(7), 1001–1011.

Jodelet, D. (1991). *Madness and social representations*. Hemel Hempstead: Harvester-Wheatsheaf.

Kang, M., Dunbar, M., Laver, S., & Padian, N. (2008). Maternal versus paternal orphans and HIV/STI risk among adolescent girls in Zimbabwe. *AIDS Care, 20*(2), 214–217.

Kirigia, J., Nganda, B., Mwikisa, C., & Cardoso, B. (2011). Effects of global financial crisis on funding for health development in nineteen countries of the WHO African Region. *BMC International Health and Human Rights, 11*(1), 4. doi:10.1186/1472-698X-11-4 Retrieved January 5, 2015, from http://www.biomedcentral.com/1472-698X/11/4

Knighting, K., Rowa-Dewar, N., Malcolm, C., Kearney, N., & Gibson, F. (2011). Children's understanding of cancer and views on health-related behaviour: A 'draw and write' study. *Child: Care, Health and Development, 37*(2), 289–299.

Leach-Kemon, K., Chou, D. P., Schneider, M. T., Tardif, A., Dieleman, J. L., Brooks, B. P., et al. (2012). The global financial crisis has led to a slowdown in growth of funding to improve health in many developing countries. *Health Affairs, 31*(1), 228–235.

Meintjes, H., & Giese, S. (2006). Spinning the epidemic – The making of mythologies of orphanhood in the context of AIDS. *Childhood, 13*(3), 407–430.

Moscovici, S. (1973). Foreword. In C. Herzlich (Ed.), *Health and illness: A social psychological analysis* (pp. ix–xiv). London: Academic Press [for] the European Association of Experimental Social Psychology.

Nyamukapa, C., Gregson, S., Wambe, M., Mushore, P., Lopman, B., Mupambireyi, Z., et al. (2010). Causes and consequences of psychological distress among orphans in eastern Zimbabwe. *AIDS Care, 22*(8), 988–996.

Nyberg, B. J., Yates, D. D., Lovich, R., Coulibaly-Traore, D., Sherr, L., Thurman, T. R., et al. (2012). Saving lives for a lifetime: Supporting orphans and vulnerable children impacted by HIV/AIDS. *JAIDS Journal of Acquired Immune Deficiency Syndromes, 60*, S127–S135.

PEPFAR. (2012). *Guidance for orphans and vulnerable children programming*: U.S. President's emergency plan for AIDS relief. Retrieved January 15, 2013, from http://www.pepfar.gov/documents/organization/195702.pdf

Skovdal, M. (2012). Pathologising healthy children? A review of the literature exploring the mental health of HIV-affected children in sub-Saharan Africa. *Transcultural Psychiatry, 49*(3–4), 461–491.

Skovdal, M., & Abebe, T. (2012). Reflexivity and dialogue: Methodological and socio-ethical dilemmas in research with HIV-affected children in East Africa. *Ethics, Policy & Environment, 15*(1), 77–96.

Skovdal, M., & Andreouli, E. (2011). Using identity and recognition as a framework to understand and promote the resilience of caregiving children in western Kenya. *Journal of Social Policy, 40*(03), 613–630.

Skovdal, M., & Campbell, C. (2013). Public engagement and policymaking for care giving children of the HIV epidemic in Sub-Saharan Africa. In R. A. Smith (Ed.), *Global HIV/AIDS politics, policy, and activism: Persistent challenges and emerging issues* (Policy and policymaking, Vol. 2, pp. 107–130). Santa Barbara: Praeger.

Skovdal, M., & Daniel, M. (2012). Resilience through participation and coping-enabling social environments: The case of HIV-affected children in sub-Saharan Africa. *African Journal of AIDS Research, 11*(3), 153–164.

Skovdal, M., Ogutu, V., Aoro, C., & Campbell, C. (2009). Young carers as social actors: Coping strategies of children caring for ailing or ageing guardians in Western Kenya. *Social Science and Medicine, 69*(4), 587–595.

Skovdal, M., Campbell, C., & Onyango, V. (2013). Supporting 'young carers' in Kenya: From policy paralysis to action. *Child Care in Practice, 19*(4), 318–339.

UNAIDS. (2013). *Global report: UNAIDS report on the global AIDS epidemic 2013*. Geneva: UNAIDS.

UNICEF. (2002). *Children participating in research, monitoring and evaluation (M&E) – Ethics and your responsibilities as a manager*. UNICEF Evaluation Office. Retrieved January 6, 2010, from http://www.unicef.org/evaluation/files/TechNote1_Ethics.pdf

UNICEF. (2004). *The framework for the protection, care and support of orphans and vulnerable children living in a world with HIV and AIDS*. UNICEF. Retrieved May 27, 2008, from http://www.unicef.org/aids/files/Framework_English.pdf

UNICEF, UNAIDS, & USAID. (2004). *Children on the brink*. New York: United Nations Children's Fund.

Watts, H., Lopman, B., Nyamukapa, C., & Gregson, S. (2005). Rising incidence and prevalence of orphanhood in Manicaland, Zimbabwe, 1998 to 2003. *AIDS, 19*(7), 717–725.

World Bank. (2005). *The OVC toolkit for SSA: A toolkit on how to support orphans and other vulnerable children (OVC) in sub-Saharan Africa*. Washinton, DC: World Bank Africa Region and the World Bank Institute. www.worldbank.org/ovctoolkit

Chapter 3
Children's Experiences of Living with HIV-Positive Parents Within the Family Context of Bangladesh

Md Shahidul Islam, John Scott, and Victor Minichiello

Contents

3.1 Introduction

HIV may be particularly challenging for children in a family with HIV-positive parents (Hosegood and Madhavan 2010; Richter 2010). Studies show that HIV-infected and affected children suffer from material and psychosocial disadvantages due directly and indirectly to HIV/AIDS-related stigma (Chase and Aggleton 2001; Messer et al. 2010; Chi and Li 2013). Several studies on HIV and AIDS have

M.S. Islam, Ph.D. (✉)
School of Health, University of New England, Armidale, NSW 2351, Australia
e-mail: mislam27@une.edu.au

J. Scott, Ph.D.
School of Justice, Queensland University of Technology, Brisbane, Queensland, Australia
e-mail: j31.scott@qut.edu.au

V. Minichiello, Ph.D.
The Australian Research Centre in Sex, Health and Society La Trobe University, Melbourne, Australia

University of New England, Armidale, NSW 2351, Australia
e-mail: vminichiello56@gmail.com

P. Liamputtong (ed.), *Children and Young People Living with HIV/AIDS*, Cross-Cultural Research in Health, Illness and Well-Being, DOI 10.1007/978-3-319-29936-5_3

identified a number of risks and pressures on children's lives due to HIV infection in the family. These include the disruption or loss of parental care and support, increased poverty, malnutrition, withdrawal from school, decreased access to health care, increased participation in household activities, psychological stress, social stigma, as well as increased risks of abuse, exploitation and HIV infection (Schuster et al. 2000; Beard et al. 2010; Leeper et al. 2010; Richter et al. 2010; Chi and Li 2013; Sherr et al. 2014; Stein et al. 2014). In terms of services, HIV/AIDS has an incremental impact on children in families and communities in developing countries, including poor infrastructure and limited access to basic services, accelerate the adverse impacts experienced by children and families in a number of ways (Brown and Lourie 2000; Hosegood and Madhavan 2010). Social, economic and psychological impacts of HIV on children increase their vulnerability to HIV infection through early onset of sexual activity, commercial sex and sexual abuse (Foster and Williamson 2000; Chi and Li 2013).

At a psychosocial level, several studies have identified how children's psychological adjustments have been influenced by parental illness (Armistead et al. 1995; Schuster et al. 2000; Chi and Li 2013). Children living with HIV-positive parents tend to have poorer psychological functioning than children living with HIV-negative parents (Armistead et al. 1995; Reyland et al. 2002; Cluver and Gardner 2007). Due to the experience of the life-threatening nature of HIV, children have to endure psychosocial distress in the family (Richter et al. 2010; Chi and Li 2013). Children of HIV-positive parents may perceive themselves as tainted or contaminated because of their parents' HIV status (Harms et al. 2010; Chi and Li 2013). Consequently, children of HIV-positive parents suffer from mental distress and depression (Boyd-Franklin et al. 1995). Research has also shown that children living with HIV-positive parents face more psychological and cognitive difficulties than children living with HIV-negative parents (Reyland et al. 2002; Cluver and Gardner 2007). There is increasing evidence from the developing world that children of HIV-positive parents experience increased mental health and behavioral problems (Forehand et al. 1998; Cluver and Gardner 2007). Research also shows that children in an HIV-affected family demonstrate lower self-esteem than children in a non-HIV-affected family (Murphy et al. 2006). Brewer and Sparkes (2011) explored the experiences of parentally bereaved young people in the UK and they found that these children experienced several emotional and social difficulties with respect to fear, sadness, grief, and feelings of isolation.

At a societal level, a growing body of clinical and anecdotal evidence suggests that children in HIV-affected families are extremely vulnerable to social isolation (Strode and Barrett Grant 2001; Beard et al. 2010; Richter 2010), that may hamper their health, development and well-being. For instance, Strode and Barret-Grant (2001) reported that some HIV-positive children were excluded from schools in South Africa. Similarly, Chase and Aggleton (2001) revealed that children of HIV-positive parents were taunted by their peers and excluded from school in Zambia. Deacon and Stephney (2007) suggested that, due to fears of bullying and discrimination, caregivers were unwilling to send HIV-positive children to school. In a study conducted in Zimbabwe, Mahati and colleagues (2006) identified verbal abuse from peers as a manifestation of stigma and discrimination against affected children.

Several studies have reported that children of HIV-infected parents avoid social interaction in order to avoid situations in which they may encounter stigma (Strode and Barrett Grant 2001; Messer et al. 2010). In a qualitative study, Gossart-Walker and Nancy (1998) showed that six towards children of HIV-positive parents tend to result in them being emotionally secluded from other children.

Children in the early stages of their socialization may interpret, express and react to stigma differently to adults. For instance, children may experience stigma more deeply than adults when they find themselves in a HIV situation (Deacon and Stephney 2007). In this way, the disease changes their lives whether they are infected or one or both of their parents are infected. It disrupts their family and community relationships, and the regular visits to health facilities and social services intrude on their everyday lives (Reyland et al. 2002; Liamputtong et al. 2013). For instance, when a parent develops HIV-related symptoms, children are often given new responsibilities. In particular, children often assume responsibility for household tasks, care for younger siblings, pursue income-generating activities and provide emotional support for their parents at the expense of their own developmental needs (Deacon and Stephney 2007). Death of parents within the household often has detrimental economic consequences because of the loss of parents' income and property. This often forces them to withdraw from school in order to pay for the medical and household expenses of the family (Harms et al. 2010; Chi and Li 2013).

A number of recent studies in Africa explore the experience of children affected and infected by HIV/AIDS (Cluver and Gardner 2007; Floyd et al. 2007), but with a general tendency to research children from adult perspectives. Most of the studies on HIV-affected families focus mainly on parents (Schuster et al. 2000; Cowgill et al. 2008), with limited input from the children. There is a small but growing body of literature on the experiences of HIV-positive children. However, these are only relevant to economically developed countries (Schuster et al. 2000; Reyland et al. 2002; Gosling et al. 2004; Nöstlinger et al. 2006; Murphy and Marelich 2008). An earlier study reported on orphan experiences of parental loss (Harms et al. 2010). They emphasized the academic, physical and mental health outcomes of HIV/AIDS orphans. Further, the individual experience of orphanhood, as expressed through personal perspectives of orphaned youth, has been discussed, while children's experiences of living within HIV-affected families have been comparatively less understood.

An additional problem is that most studies on children are quantitative (Schuster et al. 2000; Reyland et al. 2002; Nöstlinger et al. 2006; Floyd et al. 2007; Murphy and Marelich 2008), rather than qualitative in design, which makes it difficult for researchers to deeply explore experiences with regards to stigma that disadvantage children and recounted from their worldviews. In order to bridge this gap, our study focuses on children so that their voices can be heard.

Whilst HIV prevalence is low in Bangladesh, the number of HIV-infected and affected children is steadily increasing. Despite this increase, research on HIV-infected and affected children has not increased proportionately. The study on which this chapter is based is the first research on HIV and its impacts on children in Bangladesh. Little is known about the vulnerabilities faced by the children in HIV-affected families in Bangladesh. In this context, this chapter aims to understand

HIV-positive or negative children's experiences of living with HIV-positive parents within the family context in Bangladesh. While, as noted above, there has been some research on the psychological impacts of illness in the family context, the chapter especially seeks to understand the *social* impacts of HIV. As such, concepts such as *stigma* and *discrimination* will be utilized to understand the experiences of the children involved in this research.

3.2 Stigma and Discrimination

The concept *stigma* is broad and difficult to define, but most definitions are associated with deviance (Liamputtong and Kitisriworapan 2012; see also Chap. 1). People who are stigmatized are regarded negatively for having violated rules, ideals, expectations or traits considered socially desirable (Alonzo and Reynolds 1995). In this way, stigma is a social experience and one which is anchored in time and space. As such, the term is useful in comprehending the particular experience of children in the context of Bangladesh.

Stigma theorists, starting with Goffman (1963), posit that stigma is a social construct which creates a powerful and discrediting social label that gradually changes how we see ourselves (the stigmatized adopting the perspective of those who have rejected them) and how we are regarded by others (Alonzo and Reynolds 1995). Stigmatized people may actually accept the norms that disqualify them from comfortable and equal participation in social interaction. This manifests in psychosocial impacts such as self-loathing or shame, and internalization of negative values or repressed anger resulting from discrimination.

While some social psychologists have declared that categorization and construction of stereotyping beliefs are normal functions of the cognitive operations of the human mind, others have argued that beliefs are shaped by social context (Crocker et al. 1998; Earnshaw and Kalichman 2013). In this way, stigma is a product of social interaction and manifests in culturally specific ways (Parker and Aggleton 2003). Goffman (1963: 3) defines stigma as discrediting attributes that are used to identify social positions or boundaries. He also describes stigma as the product of a discrepancy between 'virtual social identity' and 'actual social identity' where '*virtual social identity*' is the stereotyped attributions and social categorization of others that we expect and '*actual social identity*' is the attributes the individual actually posses. Alonzo and Reynolds (1995) have argued that HIV and AIDS are stigmatizing conditions because: they are considered to be caused by deviance and are considered to produce deviance; they are viewed as the responsibility of the individual and linked to a morally sanctionable behavior and, therefore, represent a character blemish; they are perceived as contagious and threatening to the community; they are associated with an undesirable and unaesthetic forms of death; and in some countries they are still not well understood by the community and viewed negatively by healthcare providers.

Aggleton and Parker (2005: 18) also contend that "power stands at the heart of social life and is used to legitimize inequalities of the status within the social structure". They emphasized that stigmatization and discrimination should be conceptualized as a social process of power and domination. In their view, HIV/AIDS-related stigmatization and discrimination should be understood in the broader context of the political economy of social exclusion of a particular society (Aggleton and Parker 2005). Link and Phelan (2001) argue that social, economic and political power relies on stigma. In this chapter, we will show that such political activity does not just occur at the broader institutional level of states, but is also rife in the context of families and that children are impacted by such activity.

These theoretical and conceptual explanations suggest that to understand HIV stigma within a particular society, we should first stress an understanding of the social processes that mark the construction of HIV stigma within that particular socio-cultural context (Earnshaw and Kalichman 2013). Although stigma is a global phenomenon, it is inextricably linked to the social and cultural context of HIV-positive individuals where they live. For example, socio-cultural beliefs, norms, values, and morals of community members have a major role in shaping stigma and discrimination. In Bangladesh, the implications of HIV stigmatization are particularly detrimental due to a rigid and hierarchical socioeconomic system, strict cultural norms and values, clear gender divisions, and religious ideologies which emphasize physical purity (Ullah 2011). For example, while studies in western contexts have revealed that HIV-positive individuals who are infected with the virus via injecting drug use faced significant stigma (Alonzo and Reynolds 1995; Herek et al. 2002; Clark et al. 2003), in a Bangladeshi context, the social emphasis has largely been focused on sexual immorality, rather than illicit activities (e.g., drug use) (Ullah 2011).

Managing stigma involves developing strategies to avoid or minimize negative attributions. Indeed, one way to manage stigma is denial or attempts to conceal a stigmatized identity, which might be possible with HIV as outward signs of infection with the virus may not be readily visible or possible to associate with HIV. Stigma may cause family members to be secretive with each other, be it husband and wife or parent and child, so as to conceal a spoiled identity and protect self-esteem or protect others negative impacts associated with stigma. Stigma may also limit access to broader or extended familial or social networks, either through desire to conceal the stigma or because of social discrimination associated with the stigma. The stress of managing stigma can be emotionally exhausting may lead to strains in family relations and mental health problems, such as stress, anxiety and depression (Kimberly and Serovich 1999; Guoping et al. 2007). Concealment of stigma can also reduce access to social support networks and also risks the hostility or intimate others when the condition is voluntarily or involuntarily revealed (Alonzo and Reynolds 1995). In this way, strategies to manage stigma associated with HIV and AIDs may further erode the social capital that can be sourced from networks. For example, trust, an important aspect of social capital, especially intimacy and bonding, is challenged by the need to conceal stigma (See also Chaps. 2, 4, 6, 9, and 14 in this volume).

3.3 The Study

We used a qualitative research design informed by principles of grounded theory for this study. We recruited the participants with the support of two self-help groups of HIV-positive people, in two settings namely Khulna and Dhaka in Bangladesh. Participants were selected through theoretical sampling procedures. Children of HIV-positive parents provided the pool of potential child participants. We recruited a total 19 children, either HIV-positive or – negative, between ages 10 and ≤18 years if they were aware of their parent's HIV infection, had regular contact with their parent/s, and they were permitted by their parents to participate as participants in the study. If the parents had more than one child who met the eligibility criteria, the child who was HIV-positive was selected to participate as very few HIV-positive dyads were found.

Given that participants comprised a stigmatized group who had experienced disadvantage and discrimination, we took the care to protect the confidentiality of those participating in the study. Prior to conducting this study, we obtained ethical approval from the Human Research Ethics Committee, University of New England, Australia. We provided the information sheets about the study to the self-help groups and our contact details. For ease of understanding, we translated the information sheets into Bangla language. The organisations disseminated information about the objectives and purpose of our study among prospective participants. After confirming the participants' willingness to participate, the staff of the organizations contacted the first author with the details of the potential participants, so that a time, date and place for the interview could be arranged. The first author visited the office of the organizations at the participant's chosen date and time. After being introduced by the staff of the organizations, the first author briefed the potential participants about the research. If he/she agreed to participate, the interview was organized. The consent of parents as well as children was sought regarding the interview arrangements. We permitted a counselor from the respective organization rather than a parent to accompany the child if this was requested by the child. All the interviews were held in the offices of those organizations. The interviews were audio-recorded, following consent. All interviews were conducted in secure, private locations which allowed for confidentiality. Informants' names were replaced by pseudonyms. Data was organized and analyzed through qualitative data analysis software Nvivo 9. Our basic technique was to read the transcripts line by line and then code the node by using a key word, phrase, clause or concept found in the text or in the meaning of the text of the transcripts. An interlinked relational network was then developed in logical combinations, as a tool for the identification of common themes.

The sample consisted of ten female and nine male children. There were four HIV-positive children, all of whom had been infected via their parents. The range of age for children was 10–18 years and the average was 14 years. For children, the average years spent in education were 7.8. Seventeen children were studying at the time of the interviews.

3.4 Children's Experiences of Social Stigma and Discrimination

Almost all the children remarked that they directly and indirectly experienced stigma and discrimination through the attitudes and behaviors of community members, peers and school mates because of their own and their parents' HIV status. They illustrated a number of manifestations of stigma and discrimination, including derogatory remarks, neglect, abuse, rejection, humiliation and bullying.

The children had to endure their parents being called *kharaplok*[1] (literally translated as 'bad person') for having HIV contraction by *kharapkaj*[2] (literally translated as 'bad practices'). This provided something of a contrast with western attitudes to illness where children, assumed to lack rationality, are adjudged 'innocent' of their circumstances (Fitzpatrick 1991). The stigma of HIV was so powerful as to affect all members of the immediate family, regardless of their perceived 'blame' for contracting the virus. Nonetheless, people in the community did not use the terms *kharapkaj* and *kharaplok* against the children as they were not perceived to be old enough to be having sexual relations. This is in line with Bangladeshi social norms which see children as asexual (particularly the girls) until they are ready to marry at 18 years of age (for girls) and 21 for boys (Caldwell et al. 1999). However, while this is the case, the children were associated by proxy with individuals with poor character and integrity. This showed how the morally polluting character of stigma could be very powerful, affecting mot just the supposed deviant but those they were socially intimate with. In this way, stigma was manifest in social interactions. This is evidenced by the abuse, mockery and harassment they were subjected to. For example, Asif indicated that community members described his father as *kharaplok* and the disease as *kharaprog* (literally translated as 'bad disease') when their HIV status was disclosed.

> People told me that my father is a kharaplok. They said he did kharapkaj, therefore, he had contracted kharaprog. I feel bad at that time. I would not hear this kind of kharapkotha (literally translated as 'bad words') if my father had not had this disease. (Asif, male child, HIV-negative)

Putul (female child, HIV-negative) described how she faced insults and hostility from peers due to her parents' HIV status. Notably, she remarked that her school mates taunted and teased her about her parents being HIV-positive.

> In my school, when I had a quarrel with someone, they reminded me sarcastically of my situation. They would say, 'Why do you become so emotional? You are an orphan. Your father has died with kharaprog. Your mother is sick.

---

[1] In the context of sexuality, men who have been engaged in sexual relations outside of a heterosexual marriage are considered *kharaplok*.

[2] When other people referred to *kharapkaj* they specifically implied sexual promiscuity or, more particularly, that people had extramarital relations with sex workers.

Children of HIV-infected parents discussed their exclusion from neighborly contact, such as playing with their peers, and from communal facilities and occasions (e.g. marriage ceremonies and community festivals, as well as attending school). Several children felt isolated and were treated like 'untouchables' within the community. For instance, Puja (female child, HIV-positive) described how neighbors retreated from them after learning that HIV had affected her family.

> People did not talk with us and did not come to our house. Whenever they saw us, they kept distance from us. They did not allow their children to play with us.

Himu (male child, HIV-negative) indicated that his parents' HIV-positive status also had an adverse affect on his acceptance in the community. For example, he noted that his peers assumed that he too was HIV-positive and subsequently relegated him to isolation, physically abused him and exacerbated his fears about the future.

> Our neighbor behaved very rudely. No-one visited us and people told us to leave our house. We moved house, but the same thing happened. No-one would talk or play with us. If we had arguments with other children, their parents would hit us and say kharapkotha to me. They told me, 'Your mother has already died; your father will also die; we will see what you will do then.' I felt very upset after hearing this.

The children described, as their parents had, how people in the community perceived HIV as a highly contagious and transmissible disease. As a consequence, the children were excluded and harassed by their neighbors and peers because it was assumed that they were also HIV-positive. For example, Rafik (male child, HIV-negative) indicated that people presumed that if a parent was HIV-positive, the whole family was also infected. He further described that he was mistreated in the community for being associated with an HIV-affected family.

> I have faced problems in my community before due to HIV. People thought as my mother is infected with HIV, we are also infected with this disease. When I was a child many children did not play with me. Someone said, 'Your mother has kharaprog; you also have kharaprog, don't come to us and don't play with our children'.

The children mentioned that when they were at school they were treated poorly, differently and discriminated against by their classmates due to their parents' HIV status. For example, Asif (male child, HIV-negative) indicated that classmates actively rejected and abused him.

> Students sometimes use abusive words in school. They say that my father has a kharaprog. He is a kharaplok. So, you got kharaprog. I feel bad at that time. I would not hear this kind of kharapkotha if my father had not had this disease.

Such isolation from informal social networks (peers) and formal social institution (educational) had negative impacts on the children's socialization (Pufall et al. 2014; Qiao et al. 2014). In terms of reactions to these circumstances, one response was to impose self-seclusion, thus exacerbating their isolation. All the children noted that they secluded themselves in order to prevent outsiders from knowing that their family had been affected by HIV. Due to feelings of shame associated with having HIV-positive parents and the negativity some experienced in their communities, the children became reluctant to approach friends or attend social gatherings for fear of rejection and/or abuse. Given the limited social networks of children and their close attachment to parents, feelings of shame for their parent's condition were readily transferred and amplified. For example, Sami (male child, HIV-negative) articulated that he preferred not to leave the house due to the negative comments others made about his mother. Similarly, Mala (female child, HIV-negative) told us that she was anxious about confiding to her friends about her parents HIV status. As a consequence, she attempted to distance herself from her friends.

> I don't talk about my parent's disease with my few friends and I try to keep distant from them and don't invite them to my house. After my mother's death, I prefer to be alone.

Some children also felt nervous and apprehensive about interacting with community members because they would be asked about their parents' HIV status. So much of the child's identity is closely bound to that of the parents that there were limited opportunities to construct social networks or narratives to counter the stigma they encountered. Putul (female child, HIV-negative), for instance, indicated that she actively avoided social gatherings due to the endless focus on her parents' HIV status.

> How can I get to know others? When I introduce myself, they ask my father's name. If I say my father's name, they just turn their faces showing some hatred. So I don't feel any interest to meet with others.

Children in rural Bangladesh experience more confinement because of the integrated socio-cultural nature of the society. In rural areas people reside very closely in clusters of houses and they interfere in every aspect of each others' lives being highly socially integrated (Aziz 1979). In some sense, the gemeinschaft qualities of such settings, which have been associated with social capital in western contexts (Toennies 1961; Tonnies 2001), can make it difficult to escape social stigma, the very closeness of such communities precipitated by strong normative structures which those with HIV were perceived breached. In communal gossip and meddling, children are normally procured to illicit information on family affairs. As a consequence, children of HIV-positive parents seclude themselves for two reasons. Firstly, they do not like to be asked about their parents' HIV status, and secondly, they do not like to disclose family secrets. Self-imposed isolation becomes a strategy to protect the status of family members.

3.5 Impacts of Stigma on Self

All the children were able to express and articulate their thoughts and feelings after finding out their own and/or their parents' HIV status. They cited numerous instances across a range of social situations in which their parents' HIV-positive status negatively affected their mental and psychological well-being, and in some cases, changed the interactions with their families and neighbors. These sentiments and experiences are described below and we have tried to use the voices of the children as much as possible to highlight how HIV has impacted on their everyday life.

All four HIV-positive children described feelings of sadness after being diagnosed with HIV. They noted that, as they aged, they began to better understand how they had contracted HIV (in utero) and the salience of being HIV-positive. For example, Adil (male child, HIV-positive) explained his mental and psychological condition after being diagnosed with HIV.

> I am HIV-positive by birth. I could not understand when I was very young. When I came to understand day by day that I was suffering from HIV, I felt very sad.

Puja (female child, HIV-positive) also indicated that she felt very unhappy when she became aware of her HIV-positive status.

> I felt very upset when I became aware of my HIV-positive status. At first, I could not understand but gradually I could understand. I saw my mother suffering miserably, so I felt very unhappy.

Children of HIV-infected parents often worried about what would happen to them if their parents died. They were particularly concerned with how they would feel, what they would do and who would care for them upon the death of one or both of their parents. For example, being a HIV-positive child of a single parent, Puja (female child, HIV-positive) felt worried about her mother's illness.

> When my mother gets sick, I feel very upset. I think that if mother dies, who will care for me?

The children's anguish increased as their parent's health deteriorated. The all-encompassing grief which Sabina (female child, HIV-negative) felt about her mother being ill is captured below.

> My father died. We have only mother with us. If she dies who will look after us? How will we survive without her? So I feel scared and anxious when I think something bad might happen to my mother.

The grief which the children felt in the present and for the future altered their sense of identity. The ability to visualize one's future is a central aspect of identity. This is amplified within Bangladeshi society where status is closely informed by familial bonds, in which an individual's worth is based on lineage, heredity and social positioning (Amin 1998). Without the relative predictability of these aspects of social identity the children became occupied by the uncertainty of the future.

3.6 Impacts of Stigma on Parent-Child Relations

Several children elaborated on their relationships with their parents after HIV had been diagnosed in their family. From their narratives, it is clear that the parent – child relationship began to change after the parents were diagnosed with HIV. When the children were discussing the changes in their relationship with their parents, they emphasized that HIV had affected family interaction. Several indicated that having HIV-positive parents sometimes threatened their relationship with their parents. For instance, Rina (female child, HIV-negative) told us that due to her mother's HIV status, her subsequent physical limitations and increased separation due to hospitalization changed the family routines.

> My mother always looked after the family, but when she became sick she could not care for us. Our family became disorganized and there was no discipline. Although my aunty looked after us, we missed our mother, especially when she went to Dhaka for treatment. Then we were very sad and my brother cried a lot.

After having been diagnosed with HIV, several parents refrained from interacting with their children. This phenomenon is in line with the belief in Bangladeshi society that HIV is highly contagious (Ullah 2011; Hasan et al. 2012). Because of this, children were deprived of affection, love and sympathy. For example, Sohel (male child, HIV-negative) explained that his father rarely talked with him after being diagnosed with HIV and made a deliberate effort to distance himself. He also noted that once he became aware that his father was HIV-positive he also alienated himself from his father and refused to use anything his father had touched.

> My parents always cried after my father's HIV diagnosis. Sometimes, my father and mother quarreled with each other. He did not talk much. I did not talk much with him at that time. Rather I talked with my mother most. My father just cried and slept. His physical condition was not good at that time and he could not work properly. I could not touch father's things due to his illness. He used a separate plate to eat from, and glass to drink from.

Children had unpleasant interactions with their parents in relation to their parents' HIV status. In particular, their narratives indicated that parental HIV contraction inhibited some children from experiencing a 'normal' childhood. In the course of the conversation, Sohel (male child, HIV-negative) spoke about his experience of emotional distance and difficulty communicating with his father when he became aware of his father's HIV status.

> I was too young to describe all the events. My mother was crying very much at that time. My father came back from India. Usually when he came home from India he brought new clothes and games for me and my brother, and gifts for my mother and our cousins and relations. But when he came back the last time, after being diagnosed with HIV, he didn't bring anything and he didn't hug or kiss me as usual. I couldn't understand.

Some children indicated that, after being diagnosed, their parents were unable to support their daily needs. For example, Imran (male child, HIV-negative) articulated that he missed their parents' academic support and how it affected their relationship.

> I did not spend much time with my father after he became sick. He could not help me with my study. When he stays at home he sleeps most of the time.

For several children, their parents passing affected them mentally and emotionally. The children remembered and missed their mothers and fathers who had died from HIV/AIDS. In Bangladesh, mothers are generally responsible for the social, emotional and daily care of the family (Amin 1998; Islam et al. 2014). As such, the effect of a HIV-positive mother is more significant for the maintenance of family structure than an HIV-positive father. Similarly, the effect of the mother's death has a more severe or holistic effect on the family than a father's death. The mother's death had the most adverse impact on the children's education. It led to school absenteeism, and in some cases, children left school altogether. Mala (female child, HIV-negative) described how her mother's death had a negative effect on her and her brother's experiences of study. For instance, she explained that without her mother she was not as academically attentive or successful as she could have been. She also indicated that the family had separated since her mother's death resulting in separated living arrangements for her and her brother.

> The disease has broken our family. If my mother was alive, my brother would not be separated. She would manage to keep us united. Actually mother is the most valuable thing in this world. We can realize this because we don't have a mother. She would motivate and care for us. Now I have to do the family chores and can't spend time on study.

Considering that the mother is the source of social and emotional support, children who had lost their mothers felt emotionally incomplete as they did not feel they had someone to confide in. For example, Hira (female child, HIV-negative) indicated that she missed her mother very much as there were many things she could not share with her father.

> My heart was broken when my friends talked about their mothers. Only the sufferer can realize the sorrow of a motherless girl. Mother prepared different interesting foods. I missed those foods. I cannot share and talk openly with my father like I could with my mother. Still we are lucky to have our father amidst us. I have lost one so I can realize the importance of the other. Today my mother is not alive so I rely on my father very much.

The death of the father also adversely affected the lives of several children. Considering that Bangladeshi fathers are most often the main (and sometimes the only) source of family income, the death of the father brings with it severe economic hardship and a significant reduction in opportunities (Caldwell et al. 1999). The data show that it was the daughters' privileges and lifestyles which were most severely impacted by the death of their fathers.

> I got disheartened at my father's death. Who doesn't feel distressed if their loved one passes away? I remember my father always. Other children's fathers buy many things for them. They can get their desirable things from their fathers. I cannot get anything because I am fatherless and my mother is also unwell. (Putul, female child, HIV-negative)

The death of the father also left Sabina (female child, HIV-negative) with emotional scars. Sabina recounted how it felt to use the word *abba* (dad) and the cognitive and emotional effect it had on her when she reminisced about him.

> Everybody has a father. We don't have father. We cannot say abba. If my father was alive we would get a lot of things from him.

Putul (female child, HIV-negative) indicated that as a girl she was worried about her future because females in Bangladesh's patriarchal society face many problems (Sultana 2010).

> We will not face many problems if my brother looks after us well. Several boys his age are running families in our society. There are a lot of opportunities for him to do. I cannot work in all occupations as a girl. In our society women are not allowed to do some jobs. It is really tough to live alone for a girl in a society like ours. I could face a lot of danger.

3.7 Impacts of Stigma on Social and Economic Welfare

From a practical perspective, the early loss of parents prevented transferal of social and work related skills and knowledge. In this way, the marginalizing aspects of stigma, described above, impeded formal and informal aspects of the socialization of children. Adil (male child, HIV-positive), who contracted HIV from his parents, mentioned that his education had ceased since he learned that he was HIV-positive. He indicated that going to school was a hopeless venture as he was occupied with the thought of imminent death in addition to being different from other children.

> The disease changed our lives drastically. It caused the death of my mother and younger brother. The happiness of our family had been destroyed. I don't go to school any more as there is no purpose because I will die. Other children of my age go to school as they have a mother and father and they have no disease like us. They have no stress.

The education of children with HIV-positive parents was identified as one of the important concerns for this research. Parental illness reduced the children's opportunity for education. All children described the effects of their parents' HIV on their studies. They described a number of ways it affected their studies and education. These included depression, a lack of motivation and interest in their schoolwork, falling behind in their studies and withdrawing from school. From the narratives, it is also clear that children of HIV-infected parents often experienced a high level of disruption in schooling for various reasons including economic hardship, restriction from attending school, their worsening physical condition in the case of HIV-infected children, and household responsibilities, such as looking after sick parents and younger siblings.

Children recalled how they were forced to cease their study at a young age. Several children indicated that they abandoned their studies because their parents could no longer afford to keep them in school. In most instances, daughters of HIV-infected parents were denied their education as a consequence of the cultural expectation that they maintain the household (Pradhan et al. 2006). For example, Mala (female child, HIV-negative) reported that her education was hampered by her household responsibilities as both parents were HIV-positive. Her mother's illness eventually compelled her to stop her schooling.

> HIV affected our life severely. I lost my mother. My father is ill now. Because of the disease I had to cease my study. I could have completed my schooling by this time. It has ruined my life.

As the health of the parents declined, the children had to take on an increasing role as carers and household managers (Pradhan et al. 2006). This prevented them from continuing their schooling. For example, being a single child, Dev (male child, HIV-negative) had to take a parental role in the family as he had to care for his sick parents and manage the household, and therefore, he could not continue his studies.

> I stopped my study due to my father's illness. I moved with my father to different places for his treatment. So I could not attend the final exam because we were in India.

Several children described how their parents' HIV-positive status affected them psychologically, and therefore, they could not concentrate on their studies. For instance, after becoming aware of his father's HIV-positive status Asif (male child, HIV-negative) lost interest in his studies as he believed that he would not be able to continue with his schooling. Nonetheless, he felt that he would have to take the role of breadwinner for his family as his father could not work due to his physical disability.

From their narratives, it is clear that children's academic success was hampered by having an HIV-positive parent. For example, Sami (male child, HIV-negative) indicated that he fell behind in his studies due to his mother's illness.

> My study was hampered due to my mother's illness. I could not concentrate on study very much at that time. My result (grade) was deteriorating compared with the previous year.

Although childhood education is very important for personal development and acquiring gainful employment to maintain basic needs for the future, this can be impeded by long-term school absenteeism due to increased household responsibility in early life (Alkenbrack et al. 2004; Pradhan et al. 2006). While some children, like Puja, could not attend school regularly, several could not go to school at all. For instance, Rupa (female child, HIV-positive) could not go to school due to on-going sickness.

> I cannot go to school regularly because I am often sick and then my mother does not allow me to go to school. I don't have the strength for studying.

At a work related level, Mukul (male child, HIV-negative) indicated that he felt nervous about his future and that of his three siblings after his father was diagnosed with HIV. As the eldest son, within a Bangladeshi context, he would become solely responsible for the health and well-being of the remaining family members as well as maintaining the family's business and assets after his father's death. The thought of taking on these responsibilities unnerved him as he felt incapable of meeting his family's needs and was not accustomed to the agricultural activities needed to maintain the family business.

> My father was the only earner in our family. I thought who would run the family if he died? I was the eldest child but was too young to work the land and look after a big family. I felt very worried at that time.

Within the Bangladeshi context, daughters of parents with HIV faced more difficulties than the sons, reflecting their greater reliance on patriarchal supports (Sultana 2010; Islam et al. 2014). For instance, Putul (female child, HIV-negative), a daughter of a single parent, felt worried about her economic security and feared having to resort to begging to support herself.

> My father is no more. I get scared thinking if mother dies, then what will happen to me? How will I cope alone? I don't know what is in my destiny in absence of mother. We don't have much money. Most probably I will have to beg from others. Sometimes I shiver thinking of this.

It is clear that the degree of future certainty and security for Bangladeshi children is dependent on their gender. As boys are held in higher esteem than girls, their social and economic capital is of higher value, and we will discuss the impact of gender later in the chapter.

The impact of parental HIV-positive status on children cannot be explained only by the disease itself, as a number of other factors can affect children negatively. However, the children's narratives indicated that their parents' HIV-positive status resulted in significant reduction in economic opportunities and security. The children also compared their new lives to those of other children in their community and noticed the clear disparities between them. Notably, several children compared their parents' present economic condition with that prior to their HIV diagnosis. They stated that their parents had greater economic security prior to learning they had HIV. For instance, Sohel (male child, HIV-negative) articulated that his family had been quite wealthy due to profits from his father's business.

> Before he had the disease my father had a very good income from his business. He was generous and gave gifts to everyone. Now we are in a bad situation.

Mukul (male child, HIV-negative), his family's first child and eldest son, mentioned the privileges and the opportunities that had been available to him during his childhood. He indicated his parent's robust economic circumstances prior to contracting HIV.

> I was the first child and got the most privileges, even more than my brothers and sisters. I had lots of toys and clothes. I also had a private tutor to support my studies.

3.8 Discussion and Conclusion

Children were exposed to several traumas including family disruption, conflict and mental disorder. The results show that parental HIV-positive status increases children's vulnerability, abuse, exploitation and neglect, and these circumstances are largely a product of the stigma associated with the virus. In addition, parents seemed to be engaged deeply with their own health, making them mentally and physically unavailable to their children. These challenges place immense pressure and strain on the family's ability to perform as a unit of socialization, economic support, nurturing and care. In addition to the stigma attached to HIV, unpredictable events resulting from illness interrupted consistent parenting within the family environment. Research indicates that the existence of HIV in the family decreases a parent's ability to provide a consistent environment (Gossart-Walker and Nancy 1998; Richter et al. 2010). In a study which examined the impact of HIV-related stigma among HIV-infected mothers with young children, Murphy et al. (2006) suggested that mothers who experienced high levels of stigma had lower physical, psychological, and social functioning. Further adolescents who perceived high levels of stigma because of their mother's HIV status were more likely to participate in delinquent behavior (Murphy et al. 2006). However, this was not found amongst the Bangladeshi children in this study. Considering the social hierarchy and the strict demand on children to respect their communities, children may repress their rage and anger about HIV in the family as it would not be socially acceptable to express such emotions publicly, if at all. Without a doubt, there are complex human right issues (see also Chap. 16) involved with children affected by HIV that require urgent attention, and in particular to reducing the discrimination they face and access to education and other social and community opportunities.

The children's experiences indicate that they were overshadowed by the socio-economic and socio-cultural consequences of their parents' HIV status. Through their eyes, we can see that they felt high levels of psychological distress after learning of their parents' HIV diagnosis. While the experience of distress associated with a life threatening condition might be considered relatively normal, the experience of stigma upon the family network amplified the experience of distress and also prevented access to social resources which might have mediated such effects. The children were overwhelmed with anticipatory grief as they lived with the possibility of losing one or both of their parents and the potential impact this would have on their lives. Mostly, they thought about who would care for them when their parents died and felt anxious about their future lives. This was primarily the case for single children and children whose parents both had HIV. Likewise, single female children were particularly scared about the negative consequences of parental HIV on their futures. Female children were worried about their future lives and the numerous obstacles they would face as women in a society where patriarchy is the social norm. As such, girls were very much aware of the social and economic restrictions on females and how HIV would exacerbate these. The results further indicate that the eldest children worried about having to take on family responsibilities due to parental illness, disability and death particularly during adolescence. This is particularly important in the Bangladesh context as the eldest children are responsible for caring for younger siblings and family members (Amin 1998).

It is important to note, however, that the effect of HIV on children differs according to their family's epidemic contexts (i.e., children's HIV status, being a child of one versus two HIV-positive parents, family structure, parental death and whether the children lost their mother or father) and their family's income. Our findings indicate that children were most affected by the family's economic crisis (Brown and Lourie 2000). This was confirmed through their constant referral to the differences between their past and present lives. Their stories also confirm that most of the children were deprived from childhood opportunities and facilities due to parental economic incapacitation. This was borne out by the frequent references children made to how little they had in comparison to their peers. Exclusion and marginalization from informal and formal networks for socialization impaired the social development of the children and this was reflected in their anxieties.

Clearly, parental HIV contraction had a negative effect on children's experience of childhood and academic achievement. As indicated by some studies from developing countries, children of HIV-positive parents experience lower school enrolment and attendance, and higher rates of school dropouts (Deacon and Stephney 2007; Operario et al. 2008). For many HIV-positive children, education ceased as they believed that going to school was a pointless venture. The school environment was also a source of stigma and discrimination, experienced in interaction with both peers and teachers. Compounding the poor school attendance by children of HIV-positive parents is the need for daughters to take on the family maintenance and caring roles of the mother in the household, meaning many drops out of school (Cluver and Gardner 2007). Considering that mothers in Bangladesh are mostly responsible for family maintenance, the HIV-positive status of mothers brings significantly negative impacts on daughter's lives and life opportunities. Parents were unable to provide adequate educational opportunities, support, care and daily maintenance for their child due to deteriorating health (Strode and Barrett Grant 2001). In this way, stigma, while defined according a cultural norms, had material effects for those who were defined as members of the family, be they ill or other. The stigma associated with HIV was highly polluting of character and could inhabit the space of a family unit. A status as child did not render the children 'innocent' and invulnerable to the political effects of stigma.

Our results indicate that children were rejected and discriminated against directly and indirectly by peers and community members because of their parents' HIV-positive status. In a study of children affected by HIV/AIDS aged 10–17 years, Surkan and colleagues (2010) suggested that children were discriminated against simply for living within an HIV-affected family. Our results further indicate that children were accused by others of having HIV, although there was no public evidence to substantiate such claims. As a consequence, children were often mistreated and insulted by others in their community. In this study, the voices of these children describe some unusual aspects to HIV stigma that make normal social interaction difficult. For example, people held negative attitudes like *kharaplok* and *kharapkaj* towards parents which created problems for children when negotiating public encounters. Such stigma makes social interaction extremely problematic for children affecting formalized socialization in areas such as schooling and informal forms of socialization such as interaction with peers and the broader community. The fact that many of the participants resided in what could be considered close-knit social settings amplified rather than lessened the experience of stigma. The research of Mahati et al. (2006) also suggested that children were verbally abused and blamed for their parents' HIV status in what could be characterized as tightly integrated social setting. As a result of stigma, thinking about the negative consequences, children always tried to keep their parents' HIV news secret from their friends and school mates (Gossart-Walker and Nancy 1998). As having an HIV-positive parent is perceived negatively in Bangladesh, isolation from the community only increases children's vulnerability and marginalization (Islam et al. 2014). It is interesting to note here that a primary strategy to resist stigma in a close-knit community is to self-impose isolation from the community and limit social interaction, given that social interaction is the source of stigma.

To this end, schools could play a vital role in creating awareness among students about HIV and AIDS. In addition to biomedical information, school curricula should incorporate social and behavioral aspects of HIV/AIDS so that children receive a clear and solution-focused message about stigma and discrimination faced by PLHIV and their children. Mass media can also play a positive role in changing people's attitudes toward PLHIV and especially towards their children. In addition, religious leaders could be included in the process of implementing education, social support or income generation programs to increase the acceptability of the initiatives in Bangladeshi society. This is especially important, as it was clear much of stigma associated with HIV derived from moral frameworks, based on understandings of 'good' and 'bad' thoughts and practices. Multiple levels of community engagement and social support can further reduce and help PLHIV and their children to overcome stigma and discrimination.

The deteriorating impact and assault of the HIV virus on the human body are medically well understood and described (Lee et al. 2006; Desmond et al. 2014; Stein et al. 2014). However, what this chapter shows is that HIV can also cause what we call a 'social assault' (Kalichman et al. 2003) on HIV individuals and their families and cause deteriorating interactions and relationships in families. The cause of this is discrimination, fear, misplaced 'morality' and intolerance (Khan et al. 2009; Islam et al. 2014; Sherr et al. 2014). The preventative cure is to educate society so that they do not add to the physical burden already caused by a virus attacking the human body and spirit. The normalization of HIV as any other illness, caused because of multiple reasons and risk factors, should be a priority of all governments. Yet, at this point in time, the impact of how some societies impute case and personal responsibility for HIV comes with a huge cost to families, including children.

Acknowledgements We express our gratitude to the participants for sharing their experiences. The first author would like to acknowledge the financial support received from University of New England, School of Health.

References

Aggleton, P., & Parker, R. (2005). *HIV-related stigma, discrimination and human rights violations: Case studies of successful programmes*. Geneva: UNAIDS.

Alkenbrack, S., Chettra, T., & Forsythe, S. (2004). *The social and economic impact of HIV and AIDS on families with adolescents and children in Cambodia*. Phnom Penh: Ministray of Social Affairs Veterans and Youth Rehabilatation, Cambodia.

Alonzo, A. A., & Reynolds, N. R. (1995). Stigma, HIV and AIDS: An exploration of stigma trajectory. *Social Science & Medicine, 41*(3), 303–315.

Amin, S. (1998). Family structure and change in rural Bangladesh. *Population Studies, 52*, 201–213.

Armistead, L., Klein, K., & Forehand, R. (1995). Parental physical illness and child functioning. *Clinical Psychology Review, 15*, 1–14.

Aziz, K. M. A. (1979). *Kinship in Bangladesh*. Dhaka: International Centre for Diarrhoeal Disease Research, Bangladesh.

Beard, J., Biemba, G., Brooks, M. I., Costello, J., Ommerborn, M., Bresnahan, M., Flynn, D., & Simon, J. L. (2010). Children of female sex workers and drug users: A review of vulnerability, resilience and family-centred models of care. *Journal of the International AIDS Society, 13*(Suppl 2): (S6), 1–8. doi:10.1186/1758-2652-13-S2-S6.

Boyd-Franklin, N., Steiner, G. L., & Boland, M. G. (1995). *Children, families and HIV/AIDS: Psychosocial and therapeutic issues*. New York: The Guilford Press.

Brewer, J. D., & Sparkes, A. C. (2011). Young people living with parental bereavement: Insights from an ethnographic study of a UK childhood bereavement service. *Social Science & Medicine, 72*(2), 283–290.

Brown, L. K., & Lourie, K. J. (2000). Children and adolescents living with HIV and AIDS: A review. *The Journal of Child Psychology and Psychiatry, 41*(1), 81–96.

Caldwell, B., Pieris, I., Khuda, B., Caldwell, J., & Caldwell, P. (1999). Sexual regimes and sexual networking: The risk of an HIV/AIDS epidemic in Bangladesh. *Social Science & Medicine, 48*(8), 1103–1116.

Chase, E., & Aggleton, P. (2001). *Stigma, HIV/AIDS and prevention of mother-to-child transmission: A pilot study in Zambia, India, Ukraine and Burkina Faso*. London: Panos Institute, United Nations Children's Fund.

Chi, P., & Li, X. (2013). Impact of parental HIV/AIDS on children's psychological well-being: A systematic review of global literature. *AIDS and Behavior, 17*, 2554–2574.

Clark, H. J., Lindner, G., Armistead, L., & Austin, B. J. (2003). Stigma, disclosure, and psychological functioning among HIV infected and non-infected African-American women. *Women and Health, 38*, 57–71.

Cluver, L., & Gardner, F. (2007). Risk and protective factors for psychological well-being of children orphaned by AIDS in Cape Town: A qualitative study of children and caregivers' perspectives. *AIDS Care, 19*(3), 318–325.

Cowgill, B. O., Bogart, L. M., Corona, R., Ryan, G., & Schuster, M. A. (2008). Fears about HIV transmission in families with an HIV-infected parent: A qualitative analysis. *Pediatrics, 22*(5), e950–e958.

Crocker, J., Major, B., & Steele, C. (1998). Social stigma. In D. T. Gilbert, S. T. Fiske, & G. Lindzey (Eds.), *The handbook of social psychology* (pp. 504–553). New York: The MacGraw Hill Companies.

Deacon, H., & Stephney, I. (2007). *HIV/AIDS, stigma and children*. Cape Town: HSRC Press.

Desmond, C., Bruce, F., Tomlinson, M., Marlow, M. B., Aber, J. L., Quifki, R., et al. (2014). Modelling the long-term impacts on affected children of adult HIV: Benefits, challenges and a possible approach. *AIDS, 28*(Suppl 3), S269–S275.

Earnshaw, V. A., & Kalichman, S. C. (2013). Stigma experienced by people living with HIV/AIDS. In P. Liamputtong (Ed.), *Stigma, discrimination and living with HIV/AIDS* (pp. 23–38). Dordrecht: Springer.

Fitzpatrick, T. L. (1991). Innocent until proven guilty: Shallow words for the falsely accused in a criminal prosecution for child sexual abuse. *University of Bridgeport Law Review, 12*, 175–208.

Floyd, S., Crampin, A. C., Glynn, J. R., Madise, N., Mwenebabu, M., Mnkhondia, S., et al. (2007). The social and economic impact of parental HIV on children in northern Malawi: Retrospective population-based cohort study. *AIDS Care, 19*(6), 781–790.

Forehand, R., Steele, R., Armistead, L., Morse, E., Simon, P., & Clark, L. (1998). The family health project: Psychosocial adjustment of children whose mothers are HIV infected. *Journal of Consulting and Clinical Psychology, 66*(3), 513–520.

Foster, G., & Williamson, J. (2000). A review of current literature of the impact of HIV/AIDS on children in sun-Saharan Africa. *AIDS, 14*(Suppl. 3), S275–S284.

Goffman, E. (1963). *Stigma: Notes on the management of spoiled identity*. New York: Simon and Schuster.

Gosling, A. S., Burns, J., & Hirst, F. (2004). Children with HIV in the UK: A longitudinal study of adaptive and cognitive functioning. *Clinical Child Psychology and Psychiatry, 9*(1), 25–37.

Gossart-Walker, S., & Nancy, E. M. (1998). Support groups for HIV-affected children. *Journal of Child and Adolescent Group Therapy, 8*(2), 55–69.

Guoping, J., Li, L., Chunqing, L., & Sun, S. (2007). The impact of HIV/AIDS on families and children: A study in China. *AIDS, 21*(Suppl 8): (S157), 1–10. doi:10.1097/01.aids.0000304712.87164.42.

Harms, S., Jack, S., Ssebunnya, J., & Kizza, R. (2010). The orphaning experience: Descriptions from Ugandan youth who have lost parents to HIV/AIDS. *Child and Adolescent Psychiatry and Mental Health, 4*(6), 1–10.

Hasan, M. T., Nath, S. R., Khan, N. S., Akram, O., Gomes, T. M., & Rashid, S. F. (2012). Internalized HIV/AIDS-related stigma in a sample of HIV-positive people in Bangladesh. *Journal of Health, Population, and Nutrition, 30*(1), 22–30.

Herek, G. M., Capitanio, J., & Widaman, K. (2002). HIV-related stigma and knowledge in the United States: Prevalence and trends, 1991–1999. *American Journal of Public Health, 92*, 371–377.

Hosegood, V., & Madhavan, S. (2010). Data availability on men's involvement in families in sub-Saharan Africa to inform familycentred programmes for children affected by HIV and AIDS. *Journal of the International AIDS Society, 13*(Suppl 2), S5, 1–7. http://dx.doi.org/10.1186%2F1758-2652-13-S2-S4.

Islam, S., Minichiello, V., & Scott, J. (2014). Children living in HIV family: A review. *Journal of Child & Adolescent Behavior, 2*(170), 1–7.

Kalichman, S. C., DiMarco, M., Austin, J., Luke, W., & DiFonzo, K. (2003). Stress, social support, and HIV-status disclosure to family and friends among HIV-positive men and women. *Journal of Behavioral Medicine, 26*(4), 315–332.

Khan, S. I., Hussain, M. I., Parveen, S., Bhuiyan, M. I., Gourab, G., Sarkar, G. F., et al. (2009). Living on the extreme margin: Social exclusion of the transgender population (Hijra) in Bangladesh. *Journal of Health, Population and Nutrition, 27*(4), 441–451.

Kimberly, J., & Serovich, J. (1999). The role of family and friend social support in reducing risk behaviors among HIV-positive gay men. *AIDS Education and Prevention, 11*, 465–475.

Lee, G., Gortmaker, S., McIntosh, K., Hughes, M., Oleske, J., & Pediatric AIDS Clinical Trials Group Protocol 219C Team. (2006). Quality of life for children and adolescents: Impact of HIV infection and antiretroviral treatment. *Pediatrics, 117*(2), 273–283.

Leeper, S. C., Montague, B. M., Friedman, J. F., & Flanigan, T. (2010). Lessons learned from family-centred models of treatment for children living with HIV: Current approaches and future directions. *Journal of the international AIDS Society, 13*(Suppl)(S3), 1–11.

Liamputtong, P., & Kitisriworapan, S. (2012). Deviance, difference and stigma as social determinants of health. In P. Liamputtong, R. Fanany, & G. Verrinder (Eds.), *Health, illness and well-being: Perspectives and social determinants* (pp. 242–256). Melbourne: Oxford University Press.

Liamputtong, P., Haritavorn, N., & Kiatying-Angsulee, N. (2013). AIDS support groups and women living with HIV/AIDS in central Thailand. In P. Liamputtong (Ed.), *Stigma, discrimination and living with HIV/AIDS* (pp. 377–397). Dordrecht: Springer.

Link, B. G., & Phelan, J. C. (2001). Conceptualizing stigma. *Annual Review of Sociology, 27*, 363–385.

Mahati, S. T., Munyati, S., Chitiyo, G., Mashange, W., Chibatamoto, P., & Mupambireyi, P. F. (2006). *A qualitative assessment of orphans and vulnerable children in two Zimbabwean districts*. Cape Town: HSRC Press.

Messer, L. C., Pence, B. W., Whetten, K., Whetten, R., Thielman, N., O'Donnell, K., et al. (2010). Prevalence and predictors of HIV-related stigma among institutional- and community-based caregivers of orphans and vulnerable children living in five less-wealthy countries. *BMC Public Health, 10*(504), 1–7.

Murphy, D. A., & Marelich, W. D. (2008). Resiliency in young children whose mothers are living with HIV/AIDS. *AIDS Care, 20*(3), 284–291.

Murphy, D. A., Laine, A. E., & Lisa, G. (2006). Correlates of HIV- related stigma among HIV-positive mothers and their uninfeted adolescent children. *Women & Health, 44*(3), 19–42.

Nöstlinger, C., Bartoli, G., Gordillo, V., Roberfroid, D., & Colebunders, R. (2006). Children and adolescents living with HIV positive parents: Emotional and behavioural problems. *Vulnerable Children and Youth Studies, 1*(1), 29–43.

Operario, D., Pettifor, A., Cluver, L., MacPhail, C., & Rees, H. V. (2008). Parental death during school-aged years and completion of compulsory school education among young people in South Africa. *Journal of Research on Adolescence, 18*(1), 173–186.

Parker, R., & Aggleton, P. (2003). HIV/AIDS-related stigma and discrimination: A conceptual framework and implications for action. *Social Science & Medicine, 57*, 13–24.

Pradhan, B., Sundar, R., & Singh, S. (2006). *Socio-economic impact of HIV and AIDS in India*. New Delhi: United Nations Development Programme.

Pufall, E. L., Gregson, S., Eaton, J. W., Masoka, T., Mpandaguta, E., Andersen, L., et al. (2014). The contribution of schools to supporting the well being of children affected by HIV in eastern Zimbabwe. *AIDS, 28*(Suppl 3), S379–S387.

Qiao, S., Li, X., Zhao, G., Zhao, J., & Stanton, B. (2014). The role of perceived social support in loneliness and self-esteem among children affected by HIV/AIDS: A longitudinal multilevel analysis in rural China. *AIDS, 28*(Suppl 3), S369–S377.

Reyland, S. A., McMahan, T. J., Higgins-Delessandro, A., & Luthar, S. S. (2002). Inner-city children living with an HIV-seropositive mother: Parent-child relationships, perception of social support, and psychological disturbance. *Journal of Child and Family Studies, 11*(3), 313–329.

Richter, L. (2010). An introduction to family-centred services for children affected by HIV and AIDS. *Journal of the International AIDS Society, 13*(Suppl 1), 1–6.

Richter, L., Beyrer, C., Kippax, S., & Heidari, S. (2010). Visioning services for children affected by HIV and AIDS through a family lens. *Journal of the International AIDS Society, 13*(Suppl I1), 1–3.

Schuster, M. A., Kanouse, D. E., Morton, S. C., Bozzette, S. A., Miu, A., Scott, G. B., et al. (2000). HIV-infected parents and their children in the United States. *American Journal of Public Health, 90*, 1074–1081.

Sherr, L., Cluver, L. D., Betancourt, T. S., Kellerman, S. E., Richter, L. M., & Desmond, C. (2014). Evidence of impact: Health, psychological and social effects of adult HIV on children. *AIDS, 28*(Suppl 3), S251–S259.

Stein, A., Desmond, C., Garbarino, J., Van IJzendoorn, M. H., Barbarin, O., Black, M. M., et al. (2014). Predicting long-term outcomes for children affected by HIV and AIDS: Perspectives from the scientific study of children's development. *AIDS, 28*(Suppl 3), S261–S268.

Strode, A., & Barrett Grant, K. (2001). *The role of stigma and discrimination in increasing the vulnerability of children and youth infected with and affected by HIV/AIDS*. Pretoria: Save the Children, UK.

Sultana, A. (2010). Patriarchy and women's subordination: A theoretical analysis. *The Arts Faculty Journal, 4*, 1–18.

Surkan, P. J., Mukherjee, J. S., Williams, D. R., Eustache, E., Louis, E., Jean-Paul, T., et al. (2010). Perceived discrimination and stigma toward children affected by HIV/AIDS and their HIV-positive caregivers in central Haiti. *AIDS Care, 22*(7), 803–815.

Toennies, F. (1961). Gemeinschaft and gesellschaft. In T. Parsons, E. Shils, K. D. Naegele, & J. R. Pitts (Eds.), *Theories of society: Foundations of modern sociological theory*. New York: The Free Press.

Tonnies, F. (2001). In J. Harris (Ed.), *Community and civil society* (J. Harris, & M. Hollis, Trans.). Cambridge: Cambridge University Press.

Ullah, A. K. M. A. (2011). HIV/AIDS-related stigma and discrimination: A study of health care providers in Bangladesh. *Journal of the International Association of Physicians in AIDS Care, 10*(2), 97–104.

Chapter 4
Adolescents Living with HIV: Emerging Issues in Public Health in South Africa

Nataly Woollett

Contents

4.1 Introduction

Today, 1.8 billion adolescents stand at the challenging crossroads between childhood and adulthood (UNFPA 2014). Nine out of ten of these young people live in the developing world and face especially profound challenges, from obtaining an education to simply staying alive. Adolescents are vacillating in a developmental stage that bridges childhood and adulthood; a time of increased flux. At no other time except infancy do human beings undergo so much development in such a short period. During adolescence, children gain 50 % of their adult body weight, become capable of reproducing, and experience an astounding transformation in their brains (UNICEF 2011). All these changes occur in the context of rapidly expanding social spheres. Although there have been tremendous strides made in children's health

N. Woollett (✉)
Wits Reproductive Health and HIV Institute (WRHI), University of Witwatersrand, PO Box 18512, Hillbrow 2038, Johannesburg, South Africa
e-mail: nwoollett@wrhi.ac.za

P. Liamputtong (ed.), *Children and Young People Living with HIV/AIDS*, Cross-Cultural Research in Health, Illness and Well-Being,
DOI 10.1007/978-3-319-29936-5_4

outcomes, the paucity of attention and resources devoted to adolescents is threatening to limit the impact of these efforts on the teen years.

Adolescents living with HIV are an emerging group in the global HIV/AIDS epidemic. An estimated 3.4 million children are living with HIV, more than 90 % in sub-Saharan Africa (UNAIDS 2011). Recent data indicate that 2.5 % of 2–14 year old children and 8.7 % of 15–24 year olds in South Africa are HIV-positive (Shisana et al. 2009). Prevalence amongst women is still nearly double that of men and intergenerational sex for young girls 15–19 years has escalated significantly over time, not diminished (Shisana 2014). As the HIV epidemic has matured, youth have become one of the most affected groups in South Africa. HIV incidence remains highest among 15–24 years olds, with approximately 40 % of horizontal transmission occurring within this age group (UNAIDS 2008). Furthermore, as access to highly active antiretroviral therapy (HAART) improves globally, the population of vertically-infected adolescents is expected to grow (Ferrand et al. 2009; Lowenthal et al. 2014). Large numbers of children with slowly progressing disease, infected before PMTCT interventions became widely available, are presenting for the first time in adolescence, having lived with untreated HIV for a decade or more (Bernays et al. 2014). While youth aged 10–19 accounted for 1 % of the total number of patients receiving HAART in South Africa in 2008, this proportion will grow to approximately 5 % by 2020, mainly as a result of vertically-infected children surviving into adolescence (Jaspan et al. 2009). Moreover, South Africans between 13 and 19 years comprise roughly 30 % of the population (STATS SA 2010, 2014), so treatment and care for HIV-positive adolescents will become increasingly important over the next decade.

Although most adolescents navigate this challenging developmental stage successfully, it can be especially difficult if there are other stressors to overcome, including HIV. HIV-positive adolescents are affected by the HIV epidemic in a multitude of ways. They have to deal with their own mortality and uncertain futures, they suffer trauma and grief as they watch their parents and family members die, many lose siblings and their home at the event of a parents' passing as siblings are displaced to various family members and areas in the country. Many adolescents are highly mobile which leads to inconsistent schooling, and in the South African context, increased teen pregnancy and high sexual risk taking behavior, many experience elevated exposure to violence. Most adolescents are stigmatized and discriminated against and many live in increasingly poor households with high food insecurity, some get exploited for the child care grant, and especially, there is increased risk for poor mental health outcomes (Mellins et al. 2006, 2009b; Cluver et al. 2008, 2011b; Domek 2009; Jaspan et al. 2009; Ferrand et al. 2010; Bernays et al. 2014; Lowenthal et al. 2014). In addition to these considerable challenges, adolescents who are perinatally-infected have lived with the virus and its consequences for much longer than adolescents who are behaviorally-infected, creating a divergent group among the adolescent population in South Africa. These complications will be explored in this chapter.

4.2 A Theoretical Framework to Understanding Adolescent Health and Development: Bronfenbrenner's Ecological Model of Human Development

Approaches to understanding human development rely heavily on Bronfenbrenner's ecological model of 1979. In his original theory, Bronfenbrenner postulates that in order to understand human development, the entire ecological system in which growth occurs needs to be taken into account. This system is composed of five socially organized subsystems that support and guide human development. Each system depends on the contextual nature of the person's life and offers an ever-growing diversity of options and sources of growth. Furthermore, within and between each system are bi-directional influences. These bi-directional influences imply that relationships have impact in two directions, both away from the individual and towards the individual. As we potentially have access to these subsystems we are able to have more social knowledge, an increased set of possibilities for learning problem solving, and access to new dimensions of self-exploration (Bronfenbrenner 1979).

Bronfenbrenner's model of human development (Fig. 4.1) starts with an initial mapping of the settings where most social interactions occur; those settings where we interact with others on a face-to-face basis. From this micro-level analysis, it is possible to explore how we are influencing those around us and how we are concurrently being influenced. But if the mapping of human development ended at this point, the scope of shaping on our development would be unfortunately incomplete. Other questions would endure: How does the relationship between and among our experiences in different settings where we interact with other people impact our development? What is the impact on our development when significant events and interactions occur in environments that we do not occupy but someone in our circle of family or friends does? Most importantly, in what ways does an increasingly complex and interconnected cultural, political and economic world reach into our lives in ways that effect our development? Bronfenbrenner answered these questions by creating a model that exposes how our development is inseparable from our environment throughout our lives. After explaining the multiple interconnected and interlocked rings of influence surrounding us as developing individuals, Bronfenbrenner helps decode the complex ways these rings of influence advance and restrain our development. Ecological models of development require that we genuinely consider the impact of the social world on the development of the individual (Bronfenbrenner 1979).

Initially, individuals are born with a host of biological characteristics and traits ranging from their sex to their health and personality type—this is the individual level of Bronfenbrenner's model. From there, we advance to the microsystem and this includes our family, friends, and environments where we interact most with others, including school, the health system we utilize and so on. Most people regularly move through various settings that constitute their microsystem (e.g. from home to school, to recreational environments with peers, to clinics to receive

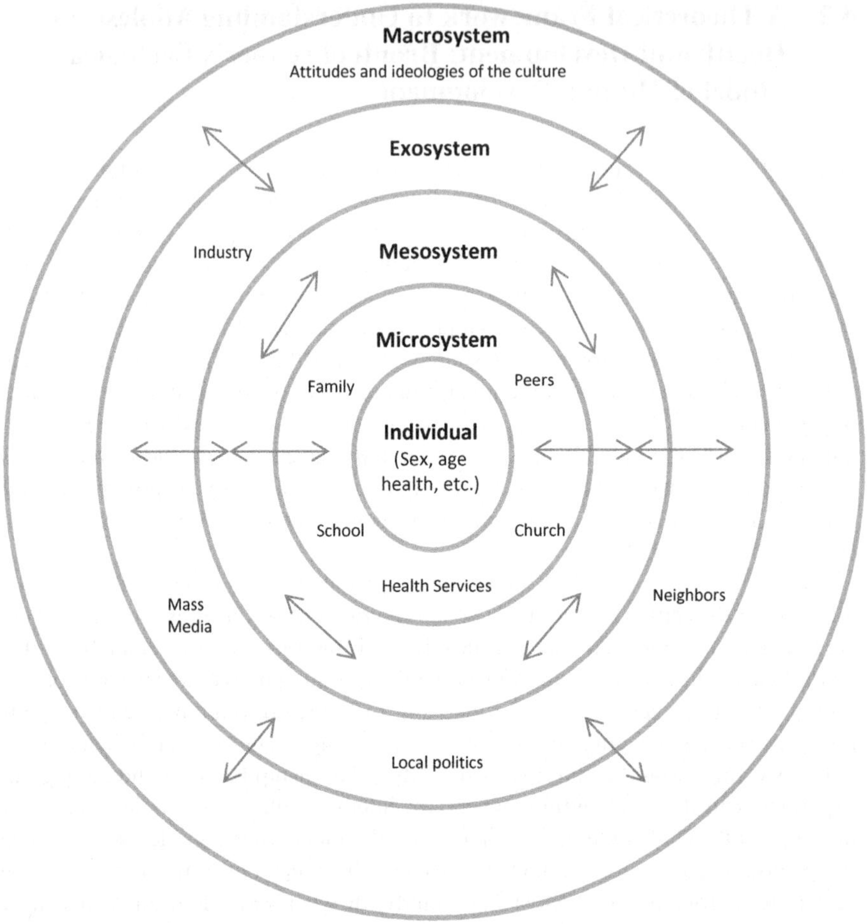

Fig. 4.1 Illustration of Bronfenbrenner's ecological framework for human development

treatment and so on). Bronfenbrenner's mesosystem captures the idea that individuals develop by interacting and relating to others within multiple settings in their microsystem (e.g. familial, academic, recreational and health settings). As people must learn to simultaneously manage experiences in more than one setting, a synergy is created across settings that affect the developing person. This is the mesosystem which captures the developmental importance produced by the connections across settings (Bronfenbrenner 1979).

The mesosystem has important considerations on adolescent development. An adolescent typically experiences the behavioral expectations of more than one important adult in their lives; for an HIV-positive adolescent, this might be their primary caregiver and their treating doctor or nurse, and in more than one setting, e.g. home and the clinic. Caregivers and nurses/doctors must interact with each other so that their independent interactions with the adolescent communicate identical expectations about disease management at home that can impact health, adherence, nutrition and sexual risk taking behavior, and so on. Likewise, what occurs in the health setting (e.g. lack of agency, medication stock-outs, poor service delivery) influences an adolescents' behavior at home.

The exosystem also assumes a linkage between two or more settings. But unlike the mesosystem, the developing individual does not partake directly in one of those settings. Initially, it might seem both obvious and developmentally inconsequential that the people who populate our lives have experiences in settings that do not include us. However, our experiences are interrelated and the systems influence each other. If a caregiver loses their job, the adolescent in their care may experience an increase in poverty that has a significant impact on their development. Similarly, an adolescent's interactions at school may indirectly influence interactions in the home setting. A poor report card, interactions with peers, stigma experienced at school are all interactions that are outside of the caregivers experience but have a major influence on the home environment. The impact of the exosystem on our development can be overwhelmingly powerful and examples occur across the lifespan. If the young people lose their primary caregiver, they have to move somewhere else, their microsystem tends to change and home life is highly impacted. If they are unable to receive their ARVs at a clinic as a result of stockouts, they miss out on schooling by having to return to clinics and experience increased stress which impacts everyone living at home. The context and processes of human lives are powerfully shaped in the exosystem through the decision-making authority of legislative bodies at the local, state and national levels (Bronfenbrenner 1979). Although the developing adolescent is not likely to interact with the Minister of Health, that ministry's decision to create fixed does combinations for HIV-positive youth would impact the adolescent in a myriad ways; from increased adherence to medication, to improved health outcomes, to improved schooling and increasingly safer sexual behavior and so on.

The macrosystem is Bronfenbrenner's overall term for cultural patterns in society. This component of the model reflects the understanding that any explanation of human development must locate knowledge about people in the pervasive cultural context in which they find themselves. Like the exosystem, the macrosystem is external to the individual and highly influential on development. This system tends to be most imperceptible when the focus is on one individual (Bronfenbrenner 1979). For example, in a society structured through a complex linking of capitalism, privilege and patriarchy, individuals can be expected to be over- or underprivileged based on race, class, gender and other divisions indicative of a society characterized by a set of hierarchies. Thus, any unequal power relation that exists in the macrosystem can be expected to imitate the human experience on the micro, meso- and exosystems.

A final system, the chrono-system, that threads through the entire system, takes into account history and the time that shapes one's development. For HIV-positive adolescents living in South Africa, this might involve the generation they are currently borne into with its consequent political systems and social inventions, and the era of AIDS denialism in South Africa in the early part of this century which is their inheritance.

Bronfenbrenner's model is a useful framework in explaining the systemic links between contexts and how this impacts individuals. Adolescents who are HIV-positive face multiple risks that can be compounded or protected against depending on the impacts of these various systems of influence and how they navigate them.

4.3 Salient Issues and HIV-Positive Young People

4.3.1 Mental Health

Studies in both more and less developed countries show that just under half of all PLWHA have a diagnosable mental disorder and in some instances a threefold higher rate of mental disorder (Freeman et al. 2007; Myer et al. 2009; Lazarus et al. 2009; Thom 2012). The reasons for this are complex but include pre-morbid mental conditions, the effects of the virus on the central nervous system, the psychological impacts of living with HIV/AIDS, side-effects of medication and results of social stigma and discrimination (Freeman et al. 2007). Mental health disorders have been shown to occur with increased frequency among HIV-positive children and adolescents. Studies conducted primarily in the United States have shown that HIV-positive children and adolescents display a higher rate of behavioral, social, and emotional problems, such as attention-deficit hyperactivity disorder, depression, oppositional defiant disorder, adjustment disorder, post-traumatic stress disorder and anxiety, relative to their uninfected peers (Mellins et al. 2002, 2006, 2009a, b). These problems are also evident in adolescents but in addition include suicidality and alcohol abuse later in development (Mellins et al. 2002, 2006, 2009b). While the virus itself or an opportunistic infection, such as one causing meningitis or encephalitis, may lead to neurodevelopmental impairments that affect mental and psychomotor development, it appears that the social context of HIV (such as familial disruption, poverty, stigmatization, orphanhood and so on) may play a greater role in the higher prevalence of mental health problems among this population (Domek 2009; see also Chap. 12 in this volume). As a consequence of the combined neuropathological effects of HIV and the environmental context, the most common psychiatric disorders found amongst HIV-positive adolescents are depression, severe anxiety and post-traumatic stress disorder (PTSD) (Williams et al. 2007; Thom 2012; Lowenthal et al. 2014). There is evidence to support that these same mental health issues are pervasive for HIV-infected adolescents in South Africa (Cluver et al. 2007, 2008, 2009; Thom 2009), but more research is required to understand the mental health problems of HIV-infected youth in this region. The emotional effects of coping with HIV infection can be severe, and the frequency of psychiatric admissions among HIV-infected adolescents is significantly higher compared with that in the general paediatric population in high-income countries (Gaughan et al. 2004). These mental health needs typically receive very little attention both in South Africa and generally in low- and middle-income countries (Patel 2007; Thom 2009). Poor mental health is strongly related to other health and development concerns in young people, notably lower educational achievements and neurocognitive delay, substance abuse, violence, and poor reproductive and sexual health (Domek 2006). Key challenges to addressing mental-health needs include the shortage of mental-health professionals, the fairly low capacity and motivation of non-specialist health workers to provide quality mental-health services to young people, and the stigma associated with mental disorder (Patel 2007). Reaching adolescents during this developmental period thus serves a preventive function regarding long standing adult disease burden. But more importantly, it can help this age group navigate a predictably difficult period in terms of developmental risk and mental health.

Worldwide, HIV/AIDS and depression are the leading causes of disease burden for young people (those aged 10–24 years) (UNICEF 2011). Major depression is highly prevalent among HIV-positive patients, ranging between 18 % and 81 % depending on the population studied and the methodology of the study (Arseniou et al. 2013). Half of the newly acquired HIV infections occur in young people, with most of those affected living in developing countries. In developed countries, mental disorders are at the forefront of disease burden in young people (UNICEF et al. 2008). Studies show that psychosocial issues form a great burden of disease for young people, including intentional and unintentional injuries, mental disorders, tobacco, alcohol and other substance use, and unprotected sexual intercourse (Tylee et al. 2007). HIV-positive adolescents confront many extra challenges including concerns about medication regimens, doctor's appointments, life expectancy, social upheaval, disclosure, adherence, transmission of the virus to others (Murphy et al. 2003; Williams et al. 2006; Merzel et al. 2008; Rudy et al. 2009). Autonomy and peer relationships are typically complicated by fears of stigma and complexities in disclosure to partners (Cluver et al. 2008; Li et al. 2010). As children age into adolescence, a normative stage of 'desire to fit in', sexual and drug experimentation, as well as a time when non-adherence becomes more prevalent, issues related to the transmission of HIV, including ART resistant strains of the virus become a public health concern (Remien et al. 2007).

Among 15–19 year olds worldwide, suicide is the second leading cause of death, followed by violence in the community and family (UNICEF 2011). Violence and injuries are the second leading cause of death and lost disability-adjusted life years in South Africa (after HIV/AIDS) (Seedat et al. 2009). The overall injury death rate of 157·8 per 100,000 population is nearly twice the global average (Seedat et al. 2009). Violence or the fear of violence can pose formidable barriers to HIV prevention, care, and treatment, limiting individuals' ability to learn their status and adopt and maintain protective measures ranging from negotiating safer sex to remaining in school (Gardsbane 2010; WHO and UNAIDS 2010). HIV and intimate partner violence (IPV) have been viewed as sharing common structural drivers, such as gender inequality and poverty. Consequently, more effective and sensitive care for adolescent victims of violence is needed (UNICEF 2011). Gender-based violence (GBV) against children and adolescents is unfortunately increasingly pervasive in South Africa (Kaminer and Eagle 2010). An evaluation of GBV programs in sub-Saharan Africa showed that children constitute a significant portion of GBV survivors seeking services but that they are underserved by adult-oriented services (Keesbury et al. 2010). Violence, its dynamic of power and control, and the fact that young women are targets of GBV obviously impacts on teen pregnancy rates (where young girls are unable to negotiate condom use) and consequent child and maternal mortality and morbidity. The national teen pregnancy rate is currently 12 % but this number shoots up to 60 % in certain districts of South Africa (Jamieson et al. 2011). The risk of dying from pregnancy-related causes is much higher for adolescents than for older women (Keesbury et al. 2010). In addition, adolescents engaged in high levels of transactional sex are poorly educated regarding sexual reproductive health and have poor access to contraception (Cluver et al. 2011a, b). Thus, violence is a significant risk faced by young people in South Africa, particularly for those living with HIV (see also Chap. 9 in this volume).

Alcohol and illicit drug use are highly prevalent among youth living with HIV (Murphy et al. 2001; Naar-King et al. 2006) and have been associated with increased sexual risk (Naar-King et al. 2006), poor adherence to medications (Murphy et al. 2001; Naar-King et al. 2010), and increased exposure to violence (Parry et al. 2010). Alcohol usage is consistently *associated* with prevalence and incidence of HIV and almost to the point of *causality*. There is now conclusive evidence of a causal linkage between heavy drinking patterns and/or alcohol use disorders and the worsening of the disease course for HIV (Morojele et al. 2004; Parry et al. 2010). The burden attributable to alcohol use in South Africa in 2004 has been estimated to be 1.3 million years in terms of years lost though premature death caused by alcohol and years lived with an alcohol-related disability (or just over 6 % of all years lost from all causes) (Schneider et al. 2007). Of all years lost through death and disability that can be attributed to alcohol, 10 % for men and 28 % for women can be directly attributed to alcohol's impact on the progression of HIV in infected adults (Schneider et al. 2007; Parry et al. 2010). Although evidence is scarce regarding HIV-infected youths' use of alcohol and substances in South Africa and the impact on HIV progression, it is probable that their progression would match those of adults with the potential of an increase as drugs and alcohol are typically experimented with at this developmental stage.

4.3.2 Orphanhood and Bereavement

It is predicted that by the year 2010 there were 25 million orphans in the world as a result of AIDS (the term orphan is typically defined by the UN definition—i.e., loss of one or both parents among children up to the age of 18 years (UNAIDS 2004). The orphanhood epidemic has matured alongside the HIV epidemic (see also Chaps. 2, 3, and 16 in this volume). Thus, more than 50 % of AIDS orphans are adolescents (Lowenthal et al. 2014). In South Africa, the overall level of orphanhood in 2012 among those 0–18 years of age and younger was 16.9 % (maternal, 4.4 %; paternal, 9.3 %; double, 3.2 %) (Shisana 2014).

HIV is a disease that affects systems at the household level. Having inherited the virus from a parent, perinatally-infected HIV-positive adolescents are more likely to be orphaned and have changing or absent guardianship, which could lead to being isolated through neglect or separation from other family members (Holborn and Eddy 2011). They inherit the consequent responsibility for welfare of younger siblings or other ill and ageing family members, increased stigma and discrimination as a result of bereavement, the fear of being viewed as abnormal, and confrontation of mortality and an uncertain future. Adolescents have to negotiate the complex demands of treatment, social pressures, and vulnerable health within the context of bereavement and disrupted care, without having necessarily developed the skills to manage these circumstances. It is important not to underestimate the potential psychological effects of the awareness of their limited mortality on their well-being, which might be both reinforced through witnessing HIV-related deaths within the household or through taking treatment—a daily reminder of their own infection. These adolescents are more likely to have lower educational achievements and consequently less chance of gaining economic independence, as little financial support for school fees exacerbates the risks of interrupted school attendance and the existing learning disadvantages that they might face through HIV-related cognitive impairment (Bernays et al. 2014). Compounded by a cycle of poverty, these interconnecting factors shape the ability of these adolescents to manage their health and prepare for adult life.

Many adverse outcomes of being orphaned have been reported, including loss of effective guidance and supervision, inconsistent care, psychological distress and poor mental health, loss of educational opportunities, impoverishment, increased sexual vulnerability, and high rates of risk taking (Lowenthal 2004). Studies from African countries have found that compared with non-orphans, children and young people who have lost at least one parent to AIDS have more unmet basic living needs, and more psychological problems including negative mood and pessimism (Makame et al. 2002; Richter 2003; Atwine et al. 2005; Remien et al. 2007; Cluver et al. 2009; Petersen et al. 2010). They are often exploited by new caregivers and have to survive with limited resources (Remien et al. 2007). In addition, being orphaned as a result of HIV/AIDS has more severe consequences than being orphaned as a result of non-AIDS related death (Cluver et al. 2011a, b). Cluver and colleagues (2011a, b) report that children and adolescents orphaned by AIDS were 117 % more likely to be suffering from post-traumatic stress disorder than children and adolescents whose parents were alive, and also 67 % more likely than children and adolescents orphaned by other causes, including homicide, suicide and cancer. AIDS orphaned children and adolescents were more likely to be engaged in economic activities and go to bed hungry on a daily basis (Delva et al. 2009). There was higher prevalence of HIV infection among orphans compared with non-orphans and orphans of non-AIDS causes, higher rates of sexual behavior among orphans, earlier sexual debut, increased risk of intergenerational sex, increased poverty, significant mental health problems (including PTSD, depression and anxiety), care giving stressors and increased family violence (Cluver et al. 2008, 2011a, b, 2012).

Orphanhood and its consequent loss creates significant additional stress on the developing adolescent. Loss is highly complex and dependent on developmental stage, resilience, quality of care, and social support networks, and often includes a progression of experiences from the onset of a parent's or caregiver's illness, through to the aftermath of death. For several reasons, AIDS-related bereavement is likely to be especially complicated and difficult to endure. Understandings of bereavement and grief among African children, and adults' responses to orphans' psychological difficulties, remain underdeveloped (Wood et al. 2006). Timing and mode of transmission may be important factors to consider as perinatally/vertically-infected adolescents may experience different psychological challenges given that they have lived with HIV for a significantly longer period, compared with adolescents infected behaviorally/horizontally. Many adolescents who contracted the virus from their mothers are orphaned by the time they reach adolescence. HIV-positive adolescents and their caregivers may experience multiple losses and children often live in households where other members are infected and may become involved in the care of terminally ill members of the household. Resultantly, at a tender age, they have had a fair dealing with death and grief.

There are many cultural taboos around death, and talking about death and people who have died. It is important to be aware that children and adolescents of different ages have different understandings of death. Only gradually do they develop an understanding that death is permanent and final; most adolescents will understand that death is permanent and final. They realize that all people eventually die, but tend to see their own death as happening at some distant time in the future. Adolescents are at a time in their lives where they need to become independent and to cope on their own. It may be particularly difficult for them to acknowledge their loss or to express it in ways they feel appropriate. They may also have difficulty seeking support, especially from adults, but sometimes even from peers, for fear of seeming weak. It might be worth noting too that often messages about the death of a loved one who died of HIV/AIDS can have a longstanding impact on HIV-positive children and adolescents and the process of disclosure. If they were told their parent died of HIV and later on their status is disclosed to them, depending on their developmental age, this disclosure can feel completely overwhelming and unmanageable. In other words, bereaved children and adolescents should also be told the truth about death as it aids in knowing the facts of disease. The death of a caregiver can set off a chain of losses for the child, including loss of a home, education and financial security. Much of the grief surrounding HIV/AIDS is quite normalized in communities and these children/adolescents often do not receive much support with their losses (which are enduring). Adolescents might miss their parent who died for the remainder of their lives and have complex and unresolved feelings about the loss, the family disruption, and their HIV status that have never been adequately or compassionately managed by the adults around them. Unresolved grief can lead to traumatic bereavement symptoms (such as post-traumatic stress disorder (PTSD)—hypervigilence, avoidance, dysregulation, re-experiencing, increased stress and hyperarousal) and depression if not dealt with. Unresolved grief can also affect the capacity of remaining caregivers to provide adequate care (Thom 2007). While many orphaned teenagers desire direct communication with adults about parental illness and death, adults themselves—whether the sick parent, other relatives in the household or a caregiver following parental loss—are often ill-equipped to identify and manage children's distress positively (Wood et al. 2006; Lowenthal et al. 2014).

Orphans and vulnerable children are at increased risk for mental health problems as a result of the typical contexts of emotional deprivation and stigma of their upbringings, and lack of attention given to their mental health outcomes. The psychosocial consequences of orphanhood are severe and place children and adolescents orphaned by AIDS at a greater risk for psychological distress and behavioral problems, making the rapidly growing number of children and adolescents orphaned by AIDS a major cause of concern (Domek 2009; see also Chaps. 2, 3, and 16 in this volume).

4.3.3 Stigma

A major distinction between HIV/AIDS and other chronic or terminal illnesses is the stigma associated with the disease (see Chaps. 1, 2, 3, 6, 9, and 14 in this volume). This stigma often stems from lack of knowledge about HIV and how it is transmitted; which can adversely affect adolescents and their caregivers in ways that have long-term negative psychological and social consequences (Close 2003). HIV-positive patients often have to endure the stigma and discrimination they feel from the community or service providers, but also, especially during adolescence, experience 'self-stigma' (or 'internalized stigma') where an individual takes on the perceived stigma of others and stigmatizes themselves. Internalized stigma has a large effect on the pediatric population through its influence on caregiver's decisions to disclose. If parents or caregivers have internalized the stigma and negative views of HIV/AIDS, their likelihood of telling the child or adolescent about his or her diagnosis decreases significantly, and if adolescents internalize the stigma regarding their diagnosis, they are more likely to become depressed and engage in denial regarding their HIV status (Close 2003). This may create fear in adolescents disclosing their status to others and they may feel shameful regarding their HIV diagnosis. Obviously, these factors have an enormous influence that can have a negative impact on interpersonal relationships, self-esteem and the practice of safe sex where honestly talking about sexual transmission and protection is crucial.

To safeguard a child or adolescent from experiencing stigma, caregivers often practice 'stigma management' and delay disclosing the child's diagnosis to the child/adolescent as a result of shame, guilt, and fears of inadvertent disclosure to community (see also Chaps. 5, 6, and 17). This is evident when between 25 and 90 % of school-aged HIV-positive children and adolescents are unaware of their own status (Close 2003) regardless of going to the clinic every 3 months to pick up treatment. However, many children and adolescents are being sensitized to HIV and ART through life orientation classes at school and through the media, so inadvertently they start to 'figure it out' on their own. They, thus learn about their status outside of the home. Unfortunately, as the family system has not been honest, stigma leads to an atmosphere of secrecy within the family that the adolescent often senses. Adolescents become acutely aware of their family's feelings towards their diagnosis, through observing their family's interactions with other adults and how they discuss or avoid the topic of HIV in their presence. Labeling the diagnosis as a secret that cannot be discussed only serves to increase the stigma and by adolescence, many HIV-positive children have internalized stigma to a degree that disastrously impacts their self-esteem and identity formation. Self-stigma thrives in environments of secrecy. When families are open, children and adolescents have increased support and with honestly, comes improved disease management as well as increased self-esteem and help seeking behavior.

On the other hand, exposure to stigma has a profound effect on adolescents growing up with HIV. Their HIV status often physically manifests with visible scars of skin disease, a smaller and physically weaker physique than their peers and having delayed puberty. As is common among young people, the desire to conform with peers could inadvertently lead them not only to stop treatment, but can also instil in them a pronounced sense of social isolation by being marked out as different, which creates a heavy psychological burden (Bernays et al. 2014). Hence biomedical interventions to address HIV in isolation are profoundly insufficient and do not meet the challenges of treatment adherence that this population faces.

4.3.4 Adherence

The introduction of highly active antiretroviral therapy (HAART) in 1996 in the international community qualitatively changed the HIV treatment landscape. Although it took a little longer for HAART to arrive in South Africa, the national antiretroviral treatment program in South Africa commenced in 2004 (years of denial, blaming, moralizing and inaction finally came to an end in the watershed year of 2003, when the South African Government approved a national program to make antiretroviral drugs publicly available to all HIV-infected people who qualified for treatment) and today South Africa has one of the largest antiretroviral programs in the world. There is, however, growing concern about ARV adherence, the development of drug-resistant HIV and drug failure. Even more troubling from a public health perspective, a drug-resistant mutant strain of HIV caused by non-adherence can be transmitted to uninfected patients, leaving newly infected and drug-naïve patients without effective treatment options (Fogarty et al. 2002). The risk of onward transmission of HIV to a sexual partner is high in adolescence (Lowenthal et al. 2014). Thus, treatment and prevention efforts should be particularly intensified in adolescence to sustain the health of young people.

Characteristics of the HAART regimens make adherence particularly difficult as these therapies require multiple drugs, sometimes as many as six (fixed dose combinations given as one pill per day are not available for children or adolescents) taken at different times of the day, some with food and some without. These medications are often taken in addition to numerous other drugs treating related ailments. Many of the HAART medications have unpleasant side effects, such as diarrhea, nausea, vomiting and peripheral neuropathy (Fogarty et al. 2002). Other characteristics of HIV treatment also make adherence more challenging—treatment is of a life-long duration, given to patients who are often asymptomatic, the high pill burden is a reminder of the stigmatized disease, and with a treatment payoff of delayed disease progression sometime in the future. Children and adolescents face the prospect of having to take ART with optimum adherence for 20 years longer on average than do adults, but fewer treatment regimens are available to them and consequently often encounter drug fatigue (Bernays et al. 2014). As opposed to other chronic illnesses and treatment adherence, HIV requires near perfect adherence to be completely effective and this is particularly difficult to achieve in adolescence. In addition, adolescents face substantial social barriers to maintaining the levels of adherence expected of them by their healthcare providers. What happens outside the clinic inevitably affect the ability of adolescents to adhere to clinical guidance. The stigma that surrounds HIV leads adolescents to take their treatment in secret which is difficult in busy school environments. Taking treatment every day of their lives is made more difficult within the context of poverty, where they might be living in crowded households with little privacy and access to food. In addition, adolescent's ability to adhere to treatment is partly dependent on the support, guidance, and information they receive from caregivers and healthcare providers and when this support is scant, especially in the case of orphans, adherence becomes increasingly challenging (Bernays et al. 2014).

Correlates of poor treatment adherence in adolescence include being orphaned, lack of knowledge, mental health problems, changes of guardianship, and absence of parental and social support (Lowenthal et al. 2014). Adherence to HAART remains problematic with this population as adolescents are often challenged with maintaining strict routines and this is often linked to mental health problems (Mellins et al. 2004; Murphy et al. 2003; Merzel et al. 2008; Rudy et al. 2009; Ferrand et al. 2010). Delayed disclosure of HIV status to the adolescent, and a resultant lack of autonomy, substantially affect adherence (Close 2003). Good adherence to an antiretroviral regimen is associated with an adolescent's knowledge of their HIV status, valuable social support, and having a strong relationship with parents (Lowenthal et al. 2014). However, even for adolescents with these apparent advantages, structural barriers of stigma and poverty still affect adherence. Since adherence means not only following dosing regimens but also being able to refill prescriptions, and since prescriptions are refilled as part of routine follow-up visits in Africa, barriers to adherence and retention overlap. Travel distance to clinic sites and associated costs, stigma and fear of disclosure, competing demands for scarce resources, religious and cultural beliefs, and unanticipated obligations and events (e.g., attending a family funeral) are key adherence barriers identified through previous research that also bear upon retention (Davies et al. 2013; see Chaps. 5, 20, and 22 in this volume).

The desire for conformity with peers during adolescence, and a fear of stigmatization, greatly affects treatment adherence. Transition of adolescents from paediatric to adult HIV care services might further disrupt adherence, because the time available for counseling is diminished and healthcare providers have little experience of addressing adolescent-specific concerns (Lowenthal et al. 2014; see also Chaps. 5, 6, and 20 in this volume).

4.3.5 *Disclosure*

With the widespread use of highly active antiretroviral therapy (HAART), the epidemic of pediatric HIV has evolved into a chronic disease of childhood and adolescence. The difference between this disease and most other chronic diseases of childhood and adolescence, however, is that it is not only a life-threatening diagnosis but also an extremely stigmatizing one, resulting in highly emotionally charged responses to disclosure of such a diagnosis to the patient. The disclosure process is made much more difficult when the person being disclosed to is a child or young person. One of the major difficulties is that one is dealing with many layers of disclosure: disclosure of HIV status to the young person; the concomitant disclosure of HIV status of the parent/s and other siblings or other family members; and having to anticipate the child's own disclosure to his/her friends, extended family and community. Approaches to disclosing the diagnosis may vary between parents and between health care providers, but one thing that has been established in many studies world-wide is that the child or adolescent needs to be informed, many suggesting sooner rather than later during the course of the illness (WHO 2011). During adolescence, disclosure of the diagnosis may also aid in preventing high-risk behavior, thereby curbing spread of the disease.

Some clinical characteristics have been shown to impact the likelihood of disclosure from systematic reviews: receiving ART, a longer duration of enrolment in clinic or on ART and the adolescent having a lower CD4 count (Vreeman et al. 2013). Numerous fears on the part of caregivers and healthcare providers were cited as barriers to disclosure. These included fear that the adolescent would disclose to others, fear of subsequent stigma or negative effects from others knowing the diagnosis, concerns for worsening the adolescent's emotional or physical health, believing the adolescent is unready or too young, feeling unprepared for questions or the disclosure process and fear of the adolescent's resentment (Vreeman et al. 2013). These fears often lead to silence and although understandable, however misplaced, desire to protect children and adolescents from knowing their HIV status results in them being confused about their future and development.

Research indicates that disclosure has a positive effect on treatment adherence. Data from five studies of children and adolescents aged 2–18 years showed a 20 % increased rate of adherence to ARV medication regimens among those whose status had been disclosed to them (Krauss et al. 2012). A study conducted in New York revealed that those adolescents who were disclosed to showed higher CD4 counts and lower viral loads (Krauss et al. 2012). Other studies suggest that HIV-infected children who know their status may be better able to seek social support, have improved coping skills and practice safer sexual practices to prevent secondary transmission (Vreeman et al. 2013). Adolescents who know their HIV status can take an active role in their care and treatment plan and can take steps to live positively to prevent new infections (see also Chaps. 5, 6, and 17 in this volume).

Healthcare providers play a significant role in assisting families with the disclosure process. Many families choose to disclose in the clinic setting so they can receive the educational support of the facility staff there. It is important to note that disclosure is a process rather than a one-time event; caregivers need to be aware of their responsibilities and create an atmosphere of asking and answering questions about the virus and living with it with an attitude and pace of information giving that is comfortable to the child/adolescent (Naeem-Sheik and Gray 2005). Caregivers might also be asked to disclose their own status, which they should be prepared for. Through basic education about the virus, how it is transmitted, and treatment options, much of the stigma surrounding HIV/AIDS can be dispelled. Through educating communities at large, families and children infected or affected by HIV/AIDS can receive much-needed support and will no longer feel alone in their struggle (Close 2003). Obviously, if this is done satisfactorily, adolescents can learn how to disclose to their friends, and later their sexual partners in ways that do not disadvantage them or their sexual partner.

The evidence that is reported in the WHO Disclosure Guidelines on HIV Disclosure Counselling for Children up to 12 years of age (2011) shows that there is little doubt that disclosure is central to the overall well-being of the child and adolescent. Thus, there is evidence of health benefits, but little evidence of psychological or emotional harm from disclosure of HIV status to HIV-positive children and adolescents. It is, therefore, alarming that most studies show that a minority of HIV-infected children and adolescents in resource-limited settings know his/her HIV status (Vreeman et al. 2013). A local study revealed that at least three quarters of children and adolescents of 12–18 years on ARV treatment were unaware of their status (Krauss et al. 2012). Delayed and suboptimum disclosure to children and adolescents of their HIV status is a common experience, leaving them to cope with their disease within an atmosphere of secrecy. In combination with children's and adolescents' low personal status in society and poor access to social resources, this secrecy curtails the opportunities that they have to discuss, learn, understand and thus accept their illness (Bernays et al. 2014; Kajubi et al. 2014).

On 1 April 2010, the *Children's Act 38 of 2005* (as amended by the Children's Amendment Act 41 of 2007) was passed into South African law. This Act guarantees the child's legal rights to participate in healthcare decisions and to clarify their right to privacy of their disclosure of HIV status. The Children's Act lowers the age at which children can consent to certain healthcare interventions in order to promote access to healthcare services. With regard to child participation, the Act states that: "Every child that is of such an age, maturity and stage of development as to be able to participate in any matter concerning that child has the right to participate in an appropriate way and views expressed by the child must be given due consideration" (p. 62). It has, therefore, become the duty and responsibility of all healthcare personnel to ensure that all interactions and interventions with the child/adolescent are practiced within a Child Rights framework (Strode 2011; Zuch 2012). It is, therefore, critical to be familiar with the legislation affecting children's health issues. The process of disclosure is a circular one that must constantly be revisited to help the adolescent enhance their understanding of the illness and associated challenges. This requires on-going, good communication between the adolescent and the caregivers, as well as with the healthcare provider, and others working with the family.

Disclosure from family to disclosure at clinic level can increase social support having an effect on a community level in decreasing the effects of stigma. Although HIV-positive adults are often loathe to engage in the disclosure process as it is a proxy for their own disclosure of HIV positivity; engaging in the process, however, models a positive role in managing the disease and living with it more openly. When healthcare providers know the status of families, they are more empowered to engage in overall systemic healthcare for the family unit. If caregivers do not have a positive attitude towards disclosure, then it is likely to filter to the adolescent and they are likely to take on the same negative attitude towards their disease. The same can be said for the healthcare system.

4.3.6 Female Sexual and Reproductive Health

Sexual identity-building in adolescence is complex and culturally specific, and sexual behaviors are shaped partly by societal norms. Ideals of masculinity and femininity may limit South African women's decision-making power in relationships and increase their risk of HIV infection (Jewkes 2006b; see also Chaps. 7, 10, and 15 in this volume). In a study focussed on young urban women in Johannesburg, South Africa, the majority of young women reported expectations of power in relationships that conform to a model of femininity marked by financial independence, freedom to make decisions, including over sexuality, and equality (Pettifor et al. 2012). The majority of young women, however, were in relationships marked by intimate partner violence, infidelity or lack of condom use. The disconnect between expectations of relationships and young women's lived realities emphasizes the need for structural changes that afford women greater economic and thus decision-making power (Pettifor et al. 2012). Social constructions of masculinity and femininity in South Africa place young men and particularly young women at increased risk of HIV infection (Jewkes et al. 2006a, b). There is a large body of literature documenting the manner in which dominant social constructions of gender lead to poor sexual health for young South Africans (Pettifor et al. 2005, 2012; Jewkes et al. 2006a, b). In fact, HIV incidence remains highest among 15–24 years olds, with approximately 40 % of horizontal transmission occurring within this age group (UNAIDS et al. 2008). So, adolescents need information to protect themselves and make informed choices about their sexual and reproductive health.

Early sexual debut, having multiple sex partners, being at high risk of sexual violence, and adolescent girls engaging in transactional sex with older men, put adolescents at especially high risk of acquiring and transmitting HIV infection

(Cluver et al. 2011a, b; Lowenthal et al. 2014; Thurman et al. 2006). A study on transactional sex conducted in South Africa highlighted that adolescents "dually" affected by AIDS orphanhood and caregiver sickness showed a threefold likelihood of experiencing severe emotional and physical abuse and, amongst girls, a sixfold likelihood of transactional sexual exploitation, compared with those in healthy families (Cluver et al. 2011a, b). The effects of familial AIDS, food insecurity, and exposure to abuse raised prevalence of transactional sex amongst girls from 1 to 57 % (Cluver et al. 2011a, b). In the teenage population in South Africa, the estimated HIV prevalence among females in 2012 was eight times that of their male counterparts, suggesting that female teenagers aged 15–19 years are more likely than their male counterparts to have sex with older sex partners (Shisana et al. 2014). Among adults aged 15–49 years, the number of new infections was 1.7 times higher in females than in males (Shisana et al. 2014). The incidence rates among young females remain concerning. The HIV-incidence rate among female youth aged 15–24 was over four times higher than the incidence rate found in males in this age group (2.5 % vs. 0.6 %) (Shisana et al. 2014). Overall, it was found that one tenth (10.7 %) of respondents aged 15–24 years reported having had sex for the first time before the age of 15 years (Shisana et al. 2014).

South Africa has very high teen pregnancy rates, approximately 30 % of teenagers in South Africa report 'ever having been pregnant', the majority, unplanned (Shisana et al. 2009; Willan 2013). Teenage pregnancy in South Africa is driven by many factors including: gender inequalities; gendered expectations of how teenage boys and girls should act; sexual taboos (for girls) and sexual permissiveness (for boys); poverty; poor access to contraceptives and termination of pregnancies; inaccurate and inconsistent contraceptive use; judgmental attitudes of many health care workers; high levels of gender-based violence; and poor sex education (Jewkes et al. 2006; Willan 2013). Awareness of and knowledge about reproductive health, HIV transmission, and contraceptive methods is poor among HIV-infected adolescents (WHO 2011). Discrepancy between the information given by health-care providers and the actual needs of HIV-infected adolescents is common, with the concerns of young people sometimes not taken into account. Healthcare providers need to recognize that young people perinatally-infected with HIV are sexually active or anticipate being so in the future (Lowenthal et al. 2014).

Young people want to know about safe sex and for those who are perinatally-infected, their main questions inevitably are whether there would even be a cure for HIV in their lifetime and whether they can become parents later on (personal interviews with youth). However, with high rates of stigma and discrimination, HIV-positive adolescents encounter difficulties disclosing their HIV status to their romantic partners and often engage in unsafe sex as a consequence. The systems of influence here between the individual, the interpersonal, the context and the society have significant impact on the HIV epidemic.

4.3.7 Medical Independence and Transition to Adult Clinics

For adolescents living with a chronic illness, transitioning to adulthood includes an important shift towards medical independence. Health service involvement decreases in adolescence at the same time that family involvement in young people's healthcare also declines. This situation can have serious implications for an adolescent's health and decision-making such as missing doses and clinic appointments and so on. Often, adolescents need to transition to a new clinic as they age as many pediatric clinics do not have funding or capacity to keep youth as they age into adulthood (Close 2003; see also Chaps. 5, 6, and 20 in this volume). In South Africa, adolescent patients are typically transitioned from pediatric clinics, where they get a great deal of investment from clinical teams, to adult clinics at the age of approximately 12 years where they are expected to navigate complex systems independently (SANAC 2011). It is unsurprising, therefore, that most of these patients are lost in these systems and their treatment and care suffers greatly. As many adolescents are not treatment literate and some do not have a sophisticated understanding of their medical histories, healthcare providers should teach adolescents to cope with specific tasks such as managing their medication, scheduling their appointments, and discussing their healthcare concerns directly with their providers. Adolescents should be thoroughly educated on HIV and feel comfortable discussing their care and treatment with healthcare providers. As adolescents transition between pediatric and adult clinical venues, healthcare providers need to have a thorough understanding of the multi-faceted issues including complicated treatment histories, complex psychosocial dynamics and development stage, in order to effectively manage adolescents living with HIV and optimize outcomes after the transfer (Agwu et al. 2013).

4.3.8 Public Health Challenges

Unfortunately, youth friendly services are not widely available in the public health sector in South Africa (SANAC 2011), and adolescents tend to get lost in adult systems of care or fall out of care as a result of their needs not being met. Better information on adolescents is needed if healthcare providers, community-level stakeholders, caregivers, and policy-makers are to respond effectively to the specific needs of this group. For adolescents living with a chronic illness, transitioning into adulthood includes an important shift toward medical independence. Youth need assistance from healthcare professionals in taking charge of their medical care and utilizing the healthcare system to their advantage. The healthcare professionals who interact with adolescents also need to be appropriate and informed of youth friendly ways of working. As long as this population is overlooked and their clinical, psychological and social needs remain poorly understood, adolescents (including those on ART) will remain one of the most vulnerable populations affected by the HIV pandemic. Our failure to address this vulnerability threatens the lives of these youth and jeopardizes the successes of pediatric HIV treatment efforts to date (Bernays et al. 2014).

Despite the substantial evidence for the burden, public-health importance, and the emerging evidence of the efficacy of psychosocial and pharmacological treatments for mental disorders in young people, health-system responses to youth mental health have been inadequate. In 2002, a systematic review and interviews with key informants showed that only 7 % of countries in the world had a clearly articulated specific child and adolescent mental health policy (Patel et al. 2007). Substantial variations exist between WHO regions and between developing and developed countries; while 78 % of countries in the high-income category have a child and adolescent mental-health policy, not one low-income country does (Patel et al. 2007). In most developing countries, very few child and adolescent mental health services or resources are available, and even fewer that specifically cater for young people. Without policies to protect adolescents, their rights are easily violated. Thus, most mental health care for adolescents and young adults is typically delivered in community and outpatient settings, often within the context of adult services (Patel et al. 2007). In addition, in South Africa, many individuals with common mental health conditions (such as depression, anxiety and PTSD) do not present for treatment, or if they do they usually present to primary care facilities, where these diagnoses are often missed. This is unfortunate, since there is good evidence that these disorders can be effectively treated and that much of this treatment can be provided by primary care clinicians (Thom 2007).

General practitioners and other primary care workers need to be educated to better engage young people, to recognize mental and substance use disorders, and to deliver simple treatments, including supportive counseling, cognitive behavior therapy, and, where appropriate, psychotropic drugs. Government departments need to work more closely together, i.e. ministries of health should be working closely with education and social service to deliver integrated responses to adolescents and fulfil their mandates to this population. Typically, there is very little inter-ministerial referral and integration of service. The key to promoting youth mental health is through strengthening of the fundamental nurturing qualities of the family system and community networks while explicitly acknowledging the rights of young people. Such action would mean recognition of families and communities as major players in determining the mental health of young people. Young people themselves must be at the centre of all policy-making, focusing on their concerns. Policies must explicitly address strengthening capacity for addressing youth mental disorders in family settings, educational settings, in primary health care and in specialist mental health care (Patel et al. 2007).

4.4 Conclusion

Adolescence is a notoriously difficult developmental stage to overcome; it is even more challenging when an individual has a chronic illness, and one as highly stigmatized as HIV, to endure. HIV-positive youth are not only undertaking the inevitable biologic, cognitive, and social developmental challenges of adolescence and young adulthood, but also undergo a myriad of physical, psychosocial and healthcare system barriers. The population of HIV-positive adolescents engaging in healthcare services is growing rapidly in the developing world (Ferrand et al. 2009) and healthcare providers need to be capacitated to manage this particular population and their care and treatment. Adherence and disclosure remain highly problematic for young people with consequent impacts on sexual reproductive health in a time fraught with experimentation and secrecy. Perinatally infected HIV-positive adolescents may have additional difficulties to navigate, having lived with the disease for a long time and withstanding the psychosocial challenges that accompany being typically orphaned (Mellins et al. 2006, 2009; Cluver et al. 2008, 2011a, b). Being mindful of and addressing some of the psychosocial stressors of this population would significantly improve the lives of adolescents and strengthening the healthcare system response to them.

The failure to address mental health problems (both in terms of prevention and treatment), including developmental and intellectual disorders in childhood and adolescents in low-resource settings is a public health issue with wide reaching consequences because such failure also impedes the achievement of basic development goals in low- and middle-income countries. Moreover, because evidence shows that a substantial proportion of mental health problems in adults originate early in life, the situation has long-lasting effects beyond childhood and adolescence (Kieling et al. 2011). Youth make up significant parts of the population in developing contexts and investment in this developmental age group would go a long way in preventing additional infection and lessening the burden on the healthcare system in adulthood. Arguably, adolescence should be seen as the gateway to adult good health.

The psychological, social, and economic consequences of ART should be considered as HIV-positive adolescents in low-income and middle-income countries are being prepared for independence and a future they have only recently been able to expect (Ferrand et al. 2009). A model that integrates HIV clinical care with sexual and reproductive health and psychological, educational, and social services will help to prepare young adults for an independent and productive future and reduce the effect of this devastating epidemic at community and societal level (Lowenthal et al. 2014). Concurrently, efforts to mobilize and strategically advocate for pediatric and adolescent HIV care, support and treatment have not been commensurate with the magnitude of the problem, need for a solution, nor inclusive of those directly affected by or living with HIV among this population. More research is required to describe this group in South Africa and provide evidence for structured intervention and policy reform.

Acknowledgements Many thanks to Shenaaz Pahad for her careful and helpful review of this chapter.

References

Agwu, A. L., & Fairlie, L. (2013). Antiretroviral treatment, management challenges and outcomes in perinatally HIV-infected adolescents. *Journal of the International AIDS Society, 16*, 1–13.

Arseniou, S., Arvaniti, A., & Samakouri, M. (2013). HIV infection and depression. *Psychiatry and Clinical Neuroscience, 68*(2), 1–14.

Atwine, B., Cantor-Graae, E., & Bajunirwe, F. (2005). Psychological distress among AIDS orphans in rural Uganda. *Social Science & Medicine, 61*, 555–564.

Bernays, S., Jarrett, P., Kranzer, K., & Ferrand, R. A. (2014). Children growing up with HIV infection: The responsibility of success. *Lancet, 383*, 1355–1357.

Bronfenbrenner, U. (1979). *The ecology of human development: Experiments by nature and design*. Cambridge, MA: Harvard University Press.

Close, K. L. (2003). Psychosocial aspects of HIV/AIDS: Children and adolescents. In *HIV curriculum for the health professional* (pp. 319–333). Houston: Baylor International Pediatric AIDS Initiative, Baylor College of Medicine.

Cluver, L., Gardener, F., & Operario, D. (2007). Psychological distress amongst AIDS-orphaned children in urban South Africa. *Journal of Child Psychology and Psychiatry, 48*(8), 755–763.

Cluver, L., Gardener, F., & Operario, D. (2008). Effects of stigma on the mental health of adolescents orphaned by AIDS. *Journal of Adolescent Health, 42*, 410–417.

Cluver, L., Fincham, D. S., & Seedat, S. (2009). Posttraumatic stress in AIDS orphaned children exposed to high levels of trauma: The protective role of perceived social support. *Journal of Traumatic Stress, 22*(2), 106–112.

Cluver, L., Orkin, M., Boyes, M. E., Gardner, F., & Meinck, F. (2011a). Transactional sex amongst AIDS orphaned and AIDS-affected adolescents predicted by abuse and extreme poverty. *Journal AIDS, 58*(2), 336–343.

Cluver, L., Orkin, M., Gardner, F., & Boyes, M. E. (2011b). Persisting mental health problems among AIDS orphaned children in South Africa. *Journal of Child Psychology and Psychiatry, 53*(4), 1–8.

Cluver, L., Orkin, M., Boyes, M. E., Gardner, F., & Nikelo, L. (2012). AIDS-orphanhood and caregiver HIV/AIDS sickness status: Effects on psychological symptoms in South African youth. *Journal of Pediatric Psychology, 37*(8), 1–11.

Davies, N. E. C. G., Homfray, M., & Venables, E. C. (2013). Nurse and manager perceptions of nurse initiated and managed antiretroviral therapy (NIMART) implementation in South Africa: A qualitative study. *BMJ Open, 3*, 1–11.

Domek, G. J. (2009). Facing adolescence and adulthood: The importance of mental health care in the global pediatric AIDS epidemic. *Journal of Developmental and Behavioural Pediatrics, 30*, 147–150.

Ferrand, R. A., Corbett, E. L., Wood, R., Hargrove, J., Ndhlovu, C. E., Cowan, F. M., Gouws, E., & Williams, B. G. (2009). AIDS among older children and adolescents in Southern Africa: Projecting the time course and magnitude of the epidemic. *AIDS, 23*, 2039–2046.

Ferrand, R. A., Lowe, S., Whande, B., Munaiwa, L., Langhuang, L., Cowan, F., Mugurungi, O., Gibb, D., Munyati, S., Williams, B. G., & Corbett, E. L. (2010). Survey of children accessing HIV services in a high prevalence setting: Time for adolescents to count? *WHO Bulletin, 88*, 428–434.

Fogarty, L., Roter, D., Larson, S., Burke, J., Gillespie, J., & Levy, R. (2002). Patient adherence to HIV medication regimens: A review of published and abstract reports. *Patient Education and Counselling, 46*, 93–108.

Freeman, M., Nkomo, N., Kafaar, Z., & Kelly, K. (2007). Factors associated with prevalence of mental disorder in people living with HIV/AIDS in South Africa. *AIDS Care, 19*(10), 1201–1209.

Gardsbane, D. (2010). *Gender-based violence and HIV* (Technical brief).

Gaughan, D. M., Hughes, M. D., Oleske, J. M., Malee, K., Gore, C. A., Nachman, S., & The Pediatric AIDS Clinical Trials Group 219C Team. (2004). Psychiatric hospitalizations among children and youths with human immunodeficiency virus infection. *Pediatrics, 113*, 544–551.

Holborn, L., & Eddy, G. (2011). *First steps to healing the South African family*. Johannesburg: South African Institute of Race Relations.

Jamieson, L., Bray, R., Viviers, A., Lake, L., Pendlebury, S., & Smith, C. (Eds.). (2011). *South African Child Gauge 2010/2011*. Cape Town: Children's Institute, University of Cape Town.

Jaspan, H. B., Li, R., Johnson, L., & Bekker, L. G. (2009). The emerging need for adolescent-focused HIV care in South Africa. *The Southern African Journal of HIV Medicine, Dec Opinion Piece, 10*(4), 9–11.

Jewkes, R., Dunkle, K., Koss, M. P., Levin, J. B., Nduna, M., Jama, N., & Sikweyiya, Y. (2006a). Rape perpetration by young, rural South African men: Prevalence, patterns and risk factors. *Social Science & Medicine, 63*, 2949–2961.

Jewkes, R., Dunkle, K., Nduna, M., Levin, J., & Jama, N. (2006b). Factors associated with HIV sero status in young rural South African women: Connections between intimate partner violence and HIV. *International Journal of Epidemiology, 35*(6), 1461–1468.

Kajubi, P., Whyte, S., Muhumuza, S., Kyaddondo, D., & Katahoire, A. R. (2014). Communication between HIV-infected children and their caregivers about HIV medicines: A cross-sectional study in Jinja district, Uganda. *Journal of the International AIDS Society, 17*, 1–8.

Kaminer, D., & Eagle, G. (2010). *Traumatic stress in South Africa*. Johannesburg: Wits University Press.

Keesbury, J., & Askew, I. (2010). *Comprehensive responses to gender based violence (GBV) in low resource settings: Lessons learned from implementation*. Lusaka: Population Council.

Kieling, C., Baker-Henningham, H., Belfer, M., Conti, G., Ertem, I., Omigbodun, O., Rohde, L. A., Srinath, S., Ulkuer, N., & Rahman, A. (2011). Child and adolescent mental health worldwide: Evidence for action. *The Lancet, 378*(9801), 1515–1525.

Krauss, B. J., Letteney, S., De Baets, A. J., Baggaley, R., & Okero, F. A. (2012). Caregiver's HIV disclosure to children 12 years and under: A review and analysis of the evidence. *AIDS Care, 25*(4), 1–14.

Lazarus, R., & Freeman, M. (2009). *Primary-level mental health care for common mental disorder in resource-poor settings: Models & practice – A literature review*. Pretoria: Sexual Violence Research Initiative, Medical Research Council.

Li, R. J., Jaspan, H. B., O'Brien, V., Rabie, H., Cotton, M. F., & Nattrass, N. (2010). Positive futures: A qualitative study on the needs of adolescents on antiretroviral therapy in South Africa. *AIDS Care, 22*(6), 1–8.

Lowenthal, E. D., Bakeera-Kitaka, S., Marukutira, T., Chapman, J., Goldrath, K., & Ferrand, R. A. (2014). Perinatally acquired HIV infection in adolescents from sub-Saharan Africa: A review of emerging challenges. *Lancet, 383*, 1–14.

Makame, V., Ani, C., & Grantham-McGregor, S. (2002). Psychological well-being of orphans in Dar El Salaam, Tanzania. *Acta Pediatrics, 91*, 459–465.

Mellins, C., BrackisCott, E., Dolezal, C., Richards, A., Nicholas, S., & Abrams, E. (2002). Patterns of HIV status disclosure to perinatally infected HIV positive children and subsequent mental health outcomes. *Clinical Child Psychology and Psychiatry, 7*, 101–114.

Mellins, C. A., Brackis-Cott, E., Dolezal, C., & Abrams, E. J. (2004). The role of psychosocial and family factors in adherence to antiretroviral treatment in human immunodeficiency virus-infected children. *The Pediatric Infectious Disease Journal, 23*, 1035–1041.

Mellins, C. A., Brackis-Cott, E., Dolezal, C., & Abrams, E. J. (2006). Psychiatric disorders in youth with perinatally acquired human immunodeficiency virus infection. *The Pediatric Infectious Disease Journal, 25*, 432–437.

Mellins, C. A., Elkington, K. S., Bauermeister, J. A., Brackis-Cott, E., Dolezal, C., McKay, M., Wiznia, A., Bamji, M., & Abrams, E. J. (2009a). Sexual and drug use behavior in perinatally-HIV-infected youth: Mental health and family influences. *Journal of the American Academy of Child and Adolescent Psychiatry, 48*, 810–819.

Mellins, C. A., Brackis-Cott, E., Leu, C., Elkington, K., Dolezal, C., Wiznia, A., Bamji, M., McKay, M., & Abrams, E. J. (2009b). Rates and types of psychiatric disorders in perinatally human immunodeficiency virus-infected youth and seroreverters. *Journal of Child Psychology and Psychiatry, 50*, 1131–1138.

Merzel, C., van Deventer, N., & Irvine, M. (2008). Adherence to antiretroviral therapy among older children and adolescents with HIV: A qualitative study of psychosocial contexts. *AIDS Patient Care and STDSs, 22*(12), 977–987.

Morojele, N. K., Kachieng'a, M. A., Nkoko, M. A., Moshia, K. M., Mokoko, E., Parry, C. D. H., Nkowane, M. A., & Saxena, S. (2004). *Perceived effects of alcohol on sexual encounters among adults in South Africa: Dimensions and associations with sexual risk behaviour*. Parow: Medical Research Council.

Murphy, D. A., Sarr, M., Durako, S. J., Moscicki, A., Wilson, C. M., & Muenz, L. R. (2003). Barriers to HAART adherence among HIV-infected adolescents. *Archive of Pediatric Adolescent Medicine, 157*, 249–255.

Myer, L., Seedat, S., Stein, D. J., Moomal, H., & Williams, D. R. (2009). The mental health impact of AIDS related mortality in South Africa: A national study. *Journal of Epidemiology and Community Health, 63*, 293–298.

Naar-King, S., Templin, T., Wright, K., Frey, M., Parsons, J. T., & Lam, P. (2006). Psychosocial factors and medication adherence in HIV-positive youth. *AIDS Patient Care & STDs, 20*(1), 44–47.

Naeem-Sheik, A., & Gray, G. (2005, November). HIV disclosure in children. *The Southern African Journal of HIV Medicine, 21*, 46–48.

Parry, C. D. H., Rehm, J., & Morojele, N. K. (2010). Is there a causal relationship between alcohol and HIV? Implications for policy, practice and future research. *African Journal of Drug and Alcohol Studies, 9*(2), 81–91.

Patel, V., Flisher, A. J., Hetrick, S., & McGorry, P. (2007). Mental health of young people: A global public health challenge. *Lancet, 369*, 1302–1313.

Petersen, I., Myezac, N., John, S., Holst, H., Bhana, A., McKay, M., Alicea, S., & Mellins, C. (2010). Psychosocial challenges and protective influences for socio-emotional coping of HIV+ adolescents in South Africa: A qualitative investigation. *AIDS Care, 22*, 970–978.

Pettifor, A. E., Rees, H. V., Kleinschmidt, I., Steffenson, A. E., MacPhail, C., Hlongwa-Madikizela, L., Vermaak, K., & Padian, N. S. (2005). Young people's sexual health in South Africa: HIV prevalence and sexual behaviours from a nationally representative household survey. *AIDS, 19*(14), 1525–1534.

Pettifor, A., MacPhail, C., Anderson, A. D., & Maman, S. (2012). 'If I buy the Kellogg's then he should [buy] the milk': Young women's perspectives on relationship dynamics, gender power and HIV risk in Johannesburg, South Africa. *Culture, Health & Sexuality, 14*(5), 477–490.

Remien, R. H., & Mellins, C. A. (2007). Long-term psychosocial challenges for people living with HIV: Let's not forget the individual in our global response to the pandemic. *AIDS, 21*(Suppl. 5), 55–63.

Reproductive Health Research Unit (University of the Witswatersrand) and Lovelife (2005). *The national survey of HIV and sexual behaviour among young South Africans*.

Richter, L. M. (2003). Poverty, underdevelopment and infant mental health. *Journal of Pediatric Child Health, 39*, 243–248.

Rudy, B. J., Murphy, D. A., Harris, D. R., Muenz, L., & Ellen, J. (2009). Patient-related risks for nonadherence to antiretroviral therapy among HIV-infected youth in the United States: A study of prevalence and interactions. *AIDS Patient Care & STDS, 23*(3), 185–194.

SANAC. (2011). *Getting to success: Improving HIV prevention methods in South Africa*. Johannesburg: South African National AIDS Council; HIV epidemic, response and policy synthesis.

Schneider, M., Norman, R., Parry, C., Bradshaw, D., Pluddemann, A., & SACRACG. (2007). Estimating the burder of disease attributable to alcohol use in South Africa in 2000. *South African Medical Journal, 97*(8), 1–9.

Seedat, M., van Niekerk, A., Jewkes, R., Suffla, S., & Ratele, K. (2009). Violence and injuries in South Africa: Prioritizing and agenda for prevention. *Lancet, 374*, 1011–1022.

Shisana, O., Rehle, T., Simbayi, L. C., Zuma, K., Jooste, S., Pillay-van-Wyk, V., Mbelle, N., Van Zyl, J., Parker, W., Zungu, N. P., Pezi, S., & The SABSSM III Implementation Team. (2009). *South African national HIV prevalence, incidence, behaviour and communication survey 2008: A turning tide among teenagers?* Cape Town: HSRC Press.

Shisana, O., Rehle, T., Simbayi, L. C., Zuma, K., Jooste, S., Zungu, N., Labadarios, D., Onoya, D., et al. (2014). *South African national HIV prevalence, incidence and behaviour survey, 2012*. Cape Town: HSRC Press.

Statistics South Africa. (2010). Report on *Mortality and causes of death in South Africa in 2008: Findings from death notification.* http://www.statssa.gov.za/publications/P03093/P030932008.pdf

Statistics South Africa. (2014). Mid-year population estimates. http://beta2.statssa.gov.za/publications/P0302/P03022014.pdf

Strode, A. E., & Slack, C. M. (2011). Using the concept of 'parental responsibilities and rights' to identify adults able to provide proxy consent to child research in South Africa. *South African Journal of Bioethics and Law (SAJBL), 4*(2), 69–73.

Thom, R. (2009). Common mental disorders in people living with HIV/AIDS. *The South African Journal of HIV Medicine, 14*(4), 8–13.

Thom, R. (2012). *HAART and mind: Common mental disorders in people living with HIV/AIDS*. Wandsbeck: The Access Series, Reach Publishers.

Thurman, T. R., Brown, L., Richter, L., Maharaj, P., & Magnani, R. (2006). Sexual risk behaviour among South African adolescents: Is orphan status a factor? *AIDS and Behaviour, 10*(6), 627–635.

Tylee, A., Haller, D. M., Graham, T., Churchill, R., & Sanci, L. A. (2007). Youth-friendly primary-care services: How are we doing and what more needs to be done? *The Lancet, 369*(9572), 1565–1573.

UNAIDS. (2004). *Children on the Brink 2004: A joint report of new orphan estimates and a framework for action*. New York: UN.

UNAIDS. (2010). *Report on the global AIDS epidemic*. Geneva: UN.

UNAIDS, UNICEF, & WHO. (2008). *Children and AIDS: Second stocktaking report*. Geneva: UNAIDS.

UNFPA. (2014). *The state of world population. The power of 1.8 billion: Adolescents, youth and transformation of the future*. New York: UNFPA.

UNICEF. (2011). *State of the world's children: Adolescence an age of opportunity*. Geneva: UNICEF.

Vreeman, R. C., Gramelspacher, A. M., Gisore, P. O., Scanlon, M. L., & Nyandiko, W. M. (2013). Disclosure of HIV status to children in resource limited settings: A systematic review. *Journal of the International AIDS Society, 16*, 1–14.

WHO. (2011). *Guideline on HIV disclosure counselling for children up to 12 years of age*. Geneva: World Health Organisation.

Willan, S. (2013). *A review of teenage pregnancy in South Africa*. Durban: Partners in Sexual Health.

Williams, S. L., Williams, D. R., Stein, D. J., Seedat, S., Jackson, P. B., & Moomal, H. (2007). Multiple traumatic events and psychological distress: The South African stress and health study. *Journal of Traumatic Stress, 20*(5), 845–855.

Wood, K., Chase, E., & Aggleton, P. (2006). 'Telling the truth is the best thing': Teenage orphans' experiences of parental AIDS-related illness and bereavement in Zimbabwe. *Social Science & Medicine, 62*, 1923–1933.

Zuch, M., Mason-Jones, A. J., Mathews, C., & Henley, L. (2012). Changes to the law on consent in South Africa: Implications for school-based adolescent sexual and reproductive health research. *BMC International Health and Human Rights, 12*(3), 1–5.

Chapter 5
Living Optimally with HIV: Youth Experience in a Metropolitan Canadian City

Michelle Di Risio, Peri J. Ballantyne, and Stanley Read

Contents

5.1 Introduction

In a global context, HIV/AIDS has had a serious impact on youth, ravaging families and leaving millions of children to face adolescence as AIDS orphans (UNAIDS 2008). Further, it is currently estimated that, globally, 5.4 million young people

M. Di Risio (✉)
Leslie Dan Faculty of Pharmacy, University of Toronto,
144 College Street, Toronto, ON M5S 3M2, Canada
e-mail: michelle.dirisio@utoronto.ca

P.J. Ballantyne
Leslie Dan Faculty of Pharmacy, University of Toronto,
144 College Street, Toronto, ON M5S 3M2, Canada

Department of Sociology, Trent University,
1600 West Bank Drive, Peterborough, ON K9J 7B8, Canada
e-mail: periballantyne@trentu.ca

S. Read
Division of Infectious Diseases, The Hospital for Sick Children,
555 University Avenue, Toronto, ON M5G 1X8, Canada
e-mail: Stanley.Read@sickkids.ca

P. Liamputtong (ed.), *Children and Young People Living with HIV/AIDS*,
Cross-Cultural Research in Health, Illness and Well-Being,
DOI 10.1007/978-3-319-29936-5_5

aged 10–24 are living with HIV and an estimated 780,000 youth aged 15–24 are newly infected with HIV, with 97 % of the new infections occurring in low- and middle-income countries (UNAIDS 2013). In developed world settings, youth prevalence rates vary widely, and youth are a concerning component of the HIV-positive population. For example, in the United States, individuals aged 13–24 were estimated to represent 17 % of the population, but accounted for 26 % of newly diagnosed HIV/AIDS cases in 2010 (Centres for Disease Control and Prevention 2014). In the United Kingdom, individuals aged 15–24 were estimated to represent 12 % of all persons with HIV up to the end of 2012 (HPA Communicable Disease Surveillance Centre and the Scottish Centre for Infection and Environmental Health 2013). In Canada, youth represent a small proportion of the total number of reported HIV/AIDS cases. As of December 31, 2008 the Public Health Agency of Canada reported that of 67,442 positive HIV tests, 957 (1.4 %) were among youth aged 15–19 years, while 15,624 (23.1 %) were among individuals aged 20–29 years. Of 21,300 AIDS cases, 74 (0.3 %) were among youth aged 15–19 years and 3287 (15.4 %) were among individuals aged 20–24 years (Public Health Agency of Canada 2010).

These prevalence rates, along with risk behavior information about HIV transmission among youth, gives cause for concern. Canadian studies suggest that youths' susceptibility to HIV is related to many factors, including risky sexual behavior, substance abuse, poverty, perceptions that HIV is not a threat and lack of awareness of modes of HIV transmission (Council of Ministers of Education, Canada 2003; Canadian Association for Adolescent Health 2006; Public Health Agency of Canada 2010). Furthermore, it has been suggested that youth who become HIV-infected face unique illness-related stressors including social stigma, secrecy, isolation, complex disclosure issues, and multiple losses, particularly among perinatally-infected youth. Many families affected by HIV/AIDS confront accompanying social issues, such as an impoverished home environment, homelessness, substance abuse, and inadequate access to medical, social, and educational resources (Orban et al. 2010; see also Chap. 3 in this volume). The health community's concern about these risks is evident given that most HIV/AIDS research including youth in developed countries is focused on such higher-risk populations (Belzer et al. 1999; Murphy et al. 2001, 2003; Flicker et al. 2005; Veinot et al. 2006; Public Health Agency of Canada 2007; Mellins et al. 2009; Nichols et al. 2014).

Little research has examined the consequences of HIV-positive status for youth in stable social contexts. Such a focus, taken here in the current chapter, illuminates the general challenges of concurrently negotiating the developmental tasks of adolescence and serious chronic disease – outside the particular and complex problems of HIV-positive 'at risk' youth. It also highlights the positive outcomes possible – of living well with serious disease (see also Chap. 6 in this volume).

5.2 Theoretical Framework

Being HIV-positive occurs in the context of, and is influenced by a series of related phenomenon: the timing of diagnosis, when (or whether) treatment is initiated; and when the HIV-positive status is disclosed or becomes known to the infected person. In turn, the ordering, timing and context of diagnosis, treatment, and disclosure has implications for understanding the impact of the disease on an HIV-positive person's self and identity (see also Chaps. 7 and 17 in this volume).

A substantial body of conceptual and empirical research has considered the implications of chronic illness on a person's sense of self and identity. In this literature, *identity* is a term that reflects a person's sense of relationship to others; assuming a configuration of previous relationships and roles, identities influence and shape the evolving *self* (Charmaz 1987). The literature centers on the problematization of the self-in-chronic disease where a diagnosis results in modifications to self-concept. This involves the management of chronic illness 'interruptions', the deferral of preferred identities and 'real' self to the contingencies of the illness; learning about chronicity and acceptance of intrusive illness – demanding continued attention, allotted time, and forced accommodation (Charmaz 1997) – that is, acknowledgement of the permanent, sometimes degenerative, and uncertain nature of the course of one's illness. Intrusive illness has spiralling effects with consequences for valued pursuits and self-images and interpersonal relationships (Charmaz 1997). In this sense, chronic illness has been described as producing "biographical disruption" (Bury 1982: 167); its management requiring biographical work involving "recapturing the past, examining the present, and projecting into the future" (Corbin and Strauss 1988: 70). In the context of chronic illness, new life course trajectories are framed by the (non)/containment of illness and the management of its disclosure to others. Thus, the dialectical self is produced – contrasted between the compromised physical self and the monitoring self – one's own emerging relationship with their object body and with the management of uncertainty (Charmaz 1997).

An early body of research examined the effects of an HIV-positive diagnosis on identity management and re-negotiation. For example, Chidwick and Borrill (1996) focused on the identity effects and self-management strategies of living with HIV as a terminal disease. Earlier detection of HIV and effective early intervention created new identity challenges related to the emerging experience of HIV-positive status as a chronic condition rather than a fatal one (Gallo 1996; Battles and Werner 2002; Siegel and Lekas 2002; Giacomet et al. 2003). Brashers et al. (1998) described the revival experiences of persons who were once reconciled to their death from HIV/AIDS, but who, as a result of dramatic treatment responses, came to anticipate living with HIV. Identity challenges included ambiguity about the durability of treatment response and ultimate survival, and in the face of uncertainly, renegotiation of hope and future orientation, social roles and identities, interpersonal relations and quality of life. In this new context, those living with the virus were confronted with the task of incorporating their HIV-positive status into their identities and self-concepts (Baumgartner 2007).

In this chapter, we focus on the implications of living as HIV-positive from childhood and into adolescence, in a setting where there is reasonable access to treatment, and thus, of *living with* the virus. We highlight the novelty of the sample – HIV-positive adolescent living in highly supportive personal and social environments – and of the opportunity to learn about these youths' negotiations of themselves through the contingencies of HIV and adolescence. It is notable that most of the youth in the sample became HIV-infected early in life when early antiretroviral medicines were emerging, or after there were established therapies for HIV infection; disclosure *followed rather than preceded* treatment; and, surveillance and treatment of HIV-positive status was ongoing and normalized *before* disclosure of HIV-positive status imposed a need to contemplate its meaning for one's life. While the sample is not representative of the 'at risk' HIV-positive youth described previously, we provide a positive narrative regarding the potential outcomes of living with HIV that all nations grappling with HIV and AIDS might aim to achieve.

5.3 The Study

A convenience sample of youth who met eligibility criteria for the study was identified from patient-files at a pediatric HIV/AIDS clinic who provide treatment to HIV-infected youth until they are 19 years old. The clinic is set in a metropolitan urban setting where the cost of antiretroviral therapy is not insured in the public health plan, but where pediatric HIV/AIDS patients in the clinic have their medications covered through private health insurance, enrolment in a pharmaceutical trial, or provincial government insurance (available to some low-income families). All participants were actively receiving routine HIV-related health care services when recruited to the study, and had access to other medically necessary health care through the Ontario Health Insurance Plan (OHIP).

HIV-positive youth were eligible for participation in the study if they met the following criteria: (1) aged 13–19 years old; (2) ability to read, write and converse in English; (3) currently prescribed highly active antiretroviral therapy (HAART); (4) caregivers or legal guardians do not take full responsibility for the youth's drug management; (5) had been prescribed anti-retroviral medicines for ≥1 year. The fourth criterion was implemented so as to eliminate HIV-positive adolescents who were highly adherent to their drug regimen because their parents and/or legal guardians managed their daily regimes. The fifth criterion was applied to increase likelihood that medication regimes had been stabilized.

The study was given ethics approval by the Hospital for Sick Children (HSC), and the University of Toronto, both in Toronto, Canada. Following HSC protocol, capacity rather than age is the basis of a minor's eligibility to consent to participate in research. Capacity is based on an ability to understand the elements of the information relating to the decision to participate and the consequences of participation.

In this study, a single clinic staff member explained its general objectives to adolescents who had been previously assessed as having capacity by their HIV/AIDS physician. Interested adolescents were introduced to the interviewer (MD) – a graduate student without ties to the clinic – who described the study in detail and obtained final informed consent from those who volunteered to participate. Sixteen youth were identified as meeting all of the eligibility criteria; after being briefed about its purpose, seven declined to participate, and a final sample of nine youth was achieved.

We conducted a time series of in-depth interviews – with interviews undertaken over a period of approximately 4 months for each participant. Initial interviews were organized loosely around a semi-structured interview guide, and sought to apprehend each youth's health history, their current living arrangements including the daily management of antiretroviral therapy, general health status; HIV disease knowledge; their current social roles and experiences, and youths' perceptions and expectations of the future. Follow up interviews picked up from earlier ones, documenting the youths' ongoing relationship with themselves, with family members, and with peers and others, around the general theme of living as an HIV-positive person.

All interviews were audio-recorded and transcribed verbatim immediately following each interview. Preliminary data analysis, i.e. an evolving outline of response-types occurred concurrently with the collection of interview data. The interviewer (MD) performed a 'constant comparison' (Glazer and Strauss 1967) of new/emerging interview content with previous interview accounts – seeking to broadly and specifically depict adolescents' experiences with HIV in this study's particular location.

5.4 The Participants and Social Context

The mean age of the nine HIV-positive adolescents was 15 years. Five males and four females were included in the study. They were predominantly members of ethnic and racial minority groups (five African-Canadians, one Latino and three Caucasian). Four of the nine participants had immigrated to Canada; three from developing countries.

The early stage of initial interviews focused on health history; eight adolescents spontaneously revealed that they had been infected with HIV via maternal transmission; one youth had been infected by a needle while being treated for a minor injury in a hospital (in their country of origin). Of the adolescents who contracted HIV via maternal transmission, seven of eight had their status disclosed to them when they were between the ages of 10–12 years; one reported being aware of their HIV-positive status since their earliest memory. The youth who had been infected by a needle became aware of their HIV-positive upon diagnosis, at approximately age 9.

Approximately half of the participants had been on HIV medication 'since birth'. All were on antiretroviral regimes at the time of the study, with the number of medication doses (i.e. one tablet/capsule or injection = 1 dose) per day ranging from 2 to 10. Most of the participants did not regularly take other prescription medication for HIV (other than antiretrovirals) or for any other medical condition. The broader study from which the current analysis is derived included a systematic analysis of anti-retroviral adherence levels of the study participants. The measurement of adherence, and adherence rates has been reported elsewhere (Di Risio 2008); in general, however, except in two cases, these youth had very high adherence rates (≥94 %) – unlike those typically found in other HIV/AIDS medication adherence studies (Belzer et al. 1999; Murphy et al. 2001, 2003; Hosek et al. 2005; see also Chaps. 4 and 22 in this volume).

It was noted that this youth sample is not representative of the HIV-positive adolescent 'at risk' population described previously. None of the participants had drug and/or alcohol addictions, were homeless or contracted the virus via illicit drug use or sexual relations. Moreover, all participants were living at home with other family members; they were actively seeking health care services; and were enrolled in school.

5.5 The HIV-Positive Adolescent Identity and Performance of One's Self

In the current study, adolescent participants reported having no obvious medical symptoms of HIV. While the participants were aware that they could get sicker than others because of their HIV-positive status, they did not physically feel ill, and saw themselves as healthy persons. Thus, they did not perceive themselves as having a chronic illness (although they recognized the chronic nature of their HIV-positive status in 'objective terms'). For the most part, they described very positive self-concepts:

> ...like at school, I don't really feel different because I can do pretty much everything that everyone else does and having HIV doesn't affect me really...it doesn't affect my outside appearance or what I can do and what my brain can do...like it doesn't effect how I do in school or anything like that... [Jane, aged <15]
>
> I just deal with it. I am just...you know...'it's life...some people can't eat; I have HIV... [Bridgette, F 15+] ...I feel healthy so I don't really think about it. [Bridgette, aged 15+]

Being asymptomatic and experiencing minimal side effects from their daily pharmaceutical regimes influenced their positive self-assessments. And, participants described their ease at managing side effects, when they were experienced – providing a sense of control over the situation:

> I sort of get very drowsy...and have dizziness but...when you are sleeping, it doesn't really matter...it kind of rocks me to sleep (laughing). [Bridgette, aged 15+]
>
> ...the Kaletra kind of makes my stomach hurt...and I tried taking the Kaletra with some food ...like something that will make it go down smoothly like yogurt or apple sauce...that kind of helps a bit... [Mary, aged <15]

Although the participants claimed that HIV has had minimal impact on their lives, when pressed, they did describe a variety of ways they negotiated their HIV-positive status, showing that they recognized HIV as a highly stigmatized medical condition (Wiklander et al. 2013):

> You have to be more secretive. Like you have to know how to like keep things a secret better... it's not like you are going to meet someone and be like, "Hi, I have HIV, how are you?... It's like something you have to trust people to eventually tell them so that is pretty much it. So you just have to be careful what you say at times. [Jane, aged <15]
>
> I know that I have HIV and sometimes I have to be careful so I don't just end up saying that to someone else when I am outside because I have to be, I have to think. [Toby, aged <15]

Some comments indicated concern about social rejection (i.e. not be accepted by friends). Others showed a desire to pass as normal and not be given 'special 'treatment' if their HIV-positive status was revealed:

> It is kind of difficult because you are different from other kids, you are not different but it's just because you have HIV its like other kids, if you tell friends or anything they won't like accept you. [John, aged <15]
>
> I think they would understand...it's just that I feel that I am going to get this special treatment ...like they would make sure that I eat right and make sure that nothing would happen to me ..like because when my mother passed away I got special treatment from my friends...I want them to still be themselves. [Mary, aged <15]

Participants also described using certain 'coverage' strategies (Liamputtong et al. 2015) to manage and account for their daily use of medicines that they sometimes needed to take in the presence of friends (at home) or acquaintances at school:

> I just tell them I take vitamins or whatever and I will be right back in a second and then I come back. [Sonny, aged <15]
>
> If they ever come over to sleep at my house I tell them the reason I take medication is because I have a heart problem or I have asthma. I just make up some kind of condition. [Mary, aged <15]

The youth all confronted the issue of whether and when to disclose their HIV-positive status to others. Of the nine participants, four had not disclosed their HIV-positive status to anyone outside their families, explaining their decision-making:

> If I wanted to tell someone at school I have the option to but I just don't feel that I have to tell people because I don't think it's important. Like they don't really need to know, to know me. [Jane, aged <15]
>
> Right now, I'm not too open about this virus. People are so ignorant about it...and I just keep it to myself and to my family. I am not ready to open, like tell people I have it because I am afraid of what they are going to think. [Tessa, aged 15+]

On the other hand, after careful deliberations, five participants had disclosed their HIV-positive status to a selected friend or friends:

> I just felt I needed someone to talk to about it that is my own age. [John, aged <15]
>
> I just felt that he was ready because like he, he is a little older than me and I have known him for a really long time and I knew I could trust him with it. [Jane, aged <15]
>
> I started going to sleepovers and I would have to take my meds and I am not NOT going to tell them because they would ask me 'why do you take medicine'...like I told them, and that was all... [Fred, aged <15]

If they need to know then I would tell them but if there is no need to know, then there is no point in telling them. I think one time I told a grade 8 teacher because we were going on a trip overnight for four days and I said 'yeah, I take pills for HIV' and they were okay with it. [Fred, aged <15]

Thus, living well with HIV was accomplished through both the careful management over keeping their status confidential, and careful decision-making about the disclosure to a trusted other (see Chaps. 6, 17, and 20 in this volume). The youth in this study described their ease at managing these aspects of their HIV status, and persuasively asserted that having HIV did not impact their everyday lives and that they rarely thought about their condition:

It's not something that I will be whining over for the rest of my life…I won't say "oh I have HIV (said with a tragic voice) and feel really sad about it and I feel like I am going to die soon." I don't really think about it because I know that HIV isn't me, it is just what I am infected with. [Toby, aged <15]

These results coincide with those of Flicker et al. (2005) who found that among perinatally-infected adolescents, being HIV-positive was a relatively small part of their identity and adolescents were found to rarely reflect upon being HIV-positive (see also Chap. 6). In the current study, although medication-taking and hospital visits could remind adolescents of their condition of being HIV-positive, for the majority, these activities were 'normalized' even before they knew they had HIV:

I remember every time I take my medicine but to me I seem healthy and I am like other people. I don't feel any different. [Tessa, aged 15+]

Well, I actually just live my life normally…I see that now all I am doing is taking medicine the morning and night and just for my check up every two months… [Toby, aged <15]

This is not to suggest that their own disclosure experience, that moment when a family member or doctor revealed the HIV-positive status to the participants, was not traumatic. Some participants described their reactions of shock, anger, disappointment, loneliness, confusion, fear and nervousness when their disease status had been disclosed to them:

I didn't really know what to feel because it was a really big shock and I was really wondering what I am going to feel because I didn't actually feel like really sad or upset about anything. I was just shocked. [Toby, aged <15]

I was very angry, disappointed, mad. I felt like it was my parents' fault and I felt alone – why did it have to be me? [Mary, aged <15]

I felt confused…just so many questions were going through my head. I was scared… [Tessa, aged 15+]

However, others described being more circumspect at the time of 'the reveal', where their by-then-normal routines of medicine-taking and clinic visits suddenly made sense:

I was ten or eleven around the time where I really…like doctors and my mom really started to explain to me what HIV was and I think that was like the period in my life where really I started to understand like holy shit you know I have HIV and it was just like at that time it was more of a I guess a shock in a sense I really had it in the back of my head that I already knew there was something different. [Bridgette, aged 15+]

> I didn't really react much because I suspected something…I already knew I took medicine and stuff like that… [Jane, aged <15]
>
> I didn't think it was that big of a deal like I know I got it and everything so but nothing changed in my personal life or anything else. [Fred, aged <15]

Ultimately the study participants expressed acceptance and coming to terms with an HIV-positive identity:

> I try to live as if I don't have it… [Mary, aged <15]
>
> I guess I didn't have much of a choice but it is something I have to live with. [Tom, aged 15+]

Thus, at the time of interviews for this study, their HIV-positive status was well integrated into the participants' self-concepts and daily performances of their selves; and despite having to retain secrecy, and/or to manage disclosure, they described themselves as normal and healthy adolescents (see also Chap. 6 in this volume).

5.6 Social Structural Context Supporting Adolescents' Disease Management

The social structural context of these adolescents' lives supported their disease- and drug- management successes, and for most of the study group, positive health-self assessments. In this section, we discuss support related to accessing and using antiretroviral medicines; having role models for HIV, and living in a positive HIV-positive social environment, where educational programs and services about HIV/AIDS helped to normalize their own experiences; and where the youths' self-perceived 'expertise' around HIV/AIDS gave some adolescents a sense of purpose and responsibility to educate others.

First, considering the cost of drugs, and participants' access to pharmaceutical treatment, none of the participants paid out-of-pocket the full cost of the HIV medications (Most reported that their families were only required to pay the dispensing fee for their medications.) Participants either had the cost covered via private health insurance or a drug eligibility card, or they were enrolled in a clinical trial, where they were provided with the study medicine(s) (Di Risio 2008).

Among other studies examining HIV drug adherence among youth from developed nations, access to or the cost of medications was not consistently examined, and cost-barriers to treatment could not be assessed (Belzer et al. 1999; Murphy et al. 2001, 2003; Pugatch et al. 2002; Hosek et al. 2005; Rao et al. 2007). However, many of the HIV-positive adolescents in the study conducted by Veinot et al. (2006) in Ontario, Canada viewed prohibitive cost of treatment as contributing to their lack of HIV drug adherence. Among the participants in Veinot et al. (2006), 69 % had a history of street involvement; the authors suggested these individuals are less likely to be linked to health, financial and social services that support access to health care and medications for those in need. It seems an understatement to suggest then, on the basis of our own findings, and those of Veinot et al. (2006), that unimpeded access to antiretroviral medication and other necessary medicines is a pre-requisite for the kind of positive narratives about living as an HIV-positive person, such as we observed among the participants in our study.

A second level of support available to the participants in our study was the availability of role models – usually, parents who were also HIV-positive (in seven of nine cases in the current study), and who were, along with their adolescent child, responsible for the management of their HIV-positive status on a daily basis:

> My mom has the same medications so if one forgets the other one remembers type of thing…it is because my mom…I see my mom take it and that is how…like seeing her is a reminder that I have to take it… [Bridgette, aged 15+]
>
> Basically, my mom will be like 'did you take your medicine?' and I will be like 'oh well, I have to take it.' They just call sometimes and if they don't remember I will remember and if I don't remember, they remember. [Fred, aged <15]

Thus, living with an adult who provides daily support for HIV therapy, and/or who is also HIV-positive helped to normalize these adolescents' routine on-going medication use.

Support for these HIV-positive youth was also available from several sources within their communities. Some spoke specifically about their long-term and positive experiences as a pediatric patient at the Hospital for Sick Children:

> I just came in and it didn't really bother me because I liked coming here....it is really fun here. Yeah…(laughing) [Toby, aged <15]
>
> It was a pretty good experience to me. I think I took (disclosure) it very positively because I remember taking…like a bunch of medical tests and stuff like that and just like I just really enjoyed it and I still do. I mean, I had – you know like pregnant ladies they have the eco-gram thing. I had that on my heart, so I saw my heart pumping and stuff like that… and it was like 'that is so cool' (laughing). [Bridgette, aged 15+]

Most of the participants also either previously or currently attended an HIV support group (see Chaps. 6 and 20), and described how they were able to be open about their HIV status with others; and to be comforted knowing other HIV-positive adolescents:

> I go to Leading the Way group…because you get to meet with other people that are infected or affected with HIV/AIDS and just getting to talk to them. It really helps. [Jane, aged <15]
>
> It did help in a way (going to the Teresa Group)…like I wasn't the only person that had it and like, it's not awkward about it you know being so open. [Tessa, aged 15+]
>
> I am going to camp this year again so I don't feel that much alone because I know there are kids like me out there and like now I know you can still have a family, have kids so I don't feel that much angry and alone or disappointed as when I was a little kid. [Mary, aged <15]

Finally, the adolescents also benefited when, in the setting of their schools or in other social environments, they came to recognize themselves as having significant expertise about HIV/AIDS. One adolescent described having evolved into a person who is non-judging, a 'teacher of HIV/AIDS' who could provide information and insights about HIV/AIDS to others with less knowledge; and who saw themselves as having a responsibility to help the educators 'get it right':

> Most people…they don't know, like for example, friendly facts you know like breast milk is the one thing that has the most HIV count in it. [Bridgette, aged 15+]
>
> I had this very long discussion with two of my very good friends. And I was just telling them …for a woman…it is much harder for her to contaminate a man than for a man to contaminate a woman because… [Bridgette, aged 15+]
>
> I am not going to judge people and I guess that in a sense this was probably in my nature but I think that HIV really pushed it a bit further because I have seen people sick. I have seen people you know at their worse moments I mean like I have seen kids that it was not their best day… and you know…it didn't matter. I don't know…I think that kind of changed me… [Bridgette, aged 15+]

The youths' moral- and knowledge- capital and the claim of having responsibility to educate others or correct people's misconceptions about living with HIV/AIDS may have helped minimize the burdens of their HIV-positive status.

In this section, we discussed four distinctive types of structural support that enhanced these youths' capacity to live 'normally' with HIV: ready access to antiretroviral medicines; having role models for HIV and the ongoing medication management: having the availability of high quality and accessible hospital/health care and support group services; and living in a positive HIV-positive social environment where educational programs and services about HIV/AIDS helped to normalize their own experiences; and where the youths' self-perceived 'expertise' around HIV/AIDS gave some adolescents a sense of purpose and responsibility to educate others.

5.7 Expected Future Identity and Role Challenges

At the time of completing interviews for the study, for all but one of the youth, disclosure experiences – involving disclosing their HIV-positive status to others – had been confined to their relationships with friends and peers or adults who played a significant role in their lives. Among those who had chosen to reveal their status to selected friends, none had experienced rejection on the basis of their disclosure.

However, the youth also made specific reference to imminent and anticipated future challenges in the negotiation of intimate and sexual relationships:

> It (HIV) started affecting me really in the teenage years with just high school and stuff…it's pretty much the sex thing…just in case like the condom breaks or something like that. [Sonny, aged <15]
>
> I see all my friends are out with girls and what not and doing whatever and I can't really do that because I don't want to like do some random things with a girl and you know get her sick or whatever…I would rather be like in a relationship before I just go around with somebody, fool around with some random girl…and then something happens and she can probably sue me for manslaughter because she didn't know about my status. [Tom, aged 15+]
>
> I really have to trust a person in order to have any like any sexual relations with them because it's kind of far fetched but up to a certain extent you know like I can contaminate them and you like they could get very sick. [Bridgette, aged 15+]

The adolescents recognized the challenge of revealing their HIV-positive status to potential sexual partners:

> I have the obligation of telling him which…which it's like the complete other side of it… like you know, keeping it to myself is the easy part…you know, having to say it to other people is the hard part. [Bridgette, aged 15+]
>
> Because like…if I want to ever get married it's going to be like a really tough topic to bring up with my husband or my boyfriend or something like that. [Mary, aged <15]
>
> I could be trying to get married or something like that and I tell them and like they might think it is a big deal, they might not…but I will deal with that when it comes. [Fred, aged <15]
>
> I have to tell someone that I have HIV before we start dating and everything. [Case Toby, aged <15]

The one adolescent who had revealed her status to a new partner described this as a positive experience:

> I lost my virginity to which was the like biggest thing of my life… he immediately did not care he kind of looked at me he was like really? He was like no way and I was like I am telling you…He was concerned about me as everybody was but he, he really didn't care he was like holy shit like wow that is so weird you don't look like it you know. Yeah I was like I don't. He was like are you healthy? I was like yeah. He was like are you sick? I was like no. He was like ok that is good… [Bridgette, aged 15+]

While the youth perceived that managing their HIV status in the context of intimate relationships and sexuality was manageable, they viewed their major challenge as confronting others' fears about the disease, and the general social stigma of HIV. For this reason, several of the adolescents continued to hide their status.

When asked where they saw themselves in 5 or 10 years, all study participants anticipated futures involving the completion of education, the development of careers, and marriage and child-bearing:

> I want to be at 27 getting very, very seriously prepared to have children cause that is my goal. [Bridgette, aged 15+]
>
> I am going to get a job as a mechanic on cars and stuff. I might go back to a trade school to learn, like welding…or something like that. [Sonny, aged <15]
>
> Hopefully starting a family or working on my career. This is what I will be doing. [Sonny, aged <15]
>
> Living happily ever after like with my husband and kids and my dad. Living in a good home and my little sister she'll probably still be in college so like when I am 25 I will be working and stuff and I am still going for my dream (singing). [Mary, aged <15]

In summary, we found that their HIV-positive status was well integrated into these youths' self-concepts and daily performances of their selves. While comfortable with themselves, these youth described their efforts to control the disclosure of their HIV-positive status to others; none of those who had reported any negative consequences. For the most part, participants in this study had not experienced major disruptions at school or in family and social relationships, and this may have led them to minimize the impact of their HIV-positive status in their stories about how they lived their everyday lives. Four distinctive types of structural support enhanced these youths' capacity to live 'normally' with HIV: ready access to antiretroviral medicines; having role models for HIV; the availability of high quality and accessible hospital/health care and support group services; and living in a positive HIV-positive social environment. Finally, the youth anticipated future challenges related to the management of the stigma of HIV, and particularly around the negotiation of intimate and sexual relationships. None saw these challenges as insurmountable, and all anticipated futures involving completing of education, careers, marriage and children.

5.8 Discussion

In this chapter, we describe the experiences of a select sample of HIV-positive youth whose intact adolescent identities contrast sharply with the expected identity challenges of persons living with serious, chronic condition. Our focus on youth whose HIV-positive diagnosis and treatment initiation occurred at very early ages provided an opportunity to learn about youths' negotiation of HIV-positive adolescent identities and experiences in the context of established medical and social support.

Since the mid-1990s, HIV/AIDS has transitioned from a rapidly debilitating and fatal illness to a chronic condition, like diabetes or asthma, because of the development of potent antiretroviral combination therapies (Battles and Werner 2002; Gifford and Groessl 2002). To emphasize the novelty of this phenomenon, we apply the concept of the 'pharmaceutical person' (Martin 2006; Ballantyne et al. 2011) to the participants and to other people like them – who are living with HIV because of the availability of effective pharmaceutical treatment. In being an HIV-positive 'pharmaceutical person', the problems of living become those related to assuring the continual appropriate use of medicines, living with adverse effects of medication, and on-going negotiation of identity and self in social settings where HIV remains a highly stigmatized condition.

Charmaz (1987, 1997), Corbin and Strauss (1988), Bury (1982) and others have problematized the phenomenon of the self-in-chronic illness, where a diagnosis results in modifications to self-concept, and 'biographical disruption' (Bury 1982). This involves the management of chronic illness 'interruptions', the deferral of preferred identities and 'real' self to the contingencies of the illness, and acknowledgement of the permanent, degenerative, and uncertain nature of the course of one's illness. However, the participants in our study had been HIV-positive since birth or very early in their lives; most of the adolescents had generally not been unwell at any time in their lives. While most suspected 'they had something' due to their ongoing use of medicines [from earliest memory or from childhood] and regular medical assessments at the Hospital for Sick Children, that most of the participants had no 'medicines-free' referent in their memories of self and everyday self-practices may account for their casual descriptions of their lives as HIV-positive teens. These adolescents' experiences are in contrast to people experiencing other chronic illnesses in adolescence or adulthood where later onset means that post-diagnosis life is compared to a pre-illness state of 'normalcy' (Gallo 1996; Brashers et al. 1998; Battles and Werner 2002; Gifford and Groessl 2002; Siegel and Lekas 2002; Giacomet et al. 2003).

These adolescents' experiences are also unlikely to be typical for other HIV-positive youth. For example, HIV-positive adolescents in South Africa were found to have had difficulty incorporating a chronic stigmatizing illness into a healthy identity, so that a mental health promotion program was recommended to strengthen protective influences at the individual, interpersonal, community and policy levels (Petersen et al. 2010). In the current study, youths' positive HIV-positive self-concepts were suggested to be reflective of the HIV-supportive social and political context, where youth benefited from HIV-positive health care policy, and positive social and educational policy contexts where public discourse about HIV is normalized, and HIV education promoted. Even within Canada, Veinot and Harris (2011) found rural/urban variation in social and political resources for HIV/AIDS minimizes the likelihood of such support.

Any sense of threat to these youths' positive HIV-positive identities was anticipated as potentially emerging around the negotiation of intimacy and sexuality. Given that most of the participants were sexually inexperienced, the youth claimed that their HIV-positive status has had little impact on their lives, and minimized the burden of managing the stigma of their condition, and negotiating disclosure. While the participants' anticipated that this aspect of their future selves could be challenging, their discussions reflected that they anticipate more of a 'bumpy ride' than an insurmountable barrier to their expected futures of coupling, having families, and establishing careers. Evangeli et al. (2014) had similar study findings where perinatally-infected young adults in the United Kingdom expressed wanting to become parents even though they had been infected since birth and grew up HIV-positive.

The participants' positive current and future self-assessments reflect the notion of the self in post-traditional society – as a negotiated, reflective, evolving project, where the natural human body is modifiable through technological inventions like pharmaceutical drugs (Giddens 1991; Braidotti 2013). Further, the youth in our study can reasonably anticipate new 'ways of living' that may improve on treatments that currently involve a twice-daily medicine regime (although, for one youth, poor outcomes from his oral medication regimes has devolved to twice daily subcutaneous injections): as one youth stated in response to our question about the future, "*I see myself waiting for a cure…* [Tessa, aged 15+]

5.9 Conclusion

We wish to conclude with a caution, to emphasize the reality that there remains a great deal of uncertainty about the long-term outcomes of antiretroviral use, that no data yet exists to produce an estimated life expectancy for the long-term HIV-positive population; and that the current study involved a selected group of adolescents whose experiences do not represent a cross-section of HIV-positive youth.

Nonetheless, on the basis of interactions with eight of nine youth who have been HIV-positive and under treatment for most of their lives, we are able to describe positive chronic illness identities emerging from the successful management of 'healthy' chronically infected bodies; we depict these youths as 'pharmaceutical persons' – actively negotiating their health on an on-going basis through continuous use of medications; and continual medical monitoring of their selves, by themselves, their families, and their health care professionals.

We reiterate that while this sample is not representative of the 'at risk' HIV-positive youth described in previous studies, we provide a positive narrative regarding the potential opportunities of life with HIV that all nations grappling with growing youth prevalence rates might aim to achieve.

References

Ballantyne, P., Mirza, R. M., Austin, Z., Boon, H. S., & Fisher, J. A. (2011). Becoming old as a "pharmaceutical person': Negotiation of health and medicines by Canadian immigrant and non-immigrant older adults. *Canadian Journal on Aging, 30*(2), 169–184.

Battles, H. B., & Wiener, L. S. (2002). From adolescence through young adulthood: Psychosocial adjustment associated with long term survival of HIV. *Journal of Adolescent Health, 30*, 161–168.

Baumgartner, L. M. (2007). The incorporation of the HIV/AIDS identity into the self over time. *Qualitative Health Research, 17*(7), 919–931.

Belzer, M. E., Fuchs, D. N., Luftman, G. S., & Tucker, D. J. (1999). Antiretrovial adherence issues among HIV-positive adolescents and young adults. *Journal of Adolescent Health, 25*, 316–319.

Braidotti, R. (2013). *The posthuman*. Hoboken: Dordrecht Wiley.

Brashers, D. E., Neidig, J. L., Reynolds, N. R., & Haas, S. (1998). Uncertainty in illness across the HIV/AIDS trajectory. *Journal of the Association of Nurses in AIDS Care, 9*, 66–77.

Bury, M. (1982). Chronic illness as a biographical disruption. *Sociology of Health and Illness, 4*(2), 167–182.

Canadian Association for Adolescent Health. (2006). *Sexual behaviour and lack of knowledge threaten health of Canadian teens*. Available at: http://www.acsa-caah.ca/ang/pdf/misc/research.pdf. Accessed 25 Aug 2014.

Centres for Disease Control and Prevention. (2014, March 2014). *CDC HIV/AIDS fact sheet. HIV/AIDS among youth*. Available at: http://www.cdc.gov/hiv/pdf/risk_youth_fact_sheet_final.pdf. Accessed 10 Aug 2014.

Charmaz, K. (1987). Struggling for a self: Identity levels of the chronically ill. *Research in the Sociology of Health Care, 6*, 283–321.

Charmaz, K. (1997). *Good days bad days: The self in chronic illness and time*. New Brunswick: Rutgers University Press.

Chidwick, A., & Borrill, J. (1996). Dealing with a life-threatening diagnosis: The experience of people with human immunodeficiency virus. *AIDS Care, 8*, 271–284.

Corbin, J., & Strauss, A. (1988). *Unending work and care: Managing chronic illness at home*. San Franciso: Jossey Bass.

Council of Ministers of Education, Canada. (2003). *Canadian youth, sexual health and HIV/AIDS study*. Factors influencing knowledge, attitudes and behaviours. Council of Ministers of Education. Available at: http://www.cmec.ca/Publications/Lists/Publications/Attachments/180/CYSHHAS_2002_EN.pdf. Accessed 25 Aug 2014.

Di Risio, M. (2008). *Understanding the barriers and facilitators to HIV drug adherence among adolescents*. Unpublished Master's thesis, Leslie Dan Faculty of Pharmacy, Toronto, The University of Toronto, Toronto.

Evangeli, M., Greenhalgh, C., Frize, G., Foster, C., & Fidler, S. (2014). Parenting considerations in young adults with perinatally acquired HIV. *AIDS Care, 26*(7), 813–816.

Flicker, S., Skinner, H., Read, S., Veinot, T., McClelland, A., Saulnier, P., & Goldberg, E. (2005). Falling through the cracks of the big cities. Who is meeting the needs of HIV-positive youth? *Canadian Journal of Public Health, 96*(4), 308–312.

Gallo, R. C. (1996). AIDS as a clinically curable disease: The growing optimism. *AIDS Patient Care and STDs, 10*, 7–9.

Giacomet, V., Albano, F., Starace, F., deFranciscis, A., Giaquinto, C., Castilli Gattinara, G., Bruzzese, E., Gabiano, C., Galli, L., Vigano, A., Caselli, D., & Guarino, A. (2003). Adherence to anti-retroviral therapy and its determinants in children with human immunodeficiency virus infection: A multi-centre, national study. *Acta Paediatra, 92*, 1398–1402.

Giddens, A. (1991). *Modernity and self-identity: Self and society in late modern age*. Cambridge: Polity Press.

Gifford, A. L., & Groessl, E. J. (2002). Chronic disease self-management and adherence to HIV medications. *Journal of Acquired Immune Deficiency, 31*, S163–S166.

Glaser, B., & Strauss, A. (1967). *The discovery of grounded theory. Strategies for qualitative research*. Chicago: Aldine.

Hosek, S. G., Harper, G. W., & Domanico, R. (2005). Predictors of medication adherence among HIV-infected youth. *Psychology, Health & Medicine, 10*(2), 166–179.

HPA Communicable Disease Surveillance Centre (HIV and STI Department) & the Scottish Centre for Infection and Environmental Health. (2013). Unpublished National HIV data surveillance tables; December 16, 2013. Available at: http://www.hpa.org.uk/Topics/InfectiousDiseases/InfectionsAZ/HIV/HIVData/#1._National_HIV_Surveillance_Data_Tables. Accessed 1 Aug 2014.

Liamputtong, P., Haritavorn, N., & Kiatying-Angsulee, N. (2015). Local discourse on antiretrovirals and the lived experience of women living with HIV/AIDS in Thailand. *Qualitative Health Research, 25*(2), 253–263.

Martin, E. (2006). The pharmaceutical person. *Biosocieites, 1*, 273–287.

Mellins, C. A., Elkington, K. S., Bauermeister, J. A., Brackis-Cott, E., Dolezal, C., McKay, M., Wiznia, A., Bamji, M., & Abrams, E. J. (2009). Sexual and drug use in perinatally HIV-infected youth: Mental health and family influences. *Journal of American Academic Child Adolescent Psychiatry, 48*(8), 810–819.

Murphy, D. A., Wilson, C. M., Durako, S. J., Muenz, L. R., & Belzer, M. (2001). Antiretroviral medication adherence among the REACH HIV-infected adolescent cohort in the USA. *AIDS Care, 13*(1), 27–40.

Murphy, D. A., Sarr, M., Durako, S. J., Moscicki, A. B., Wilson, C. M., & Muenz, L. R. (2003). Barriers to HAART adherence among human immunodefiency virus – Infected adolescents. *Archives of Pediatric Adolescent Medicine, 157*, 249–255.

Nichols, S. L., Lowe, A., Zhang, X., Garvie, P. A., Thorton, S., Goldberger, B. A., Hou, W., Goodenow, M. M., & Sleaseman, J. W. (2014). Concordance between self-reported substance use and toxicology among HIV-infected and uninfected at risk youth. *Drug and Alcohol Dependence, 134*, 376–382.

Orban, L. A., Stein, R., Koenig, L. J., Conner, L. C., Rexhouse, E. L., Lewis, J. V., & LaGrange, R. (2010). Coping strategies of adolescents living with HIV: Disease specific stressors and responses. *AIDS Care, 22*(4), 420–430.

Petersen, I., Bhana, A., Myeza, N., Alicea, S., John, S., Holst, H., McKay, M., & Mellins, C. (2010). Psychosocial challenges and protective influences for socio-emotional coping of HIV-positive adolescents in South Africa: A qualitative investigation. *AIDS Care, 22*(8), 970–978.

Public Health Agency of Canada. (2007). HIV/AIDS Epi Update. November 2007. Available at: http://www.phac-aspc.gc.ca/aids-sida/publication/epi/2010/4-eng.php. Accessed 1 Aug 2014.

Public Health Agency of Canada. (2010). HIV/AIDS Epi Update. July, 2010. Available at: http://www.phac-aspc.gc.ca/aids-sida/publication/epi/2010/4-eng.php. Accessed 1 Aug 2014.

Pugatch, D., Bennett, L., & Patterson, D. (2002). HIV medication adherence in adolescents: A qualitative Study. *Journal of HIV/AIDS Prevention & Education for Adolescents & Children, 5*, 9–29.

Rao, D., Kekwaletswe, T. C., Hosek, S., Martinez, J., & Rodriguez, F. (2007). Stigma and social barriers to medication adherence with urban youth living with HIV. *AIDS Care, 19*(1), 28–33.

Siegel, K., & Lekas, H. M. (2002). AIDS as chronic illness: Psychosocial implications. *AIDS, 16*(Suppl 4), S69–S76.

UNAIDS. (2008). 08 Report on the global AIDS epidemic. Joint United Nations Programme on HIV/AIDS (UNAIDS). UNAIDS/08.25E/JC1510E. Available at: http://www.unaids.org/en/media/unaids/contentassets/dataimport/pub/globalreport/2008/jc1510_2008globalreport_en.pdf. Accessed 25 Aug 2014.

UNAIDS. (2013). Global report. UNADIS report on the global AIDS epidemic 2013. Available at: http://www.unaids.org/en/media/unaids/contentassets/documents/epidemiology/2013/gr2013/unaids_global_report_2013_en.pdf. Accessed 15 Aug 2014.

Veinot, T. C., & Harris, R. (2011). Talking about, knowing about HIV/AIDS in Canada: A rural-urban comparison. *The Journal of Rural Health, 27*, 310–318.

Veinot, T. C., Flicker, S. E., Skinner, H. A., McClelland, A., Saulneir, P., Read, S. E., & Goldberg, E. (2006). "Supposed to make you better but it doesn't really": HIV-positive youths' perception of HIV treatment. *Journal of Adolescent Health, 238*, 261–267.

Wiklander, M., Rydstrom, L. L., Ygge, B. M., Naver, L., Wettergren, L., & Erksson, L. E. (2013). Psychometric properties of a short version of the HIV stigma scale, adapted for children with HIV infection. *Health and Quality of Life Outcomes, 11*(195), 1–7.

Public Health Agency of Canada. (2010). HIV/AIDS Epi Update, July 2010. Available at: http://www.phac-aspc.gc.ca/aids-sida/publication/epi/2010/ [illegible]

[illegible]

Chapter 6
"There's More to You Than Just This Virus": Young People Growing Up with Perinatally-Acquired HIV in Australia

Asha Persson, Christy E. Newman, and Angela Miller

Contents

6.1 Introduction

> I've always known that this is what I have and, yeah, taught to be proud of it and not hide it away, and who cares what other people think? (Dylan, 19 years old)
>
> I don't really see any difference between having HIV and not having it. It seems like you're the same as everyone else. (Tara, 13 years old)

These remarks from two young people are startling in the way they upend the kind of HIV narratives we are accustomed to. HIV has become so culturally entwined with bleak notions of shame, disgrace and otherness or, to use Goffman's (1974) legendary expression, 'spoiled identities', that it is almost impossible to think about HIV without also thinking about stigma (see also Chaps. 1, 3, 4, 9 and 14 in this

---

A. Persson (✉) • C.E. Newman
Centre for Social Research in Health, UNSW,
Goodsell Building, Level 3, Sydney, NSW 2052, Australia
e-mail: a.persson@unsw.edu.au; c.newman@unsw.edu.au

A. Miller
Previously the Paediatric HIV Service, Sydney Childrens Hospital,
High Street, Randwick, NSW 2031, Australia
e-mail: ange_76@yahoo.com

P. Liamputtong (ed.), *Children and Young People Living with HIV/AIDS*,
Cross-Cultural Research in Health, Illness and Well-Being,
DOI 10.1007/978-3-319-29936-5_6

volume). There is no shortage of literature that testifies to the realities of stigmatization. Even as medical science has transformed HIV into a manageable chronic condition that makes it possible to live life like any other person, research show that early discourses of the virus as dangerous, dirty, contagious and deviant are so embedded in the cultural imaginary that an HIV diagnosis still retains the power to generate self-stigmatization (Flowers et al. 2006; Flowers 2010; Persson 2013). But what if you were born with HIV? What if you had known since you were young that you were HIV-positive? What of stigma then? What would it mean in that context? And how would it shape your life and your sense of self, particularly in a low-prevalence country like Australia where HIV is an extremely rare disease among children? Is stigma, as the international literature suggests, an inescapable and essential presence in their lives, which radically sets them apart from other children and young people? This is what we explore in this chapter.

6.2 Background and Theoretical Context

Young people with perinatally-acquired HIV are an emerging sub-population in the global epidemic. In high resource countries, and increasingly elsewhere, advances in the treatment of pediatric HIV have changed the epidemic among children from one of almost certain mortality in their first decade to one of long-term survival with a chronic disease (Mofenson and Cotton 2013; Sohn and Hazra 2013). At the end of 2013, about 3.2 million children under 15 years and 2.1 million adolescents were estimated to be living with HIV (UNAIDS 2014). In Australia, where our research took place, this population is very small. Highly effective prevention strategies, in place since 1994, have reduced the rate of transmission from mother to child to 1 % (McDonald et al. 2009; Miller et al. 2013). Combined with low prevalence of HIV generally, a child being born with HIV in Australia today is an extremely rare event. The current population of young people growing up with HIV is approximately 80, about half of whom were born in Australia and half in sub-Saharan and other high prevalence countries. Due to effective treatment, these young people are generally healthy and "indistinguishable outwardly" from their HIV-negative peers (Miller et al. 2013). While their small numbers and survival are signs of tremendous success, it also means that these young people are growing up as a culturally invisible and often socially isolated group of individuals.

Young people with perinatally-acquired HIV in high resource countries can be said to share certain experiences with other children with early onset chronic conditions, such as ongoing treatment, medical visits, regular tests and episodes of illness. But there is general consensus in the literature that this population faces a multitude of medical, neurocognitive, psychiatric and psychosocial challenges that makes them "unique" among children with chronic conditions (Persson and Newman 2012; Persson et al. 2014). Although researchers differ on the pervasiveness of these challenges and their consequences for social, sexual and clinical health, they generally agree that the social stigma related to having HIV is a fundamental aspect of their disease that sets these young people apart from their peers and profoundly shapes their life experience and sense of self (Bush-Parker 2000; Fair et al. 2011; Mellins and Malee 2013).

The theme of stigma permeates the empirical research literature on young people growing up with HIV. Studies from the United States, England, Canada and Sweden found that HIV-related stigma was a destructive influence on their well-being and governed how they lived their lives. Because of perceived ignorance and prejudices towards HIV in society, most young people in these studies had not disclosed their HIV status to their friends or peer networks, because of fears that others would see them differently or even break off the friendship and ostracize them. They generally hid their HIV status from everyone except health workers to protect themselves from the risk of stigma and discrimination, from gossip and rumors, and were often told or encouraged to do so by caregivers (Fielden et al. 2006; Abramowitz et al. 2009; Vijayan et al. 2009; Dorrell and Katz 2013; Rydström et al. 2013; see also Chaps. 1, 3, 4, 9, 14 and 17 in this volume). Researchers point out that these young people come from families where, given the aetiology of perinatal HIV, one or both parents (and sometimes siblings) also have HIV. As a result, secrecy tends to be multi-generational, with families highly invested in protecting their privacy and concealing their status from extended family and the community. Secrecy thus becomes central to family dynamics, defining the official family narrative, the shaping of identities, social relationships and support (Bush-Parker 2000; DeMatteo et al. 2002; Michaud et al. 2009; Fair and Walker 2011). The imperative of secrecy in families affected by HIV has caused researchers to describe young people growing up with HIV as an isolated and hidden population (Fielden et al. 2006; Fair et al. 2012), which some suggest might contribute to the increased risk of behavioral and psychiatric problems reported by previous studies (Rydström et al. 2013).

Dorrell and Katz (2013: 8) argue that "without a change, young people will remain the recipients of both a legacy of secrecy and a legacy of shame, with open talk about HIV being controlled and presented as non-negotiable". Although well-intentioned, this statement includes two assumptions; that secrecy is essentially harmful and that stigma is internalized by children growing up with HIV. These assumptions are partly challenged by snippets of alternative narratives in the literature. Fielden and colleagues (2006), for example, noted that for some research participants, keeping HIV secret had a positive value by freeing them from being labelled as the "kid with HIV". This was echoed by parents and care providers who also participated in their study and who "stressed the need for children to feel 'normal' despite their HIV" (2006: 1051). This theme of normality is found in other studies. Young people in a Canadian study described living with perinatally-acquired HIV as "just a part of their regular routine that they rarely reflect upon" (Flicker et al. 2005: 309). Similarly, in a Swedish study, participants "did not feel that HIV was a big issue in their lives" (Rydström et al. 2013: 1361). Young people in Dorrell and Katz's own study in the UK described hospital visits and medical care as "second nature" and as a normalized part of their childhood experience and personal biography, which only became a point of difference "when comparing themselves with others" (2013: 5). (See also Chap. 5 in this volume).

None of these fleeting observations, which tend to remain unpacked, negate the realities of HIV-related stigma or the constraints of secrecy. But they do call into question whether we should take as given that young people growing up with HIV are affected by stigma in the same way that adults who acquire HIV might be, or whether we need to look closer at what stigma, normality or "being different" actually mean in their lives. Seminal theories of stigma tend to pivot on the idea that secrecy arises from internalized shame and operates to hide a "discredited identity" (Goffman 1974) and protect stigmatized individuals and their "failings" from "the threat of insult, injury, and devalorization" (Eribon 2004: 99). By concealing their identity in this way, so the argument goes, stigmatized people tend to experience their position and social interactions as "always false" (Eribon 2004: 103). "Coming out" or "disclosure", on the other hand, is privileged as therapeutic emancipation of the authentic self (see Chap. 17 in this volume). Critics have argued that little consideration is given to the potentially enabling and supportive benefits of concealment. Not everyone sees their stigmatized attribute as revealing of their real identity, or secrecy as a self-loathing betrayal of their true self. Secrecy, they suggest, can simply be a sensible tactic to avoid social disapproval of an aspect of their life that they consider as marginal in their "psychic economies" (Seidman et al. 1999: 18; Corrigan and Matthews 2003). In this chapter, we examine how these complex dynamics play out in the narratives of young people growing up with HIV.

6.3 The Study

Our chapter draws on an exploratory qualitative study that examined key issues for perinatally HIV-infected children transitioning to adolescence and adulthood. The study, the first of its kind in Australia, was conducted by the Centre for Social Research in Health at the University of New South Wales (UNSW) in collaboration with the Paediatric HIV Service at Sydney Children's Hospital, the main service for this population. Ethics approval was granted by Sydney Children's Hospital Network Ethics Committee and ratified by the UNSW Ethics Committee. The study was funded by an unconditional Gilead Fellowship and by the Australian Government Department of Health. In the first phase of the study, pediatric and adult clinicians with experience in caring for this population were interviewed to elicit their perspectives on needs and challenges as these children transition to young adulthood and adult care. Findings from these interviews have been reported elsewhere (Persson et al. 2014; Newman et al. 2014). In the second phase, 12 young people were recruited into interviews and it is these that we focus on in this chapter. Although this is a small number, it constitutes a significant proportion of the total population of around 80 young people with perinatally-acquired HIV in Australia. Our sample size can be compared with the ten young people who participated in a similar study in Sweden, a country with a perinatal population almost double that of Australia's (Rydström et al. 2013).

Participants were recruited through the Paediatric HIV Service, which has contact with most young people with perinatally-acquired HIV in Australia and many in New Zealand. Interviews were conducted face-to-face (n=8), by phone (n=2) and Skype (n=2). Given the profound need for confidentiality among families affected by HIV, study participants were given the option of being interviewed by any of the three investigators on the team to remove any barriers to participation. All but one participant elected to be interviewed by the senior social worker on the team (Angela Miller) who was trained in qualitative interview technique by the team's researchers (Asha Persson and Christy Newman), particularly how to use a semi-structured format and how to pose open-ended questions. As a long-term employee at the Paediatric HIV Service, Angela was known to participants, in many cases since they were very young. Familiarity created a safe environment for participants that proved critical to successful recruitment. We took care to de-brief regularly to support Angela in managing prior knowledge when conducting interviews and to minimize potential conflicts of interest. Asha and Christy had no prior contact with participants.

The interview schedule was developed based on the initial clinician interviews and our previous analysis of the literature (Persson and Newman 2012), as well as in consultation with the study's expert committee, which consisted of HIV clinicians and service providers with experience in working with young people with HIV. The interviews included general questions about origin, family and living conditions, and more specific questions about experiences of treatment and health care, growing up with HIV, stigma, disclosure and, where relevant, sexuality and prevention. Participants 18 years and older provided written consent, while parental consent was secured for children under 18 years, along with their own written assent.

Interviews were digitally-recorded with permission from participants and subsequently transcribed verbatim. Any potentially identifying information was removed from transcribed interviews to protect participant anonymity. Transcripts were hand-coded by Asha who has extensive experience in qualitative data analysis and checked by the other two team members. Using thematic analysis, the foundational method for qualitative analysis (Guest 2012), transcripts were read multiple times and coded according to key issues covered in the interviews, focusing on inductive identification of recurrent and divergent themes. These themes were then analysed in detail to build a contextual understanding of differences and similarities across interviews. During this process, we regularly discussed emerging themes and interpretive possibilities, subsequently workshopped with the expert committee and refined during the manuscript drafting process. We also engaged in a process of member validation by providing the draft manuscript to select study participants for feedback, thus securing their confirmation that the analysis was a valid and accurate representation of their accounts.

6.4 The Participants: Characteristics

Eight females and four males participated in the study. They ranged from 13 to 21 years old, with a median of 15 years. Four were of Anglo-Australian background, six were born in the sub-Saharan African region, one in South East Asia, and one in Southern Europe. The majority now lived in the Australian state of New South Wales. All but three participants had lost one or both of their birth parents and one girl had also lost her brother. Although six were very young when their parents passed away and had few memories of them, it was still a very emotional issue for some. Two participants were adopted and another two lived with extended family or family friends, while the rest lived with a biological parent and, in one case, also a step-parent. Seven lived with biological siblings. Six participants were the only person currently living with HIV in their family. Most had known about their HIV since an early age. Six said they had always known or had been told when very young. Five found out when they were between 8 and 12 years old. The oldest age of finding out was 14. Several described being initially shocked or scared when they found out about their condition, but had been reassured by their parents or doctor that they would be fine and had since learnt a lot about HIV. Five participants attended pediatric care and seven attended adult care services.

What most characterized their interviews was the way they shifted between narratives of stigma and everyday life, normality and difference, and at the same time weaved these themes together into lived experiences not easily accounted for by conventional theories of stigma. We now turn to an outline of these themes.

6.5 Stigma, Secrecy and Disclosure

Participants were acutely aware of the stigma surrounding HIV and thought that most people still perceived it as a "bad disease", as 13-year old Jordan put it. But they generally attributed this to ignorance and outdated knowledge in society rather than to prejudices. In their view, HIV is a misunderstood and invisible illness that does not receive the same attention and support that other illnesses do and, therefore, people take little notice of HIV because they cannot relate to it. Although some believed that young people today are better informed, several participants commented that HIV is a disease that people at school "make fun of", which they found upsetting and difficult, or else dismissed as a lack of education.

> Like at school, people joke about it. Like it reminds me. But it doesn't make me feel upset, but it's just like people don't really get, you know, they don't really get it. But they just haven't been taught so I don't really get offended by it … It's not talked about every day and, you know, it's not advertised every day, you know, like fundraisers, like cancer is always, you know, there's advertisements and there's fundraisers, and stuff like that. But yeah, not with the HIV (Daisy, 17 years old).

Few felt safe to speak up when friends or strangers made jokes or said negative or incorrect things about HIV. They dealt with those situations differently and as best they could, by keeping quiet, or playing along, or getting into fights.

> Growing up's been hard. Three schools. Got in fights and that'cause of the word [HIV]. And kicked out of school for fighting'cause people making fun of it. I didn't really like it. And I don't know, just attracts attention. When people say it, they don't really say it around me' cause ... I get angry about it. But they don't know why I get angry about it, but still, yeah, it's not like, it's not something to make fun of (Aaron, 18 years old).

For those old enough, HIV education at school was both a challenge and a revelation. It made them feel self-conscious, but also highlighted to them that they knew much more about HIV than most people do. Many found HIV education lacking and mentioned that teachers would sometimes impart outdated or, as 19-year old Dylan described it, "horribly wrong" information. Most felt unable to contest the teacher for fear of drawing attention to themselves or raising questions as to why they were so well-informed about HIV, while a few had set out to prove their teacher wrong, and others took it in their stride.

> At school, sometimes it gets talked about. So you listen and you're like, "Your information's kind of different to mine' cause you don't know as much as I know"... which is really interesting but yeah ... It's just like I've gotten used to it ... I'm fine with it during class if we're talking about it. I'll just sit there and join in the conversation and then add a few, a few of my things. Just like, "Yeah, I know this and this, and this" ... it's just like a normal day (Daisy, 17 years old).

Awareness of HIV-related stigma was also influenced by having been told by parents or by health care workers not to disclose their HIV status to others. Information was typically kept strictly within a small circle of family, health workers and, in some cases, trusted family friends. Five young people had also told one or two close friends and found it extremely supportive to have a confidante. But most were very reluctant to disclose to friends, fearing that they would be rejected or made fun of, or that the information would be posted on Facebook or other social media.

> I trust my friends and all, but I just don't wanna tell them yet ... I just get worried that, if I told them, like, you know, they'll disown me and stuff. Like if they just think differently about me ... Like, "have I caught it yet from you?" or ... "can I catch it from touching you or, you know, sharing stuff?"... I really don't think about telling someone yet (Bella, 15 years old).

Twenty-one year old Amber remarked that she was confused about the secrecy around HIV when she was younger, but now appreciates that her parents "wanted me to have as normal a childhood experience as possible, not people judging or not wanting me over to their house". She said that the reality of "why it had to be such a secret" was brought home to her when she decided to disclose to her school principal and was promptly told she would have to leave the school unless all teachers and students were informed about her status for "safety" reasons.

> I felt so violated, that my secret that I'd been keeping was about to be exploded all over my environment. I didn't want my teachers and, and kids that I didn't even know knowing about this secret that I'd been keeping for years. So I had to walk away,' cause there was no, there was no choice in my mind. I didn't want to be the circus freak at my school.

Only one participant, Dylan, had grown up being completely open and even public about his HIV, and while Dylan had encountered some ignorance, he said he had never experienced any discrimination or negative reactions. But, echoing Amber's comments, Dylan recognized that what prevents most of his peers from disclosing their HIV status is their desire to avoid having their whole persona differentiated and defined solely by the virus.

> I've always been out there in terms of: this is who I am and this is what I have. Thankfully, I have had no real bad run-ins with anyone … Like nine times out of 10 my friends, yeah, no-one gives a crap really … They know me for me and not me for the virus I have. And that's what I think people are afraid of. It's like they'll become known for the fact that they have this disease, not known for who they are. So they feel they need to hide it.

As he has gotten older, and is no longer protected by virtue of "being a kid", Dylan became more aware of how HIV-related stigma can affect people by association and therefore people he cares about. When his girlfriend became a target of rumors, he decided he needed to be "more restricted" about disclosing, because "I've seen the damaging side it can do for other people". Other older participants similarly explained that, since having taken over responsibility for making decisions around disclosure, they continued their parents' approach of being exceedingly careful and selective whom they told, primarily disclosing only on a "need-to-know basis", as 21-year old Matilda put it, often testing people's attitudes first and preparing for the worst case scenario. Although participants expressed frustration with the stigma and ignorance that forced them to keep HIV quiet, secrecy was largely presented as a normal part of their reality and an aspect of their situation they could maintain some control over.

6.6 Living with HIV: Being Normal and Different

As the young people spoke about their experiences of living with HIV and their personal aspirations, ideas about "normality" and "difference" continually folded into each other (see also Chap. 6). Some expressed concerns that HIV might constrain their job prospects, travel, relationships and ability to have children, and some spoke about an unknown future of potential ill health, which would get them down from time to time. At the same time, most of these young people articulated a strong sense of future and had many and ambitious plans for what they wanted to do in life. In most cases, HIV was not perceived to be an obstacle to fulfilling those aspirations, although for some HIV clearly shaped their sense of career direction and priorities:

> Well, if I end up being a doctor: find a cure, try and find a cure (Jordan, 13 years old).
>
> I mean [HIV] has impacted my ambitions because I want to help people and I think, I don't think I'd have that passion to be in the health sector if I wasn't [HIV] positive (Amber, 21 years old).

The literature's notion that this population is "set apart" from other young people (e.g. Bush-Parker 2000; Fair et al. 2011; Mellins and Malee 2013) was strongly articulated by three participants who described how HIV had a major impact on their lives and sense of self. Evoking Goffman's theory of "passing" and its alienating effects (1963/1974), 18-year old Aaron, who had been adopted as an orphan from overseas, spoke of living a double life:

> It's like living two lives: one is fake, another one is the real which, the real one is with HIV and the other one is with my friends, is all fake, can't talk about it ... You just think about it 24/seven. Like you'll just be looking at your friends, you're going, "Yep, you're lucky. You just don't know it. You've got your whole family there. You don't have to think about it. Go and get a girlfriend or whatever you wanted to. Go and join whatever you wanna do." And HIV's just like, there's barriers what you can do and what you can't do.

The stories of two other participants were in stark contrast, yet included the same theme of being different. Dylan and Amber grew up in Australia as part of the first generation of children surviving with perinatally-acquired HIV and were the only young people who had been completely or partially open about their HIV during their childhood or teenage years. For 19-year old Dylan, growing up with HIV had not "been a bad thing at all for me as a personal experience", but had brought with it unique opportunities to do things, meet people and make "lifetime friends because of it". Twenty-one year old Amber similarly described how HIV had given her a childhood that was both different and special and had defined her sense of self in a positive way:

> HIV's such a big part of my life that it's part of my personality, it's a part of my whole, entire life ... I can't say at all [what life would have been like without HIV]. It would have been completely different. I wouldn't see the world as I see it now. I wouldn't have met the people I've met. I wouldn't have had all the experiences I've had ... I don't want to think about what it would be like [to have grown up without HIV], because I think I would have had such a boring childhood.

But for the majority of participants, HIV was seen as a relatively minor issue in their lives with little bearing on how they saw themselves. Although they described moments of feeling upset or confused, for the most part HIV was not something they thought about, nor did it prevent them from doing or trying anything. Indeed, their interviews were replete with stories of typical teenage lives and interests, such as sport, computer games, music, drama and hanging out with friends. As 17-year old Daisy put it, "I'm like a normal teenager". This theme of "normal" flowed throughout their narratives in one way or another and was invoked time and again when asked to describe what living with HIV was like.

> Normal ... Well I [was] born this way ... [It] is just part of human, what you get, disease. You don't get to choose what you want to be (Grace, 14 year old).
>
> I don't really know how to describe it,' cause it's just like normal people ... and, yeah, I don't really see any difference between having HIV and not having it. It seems like you're the same as everyone else (Tara, 13 year old).

Being born with HIV was their reality, whether they had known it from an early or later age and, as such, HIV had become normalized, making it possible to see themselves as being the same as other people, "just with a virus in us", as Tara put it. In this way, even for those who did articulate a sense of difference, such as Dylan, being different was an intrinsic component of being normal:

> It's all I've ever known, so I don't know what it's like to live without it. So I can't answer what it's like to live with it, because I've known no different. It's been my life ... I had it since birth, since day one. It's all I've ever known ... so I don't know what it's like to really live with it because I haven't experienced what it's like without it.

In these accounts, difference and normality blend together as participants describe how HIV shapes their lives. But, importantly, none of them articulated a "spoiled identity", the hallmark of internalized stigma, as conceptualized by Goffman (1974). There was little in the interviews to suggest that their sense of self was marked by shame or reduced to their HIV status, even when HIV was seen as central and seminal to their lives. As Dylan summed up when asked what advice he would give to other young people growing up with HIV:

> Don't let it be who you are. It's not your dominating quality ... It's just something that comes along with you, good or bad ... Keep taking your medication and just live your life. Don't let it control you. Stay healthy. Keep on top of everything and you'll be able to live a rich, fulfilling, happy life.

6.7 Treatment and Its Twofold Effects

Dylan's quote hints at another compelling theme in the interviews; HIV treatment and its interplay with experiences of normality and difference. Like many of the participants, 16-year old Sabina nominated "taking tablets", rather than HIV itself, as the "only thing that really makes you different" from people who do not have HIV (see also Chap. 5).

> [Living with HIV] is not that different from normal life ... Just taking medicine, that's all (Jordan, 13 years old).
>
> [T]he last couple of years I haven't really thought about it. I haven't been like, "Oh, I have HIV," you know, it's not really like a day-to-day thing ... And like it's only when I have to take the tablets I'm like, "Oh, I have HIV." And then I'll forget about it like two minutes later. So it's not really like a, "Oh my God! Blah, blah, blah," you know (Daisy, 17 years old).

As these extracts suggest, having to take medication thematized their condition and foregrounded their sense of difference, "cause no-one else takes pills", as Aaron said: "when you take the pills, it reminds you [that] you have HIV". And at the same time, taking medication was, paradoxically, also the key that enabled and ensured normality. As Jordan said when asked what advice he would give other young people with HIV: "Just take your medicine and everything will be fine". Time and again, they stressed the importance of medication, a message they had thoroughly imbibed from parents and clinicians.

> Like the doctors are there to help and the nurses are there to give you the medication that you need and to keep healthy. If you do the right thing, you're gonna live a normal, healthy life, and you're not gonna feel like you have HIV. And, it's just a disease that's inside you, but you can live through like a normal human (Olivia, 15 years old).
>
> [The doctor] told me, if you do take them, you know, you'll still be able to live a healthy, normal life, you know. Just one tablet a day, and it'll be worth it' cause, you can have children, have a family, you know, grow up (Daisy, 17 years old).

This theme was common among the younger teenagers, who were all on treatment, except for Bella who had not yet started. Most were aware that much was at stake if they did not take their tablets, but it was also an abstract scenario which they preferred not to think about. For older participants who had been on a variety of treatment regimens since birth, this scenario was more real and also more complicated. Their long treatment histories and the serious side effects of early HIV drugs had been tough on their bodies and had made the virus resistant to some medications. This meant their treatment options were more limited and that recent, easier regimens were not necessarily available to them. "Normal" took on a different twist in their stories.

Twenty-one year old Matilda had stopped taking her medication some months before her interview because of unpleasant side effects, which she felt were an intolerable disruption to her ability to go about her everyday life (see Chap. 22 in this volume). Despite a critically low CD4 count and several stints in hospital due to opportunistic infections (which had also left her with quite a challenging disability), Matilda insisted that "in myself, I feel fine, I feel normal" and that she managed by "pushing through". She explained that her doctor was desperately trying to persuade her to resume treatment by "lecturing" her about the dire consequences of not doing so. Although she found this upsetting and was realistic about the likelihood of those consequences, including further infections and potential death, she argued that "I push it out of my mind most days" and that "something needs to click in my head before I start taking tablets again". The intricate balance between treatment and normality was starkly brought home to 19-year old Dylan who said he paid a heavy price when he stopped taking his medication while going through a turbulent period and when, to modify Maynard's phrase (2006), the pull of a *different* kind of normal became too tempting:

> Yeah, so what happened was I guess I kind of, teenage years, a bit rebellious, kind of got sick and tired of taking medication and stopped taking it ... And then it all fell to bits and I ended up turning resistant to that medication ... I was really, really sick ... I guess I was just kind of fed up with taking my medication for 15 years, same routine, wake up, breakfast, pills, school, wake up ... For a while it was good until it kind of all hit me in the face ... [I] t hit me that I have to put in the effort and really have to sort this out. And, if I wanna do the things I wanna do later on in life, because I can't do them if I'm not healthy ... I can't do anything—I'm stuck at home feeling crap—so I have to be healthy in order to achieve what I wanna achieve. So, and the first step to getting healthy is taking my medications consistently day in, day out for the rest [of] forever.

For these young people, treatment clearly had twofold meaning. It was seen as a point of difference to other young people, but also as the key to being the same as everyone else. It had the capacity to both constrain and enable normality. Despite this dual capacity, taking tablets was in itself part of normal life for many participants. Even if they did not always find it easy, daily medication along with regular blood tests and clinical visits was a routine they had been familiar with for years:

> I have never known a life without medication … You have to go and get your medication at the sexual health centre and it's just, it's normal now. A life without doctors' appointments would be, feel weird to me (Amber, 21 years old).

It was also a routine that, in many cases, helped them feel loved, cared for and supported by parents and health care professionals. Although some teenagers complained about parents "nagging" them about their medication, doctors asking "annoying" questions, and the drudgery and sometimes intimidating experience of attending medical appointments, they also recognized that the adults in their lives were looking after their best interests and many expressed fondness for their health care providers and thought they did "amazing jobs", as Olivia put it.

6.8 Camp: The Power of Peers

The need to keep HIV secret brought with it contrasting realities. Not being branded as the "kid with HIV" or, worse, the "circus freak", gave participants the capacity to engage with life freely, blend in with their friends, and shape their own identities. But secrecy also meant they were dependent on only a few people for all of their support and communication in relation to their HIV, which mostly meant one or two family members. Although this reliance, particularly on parents, had led to strong bonds for some, it could also be difficult for those who did not get along with their parents or who were the only one with HIV in their family. The isolation many felt in relation to their condition became apparent when they described how much "Camp" meant to them. In Australia, there are three annual residential camps for families affected by HIV and for HIV-positive children under 18 years, which are organized by the Paediatric HIV Service and funded by donations. All participants in this study had attended Camp, often over many years, and the importance of this experience was one of the most striking and consistent themes in the interviews. Some nominated Camp as the only positive aspect of having HIV, as Aaron said: "nothing comes great with [HIV] except Camp". Several participants emphasized that Camp had been crucial to their well-being:

> It's probably one of the things that saved me from like going mentally crazy. Like coming to a place where you know everyone knows how, what you're going through and how you're feeling. And no-one judges you. No-one's, you know, everyone's just one person. They're all together and everything all the time and support you (Daisy, 17 year old).

Like Daisy, many mentioned that Camp was the only environment in their life where everyone knew they had HIV, where secrecy was not the norm and no-one treated them "any different just because you have an illness that can't be cured yet", as 16-year old Sabina said. But to most participants, Camp was so much more than a safe and non-judgemental space. It was also a unique setting for sameness and understanding arising from the fact that, as Amber put it, "you have the same virus running through your body". Participants described the closeness and empathy among their peers as an "unspoken bond" and Camp as the invaluable place where they could come together to learn, talk and cry about HIV, even make fun of it together, where "nothing's taboo" or "off limits", as Dylan noted, and where they could just "muck around as kids". A couple of older participants also noted that it was a place where they felt safe to pursue a sexual relationship with their peers. The following quote by Amber captures the critical role played by Camp when growing up with a disease as rare and socially hidden as HIV:

> I would have felt so isolated and alone in this virus, because knowing that somebody else knows exactly how you're feeling is priceless. And, if I didn't have that, I would feel a longing to meet someone who was like me and understood me and, without actually having to say, "I understand," because you just do … It is very unspoken the majority of the time. It's not like we all sit around talking about HIV the whole time … Oh, such an important, such a pivotal point in my, my life, having people around you that understand and being able to cry, and remember people in the past, and be able to talk about medicine and side effects without having to explain. It was the one time of the year where you felt normal, where you felt like part of something … It's just about having someone there for you that "gets" you and, as much as doctors and parents try and understand that, they won't ever understand more than someone who's gone through it themselves.

In their stories, Camp emerged as a place where, paradoxically, the participants could be at once normal and different; where having HIV was a shared experience and where losing your parents and being from another country were commonplace, yet also part of the less than ordinary experiences bringing them together. In this sense, Camp worked to reinforce both a sense of normality and uniqueness (see Chap. 19). Turning 18, the age when they are no longer eligible to attend Camp, was difficult and disorienting for the "first generation of Camp kids", as Dylan called them:

> We were such a tight-knit bunch. We'd grown up with each other. To lose it all, when you turn 18, is a really big thing … Over like 13, 14 years, you've formed such a tight little family that, yeah, that to lose that at 18, that's just kind of, you're a little bit lost … [We] were all just so incredibly close … you go through everything together … And, once that kind of goes, it's a big kind of thing that's missing.

Finding alternative peer support networks proved difficult for those who had graduated from Camp, or for the periods between Camp visits. "There's nothing, really", Matilda said. Available HIV support services were of little interest to them, not only because they were seen as catering primarily for gay men and older people with HIV, but because their sense of identification was strongly and uniquely tied to other young people having grown up with HIV, rather than to people with HIV in general. One older participant mentioned that she stayed in touch with her Camp-buddies across Australia via a Facebook group, while others found it was hard to maintain contact with friends in different states as the demands of young adulthood took over. Indicative of the power of peers (see Chaps. 19 and 20), one interview question that animated many participants was: "What advice would you give to another young person growing up with HIV?" We end this part of the chapter with some of their answers, which centred on support and resilience: "you're not alone" (Amber), "never give up" (Aaron), "stay positive" (Bella), "keep believing in yourself" (Sabina), "be yourself, don't let [HIV] hold you back" (Marcus), "you can still do everything" (Daisy), "*there's more to you than just this virus* and there's more to life than just this virus. So live it and don't let it live you" (Dylan, 19 years old).

6.9 Conclusion

The young people who participated in this study described HIV as a disease that is still stigmatized, misunderstood or ignored by society. For that reason, most kept their HIV status secret, including from close friends, a practice imparted by parents and carers. This finding is consistent with the literature (Bush-Parker 2000; DeMatteo et al. 2002; Fielden et al. 2006; Abramowitz et al. 2009; Michaud et al. 2009; Vijayan et al. 2009; Fair and Walker, 2011; Dorrell and Katz, 2013; Rydström et al., 2013). But our analysis also departs from this theme and contributes a different perspective on experiences of stigma in this population. As mentioned in the introduction, Dorrell and Katz (2013: 8) refer to a "legacy of secrecy and a legacy of shame" among young people with perinatally-acquired HIV. This rendering echoes seminal theories of stigma that equate the practice of concealment among stigmatized people with an urge to hide one's perceived failings or "spoiled identity", a practice with critical consequences for social interactions and selfhood (Goffman 1974). As Eribon (2004: 99) writes about the stigma of homosexuality: "Such an effort at disguise, such an obligation to lie, even to those to whom one is close, to one's relatives, produces an "intolerable" strain, which cannot fail to have profound effects on an individual personality, on a given subjectivity". Those "effects", according to Eribon, are typified by withdrawal, alienation, constant hyper-vigilance against discovery, and self-exclusion from social situations to prevent feelings of pretence and falsehood. But this interpretation of stigma and secrecy does not fit easily with the accounts of the young people in our study.

Our participants provided many accounts of feeling "different", including one young man who spoke of living two lives, one "fake" and one "real". But we observed no indications of actual shame in these accounts. In fact, the assumed connection between secrecy and shame seemed absent in their stories. The "legacy of secrecy" certainly held true, which makes sense given the aetiology of perinatal HIV: for these young people, HIV is not solely their secret to share or withhold—it is also their mother's and sometimes their father's. But nor is the stigma necessarily theirs to "carry" or "internalize", as some might assume about the experience of growing up with HIV. Although they were highly conscious of the stigma surrounding HIV, our study suggests that this stigma was not interiorized in the same way it might be for adults. The fact that their HIV infection happened before their story began, rather than being about the kind of life they have lived or any socially stigmatized action on their part, seems to decouple it from the biographical disruption (Bury 1982) and the powerful social narratives around culpability, shame, regret and anger that can make an adult diagnosis so traumatic. In other words, their infection is part of their pre-history, not the story of their life as *they* have lived it. In this sense, HIV is "theirs" in a very different way to that of a person diagnosed as an adult in terms of how it is embodied and the meanings attached to it. It should also be noted that this is a uniquely supported population who, whether aware of their HIV from an early or later age, has grown up with considerable support from primary carers and health care providers, and with particular value invested in helping them develop a positive self-image. This care and attention to both the physical and mental well-being of these children and young people appear to have shaped their sense of themselves as unique, as not being the same as other children. And by the same token, it has also shaped their sense of possibility and permission with regards to living a normal life with HIV.

Despite, or perhaps because of, this lack of internalized stigma, there was a sense of frustration among these participants that society had such a different view of something which to them was relatively normal. HIV was neither a discrediting "attribute" nor a defining characteristic, but rather an aspect of their reality that could be integrated into everyday life. Taking medication and not telling people about HIV were part of the work and care required to maintain this normality and to prevent the outside world and friends from turning their HIV status into something "abnormal" or shameful. And yet to construe this experience of protecting normality as evidence of an apparent binary between a "true" self and a "false" self would likely make little sense to most of them: in their view, kids with HIV are the same as any others, they simply have to do a few things their friends may not, such as take medicine, visit the clinic, have blood tests, and keep secrets. This finding echoes a less common and undeveloped theme in the literature, which suggests that HIV can be perceived by this population as a relatively small part of their life and identity (Flicker et al. 2005; Rydström et al. 2013). But, as Fair and Albright (2012) argue, it is the tension and "cognitive dissonance" between *realities*—between the stigma of HIV and the normality of their everyday lives—that has the greatest impact on young people growing up with HIV.

It is possible that stigma becomes a more immediate experience for this population as they enter young adulthood, particularly as they start to negotiate sexual relationships and possible rejection by potential sexual partners (Fair and Albright 2012; Newman et al. 2014). This issue has not been covered in this chapter, but will be discussed in a forthcoming publication. But briefly here, most participants in this study did not see HIV as an obstacle to dating or sex now or in the future, and some already had experiences of significant and intimate relationships. They were, however, acutely aware that certain steps had to be taken, foremost disclosure and safety, which were seen as critical but far from easy given the sexual culture and general ignorance about HIV among young people. This loomed as a concern for the younger participants, while older participants reported mostly positive experiences of negotiating this terrain. Research also suggests that feelings of stigma can increase with transition from paediatric to adult care services where most individuals have acquired HIV through behavioral practices, which can reframe the meaning of HIV infection (Dowshen and D'Angelo 2011; Wiener et al. 2011). There was little in the interviews to suggest this, although transition to adult services was sometimes seen as difficult for other reasons, which is another issue we examine in our forthcoming article. Of far more concern among the participants in relation to the transition to adult care was the loss of entitlement to connect to peers through organized Camp activities for people under 18.

The importance of peers was a compelling finding and one that resonates with the few studies that have touched on this issue. They similarly noted that contact with peers has a positive effect on young people's ability to manage their condition and enhances their sense of support, mental well-being and confidence. A major reason for this is the ability to be open about their HIV status and to share their experiences with each other (Fielden et al. 2006; Lam et al. 2007; Fair et al. 2012). What our analysis adds to this is the intriguing capacity of Camp to accommodate both difference and normality: to dissolve a sense of social difference and affirm normality through shared experiences and, at the same time, reinforce a sense of being part of a unique generation of children and a unique group of people with HIV. As Mellins and Malee (2013) have argued, the resilience model that is increasingly popular in research on other vulnerable youth populations has not received much attention in studies of young people growing up with HIV. We suggest that future research could usefully focus on the pivotal role of peer environments in enabling resilience in this population, including ways to sustain such support structures into young adulthood and beyond.

References

Abramowitz, S., Koenig, L., Chandwani, S., Orban, L., Stein, R., LaGrange, R., & Barnes, W. (2009). Characterizing social support: Global and specific social support experiences of HIV-infected youth. *AIDS Patient Care and STDs, 23*(5), 323–330. doi:10.1089/apc.2008.0194.

Bury, M. (1982). Chronic illness as biographical disruption. *Sociology of Health & Illness, 4*(2), 167–182. doi:10.1111/1467-9566.ep11339939.

Bush-Parker, T. (2000). Perinatal HIV: Children with HIV grow up. *Focus: A guide to AIDS research and counseling, 15*(2), 1–4. http://www.ucsf-ahp.org/HTML2/services_providers_publications_focus.html

Corrigan, P., & Matthews, A. (2003). Stigma and disclosure: Implications for coming out of the closet. *Journal of Mental Health, 12*, 235–248.

DeMatteo, D., Wells, L., Goldie, R., & King, S. (2002). The family context of HIV: A need for comprehensive health and social policies—Psychological and socio-medical aspects of AIDS/HIV. *AIDS Care, 14*, 261–278.

Dorrell, J., & Katz, J. (2013). "I knew I had something bad because no one spoke about it"—Disclosure discovery: Experiences of young people with perinatally acquired HIV in the UK. *Vulnerable Children and Youth Studies, 8*(4), 353–361. doi:10.1080/17450128.2013.774453.

Dowshen, N., & D'Angelo, L. (2011). Health care transition for youth living with HIV/AIDS. *Pediatrics, 128*, 762–771. doi:10.1542/peds.2011–0068.

Eribon, D. (2004). *Insult and the making of a gay self.* London: Duke University Press.

Fair, C., & Albright, J. (2012). "Don't tell him you have HIV unless he's 'The One'": Romantic relationships among adolescents and young adults with perinatal HIV infection. *AIDS Patient Care and STDs, 26*(12), 746–754. doi:10.1089/apc.2012.0290.

Fair, C., & Walker, S. (2011). Pediatric HIV social workers: Perspectives on disclosure. *Qualitative Social Work, 10*(4), 415–433. doi:10.1177/1473325010373527.

Fair, C., Sullivan, K., & Gatto, A. (2011). Indicators of transition success for youth living with HIV: Perspectives of pediatric and adult infectious disease care providers. *AIDS Care, 23*(8), 965–970. doi:10.1080/09540121.2010.542449.

Fair, C., Connor, L., Albright, J., Wise, E., & Jones, K. (2012). "I'm positive, I have something to say": Assessing the impact of a creative writing group for adolescents living with HIV. *The Arts in Psychotherapy, 39*(5), 383–389. http://dx.doi.org/10.1016/j.aip.2012.06.010.

Fielden, S., Scheckter, L., Chapman, G., Alimenti, A., Forbes, J., Sheps, S., Cadell, S., & Frankish, J. (2006). Growing up: Perspectives of children, families and service providers regarding the needs of older children with perinatally acquired HIV. *AIDS Care, 18*, 1050–1053. doi:10.1080/09540120600581460.

Flicker, S., Skinner, H., Read, S., Veinot, T., McClelland, A., Saulnier, P., & Goldberg, E. (2005). Falling through the cracks of the big cities: Who is meeting the needs of HIV-positive youth? *Canadian Journal of Public Health, 96*(4), 308–312. http://journal.cpha.ca/index.php/cjph/article/view/624/624

Flowers, P. (2010). HIV transitions: Consequences for self in an era of medicalisation. In M. Davis & C. Squire (Eds.), *HIV treatment and prevention technologies in international perspective* (pp. 109–125). NY: Palgrave Macmillan.

Flowers, P., Davis, M., Hart, G., Rosengarten, M., Frankis, J., & Imrie, J. (2006). Diagnosis and stigma and identity amongst HIV positive Black Africans living in the UK. *Psychology and Health, 2*(1), 109–122.

Goffman, E. (1974[1963]). *Stigma: Notes on the management of spoiled identity.* Harmondsworth: Penguin Books.

Guest, G. (2012). *Applied thematic analysis*. Thousand Oaks: Sage.

Lam, P., Naar-King, S., & Wright, K. (2007). Social support and disclosure as predictors of mental health in HIV-positive youth. *AIDS Patient Care and STDs, 21*(1), 20–29. doi:10.1089/apc.2006.005.

Maynard, R. (2006). Controlling death—Compromising life: Chronic disease, prognostication, and the new biotechnologies. *Medical Anthropology Quarterly, 20*(2), 212–234. doi:10.1525/maq.2006.20.2.212.

McDonald, M., Zurynski, Y., Wand, H., Giles, M., Elliott, E., Ziegler, J., & Kaldor, J. (2009). Perinatal exposure to HIV among children born in Australia, 1982–2006. *Medical Journal of Australia, 190*(8), 416–420.

Mellins, C., & Malee, K. (2013). Understanding the mental health of youth living with perinatal HIV infection: Lessons learnt and current challenges. *Journal of the International AIDS Society, 16*(1), 1–19. http://dx.doi.org/10.7448/IAS.16.1.18593.

Michaud, P.-A., Suris, J.-C., Phil, R., Kahlert, C., Rudin, C., & Cheseaux, J.-J. (2009). To say or not to say: A qualitative study on the disclosure of their condition by HIV-positive adolescents. *Journal of Adolescent Health, 44*, 356–362. doi:10.1016/j.jadohealth.2008.08.004.

Miller, A., Ziegler, J., & Palasanthiran, P. (2013). Paediatric HIV in Australia: 30 years of a changing landscape. *HIV Australia, 11*(1), 25–28.

Mofenson, L., & Cotton, M. (2013). The challenges of success: Adolescents with perinatal HIV infection. *Journal of the International AIDS Society, 16*(1), 18650. http://dx.doi.org/10.7448/IAS.16.1.18650.

Newman, C., Persson, A., Miller, A., & Cama, E. (2014). Bridging worlds, breaking rules: Clinician perspectives on transitioning young people with perinatally acquired HIV into adult care in a low prevalence setting. *AIDS Patient Care & STDs, 28*(7), 381–393. http://dx.doi.org/10.1089/apc.2013.0346.

Persson, A. (2013). Non/infectious corporealities: Tensions in the biomedical era of 'HIV normalisation'. *Sociology of Health & Illness, 35*(7), 1065–1079. doi:10.1111/1467-9566.12023.

Persson, A., & Newman, C. (2012). When HIV-positive children grow up: A critical analysis of the transition literature in developed countries. *Qualitative Health Research, 22*(5), 656–667. doi:10.1177/1049732311431445.

Persson, A., Newman, C., & Miller, A. (2014, January 2014). Caring for ‘underground’ kids: Qualitative interviews with clinicians about key issues for young people growing up with perinatally acquired HIV in Australia. *International Journal of Adolescence and Youth*, published online. doi:10.1080/02673843.2013.866149

Rydström, L.-L., Ygge, B.-M., Tingberg, B., Navèr, L., & Eriksson, L. (2013). Experiences of young adults growing up with innate or early acquired HIV infection: A qualitative study. *Journal of Advanced Nursing, 69*(6), 1357–1365. doi:10.1111/j.1365-2648.2012.06127.x.

Seidman, S., Meeks, C., & Traschen, F. (1999). Beyond the closet? The changing social meaning of homosexuality in the United States. *Sexualities, 2*, 9–34.

Sohn, A., & Hazra, R. (2013). The changing epidemiology of the global paediatric HIV epidemic: Keeping track of perinatally HIV-infected adolescents. *Journal of the International AIDS Society, 16*(1), 1–8. http://dx.doi.org/10.7448/IAS.16.1.18555.

UNAIDS. (2014). *The gap report*. Geneva: Joint United Nations Programme on HIV/AIDS. http://www.unaids.org/sites/default/files/media_asset/UNAIDS_Gap_report_en.pdf.

Vijayan, T., Benin, A., Wagner, K., Romano, S., & Andiman, W. (2009). We never thought this would happen: Transitioning care of adolescents with perinatally acquired HIV infection from pediatrics to internal medicine. *AIDS Care, 21*, 1222–1229. doi:10.1080/09540120902730054.

Wiener, L., Kohrt, B.-A., Battles, H., & Pao, M. (2011). The HIV experience: Youth identified barriers to transitioning from pediatric to adult care. *Journal of Pediatric Psychology, 36*(2), 141–154. doi:10.1093/jpepsy/jsp129.

Part II
Children, Young People, HIV/AIDS, Identity and Risk

Chapter 7
Masculinities, Femininities and the Burden of Culture Among Rural South African Teenagers in the Context of HIV

Deevia Bhana

Contents

7.1 Introduction

The KwaZulu-Natal province of South Africa is regarded as the epicentre of the global HIV epidemic where almost 1.7 million people are estimated to be living with the disease (HSRC 2014). Almost 12 % of young people in the province between the ages of 15 and 24 years old are infected with HIV (HSRC 2014). Rural areas of KwaZulu-Natal, and the setting for this study, are often regarded as HIV "hotspots" with wide gender disparity in rates of infection (Ramjee and Wand 2014). Recent HIV prevalence statistics amongst rural KwaZulu-Natal teenage school learners in grades 9 and 10 was 1.4 % in males and 6.4 % in females (Kharsany et al. 2012; Karim et al. 2014; Frolich et al. 2012). According to Karim and colleagues (2014), a substantial number of female learners were infected by the age of 18 years old and overburdened with vulnerability to HIV. Moreover, the overall

D. Bhana (✉)
School of Education, University of KwaZulu-Natal, Private Bag X03,
Cnr Mariannhill & Richmond Roads, Ashwood 3605, South Africa
e-mail: bhanad1@ukzn.ac.za

P. Liamputtong (ed.), *Children and Young People Living with HIV/AIDS*,
Cross-Cultural Research in Health, Illness and Well-Being,
DOI 10.1007/978-3-319-29936-5_7

pregnancy prevalence in the same study was found to be 3.6 %. Early pregnancy has been found to correlate with risky sexual activity and increases women's vulnerability to HIV (Christofides et al. 2014). In an earlier study, Jewkes et al. (2001) found that 72 % of pregnant teenagers in South Africa reported that they were forced to have sex. The high burden that South African teenage women face under-scores the significance of addressing gender, sexuality and young people situated in defined contexts in order to respond to locally relevant HIV prevention and school-based interventions (Jewkes 2010; Karim et al. 2012). As Bell and Aggleton (2014:2) note in their study of young people in rural Uganda:

> Despite awareness of various contextual influences on young people's sexual health, there remains a tendency to design sexual health programmes that focus on individual behaviour change, including sexual health Information, Education and Communication strategies (IEC) and Behaviour Change Communication (BCC). These tend to be based on the idea that given the 'right' information, individuals' knowledge and attitudes will change, leading to required behaviour change to reduce sexual…

Against this backcloth, this chapter asks: How do rural African teenage men and pregnant teenage women conceptualize gender and sexuality within relationship dynamics? In what ways are masculinities and femininities forged to produce and contest gendered vulnerabilities to HIV? Whilst there is an emerging body of work that addresses teenage sexualities in South Africa (Bhana and Pattman 2011; Bhana and Anderson 2013; Bhana 2015), there remains a dearth of research as it relates to contextual variations in the social constitution of sexuality. This chapter examines how teenage men and pregnant teenage women located in rural areas of KwaZulu-Natal construct gender and sexuality analyzing the implications for HIV prevention.

Rural areas of KwaZulu-Natal are often under economic stress and face massive levels of structural inequalities which are both the consequences of apartheid policies and continuing levels of poverty and unemployment. The aggregate effects of these conditions have produced large scale social suffering and marginalization for rural men and particularly for rural women and girls who bear the brunt of gendered poverty and inequalities (Sideris 2004; Harrison 2008; Bhana 2010; Hunter 2010). Converging with these structural conditions and inequalities are cultural patterns based on masculine power and entitlements which circumscribe women and girls' agency (Hunter 2010). As Sideris (2004) notes, customary practices in rural South Africa, whilst open to change and changing, maintain continuity in relation to cultural traditions embedded within gendered patterns mobilized around male hegemonic power and female docility. These gender and cultural processes weave through sexual relations and have effects for the ways in which teenage Africans make meaning of gender and sexuality. The coming together of gender, sexuality and culture within teenage relationship dynamics serve to increase teenage women's vulnerability to pregnancy and HIV.

Globally, there has been recognition of the ways in which gender inequalities fuel women's vulnerability to HIV. UNAIDS (2013) reports that gender inequalities and harmful gender norms creates a burden on women and girls reducing their ability to negotiate safe sex. Studies have focused upon unequal gender relations and argued that epidemiological realities provide significant bases for continuing to focus and transform the ways in which gender inequalities fuel HIV. As Gupta and colleagues (2011:S317) argue, a comprehensive response to HIV requires attention to gender-related vulnerabilities. The elimination of gender inequalities and gendered violence is vital in comprehensive prevention strategies as well as increasing the capacity of women and girls to enhance their capabilities to protect themselves from HIV (UNAIDS 2013).

In the context of HIV in sub-Saharan Africa, research focusing on understanding gender dynamics amongst young Africans is increasing (Dilger 2003; Bhana and Pattman 2011; Muhanguzi 2011; Jewkes and Morrell 2012; Bhana and Anderson 2013; Gevers et al. 2013; Groes-Green 2013; Bell and Aggleton 2014; Corbett 2014; Bhana 2015; Harrison and O'Sullivan (2010). Such research is motivated by understanding from the viewpoints of young people, why and how gender inequalities manifest within relationship dynamics which fuel young women's disproportionate vulnerability to HIV infection. By focusing on and involving young Africans as active agents in the making of gender and sexuality, research is illuminating the gendered and cultural worlds through which teenage sexualities are forged and gender relations and power remain significant areas of development (Corbett 2014).

Studies have found that unequal gender power relations play a significant role in HIV settings and drives young women's vulnerability to disease (Jewkes and Morrell 2010; see also Chaps. 4, 13 and 15 in this volume). Dominant masculinities and acquiescent femininities, as many scholars have argued, lead to unequal relations of power and teenage women's heightened vulnerability to disease infection and risky behavior (Reddy and Dunne 2007; Jewkes and Morrell 2012). Within heterosexual relationships, gender expectations often cohere around appropriate behavior for young men and women and where women's docile and submissive behavior is often acknowledged, expected and rewarded (Harrison 2008; Jewkes and Morrell 2010). On the other hand, the appropriate behavior for young men is sexual prowess, sexual entitlement and the demonstration of and the continuing jockeying for power. As Mane and Aggleton (2001) note, gender roles and expectations lead to the construction of masculinities which place emphasis on fearlessness and sexual risks. Male gender norms affect both women's sexual health and men's health through gendered ideologies based on domination and female docility (Fleming et al. 2014). The effects of gendered ideologies result in women's inability to control and negotiate sexual relations and sexual encounters.

Harrison and O'Sullivan (2010) and others (MacPhail and Campbell 2001; Varga 2003; Shai et al. 2012) have identified how gender and sexuality coalesce producing a context where women lack the power to negotiate condom use. Condoms function symbolically to create lack of trust and intimacy whilst fuelling suspicion of infidelity and questioning and jeopardising romantic love. Bhana and Anderson (2013) also find that condom use is often eschewed by masculine prerogatives. Whilst Bhana and Anderson suggest that teenage women are highly aware of their vulnerability within sexual relations, their decisions and negotiations around condom use is situated within a network of sexual and gender relations where female subordination and ideologies of gender roles and expectations restricts choices and possibilities of condom use.

In South Africa, gender and relationship dynamics are compounded by material, social and cultural scripts which influence and have effects for the ways in which teenage men and women give meaning to sexuality (Bhana and Pattman 2011; Bhana 2015). As Varga (2003) notes, gender roles and identities in South Africa fuel gender inequalities in sexual relations. A major theme is that inequalities within relationship dynamics and teenage women's limited agency within sexual relations created gendered patterns of inequalities and vulnerability to HIV. However, whilst the literature clearly focuses on women and girls' continued vulnerability to HIV premised on social and cultural norms and male power, the notion of monolithic male power has been subverted suggesting that women can exercise a degree of agency (Jewkes and Morrell 2012; Bhana 2014). Instead of seeing African teenage women as simply docile victims of masculine power, these authors suggest that there are different forms of teenage femininities ranging from acceptance of, to critique and accommodation of masculine power leading Corbett (2014) to suggest the construction of women beyond victims and beyond heroines.

The exercise of agency and the ways in which power manifests in relationship dynamics has been the focus of a study conducted by Jewkes and Morrell (2012) in South Africa. These authors show that teenage women's ability to exercise agency was evident in their choice of and passion for boyfriends. However, whilst teenage women were against violence within intimate relations, their agency was compromized by their need to be heterosexually desired. They produced a version of femininity that tolerated violence whilst subsuming to emotions and discourses of love whilst surrendering to cultural expectations of being 'good' women. Jewkes and Morrell (2012) find further that once relationships are forged, men reproduce masculine notions of control and domination. This research, like others, highlight that it is not simply a lack of female agency or knowledge about their position within gender and sexual relations that is problematic but the normative and culturally embedded notions of femininity which lead to risky and coercive behavior (Reddy and Dunne 2007).

As Jewkes and Morrell (2012) and other research have found, femininities are often based on acquiescence to male domination, accommodation of control and violence rather than contestation (Harrison 2008; Bhana and Anderson 2013; Firmin 2013). Similarly, research too has highlighted the ways in which teenage masculinities are divergent and not homogenously based on sexual prowess and coercive relations (Bhana and Nkani 2014; Bhana 2015). Dworkin and colleagues (2013a) suggest that the increased attention to the need to address gender equality in HIV prevention has enhanced the opportunities to work with men and a focus on the masculinities has thus increased with evidence suggesting that some scope exists to transform men's notion of sexual entitlement and toxic patterns of male power (Barker et al. 2010). These variations in the construction of femininities and masculinities offer scope in addressing female vulnerability to disease. If women are not simply docile victims of male power and men are not simply sexual predators, then the possibility exists of expanding pathways of better sexual health outcomes for teenage Africans – both men and women. To do so requires attention to the range of ways in which sexualities and gender are constituted under local conditions. As Bell and Aggleton (2014) note, the development of sexual health intervention programs must be premised on and informed by the actual realities through which young people negotiate gender and sexuality.

7.2 Gender and Sexuality in Rural KwaZulu-Natal

This section focuses on the gendered and cultural context of KwaZulu-Natal through which teenage sexual cultures and patterns can be understood. Rural KwaZulu-Natal, the site from where teenage Africans in this study emerge, is often characterized as impoverished, lacking resources and contexts where food insecurity and economic marginalization continue to face poor Africans. It is also a context of high HIV prevalence rates and where loyalty to certain customary practices remains constant despite evidence of changing cultural norms (Sideris 2004; Bhana et al. 2009; Bhana 2010; Hunter 2010; Rudwick and Posel 2014). Entrenched cultural and gender ideologies continue to influence how people regulate and accommodate social norms where women's deferential conduct is still valued (Hunter 2010).

Historical processes mark the ways in which gender and generation divisions were created. Reid and Walker (2005) elucidate that in the late nineteenth century, a gendered and cultural organization saw men dominate a system of chieftaincy. Men had control over access to land and dominated the household. In rural KwaZulu-Natal, as many historical commentators have noted, male power was mobilized and legitimated with through the Chief, his headman and elder men is hierarchical order (Delius and Glaser 2002; Sideris 2004; Hunter 2010). Carton and Morrell (2012) note that young men were inducted into masculine rituals through stick fighting which was rooted in Zulu masculinity, power and in preparation for the role as heads of households and defense. Masculine power was premised upon building a homestead, accumulation capital through the acquisition of cattle and polygamy. Polygamy was linked to women's labor and economic wealth (Carton 2000).

Within this gendered social organization, women's power was minimal although their productivity in relation to agriculture was important for the household. Women who worked hard were valued and as well as those who upheld deferential conduct and respect (*hlonipha*). Cultural practices, for instance, included women adoption of chaste disposition, docile and respectful to men and older men. Within this system, deferential conduct was expected and rewarded for women who had minimal. These gendered values, were steeped in cultural practices and had effects for the social norms around sexuality. Virginity was highly valued and was linked to cultural notions of respect (*hlonipha*) and *ilobolo* (bridewealth). Virginity, as Hunter (2010) argues, increased the bride-wealth cattle whilst reinforcing pride and dignity as the very 'essence' of Zulu femininity. Related to the cultural value placed in virginity, was the practice of *umemulo* which is a ceremony that indicates that a young woman is an adult and ready to accept a boyfriend and get married. Losing one's virginity was frowned upon and especially if young women were pregnant before marriage (Delius and Glaser 2002).

Gender and cultural systems of organization are always in flux and never static and as Hunter (2005) states, Zulu tradition is not passed down or lost but at every point is contested. Thus, whilst the cultural practices that place great power in masculine prerogatives have been elucidated above, changes in the political economy, urbanization, and apartheid combined to disrupt gendered organizations. With migrant labor, many men left rural areas and women were often left to head the households whilst relying on male breadwinners and a cash economy. Hunter (2010) refers to provider masculinity as a critical dimension of Zulu identity. Provider masculinity is both key to Zulu manhood and powerful but also weakened in relation to economic impoverishment. These economic changes produced changes in sexual relations and different possibilities were created for sexual relations outside of marriage and in many instances resulted in the manifestation of toxic forms of masculinities based on multiple partnering (Delius and Glaser 2002). The production of toxic patterns of masculinities has been critiqued for producing multiple vulnerabilities for women and girls especially in rural hotspots where HIV continues to ascend.

In the context of HIV, multiple partners and masculinities based on sexual entitlements have been challenged with women critiquing men who use violence and coercive sexual practices (Hunter 2010). This is not without male challenges to women's critique. In rural areas, however, whilst contestations are possible, within the cultural norms and women's dependency of male economic provision, the ability to contest and challenge male authority is often limited. It is in this context that teenage Africans give meaning to sexuality as they contest, accommodate and reproduce narrow strictures of gender and culture. I argue that teenage men and women draw on notions of masculinity and femininity which are rooted in cultural ideals of respect (*hlonipha*) which emphasizes virginity and women's subordinate position within gender relations. The effects of the cultural organization of gender within local rural contexts are relations of domination and subordination with reduced levels of agency for teenage women in contraceptive use (which account for their pregnancy status) and greater risk to HIV. Teenage men, on the other hand, foreground culturally embedded practices that value 'polygamy' in dating practices and reinforces male power and privilege. Teenage women are not simply seen as dupes of power but actively accommodate the cultural practices which contribute to their subordination. Whilst feminist research elsewhere has highlighted teenage women's active agency in transforming their social conditions, I argue that the cultural processes through which sexuality and gender are embodied are organized in ways that reproduce male domination and risk to HIV making it difficult for teenage women to exercise choice and agency. The chapter concludes with renewed efforts to focus on teenage men and women in local rural contexts, changing ideas of masculinities and femininities and reworking the 'burden' of culture that limits agency as well as the broader structural conditions which engenders poverty and vulnerability to disease.

7.3 The Study

The analysis in this chapter draws on elements of a larger qualitative research project titled "16 turning 17 youth, gender and sexuality in the context of HIV and AIDS". Based on interviews and over 44 focus group discussions with teenagers across various schools in KwaZulu-Natal, the study aims to explore teenage South Africans opinions about and investments in gender and sexuality against the backdrop of HIV. Within this broad aim, a significant theme that arose from the perspectives of and views on sexuality were heterosexual relationships. Romantic relationships whether imagined, real or future oriented are of a central preoccupation amongst young teenagers across the globe, as Allen's (2005) study of New Zealand young people illustrate. Thus, as Harrison (2008: 176) notes, an "understanding the social construction of young people's sexuality requires attention to the range of meanings and definitions attached to sexuality and relationships".

This chapter focuses on five teenage men and six pregnant teenage women located in two rural schools in KwaZulu-Natal province in the districts of KwaMakhutha and Mgugu respectively. Teenagers in both districts rely on the child support grant of R310 per month and emerge from under-developed homesteads (in many instances made of mud and corrugated iron) as well as low cost state supported houses. In aiming to understand how sexualities are produced by teenagers under local circumstances, the project has worked with teenagers across race and class settings. This chapter focuses on pregnant teenagers and teenage men in two rural settings. Schools in KwaMakhutha and Mgugu provided access to the teenagers.

Focus group discussions were adopted by the research team which consisted of a male researcher (aged 30) at KwaMakhutha and a female researcher (aged 36) at Mgugu. Single-sex focus group discussions lasting 60–90 min were conducted with young people in the two research areas. Focus groups were conducted in school and were based on what young people thought was important in terms of relationship dynamics and included a focus on condom use. During the discussions, young people emphasized cultural dimensions sexuality. Purposive sampling was used to select teenagers. At Mgugu, only those who were pregnant at school and were willing to participate in the study formed part of the sampling.

The study adopted key ethical principles including informed consent, voluntary participation, confidentiality and the maintenance of anonymity through the use of pseudonyms. All participants provided informed consent as well as consent from their parents or guardians. Data was subjected to Braun and Clarke's (2006) system of thematic coding which involved three steps. Firstly, the entire data set was searched for repeated patterns of meaning after which different codes were produced. A thematic map was then produced and finally themes were refined in relation to the entire data set.

7.4 Gender and Relationship Dynamics

This section focuses firstly on the ways in which teenage masculinities are constructed before it addresses the ways in which pregnant teenagers account for dynamics through which their power within intimate relations are diminished. To this end, within the broader framework of gender power relations, this section goes on to illustrate the subordinate status of teenage women and the dominant constructions of male sexuality. Whilst care is taken to show agency and contestation, the rural context of KwaZulu-Natal, circumscribes and has effects for the tighter strictures on the expression of agency.

7.4.1 Multiple Partners: Playing/Proving Masculinity

Sexuality is a chief means through which masculinities are negotiated and produced (Connell 2005). In this study, not all boys proclaimed to be sexually active and yet produced versions of masculinity that were in keeping with male sexual prowess and power. When young men were asked about girlfriends, they spoke about multiple partners exaggerating their sexual feats by referring to 'less than 20' girlfriends.

Counting girlfriends is key to being identified and being recognized as a man. It also suggests being recognized as sexual and having knowledge about sex. Hegemonic forms of masculinity are key to heterosexual success and therefore the focus on heterosexual power and status must also be read as a ways to avoid appearing less of a man and lacking in sexual knowledge and sexual prowess:

> There are those that are at school, I see at school. Others stay closer to where I live but I see others when I go visiting (David).
>
> More than five. (Anton).
>
> Not too many, even though I cannot recall the exact number. But I think are less than 20, because it is not too long since I started having girlfriends… (David).
>
> Maybe seven but they do not live close to each other…. I see this one and I like her and then I see another one. In my heart, I do not love one person (Sango).

As many masculine theorists have argued, the key to proving masculinity is proving sexual conquests (Barker 2005; Hunter 2010). It is important at this point not to reproduce racist versions of masculinity which position African men as hypersexual. Spronk (2014), for instance, suggests that in much of Africa, HIV is stereotyped as stemming from and rooted in certain sexual behaviors that are associated with African 'culture'. Whilst the teenagers above valorize multiple partners and give meaning to masculinity and sexuality through sexual partnering, such statements have a social context. Amidst massive social dislocation and in the context of deep poverty, teenage men, like men around KwaMakhutha, suffer from emasculation brought about by the history of apartheid and persistent inequalities which produce fragile masculinities. Thus, as Hunter (2010) elucidates, their statements of male power are also about male weaknesses. The loss of power in the homestead and economic misery has produced weakened masculinities and the demonstration of power in the sexual arena must be seen in this light. Instead of dehumanizing African teenage men as hypersexual, there is need to understand how socio-economic and cultural conditions shape and have effects for the construction of masculinities based on proving heterosexual success with women. As Connell (2012) notes, we need to give weight to the social and cultural processes that shape masculinities and to the ways in which masculinities are actively constructed within these social and cultural processes.

At the same time, the focus group discussion above is an important means through which teenage men were constructing and proving masculinity in relation to peer influence and pressure and against being constructed as subordinate. Counting girlfriends from less than 20 to 7 and 5 must be seen in light of the group dynamics where proving masculinity is embedded within dominant notions of heterosexual success where the stigma against a masculinity that does not value heterosexual prowess has been found to be loom large in African teenage constructions of sexualities (Bhana and Pattman 2011). There is a wider gendered, social, cultural and contextual range for the ways in which masculinities are constructed and this relates to historical relations of male power and the cultural manifestations in the local area where male power continues to be valued albeit with contestation. Such contestation is particularly evident where teenage fathers are either absent or unemployed and who rely on their mothers' domestic labour for support.

....If you really love her you continue with the relationship even after having sex (Sango)

In their research on love in Africa, Cole and Thomas (2009) are critical of studies in Africa that cut off love from relationship dynamics. Instead, the focus on love was not absent in the ways in which teenage men reflected upon relationships. Masculinity was thus produced not only in relation to claims to sexual power but also in relation to love. Hence, masculinity was caught up in proving masculinity by proving, counting and demonstrating sexual conquests but also embedded within intimacy. Importantly, whilst the teenage men spoke overwhelmingly about multiple partners, there is a need to contextualize such demonstrations of power which both enable a form of masculine authority and limit it. In other words, there is nothing monolithic about teenage male power although the cultural and social conditions enable and have created vulnerabilities for the production of masculinities based on sexual conquests.

The teenage men also referred to having multiple girlfriends as '*isithembu somjolo*', or 'polygamous dating'. Holding in to cultural manifestations of male sexual prerogatives, the participants attempted to give meaning to multiple partners by reaching to polygamy. The study of African teenage men in KwaZulu-Natal province requires understanding of a range of cultural and contextual factors. On 27 July 2014, the king in KwaZulu-Natal, a ceremonial position held by King Zwelithini age 66, married his sixth wife Zola Mafu (age 28). The wedding was attended by the current president of South Africa, Jacob Zuma, who has four wives. Whilst polygamy and multiple partnering have come under increasing attack and is not a stable category, teenage men used it symbolically as a crutch (Hunter 2010) to invoke male power:

> I call it 'isithembu somjolo' (polygamy of dating) (Justin).
> Yes it is common around here lots of guys do it… (David).
> We just do it, we play, and it is like a competition. (Justin).
> That you are a man. You are the right one…a player… (David).
> I've heard them say 'indoda ibonakala ngezenzo zayo' (you see a man by his actions)…. having many girlfriends…ok it's having nice, beautiful girlfriends. And she must be a virgin… (Justin).

In his historical analysis, Hunter (2010) shows that polygamy was contested as it was produced and that whilst both men and women engaged in multiple partner relations, it was men who were able to engage in polygamous relationships bolstering their power as men and husbands and in doing so fuelling and giving meaning to Zulu culture. Like Hunter (2010), the teenage men above produce masculinities based on sexual power and prowess referring to playing manliness by having several girlfriends and referring to such heterosexual relations of the polygamy of dating. Of course, the values were coded with male power and where the idealization and cultural expectation of virginity deeply ingrained with respect was valued. This forms part of later discussion in this section. Within the wider cultural and social range in KwaZulu-Natal, the idea of male power, whilst contested, does rest with ideas of polygamy although this has now altered. King Zwelithini paid 20 cattle as brideprice for his sixth marriage. The teenage men in this study are unable to imagine and fulfill the cultural expectations associated with polygamy in the context of structural inequalities and deep poverty. Thus, multiple partners have replaced ideologies of polygamy although both are coded within male power and privilege. In Spronk's (2014) study of men in Kenya, she refers to 'modern polygamy', premised upon one-night stands and multiple partners and extramarital affairs.

7.4.2 Subordinated Femininities Within Intimate Partner Relations

In contrast to the ways in which African teenage men constructed power within relationship dynamics, when pregnant teenagers talked about becoming pregnant, they focused attention on their relative lack of power within intimate partner relationships. This section confirms the subordination and the marginalized status of many young South African women as other research has suggested (Bhana 2012). Pregnant teenage women pointed to constructions of masculine power and sexuality through which their agency was both limited and challenged.

> …my boyfriend took the first step and asked me for love, after a few months the relationship started….My boyfriend initiated sexual activities because he knows that I am shy (Kelly).
> …I mean boyfriends…They use all kinds of tricks to confuse us girls (Jane).
> My boyfriend told me that if I don't want to have sex with him it means I don't love him (Kim).

Dominant constructions of male sexuality were evident within relationship dynamics with sex initiated by teenage men. This domination stood in opposition to the construction of a femininity based on being "shy". As much of the research in South Africa illustrates, being good and 'shy' or docile has great cultural value and Zulu femininity is often valued for espousing such values (Scorgie 2002; Harrison 2008). Being shy is dichotomously opposed to women who are regarded as loose, without respect and morals and constructed as '*isifebe*' (bitch). Whilst the teenage women above lament their lack of power and criticize teenage men for 'confusing girls' by using all kinds of tricks, they too subordinate to emotional cues and notions of love. To show love is thus constructed as to agree to have sex:

> Each time we were together my boyfriend would say if I love him I must have sex with him. I ended up agreeing because I loved him and didn't want to lose him even if knew that I wasn't ready for sex (Abby).

Their agency is limited by the patriarchal conditions and cultural manifestations of femininities but at the same time they are complicit with these cultural and patriarchal structures. Like Jewkes and Morrell (2012) have found in their study, the teenage women do recognize their subordination and the ways in which power operates within relationship dynamics but their constructions of femininity encourage acceptance of rather than contesting dominant patterns of male domination and are embedded within affective dimensions of sexuality and the construction of femininity which is aligned to emotional desires and love. As Bhana and Anderson (2013) suggest, teenage women set themselves up for risky conduct as they attempt to rescue relationships in the interests of their emotional well-being:

> I remember when my boyfriend asked me for a relationship, he was nice and respectful. I told him that I was a virgin and not ready for sex. He promised to respect me and my decisions, but after the relationship started things changed. He wanted things done his way…It's many things like when and where we meet, when and how to have sex. When our relationship started, I told him that I was not ready to have sex but he begged me until I said its ok, the next month I found out that I was pregnant…. (Abby).

Much of the research in Southern Africa points to male power in initiating sex, timing of sex, and the use of contraceptives (Shai et al. 2012; Bhana and Anderson 2013; Karim et al. 2014). Whilst young women do have some level of agency, especially in choosing their partners and expressing romantic desires, like Jewkes and Morrell (2012) have found in their study, the teenage woman above notes the change in the relationship from being nice and respectful to "wanting things done his way". The data above confirms that teenage women are not simply docile and victims of force and sexual coercion but do have agency, "he begged me until I said its ok". Giving in to male desire for sex shows teenage women's complicity in and reproduction of asymmetrical relations of power.

> When I suggested that we use a condom my boyfriend refused. I think it's because he is older than me. One day he asked me if I suspect him of anything like a disease because he does not have any. (Kelly)

The use of condoms is embedded within highly charged gender relations. In the above example, the suggestion of condom use is negotiated within age discrepancies as well as the possibility of jeopardizing the relationship as condom use is not only associated with preventing pregnancy but HIV. To request the use of condoms, as the above example attests to, is to insinuate a carrier of disease and HIV which places intimate relations within mistrust suspicion and jeopardy.

7.5 Gender, Culture and Virginity

This section expands on the ways in which teenage Africans foreground virginity within highly charged gender relations through which cultural claims about a Zulu identity are made (see Hunter 2010). Despite evidence that culture is always fluid and changing, researchers note too that some constancy remains in relation to Zulu values around respect (*hlonipha*). These values are embedded within and aligned to gender and generational respect but is also tied to women's vulnerability within intimate partner relations and to HIV (Hunter 2010). Virginity, which was historically tied to brideprice and respect, still has value in the ways in which both teenage men and women give meaning to it and serve as a critical site for the reproduction of gender inequalities.

7.5.1 The Prize of Masculinity: Virgins

The idealization of virgins featured strongly in teenage men's construction of gender and sexuality. Globally, virginity ideals manifest within sexual relations (Valenti 2009). In rural KwaZulu-Natal, an ideal of virginity have historical rooting and provides a basis through which both teenage men and women accommodate cultural ideals and practices. It has been shown how bridewealth has historically been associated with virginity status and respect amongst people in KwaZulu-Natal (Hunter 2010). Chastity, respectability, female docility and hard work were valued and rewarded. Families frowned upon sex before marriage and especially in the context of teenage pregnancy as it brought shame to Zulu families and reduced the amount of cattle that could be bargained for during *ilobola* (bridewealth) negotiations. When African teenage men were asked questions about ideal girlfriends, they spoke about respect and "she must be a virgin":

> A beautiful one, a neat one and one who respects (David).
>
> The one with a good conduct who does not have multiple partners. I like a self-respecting girl…who is respectful. You know the girls that are forward and materialistic, I do not like them. I like a girl who is humble and is of good conduct (Sango).
>
> …in most cases guys look at the behaviour of his girlfriend and how she conducts herself. If he is suspicious of her, then he uses a condom (Rob).

Teenage men use virginity and the cultural and historical ideals in which it is embedded to reinvent male power and privilege. By placing high value in teenage women's chastity and virginity, a sexual double standard operates whereby teenage men's sexual activities are rendered invisible and normalized whilst teenage women are caste under the sexual and cultural gaze. Those who do not live up to respectability and 'good conduct' (Harrison 2008) are disparaged. The ideal of a 'humble', 'self-respecting', non-materialistic woman who is also 'beautiful and neat' has both cultural and material basis. In the first instance, teenage men reject those who aspire towards material goals. In doing so, they reveal the frailties that they experience in the economic world where they are unable to provide for such material aspirations. In contrast, women who are humble and self-respecting fulfill Zulu cultural ideals and through which male power is reproduced. It must be noted here that cultural ideals are fluid and unstable but the value in virginity currently does have important value especially as virginity testing has been resurrected as a cultural force to end pregnancy and HIV (Scorgie 2002).

> It's in the rural areas here. Those who live on this side (rural areas) you know when you do sex you must not use a condom....(David).

Bhana and Pattman (2011) show that rural teenage women or "farm-julias" are idealized by African township teenagers because they represent virginity, respect and chastity. They are regarded as the ideal Zulu women. In the same vein, the above data constructs teenage women in rural areas as virgins but also as sexually safe and where condom use is not required because it is assumed rural women do no sleep around. The contradiction is clear. Rural African women are engendered as virgins with respect but they are also sexualized and rendered vulnerable to male sexual gaze and where condom use is based on their respectful status suggesting that they are open to multiple forms of vulnerabilities and HIV infection. The imperative of sex with respectful rural women allows men to claim power and is critical to constructions of masculinity. Having sex with rural teenage women was justified because rural women were respectful and did not have multiple partners and where thus cleansed of sexual disease and immorality.

> When a girl throws herself at you that might be a problem, it might be AIDS or that she is pregnant and do not know who the father is and wants to give you the responsibility of being the father (Rob).

Against the respectability, chastity were women who were regarded as sexually promiscuous and marginalized and who were castigated as vectors in the spread of HIV or pregnant with someone else's child.

7.5.2 Culture, Virginity and the Contradiction of Pregnancy

When pregnant teenage women spoke about sexuality, they lamented the loss of virginity. Whilst virginity was valued and through which respect (*hlonipha*) was gauged, their pregnancy provided a contradiction to the cultural ideals aspirations and ideals. As Hunter (2010) and others (Scorgie 2002; George 2008) have noted, respectability is embedded in and forms part of Zulu identity. Women, who embody *hlonipha*, are acknowledged by the family and community and respectability and virginity produces adulation from others. Being pregnant meant defilement of claims to respectability and culture although the teenage women spoke eloquently about the practices they engaged in before falling pregnant:

> I took part in ukuhlolwa kwezintombi before falling pregnant. It was done once a month to check if we were still virgins. Every September, we went to Nongoma for Umkhosi Womhlanga (Reed Dance Ceremony). (Jenni).

All the pregnant teenagers acknowledged the high value placed on virginity and respectability but, as the previous parts of this analysis suggests, virginity is mired in deep-seated notions of sexuality and gender and through which virginity is idealized and virgins sexualized. Above the discussion turns to the cultural practices which valorizes virginity testing which occurs at the annual reed dance ceremony (*Umkhosi Womhlanga*) in Nongoma-the northern part of KwaZulu-Natal. More regularly, virginity testing is held monthly and the participant above actively participated in it.

> As a young Zulu woman, umemulo is important to me because it would be an indication to me and to the entire community that I have behaved according to the Zulu tradition. Unfortunately, for me I will not get umemulo because I fell pregnant, I am very angry at myself for falling pregnant at this age. If I give birth to a girl, I wish she could keep her virginity until 21 years of age, unlike me so that I give her umemulo (Jane).

Related to virginity idealization was the cultural practice of *umemulo*. *Umemulo* is a ceremony that celebrates the fact that a woman and maintained here virginity (usually celebrated at age 21) and also suggests that a woman is an adult and ready to get married. Virginity loss caused stress and anxiety. Cultural practices such as virginity testing and *umemulo* are chief means through which women can position themselves as humble, respectful and of good conduct and through which they can stake a claim as authentic Zulu women. The contradiction is apparent in the above discussion, however, the weight given to *umemulo* as well as a practice that could be performed in the future (if her child was a girl) suggests the constancy and the value attached to it. Significantly, cultural practices related to virginity and virginity testing was a chief means to claim power but being pregnant weakened such claims giving rise to anxieties and regrets.Yet, there were also apparent contradictions in relation to virginity and cultural practices as illustrated below:

> My mother did not want me to take part in ukuhlolwa kwezintombi [virginity testing] because of the church rules….She only encouraged me to attend church activities (Abby).

The influence of Christian beliefs and practices on Zulu life has been well documented (Hunter 2010). In the above example, it is clear that culture is unstable. Whilst virginity is valued within Christian doctrines, cultural practices are not stable and open to change and Christian beliefs frowned upon 'traditional' cultural practices. Change was also seen in relation to socio-economic conditions. The cultural practice related to *umemulo* required the purchase of goats and cows and their slaughter which many could not afford:

> Even if I did not fall pregnant, I don't think I would get umemulo because my mother earns very little and cannot afford to give me umemulo (Eva).

Whilst the teenagers in this study were pregnant, they weave into cultural and religious systems of meanings through which the high value placed on chastity is reproduced although such values sit in tension and contradiction with their pregnancy status. This does not, however, stop the idealization of virginity status and reproduces the highly gendered way in which virginity functions which serves to recreate male power and privilege.

7.6 Conclusion

Against the backdrop of HIV, I have described how pregnant teenagers and teenage African men in two rural areas in South Africa give meaning to gender and sexuality and the social and cultural processes through which these meanings are forged. In the context of economic insecurity prevalent in much of rural South Africa, the high rates of HIV prevalence and the tight cultural strictures through which gender relations and gender inequalities manifest, I have illustrated how teenage masculinities and femininities are caught up in cultural contradictions of sexuality. Teenage masculinities are embedded within the broader range of inequalities and economic frailties and their negotiation of sexuality is produced in tension with these vulnerabilities and against the backdrop of cultural norms. When teenage African men construct sexuality, they do so by relying on dominant cultural norms demanding obedience to heterosexual prowess and an expectation of women's virginity and chastity. The contradiction and sexual double standard prevails where men's sexual entitlements are expected to go unnoticed but rural women are placed under cultural gaze and demands for respectability and chastity. However, it is also these ideals which put rural women in positions of vulnerability – with teenage men constructing rural women as safe, differentiating between women who are immoral and thus making non-condom use with rural women acceptable. Pregnant teenage women refer to the pervasive forms of inequalities within relationship dynamics and do so not simply as docile victims but surrender to male domination in the interests of developing love and trust and building relationships at their own peril. Cultural ideals around virginity profoundly shaped how teenage men and women constructed sexuality suggesting both constancy in cultural norms and contradictions as pregnant teenagers lament the loss of virginity and teenage men idealize and talk about sex with safe rural women.

Given the widespread forms of inequalities that face teenage women including their inability to negotiate condom use and the cultural expectations requiring subservience, it becomes possible to understand why they became pregnant. Similarly, it is possible to understand in the context of economic and structural inequalities and wider range of cultural norms that propagate male power why young men use sexuality to demonstrate heterosexual prowess. These findings, whilst based on small sample of rural teenagers, illustrate clear links between constructions of masculinity, culture and the configuration of femininities which influence sexual health outcomes leading to unintended pregnancy and vulnerability to HIV.

As Harrison (2008) notes, in rural contexts of South Africa there is clearly a need for sexual health education programs that challenge harmful cultural and social norms and address gender power relations. Sexuality education must address and encourage young people to engage with ideals of masculinity and notions of femininity based on cultural prescriptions and widespread forms of gender inequalities. As Bell and Aggleton (2014) note, intervention programs must be driven by and informed by local contexts. In this chapter, I have suggested that addressing teenage masculinities and the investment in sexual conquests as key to masculinity making remains important. Secondly, relationship dynamics are embedded within unequal gender relations putting young women at risk and preventing effecting negotiation of condom use. Pregnant women, at the same time fuel and are complicit within relationship dynamics as they surrender to emotional needs fuelled by discourses of love and male power. Addressing the construction of femininities and proposing new ways of thinking about femininity is important. The chapter has also identified the pervasive ways in which virginity, culture and gender manifest within idealized notions of good femininity and good female conduct producing sexual double standards but also putting virgins at risk. Gender equitable relations must be at the core of sexuality education programs whilst taking heed of the local cultural conditions which gives rise to such relations. In schools life orientation programs do offer this possibility although for success these programs must be relevant to the actual lives, identities addressing the cultural and social norms through which gender inequalities are produced within rural contexts.

Acknowledgements Nozipho Mvune and Marcell Marindi are acknowledged for conducting the fieldwork upon which this study is based. This work is based on the research supported wholly/in part by the National Research Foundation of South Africa (Grant Number TTK 2007050300020).

References

Allen, L. (2005). *Sexual subjects: Young people, sexuality and education*. Basingstoke: Palgrave Macmillan.

Barker, G. (2005). *Dying to be a man: Youth, masculinity and social exclusion*. London: Routledge.

Barker, G., Ricardo, C., Nascimento, M., Olukoya, A., & Santos, C. (2010). Questioning gender norms with men to improve health outcomes: Evidence of impact. *Global Public Health, 5*(5), 539–553.

Bell, S. A., & Aggleton, P. (2014). Economic vulnerability and young people's sexual relationships in rural Uganda. *Journal of Youth Studies, 17*(6), 814–828.

Bhana, D. (2010). Here in the rural areas they don't say that women are equal! Contesting gender inequalities in the early years. *Agenda, 84*(1), 9–18.

Bhana, D. (2012). "Girls are not free"—in and out of the South African school. *International Journal of Educational Development, 32*(2), 352–358.

Bhana, D. (2014). Loving and Fearing: Township girls' agency amidst sexual risk. In C. Pereira (Ed.), *Changing Narratives of Sexuality: Contestations, Compliance and Women's Empowerment* (pp. 87–110). London: Zed Books.

Bhana, D. (2015). Sex, gender and money in African teenage conceptions of love in HIV contexts. *Journal of Youth Studies, 18*(1), 1–15.

Bhana, D., & Anderson, B. (2013). Desire and constraint in the construction of South African teenage women's sexualities. *Sexualities, 16*(5–6), 548–564.

Bhana, D., & Nkani, N. (2014). When African teenagers become fathers: Culture, materiality and masculinity. *Culture, Health & Sexuality, 16*(4), 337–350.

Bhana, D., & Pattman, R. (2011). Girls want money Boys want virgins. The materiality of love amongst South African township youth in the context of HIV and AIDS. *Culture, Health & Sexuality, 13*(8), 961–972.

Bhana, D., de Lange, N., & Mitchell, C. (2009). Male teachers talk about gender violence: "Zulu men demand respect". *Educational Review, 61*(1), 49–62.

Braun, V., & Clarke, V. (2006). Using thematic analysis in psychology. *Qualitative Research in Psychology, 3*(2), 77–101.

Carton, B. (2000). *Blood from your children: The colonial origins of generational conflict in South Africa*. Pietermaritzburg: University of Natal Press.

Carton, B., & Morrell, R. (2012). Zulu masculinities, warrior culture and stick fighting: Reassessing male violence and virtue in south Africa. *Journal of Southern African Studies, 38*(1), 31–53.

Christofides, N. J., Jewkes, R. K., Dunkle, K. L., Nduna, M., Shai, N. I., & Sterk, C. (2014). Early adolescent pregnancy increases risk of incident of HIV infection in the Eastern Cape, South Africa: A longitudinal study. *Journal of International AIDS Society, 19*(17), 85–185.

Cobbett, M. (2014). Beyond 'victims' and 'heroines': Constructing 'girlhood' in international development. *Progress in Development Studies, 14*(4), 309–320.

Cole, J., & Thomas, L. M. (2009). *Love in Africa*. Chicago: University of Chicago Press.

Connell, R. W. (2005). *Masculinities* (2nd ed.). Cambridge: Polity Press.

Connell, R. (2012). Gender, health and theory: Conceptualizing the issue, in local and world perspective. *Social Science & Medicine, 74*(11), 1675–1683.

Delius, P., & Glaser, C. (2002). Sexual socialisation in South Africa: A historical perspective. *African Studies, 61*(1), 27–54.

Dilger, H. (2003). Sexuality, AIDS, and the lures of modernity: Reflexivity and morality among young people in rural Tanzania. *Medical Anthropology Cross-Cultural Studies in Health and Illness, 22*(1), 23–52.

Dworkin, S. L., Hatcher, A. M., & Colvin, C. (2013a). Impact of a gender transformative antiviolence program on gender ideologies and masculinities in two rural, South African communities. *Men and Masculinities, 104*(6), 1029–1035.

Dworkin, S. L., Treves-Kagan, S., & Lippman, S. A. (2013b). Gender transformative interventions to reduce HIV risks and violence with Hetero-sexual men: A review of the global evidence. *AIDS and Behaviour, 17*(9), 2845–2863.

Firmin, C. (2013). Love hurts: Cheating and violence in teenage women's talk of boyfriends. *Agenda, 27*(2), 47–55.

Fleming, P. J., Lee, G. J. L., & Dworkin, S. L. (2014). "Real men don't": Constructions of masculinity and inadvertent harm in public health interventions. *American Journal of Public Health, 6*, 1029–1035.

Frolich, J. A., Karim, Q. A., Karim, S. S. A., Kharsany, A. B. M., Mlotshwa, M., Samsunder, N., & Zuma, N. Y. (2012). HIV prevalence among high School learners – opportunities for school-based HIV testing programmes and sexual reproductive health services. *BMC Public Health, 12*(1), 1471–2458.

George, E. R. (2008). Virginity testing and South Africa's HIV/AIDS crisis: Beyond rights universalism and cultural relativism toward health capabilities. *California Law Review, 96*, 1447–519.

Gevers, A., Mathews, C., Cupp, P., Russell, M., & Jewkes, R. (2013). Illegal yet developmentally normative: A descriptive analysis of young, urban adolescents' dating and sexual behavior in Cape Town, South Africa. *BMC International Health and Human Rights, 13*(1), 31. doi:10.1186/1472-698X-13-31.

Groes-Green, C. (2013). To put men in a bottle": Eroticism kinship female power and transactional sex in Maputo Mozambique. *American Ethnologist, 40*(1), 102–117.

Gupta, G. R., Ogen, J., & Warner, A. (2011). Moving forward on women's gender-related HIV vulnerability: The good news, the bad news and what to do about it. *Global public health: An International Journal of Research Policy and Practice, 6*(3), 370–382.

Harrison, A. (2008). Hidden love: Sexual ideologies and relationship ideals among rural South African adolescents in the context of HIV/AIDS. *Culture, Health & Sexuality, 10*(2), 175–189.

Harrison, A., & O'Sullivan, L. F. (2010). In the absence of marriage: Long-term concurrent partnerships, pregnancy, and HIV risk dynamics among South African young adults. *AIDS and Behavior, 14*(5), 991–1000.

Human Science Research Council (HSRC). (2014). *South African National HIV prevalence HIV incidence and behaviour survey 2012*. Cape Town: HSRC Press.

Hunter, M. (2005). Cultural politics and masculinities. Multiple partners in historical perspective in KwaZulu-Natal. *Culture, Health and Sexuality, 7*, 389–403.

Hunter, M. (2010). *Love in the time of AIDS: Inequality gender and rights in South Africa*. Pietermaritzburg: University of KwaZulu-Natal Press.

Jewkes, R. (2010). Where to for sexual health education for adolescents in Sub-Saharan Africa? *PLoS Medicine, 7*(6). doi:10.1371/journal.pmed.1000288.

Jewkes, R., & Morrell, R. (2010). Gender and sexuality: Emerging perspectives from the heterosexual epidemic in South Africa and implications for HIV risk and prevention. *Journal of the International AIDS Society, 13*(1), 6.

Jewkes, R., & Morrell, R. (2012). Sexuality and the limits of agency among South African teenage women: Theorising femininities and their connections to HIV risk practices. *Social Science & Medicine, 74*(11), 1729–1737.

Jewkes, R., Vundule, C., Maforah, F., & Jordaan, E. (2001). Relationship dynamics and teenage pregnancy in South Africa. *Social Science & Medicine, 52*(5), 733–744.

Karim, Q. A., Kharsany, A. B. M., Frohlich, J. A., Werner, L., Mlotshwa, M., Madlala, B. T., & Karim, S. S. A. (2012). HIV incidence in young girls in KwaZulu-Natal, South Africa-public health imperative for their inclusion in HIV biomedical intervention trials. *AIDS and Behavior, 16*(7), 1870–1876.

Karim, A. S. S. Q., Kharsany, A. B. M., Leask, K., Ntombela, F., Humpries, H., & Frohlich, J. A. R. (2014). Prevalance of HIV, HSV-2 and pregnancy among high school students in rural KwaZulu-Natal, South Africa: A bio-behavioural cross-sectional survey. *Sexually Transmitted Infections, 90*, 620–626.

Kharsany, A. B., Mlotshwa, M., Frohlich, J. A., Zuma, N. Y., Samsunder, N., & Karim, S. S. A. (2012). HIV prevalence among high school learners-opportunities for schools-based HIV testing programmes and sexual reproductive health services. *BMC Public Health, 12*(1), 231. doi:10.1186/1471-2458-12-231.

MacPhail, C., & Campbell, C. (2001). 'I think condoms are good but aai, I hate those things': Condom use among adolescents and young people in a Southern African township. *Social Science & Medicine, 52*(11), 331–345.

Mane, P., & Aggleton, P. (2001). Gender and HIV/AIDS: What do men have to do with it? *Current Sociology, 49*(6), 23–37.

Muhanguzi, F. K. (2011). Gender and sexual vulnerability of young women in Africa: Experiences of young girls in secondary schools in Uganda. *Culture, Health & Sexuality, 13*(6), 713–725.

Ramjee, G., & Wand, H. (2014). Geographical clustering of high risk sexual behaviors in "Hot-spots" for HIV and sexually transmitted infections in Kwazulu-Natal, South Africa. *AIDS and Behavior, 18*(2), 317–322.

Reddy, S., & Dunne, M. (2007). Risking it: Young heterosexual femininities in South African context of HIV/AIDS. *Sexualities, 10*(2), 159–172.

Reid, G., & Walker, L. (2005). Sex and secrecy: A focus on African sexualities. *Culture, Health & Sexuality, 7*(3), 185–194.

Rudwick, S., & Posel, D. (2014). Contemporary functions of ilobolo (bridewealth) in urban South African Zulu society. *Journal of Contemporary African Studies, 32*(1), 118–136.

Scorgie, F. (2002). Virginity testing and the politics of sexual responsibility: Implications for AIDS interventions. *African Studies, 61*(1), 55–75.

Shai, N. J., Jewkes, R., & Nduna, M. (2012). Masculinities and condom use patterns among young rural South African men: A cross-sectional baseline survey. *BMC Public Health, 12*, 462. doi:10.1186/1471-2458-12-462.

Sideris, T. (2004). "You have to change and you don't know how!" What it means to be a man in a rural area of South Africa'. *African Studies, 63*(1), 29–49.

Spronk, R. (2014). The idea of African men: Dealing with the cultural contradictions of sex in academia and in Kenya. *Culture, Health & Sexuality, 16*(5), 504–517.

UNAIDS, Global Report. (2013). *UNAIDS global report on global AIDS epidemic*. Geneva: UNAIDS.

Valenti, J. (2009). *The purity myth: How America's obsession with virginity is hurting young women*. Berkeley: Seal Press.

Varga, C. A. (2003). How gender roles influence sexual and reproductive health among South African adolescents. *Studies in Family Planning, 34*(3), 160–172.

Chapter 8
"Digging Your Own Grave": Ghanaian Young People's Construction of Vulnerability Within the Context of HIV/AIDS

Georgina Yaa Oduro

Contents

8.1 Introduction

> A society that pays attention to its youth paves the way for its future greatness.
>
> (Ghanaian proverb)

The health of the citizenry is important to every society, especially the youth who are seen as the future leaders. It is in this regard that nations strive to achieve full health and well-being of their members through effective health promotion and education. Although the invasion of the West African sub-region by Ebola has reduced the extreme fear, attention and stigma once associated with the Human Immuno Deficiency Virus (HIV) and Acquired Immune Deficiency Syndrome (AIDS), HIV/AIDS still occupies a serious place in the hierarchy of diseases in Ghana. It is in this

G.Y. Oduro (✉)
Department of Sociology and Anthropology, University of Cape Coast, Cape Coast, Ghana
e-mail: yaaoduro@hotmail.com

P. Liamputtong (ed.), *Children and Young People Living with HIV/AIDS*,
Cross-Cultural Research in Health, Illness and Well-Being,
DOI 10.1007/978-3-319-29936-5_8

direction that various initiatives and efforts have been put in place to control HIV/AIDS in the absence of a complete cure or vaccine for the disease through effective health promotion and education especially of the youth. The question that arises is, how do the youth who are the targets of HIV/AIDS education perceive the disease? To what extent do they see themselves as vulnerable to HIV/AIDS and how do they respond to persons infected and affected by the disease. These issues will be addressed in this chapter.

It is, however, imperative to know the socio-cultural context and nature of HIV/AIDS in Ghana as an entry into the constructions and perceptions of Ghanaian youth on HIV/AIDS. The chapter begins with a brief presentation of the Ghanaian society followed by the context of HIV/AIDS with special attention on the youth. It is then followed by a discussion of the social representation and social construction theories that frame the chapter. I then turn briefly to talk about how the study that I conducted to form this chapter and this followed by the presentation and discussion of themes that emerged from the study.

8.2 The Socio-cultural and HIV/AIDS Contexts of Ghana

The Republic of Ghana is a sovereign and unitary state, located along the Gulf of Guinea and the Atlantic Ocean, in the West Africa sub region only a few degrees north of the Equator, thereby giving the country a warm climate. Ghana is bordered by Togo to the East, Cote d'Ivoire on the west, Burkina Faso in the north, and the Gulf of Guinea and Atlantic Ocean in the south (Nukunya 1992; Assimeng 1999). The country has a population of approximately 28 million, according to the 2010 housing and population census. Ghana is generally defined as youthful with about 42 % of the population below 15 years (see Ghana Living Standard Survey 2005; MOWAC/UNICEF 2009; Oduro and Otsin 2013). As a tropical country, it experiences two key seasons (wet and dry seasons). It was the first African country to secure independence from British colonial rule in 1957. Ghana is an ethnically diverse nation with over 50 ethnic groups. The country practice four key descent systems[1] with the matrilineal Akans being the largest ethnic group and forming about 49 % of the total population. As a communal society, Ghana has a strong sense of community ownership of children, which gives credence to the saying "it takes a village to raise a child" (Nukunya 1992; Badasu 2004). In addition to the primary agents of socialization (family), Ghanaian youth also experience strong influence from religion, formal education, peers and the media. The transmission of traditional cultural norms and values by the family and community is gradually being weakened through social change and factors such as rural-urban migration, urbanization, globalization, western education and the media. It is, therefore, common to see a number of young people owning mobile phones in the midst of poverty with associated challenges (Oduro 2010). Within this picture of competing demands for

[1] These are the matrilineal, patrilineal, double unilineal and bilateral descent systems.

the attention of the youth is the HIV/AIDS virus and corresponding health education (MOWAC/Unicef 2009).

HIV/AIDS appeared on the Ghanaian scene in 1986 with six infections. It, however, spread quickly like wildfire over the years.[2] From a prevalence rate of 3.4 % in 2002, the prevalence increased to 3.6 % in 2003, and then declined to 3.1 % in 2004, declining further to 2.7 % in 2005, and then shot up in 2006 to 3.2 %, followed by a sharp drop to a prevalence of 1.9 % in 2010. It dropped further to 1.5 % in 2012, and 1.3 % in 2013 with a further decline to 0.8 % prevalence in 2014. It is estimated that about 150,000 people are currently living with the HIV virus in Ghana (HIV Sentinel Survey (HSS) 2014; Oduro and Otsin 2013; Ghana AIDS Commission [GAC] 2014). The current prevalence rate is not universal throughout the country as different regions and key groups present different rates. The eastern region out of the ten administrative regions in Ghana has consistently reported the highest prevalence rates of about 3.5 % with the northern regions reporting the lowest prevalence. Prevalence is generally higher in urban areas, mining and border towns, and along main transportation routes as well as among populations such as sex workers, transport workers, prisoners, sexual partners of people living with HIV/AIDS, and men who have sex with men and their female sexual partners (Ghana AIDS Commission [GAC] 2014).

Consistent with the African trend, HIV/AIDS is mainly a heterosexual phenomenon in Ghana with 80 % of all infections heterosexually transmitted, 15 % are transmitted from mother-to-child with the remaining 5 % being transmitted through infections from syringes and other sharp objects (Ghana AIDS Commission [GAC] 2014). Reflective of the global scene, HIV/AIDS in the country is also gendered with more females infected than males for reasons such as engaging in transactional sex, early marriages, sugar daddyism (sex with elderly men for material things), lack of power in sexual relations and other gender relations that disadvantage women and make them more vulnerable to the virus (Gupta 2000; Pattman and Chege 2003; Campbell 2003; Oduro 2010; see also Chaps. 7, 13 and 15 in this volume). The youth are also in the HIV/AIDS picture with a prevalence rate of 1.3 % among those aged from 15 to 24 years. The susceptibility of the youth to HIV/AIDS has long been identified by bodies such as the United Nations Population Fund (UNFPA 2009) when they argue that:

> Young people[3] remain at the centre of the HIV/AIDS epidemic in terms of rates of infection, vulnerability, impact, and potential change. They have grown up in a world changed by AIDS but many still lack comprehensive and correct knowledge about how to prevent HIV infection (see http://www.unfpa.org/hiv/people.htm accessed on 20/03/2012).

[2] It must, however, be noted that though the African sub region has been the most affected in terms of HIV infection, the dynamism of the disease in West Africa is different from that of Southern and Eastern Africa. West African countries have generally reported low prevalence rates compared to East and Southern African countries (UNAIDS 2013).

[3] Young people and youth are relative terms used interchangeably in different societies. It is used in this chapter to describe people between ages 14 and 19 years who are transiting from childhood to adulthood.

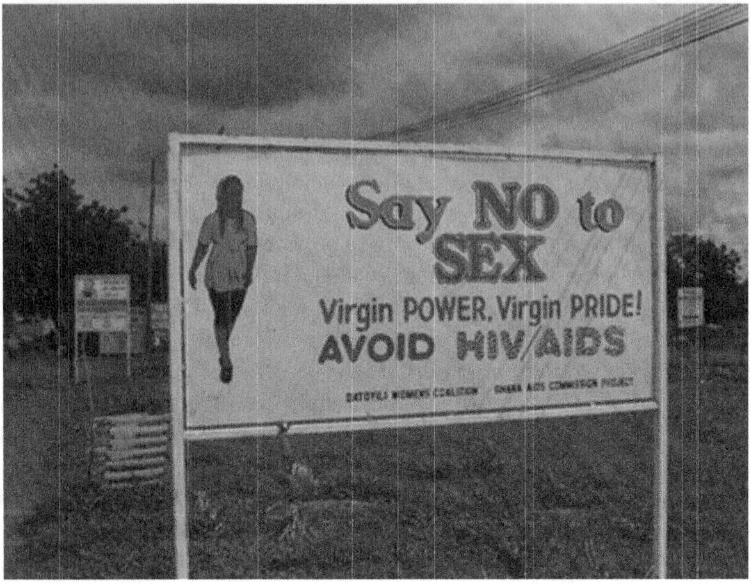
Say NO to
SEX
Virgin POWER, Virgin PRIDE!
AVOID HIV/AIDS

Fig. 8.1 An abstinence HIV/AIDS educational billboard by the road

Thus, the youth has been identified as a high risk group with HIV infection by different bodies and authors for reasons such as youth being a period of exploration, acquisition of identities, forming habits, taking risks and many more (see also Tonks 1996; Rivers and Aggleton 1999; De waal 2002; UNFPA 2009). In this regard, Ghana like many other countries, has been proactive in guarding against infection from HIV with the establishment of the Ghana AIDS Commission (GAC) in 2000 under the chairmanship of the country's President. The Commission has an oversight responsibility to co-ordinate all HIV/AIDS related activities in the country including setting targets for reducing new infections, addressing service delivery issues and individual and societal vulnerability, as well as the promotion and establishment of a multisectoral and multidisciplinary approach to HIV/AIDS control. The Commission has, therefore, been embarking on intensive health promotion and educational programs at both the formal and informal levels through mediums such as school curricula and the media among others. It is, therefore, common to come across huge billboards and other preventive educational messages by major roads and at border towns in Ghana as reflected below (Figs. 8.1 and 8.2).

Within this socio-cultural context, this chapter seeks to explore how Ghanaian youth who have been the main target of educational programs interpret the education in terms of their perception of risk and vulnerability to HIV/AIDS. The chapter further examines how the youth construct the HIV/AIDS phenomenon, their assignment of causes and consequences to HIV/AIDS infection as well as reactions and relationship with infected and affected people.

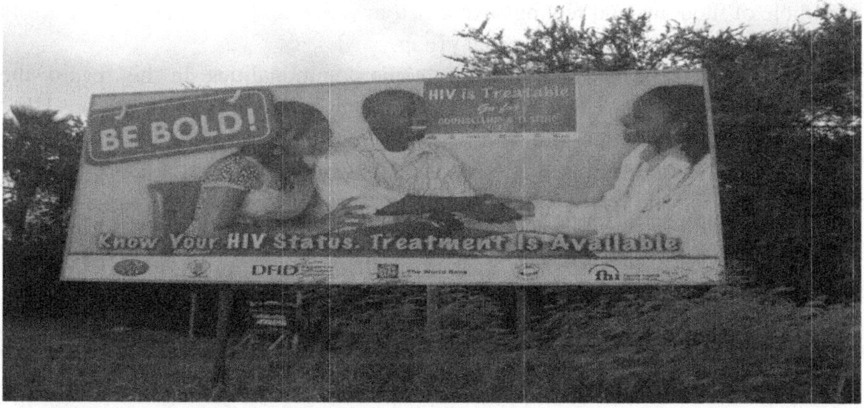

Fig. 8.2 Educational message on HIV/AIDS testing

8.3 Situating the Chapter: A Look at the Social Construction and Social Representation Theories

The chapter draws on social construction and social representation theories. Social construction is a theory of knowledge that considers how social phenomena or objects of consciousness develop in social contexts. It is often contextually defined because what determines an object or belief varies from one society to another, and even within a culture different people may likely have different notions about similar objects or issues. Social constructionism is the product of a group or society and reflects what society tells us, appreciates, upholds and accepts (Burr 2003). Thus, it is contingent on particular societies and thrives of relativities. For Berger and Luckmann (1991), knowledge is created by the interactions of individuals within society which is central to constructionism as propounded by Schwandt (2000). Social constructionism places great emphasis on everyday interactions between people and how they use language to construct their reality. It regards the social practices engaged in by people as the focus of enquiry.

Whereas social constructionism is more tilted towards the sociological perspective, social representation is more psychological in nature. Social representation is a social psychological framework used to examine concepts and ideas of societies. The theory maintains that social psychological phenomena and processes can only be properly understood if they are embedded in historical, cultural and macro social conditions. According to Moscovici (1963), social representation is a collective elaboration of a social object by the community for the purpose of behaving and communicating, such that the elaborated object becomes a social reality by virtue of the object's representation to the community. Thus, the social representation theory brings to life, the renowned sociologist, Emile Durkheim's concept of collective consciousness (Durkheim [1893] 1960). In brief, social representation is an ensemble of thoughts and feelings expressed in verbal and overt behavior of actors which constitute an object for a social group.

It is clear that the two theories have some commonalities. In this regard, the chapter will look at how Ghanaian young people make meaning of the various HIV/AIDS educational programs prevailing in the Ghanaian socio-cultural contexts from a constructionist and representational perspectives, for as Kunda (2008) argues, images, language and constructions are the products of familiar environments.

8.4 The Study

The chapter is informed by data derived from a larger study on gender relations, sexuality and HIV/AIDS education among Ghanaian youth. Data was collected over a period of 6 months in Ghana in 2008 and hence the possibility of having some views of participants changed over the last 6 years. Data was collected through creative participatory and interactive methods such as drawings, essays, focus group discussions and in-depth individual interviews (see Greene and Hill 2005; Swartz 2007; Leach 2006; Oduro 2010) from 104 young people between the ages of 14 and 19 years in a sequential manner. The essays and drawings were first held with all the participants, thereafter few of them were recruited for the focus group discussions and interviews respectively.

A combination of purposive, convenience and snowball sampling techniques were employed to recruit participants. Eighty participants were drawn from two Junior high schools from a town in Ghana's central region while the remaining 24 participants were drawn from the streets of Ghana's capital town – Accra, thus both school and street youth were involved in the study. Study questions focused on general knowledge and sources of knowledge about HIV/AIDS, perceptions and constructions about the phenomenon, notions of risk and vulnerability towards HIV/AIDS, reactions and relationship to infected and affected people, concepts of Ghanaian identity, gender roles and identities, sexual engagements and sexual pleasure as well as notions of safe and risky sex among others.

As a highly sensitive study, ethical issues were observed from the start with clearance sought from the University Faculty that housed the study and the Ghana Education Service. To ensure anonymity, pseudonyms were used to describe study participants. Participants were also voluntarily recruited without any coercion while their consents were secured, debriefing sessions were held with each participant after an activity.

Both manual and computer assisted methods were used to analyze the data. The voice data from the focus group discussions and interviews which were audio recorded were translated from the local language (Fante), transcribed and analyzed into categories, themes and patterns with the support of Nvivo 8 software while the essays were manually analyzed basing on Miles and Huberman's analytical framework (1994). The inductive approach was manually used to analyze the data from the drawings guided by Anning and Ring's framework (2004) which pays attention to the contents of the drawings rather than technical details such as lines etcetera. Utilizing that approach, the drawings were categorized into three thematic areas of 'equipments and objects', 'human beings' and 'viruses and insects or biological things'.

8.5 Young People's Constructions and Representations of HIV/AIDS

Drawing on social construction and representation theories, the youth in this study defined HIV/AIDS with sexual promiscuity, body size or physical symptoms, sharp objects, and poverty. They saw the disease as both a physical and social phenomenon. Physically, some represented HIV/AIDS by its symptoms and death. Some participants presented the disease very visually through their drawings and descriptions of emaciated and sickly looking people. Two young people, Sonia and Jamila, commented as follows:

> When one get infected with HIV, s/he can get shingles, 'ananse' and the hair can also break and drop off as the person grow *lean*. (Sonia, 15 years, school girl).
>
> ... at times one will have headache, feel pains in the head, stomach, and all over the body, you will become weak, vomit and grow *lean*. (Jamila, 16 years, school girl).

Lizzie, a 19 year old girl who lived on the streets of Accra, echoed the above perceptions as:

> When you get AIDS, you will not know because at first, you will be big but later you will grow so *lean* that people will become afraid of you. I heard they can even count your ribs.

The association between HIV/AIDS and leanness was shared by many of the young people, boys and girls as well as school and street youth. In young people's drawings was a high presence not only of leanness but also skin rashes, as illustrated in drawings in Fig. 8.3.

Figure 8.3 represent a woman with rashes and the HIV virus with the writing 'female, she has skin disease'. The drawing also indicates that AIDS is caused by a virus. Some young people were also of the view that infection with HIV/AIDS could result in a person being bedridden. Data from essays and interview also represented young people's constructs of the disease as shown in Table 8.1.

The impact of school education becomes clear as we compare the quality of data and level of the knowledge from the school and street youth. All the examples from the school youth are true while that of the street youth are wrong since having sex only once can lead to HIV infection (Ghana AIDS Commission 2014; UNAIDS 2013), and healthy looking people can also carry the virus. It is not surprising that the street youth seem to exhibit more gaps and misconceptions in their knowledge about the disease, for as MOWAC/UNICEF (2009: 155) argue, "children who are not in school and who lack parental guidance do not receive exposure to reliable information about the disease and how to prevent it".

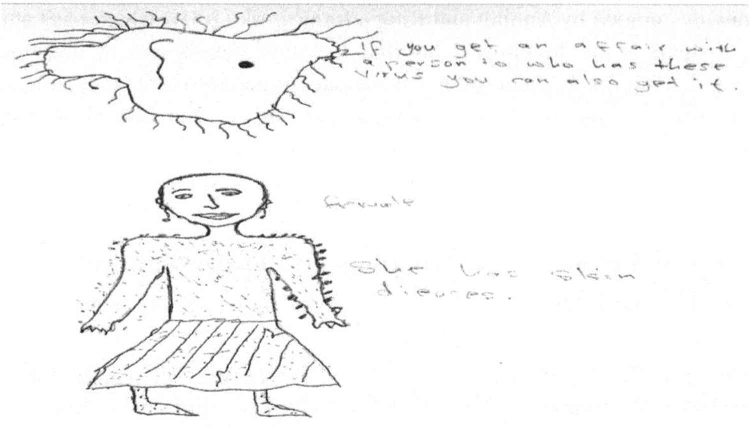
If you get an affair with a person is who has these virus you can also get it.
female
She has skin dieuses.

Fig. 8.3 An infected woman with rashes or skin disease

Table 8.1 Representations of HIV/AIDS by school and street youth

School youth	Street youth
Some people look big but they have AIDS. When you get the disease, you grow slim, then fat, and then slim again. It's on and off (Ahmed, 17 years, *Obinnim* school)	Me, I heard that you **cannot** get AIDS if you have sex only once (Tina, 14 years, street girl)
The truth is everybody is susceptible to AIDS, whether rich, poor, young or old. However, some poor people get more infection because they engage in prostitution (Moses, 15 years, *Adom* school)	Only slim people have AIDS, I mean the *chengelenge* (lean and emaciated) people (Cilla, 14 years, street girl)
HIV/AIDS is a *dangerous disease*, when you get it you will grow lean, weak and die (essay data from a school girl)	Some people steal and when they are cursed, they get AIDS. (Blakie, 18 years, street boy)
It is a *serious and wicked disease* which kill people easily (essay data from a school boy)	

Emerging strongly from the voices of the young people involved in this study was the view that HIV/AIDS was not only a physical disease but also a social phenomenon with huge ramifications. Socially, they saw HIV/AIDS as dangerous and fearful, as well as shameful and stigmatizing. In their view, the disease evokes emotions such as horror, helplessness and powerlessness in infected and affected people. To them, the powerlessness and helplessness associated with HIV/AIDS does not only affect the HIV-positive individuals but also their relatives, hence the concept of infected and affected people. The social construction of the disease reflects Xiapei He's (n.d.) assertion that,

> AIDS is not only a physical disease that destroys the human immune system and takes people's lives. AIDS as a cultural construction has also become a "social virus" that generates fear and discrimination and hampers efforts to prevent and treat the disease itself.

In general, participants perceived AIDS as a very complex phenomenon that could not be described in one word. For some, AIDS was 'bad', 'dangerous' and 'serious', not merely because it kills, but also because of the painful and deteriorating stages that the persons go through before they die. An *Akan* (refers to the majority ethnic group in Ghana, Akan is also a language) expression used in one of the essays may be used to sum up the perception of the young people: "*AIDS ye yariba bon*" [*AIDS is a bad disease*]. The mystery and fear associated with HIV/AIDS, according to Amuyunzu-Nyamongo et al. (1999: 7), relates to the variability, undefined nature and the characteristic wasting that it puts HIV/AIDS individuals through, which defies simple human understanding. The constructs and representations of HIV/AIDS by the youth also entrench stigma and discrimination (Oduro and Otsin 2013).

Another theme on representation and construction that emerged in the study relates to HIV/AIDS and poverty.[4] According to the participants, HIV/AIDS has a strong relationship with poverty. As young people from lower socio-economic contexts themselves, many were aware of how poverty could serve as a barrier to sexual abstinence and/or the practice of safe sex. According to Awusabo-Asare et al. (1999) and Anarfi (1999), most young people in poverty, especially street youth, trade sex for survival irrespective of the associated risks (see also Chap. 9 in this volume). Amuyunzu-Nyamongo et al. (1999) and De Waal (2002) have also identified poverty as a major problem for young people who have much time on their hands, and who are inclined to undertake early and risky sexual exploits. Furthermore, the high prevalence of HIV/AIDS recorded in many third world and African countries reflect the role of poverty in the spread of the disease (Radstake 2000; Campbell 2003; Bhana 2008). The poverty stance is reflected in Hope 's argument (1999: 3)[5] that:

> without a doubt, poverty and economic distress in African countries have contributed greatly to the spread of HIV and AIDS. Africa remains one of the poorest regions in the world ... poor people who contract HIV tend to develop AIDS much faster than individuals of higher socio-economic status.

While some youth argued that poverty sometimes forces people into transactional sex, others constructed AIDS as an expensive disease which drains people of money. In the words of a school youth, Sonia: "*When the poor get the disease, they are not able to manage it because they have no money for medicine and good food*". Another girl added: "*It can let you spend all your money on drugs after that you will not live longer and you can die anytime*". From this bleak scenario, it can be concluded that poverty exacerbates HIV/AIDS.

---

[4] The theme on HIV/AIDS and sex will be discussed later in the chapter. Although Ghana is described as a lower middle-income country, reality on the ground reveals a high level of poverty (although poverty is relative) with majority of Ghanaians unable to enjoy more than $2.00 a day. Majority of the workforce are in subsistence farming and trading with many children suffering from poverty, vulnerability and exclusion especially street children and other marginalized groups (MOWAC/UNICEF 2009).

[5] Hope's (1999) paper tries to establish the context of the African AIDS problem from economic, infrastructural, socio-cultural, political and human resources cost of the disease to the continent.

Furthermore, young people, particularly the school youth, demonstrated their perceptions of HIV/AIDS through drawings of some ordinary everyday objects which could predispose them to danger by contributing to infection with HIV/AIDS. Below, I discuss their representation of risk and vulnerability to sharp objects.

8.6 Causes, Consequences and Vulnerability to HIV/AIDS: Objects as Embodied Danger

The use of symbolic accounts and images in research projects with children and young people is gaining prominence for various reasons (see Pattman and Chege 2003; Greene and Hill 2005; Dillabough and Kennelly 2010; Oduro and Otsin 2013). Such imagery represents and expresses the account giver's meaning-making processes and contexts through 'unspoken words'. Young people in my study had learnt that they could acquire HIV/AIDS through piercing by sharp objects. In response to the causes and concepts of risk and vulnerability by the youth in this study, they reported feeling threatened by common everyday objects such as toothbrushes and blades used for sharpening pencils or cutting fingernails. They found anything that could lead to cuts, or the transfer of blood and other bodily fluids, risky. This was clearly reflected in the drawing of objects such as blade (42),[6] scissors (5), needle (5), knife (2), syringe (2), car (1) and toothbrush (18) (Fig. 8.4).

Young people identified the toothbrush as a common mode of infection with HIV/AIDS, as reflected in Fig. 8.5. While this might sound strange to people from

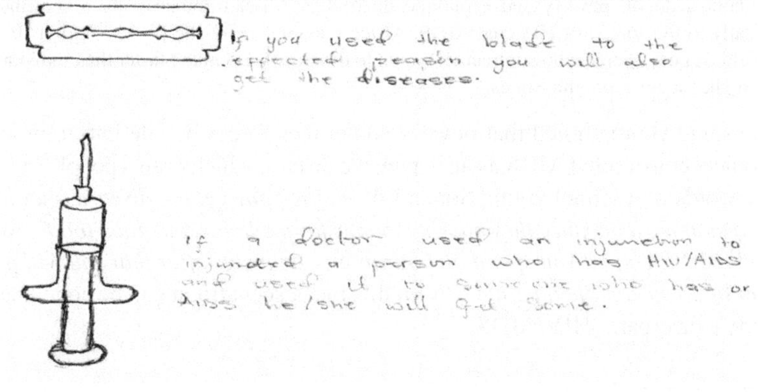

Fig. 8.4 Drawing of blade and syringe with a cautionary message. While the emphasis on the sharing of blade and toothbrush may seem odd in a western context, it is reflective of the study context, where poverty and large family sizes sometimes cause people to share blades to cut fingernails or sharpen pencils in school and sometimes share the same toothbrush among siblings

[6] 42 people drew blade in that order.

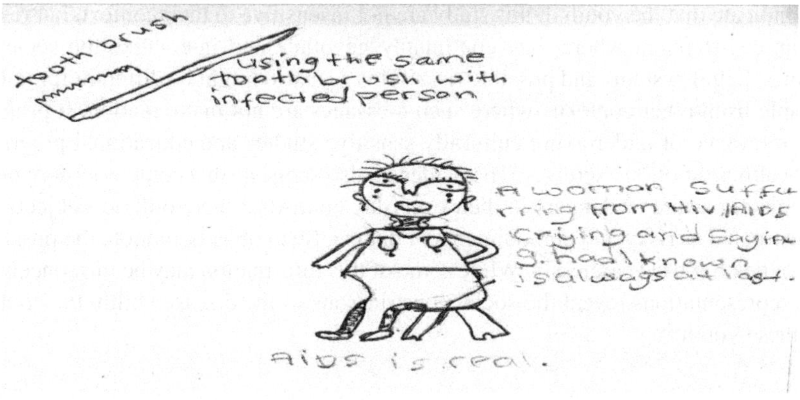
tooth brush
using the same
tooth brush with
infected person
A woman suffe
rring from HIV/AIDS
crying and sayin
g. had known
is always at last.
AIDS is real.

Fig. 8.5 Toothbrush and an infected woman

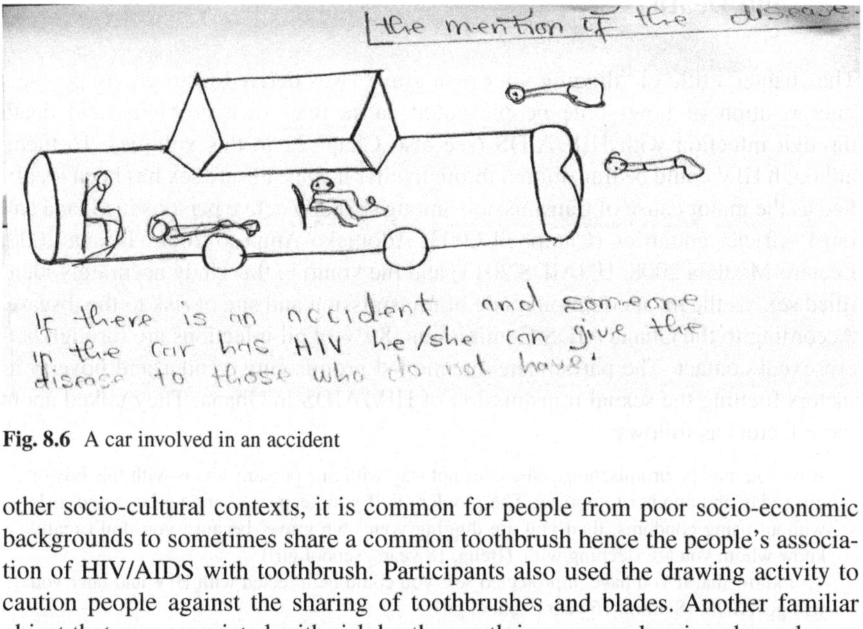

Fig. 8.6 A car involved in an accident

other socio-cultural contexts, it is common for people from poor socio-economic backgrounds to sometimes share a common toothbrush hence the people's association of HIV/AIDS with toothbrush. Participants also used the drawing activity to caution people against the sharing of toothbrushes and blades. Another familiar object that was associated with risk by the youth is car; one drawing showed a car involved in an accident (Fig. 8.6). The caption explained that, "if there is an accident and someone in the car has HIV he/she can give the disease to those who do not have it". This message implied the danger of accidental infections and the possibility of non-sexual infection, particularly through blood contamination.

The depiction of sharp objects and car accidents as possible means of catching HIV/AIDS reflects Bhana's (2008) concept of HIV/AIDS as a 'catchy' disease that invokes fear of blood and contagion. Kunda (2008: 108) argues that images do not exist in a vacuum but are the product of familiar environments. According to Kunda, people pick images that circulate within the public sphere. The representations so far indicate that the youth in this study are not insensitive to their context, but reside in an environment where they continually negotiate and internalize the society's values, belief systems and possible risks. This scenario might be different for young people from other contexts, where such messages are not in circulation. It projects the relevance of undertaking culturally sensitive studies and educational programs in health promotion exercises. The evidence also suggests that contemporary young people are aware of dangers in their everyday contexts, where ordinary objects are constructed as risky and embodiments of danger. Such objects connote the possibility of death if used carelessly. While some of this information may be misconceived, the representations reveal the social constructions of the disease within the context of these youth.

8.7 "Digging Your Own Grave": HIV/AIDS, Heterosexuality and Death

The chapter's title of "digging your own grave" was derived from young people's interpretation of how some people could cause their own problems and death through infection with HIV/AIDS (see also Chap. 22 in this volume). To them, although HIV could be transmitted through other means, unsafe sex has been identified as the major cause of transmission among sexually active persons in Ghana and most African countries (Campbell 2003; Adomako-Ampofo 2006; Bhana 2008; Leclerc-Madlala 2008; UNAIDS 2013) and the youth in this study accurately identified sex[7] as the most common mode of transmission and site of risk to the disease. According to the Ghana AIDS Commission, 80 % of all infections are through heterosexual contact. The participants mentioned promiscuity, gender and poverty as factors fuelling the sexual transmission of HIV/AIDS in Ghana. They talked about these factors as follows:

> A person may be promiscuous, s/he does not stay with one person; s/he is with this boy or girl today and another tomorrow. The problem is if you keep on changing boys and girls without using condoms, then you are digging your own grave[8] because you don't really know whom you are sleeping with. (Bella, 18 years, school girl)
>
> I know that if you have unprotected sex, you could be infected with HIV and later you will get AIDS. (Samira, 16 years, school girl)

Samira's assertion was factual and not just an opinion. Fourteen-year-old Eva added 'deep kissing' to the sexual transmission. Another girl, Anatu, explained the type of sexual transmission as heterosexual by arguing that "*when a man and a woman meet for sex and one has the disease, s/he could easily pass it on to the other*". Beebe, a 16-year-old street girl, corroborated that: "*I am told that sex is one of the commonest means by which one could be infected with AIDS, and it is how the boy and the girl*

[7] The youth used sex and unprotected sex interchangeably in their discussions.

[8] The expression "digging your own grave" refers to death.

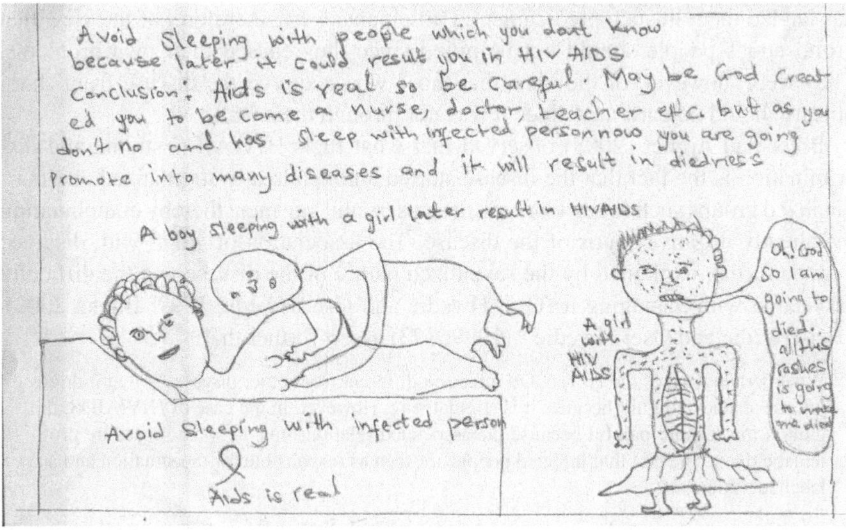

Fig. 8.7 Drawing of a boy and a girl having sex

behave in bed". Although HIV/AIDS was initially represented in America as a gay disease, due to the fact that it mainly affected a cohort of gay men (Tonks 1996; Boler and Archer 2008), UNAIDS (2013) has established its heterosexual nature, particularly in Africa. Ghana is no exception. According to UNAIDS (2013), 85% of HIV/AIDS infections in Africa are heterosexual in nature. A 17-year-old street boy, Happy, summarized the sexual nature of HIV/AIDS as: "*This whole noise about AIDS is because of sex, no sex no AIDS, but how can one stay away from sex, especially among street youth like us*". Another participant summed it up as: "*As for AIDS, it is only bad people who cannot control themselves and open their pants everywhere who get it*".

Agadzi (1989), Osei-Hwedie and Osei-Hwedie (1999), and Boler and Archer (2008) have all confirmed that the association between sex and HIV/AIDS gives the disease an immoral image, especially where it concerns pre-marital or extra-marital sex. According to Bukuluki et al. (2006), pre-marital sexual[9] activity is culturally perceived as wrong and unacceptable. In most African societies, sex among young people is, therefore, approached from a moralistic rather than a pragmatic position, complicating the image of sex in general and of AIDS in particular. The sexual construction of the disease was captured in one of the drawings as shown in Fig. 8.7.

Generally, most young people expressed no mercy for people infected with HIV/AIDS through sex with the explanation that it is their own fault and promiscuity that

[9] The practice of pre-marital sex and/or sex outside marriage is culturally frowned upon. This assumption also fail to recognize HIV/AIDS infection within marriage although the literature shows that married people are often infected by sex with an unfaithful partner, or infected from other sources (Agadzi 1989; Radstake 2000).

has landed them in such predicament. Participants were, therefore, of the view that promiscuous people should not be pitied since they caused their own problems. They were, however, of the view that those who acquired the disease from sharp objects should be pardoned since it was not through their fault.

Boler and Archer (2008) observed that what fuels HIV/AIDS stigma and discrimination is the fact that the disease started among already stigmatized and marginalized groups such as sex workers, drug users and gay men, thereby compounding the already negative status of the disease. The association of AIDS with disgrace may be further explained by the sexualized nature of the disease and the difficulty associated with managing it (Osei-Hwedie and Osei-Hwedie 1999; Bhana 2008). Osei-Hwedie and Osei-Hwedie[10] (1999: 123) assert further that:

> What perhaps makes the HIV/AIDS infection different from other diseases is that it draws intense shame and guilt because it is stigmatising. However, in the case of HIV/AIDS, the guilt is much more painful because the associated relationships, in some sense, are problematic due to the fact that infected people are seen as responsible for the situation and are labelled as deviant.

According to the youth in my study, HIV/AIDS did not bring shame on the infected individual alone, but to the whole family. Central to this perception was the notion of 'collective responsibility'[11] (Assimeng 1999; Crentsil 2007), which transforms the stigma of infection with HIV/AIDS into a shared responsibility.

Another consequence of infection with HIV/AIDS was death, according to the participants in this study. Death can, however, be viewed as a paradox in many African societies (see Chap. 20). Among some Ghanaians and Nigerians, death is traditionally believed to be pre-ordained and will come when due (Awusabo-Asare et al. 1999; Caldwell et al. 1999; Orubuloye and Oguntimehin 1999). There is an assumption that those who believe in the pre-ordination of death do not take much precaution with their lifestyle even in an era of HIV/AIDS. On the other hand, the concept of *owuo* (the *Akan* version of death) is so fearful to some people that they prefer to use euphemisms to describe it. To such people, death should be avoided at all costs, especially, death from HIV/AIDS. This school of thought believes that people sometimes bring death upon themselves earlier than expected through their own actions and one such action, according to the youth in this study, is infection with HIV/AIDS. Also, traditionally, death from ailments and causes such as leprosy, lunacy, swollen body, ulcers, suicide, accidents and execution were considered dishonorable and affected one's chances of achieving the status of an ancestor[12] (see

---

[10] Bertha and Kweku Osei-Hwedie, in a critical review of the HIV/AIDS situation in Africa, presented a thorough dimension of the problem and its possible policy implications in their paper 'The Social Context of HIV/AIDS policy in Africa'.

[11] A notion which is prevalent in traditional Ghanaian societies and operates on the philosophy that, individuals do not take credit for an offence or an achievement, rather, it is borne by the entire family, lineage or even the clan.

[12] Ancestors occupy an important place in African traditional religion. According to Assimeng (1999) and Nukunya (1992), ancestors rank high in the traditional religious hierarchy, coming after the High God or Supreme Being, Small gods or 'abosom' (Akan version of the lesser gods) and then the ancestors. They are, therefore, revered and belief in their presence are manifested in many

Nukunya 1992; Crentsil 2007). Within this traditional perception is the current image of HIV/AIDS in Ghana.

8.8 Reactions and Relationship to People Infected and Affected by HIV/AIDS

The last section of the chapter discusses the significance of young people's knowledge and construction of HIV/AIDS in their attitudes and reactions to infected and affected persons. Although the presence of antiretroviral therapy (ART) has enabled people living with HIV/AIDS (PLWHA) to live normal and longer (see Chap. 22), some Ghanaians still associate HIV/AIDS with death because of lack of easy access and limited coverage of antiretroviral therapy (ART) in the country[13] (see also Oduro and Otsin 2013). The negative status of HIV/AIDS coupled with the low access to ART continue to deter many people from undertaking voluntary counseling and testing (VCT) for the virus with the argument that knowing one's status could push one to an early death through psychological challenges. Some participants, therefore, expressed how their knowledge of HIV/AIDS would influence their relationship with people living with the virus either positively or negatively. Three different perspectives emerged on this issue, which are:

- Total rejection and/or complete dissociation,
- Compassion or display of support, love and care, and
- A conditional or contingent relationship.

(a) ***Total rejection and/or complete dissociation from HIV/AIDS***

Participants with this perception included Nina, Hoodah, Jamila and Moses, who said they would have nothing to do with people living with HIV/AIDS as argued below:

> No [*shaking the head*], I cannot relate to such persons, I will have nothing to do with them; I won't even try to get close to them. (Nina, 15 years, *Adom* School)
>
> I will not feel comfortable being close to such people, I cannot share anything with them like using the same toilet or eating from same plate, I know I will not get the disease … but me, I will not do it. (Jamila, 16 years, *Obinnim* School)

Like her two colleagues, Hoodah said she would not relate to HIV/AIDS persons unless she was unaware of their infection. Another street boy, Musa, observed: "*The truth is that although the person is my friend, I will be afraid of him, especially,*

forms, such as the putting of the first morsel of food or the first drops of water or drink on the ground and observing their presence during festivals and the celebration of rites of passage.

[13] The Ghana Health Service reported that, as at December 2007, only 13, 429 people out of an estimated 70,000 who needed treatment with ART were on the drug. Although the situation might be different now, I could not obtain an updated data but can be sure that not all infected people have access to the drug. This assertion is based on information from public discussions in the country and similar sources.

when the disease starts manifesting and he starts changing". The above quotes indicate the fear, stigma and discrimination associated with HIV/AIDS even in the presence of ART. This is not surprising because many Ghanaians still do not have access to ART after its introduction in far back 2003. Estimates indicate that only about 58 % of people living with HIV have access to ART in Ghana.[14] Although Jamila and Hoodah were certain that they would not be infected by relating and sharing some common items with infected people, they still would have nothing to do with infected people unless they were unaware of their status. The negative effect of stigma and discrimination associated with HIV/AIDS in Ghana have been recorded in studies by Radstake (2000), Crentsil (2007), Antwi and Oppong (2006), and Oduro and Otsin (2013). Boler and Archer (2008) argue strongly that it was not HIV/AIDS per se that accelerated death, but the stigma, prejudice and discrimination associated with the disease. Antwi and Oppong (2006: 323) add:

> Another challenge is stigmatisation and discrimination against people with HIV/AIDS. The PLWHA[15] have repeatedly reported subtle and sometimes overt discrimination against them at the workplace, and in the community and sometimes by health care workers.

Antwi and Oppong further assert that even some health workers in Ghana discriminate against infected persons. It was, therefore, not surprising that Jamila, Hoodah and Nina hold such strong views.

(b) ***Compassion, or display of support, love and care for HIV-infected people***

Some participants argued that they would respond to infected persons with support, love and care especially, if it emerged that they did not cause the infection. Eva and Anatu belonged to this stream. Eva noted: "*Yes, I will continue to be her friend and give her hope and comfort*". Lizzie, a 19-year-old street girl, remarked: "*Madam, there is a saying that everybody matters, so I cannot shun such a person at her most trying moment*". Anatu, a 14 years school girl, added:

> I will continue to be her friend but will be careful with what I do with her. Some things may expose me to the disease, other things will not. I can sit and converse with her. I can greet her. I will not use the same spoon with her or same sponge and so on. Also my friend has grown very weak and has no one to care for her. I will be there to serve her, to put food in her mouth. I will not neglect her.

While most boys did not express their views on this position, girls responded and were willing to show compassion, which resonates with gender perceptions about girls as caring and emotional beings (Gilligan 1982). Anatu's response was both emotional and practical. She knew her friend might need her most at this point in life and was prepared to be there for her, although with some caution. Could her behavior be the result of the impact of recent education in the country aimed at reducing stigma and discrimination? Antwi and Oppong (2006: 318) observed that

[14] See www.tradingeconomics.com/ghana/antiretroviral-therapy-coveragepercent-of-people-with-advanced-hiv-infection-wb-data.html accessed on Sunday, 11th January, 2015.

[15] It means People living with HIV/AIDS.

in November 2003, an educational campaign dubbed 'Reach out, Show Compassion' was introduced in Ghana to encourage people to show love, understanding and compassion to HIV/AIDS infected people. In 2007, a former first lady of the country urged Ghanaians to be compassionate to people living with AIDS when she delivered the following message:

> ... attempts to reduce the rate of the scourge would only be effective if they are translated into attitudinal change ... it is imperative that everyone get involved towards ensuring that stigmatization becomes a practice of the past ... Stigmatization discourages people from taking HIV/AIDS tests and disclosing their status to their partners ... this results in further spread of the disease, thereby negating our efforts at curtailing its spread. So, if by stigmatization we only worsen the situation, then we must put a stop to it. (Former First Lady, Theresa Kuffour 2007)

Furthermore, the Ghana AIDS Commission has instituted a program known as the 'Heart to Heart' campaign since 2011 to help reduce stigma and discrimination suffered by persons living with HIV/AIDS and help give HIV a human face. The campaign is led by ambassadors who are HIV-positive and on ART treatment. These ambassadors educate and share their experiences through mediums such as television, radio and at social gatherings such as churches and in schools.

(c) ***Conditional or contingent relationship***

This cohort of participants argued that their relationship with people living with HIV/AIDS would be contingent on the person's character, and how they acquired the virus. Abi and Bella, both of *Adom* school, were among this group.

> Some people are already known to be highly immoral, so if such a person gets infected with AIDS, you are not surprised; you know that they got it through sex. Some people too are unfortunate and got the disease through blood transfusion or the like, maybe through sharing of the same blade or injection. (Abi, 19 years).
>
> Maybe she got the disease by mistake for I already know this person to be well-behaved so she will continue to be my friend. (Bella, 18 years)

It was not only the school youth whose relationship would be conditional; for 18-years-old Love, in the risky context of street life, had a similar perception. To her, infection through sex was perceived as negative and immoral, while infection through blood transfusion and other such sources were acceptable, so this would define her relationship with infected and affected persons.

8.9 Conclusion

The chapter has examined how HIV/AIDS is constructed and represented by the Ghanaian youth involved in this study. It further explored where the disease is positioned in their thinking as well as their concepts of risk and vulnerability. Young people constructed the disease both socially and physically. They also showed a paradox where, through drawings and other creative methods, they reported feeling threatened by ordinary objects such as toothbrush, blade, cars and syringes and yet did not feel susceptible to HIV/AIDS through sex, because in their view, it was mostly the sexually promiscuous who are infected with HIV/AIDS. The revelation on vulnerability to everyday object might sound alien to youth from western contexts where people do not share toothbrushes or blades. The discovery, however, fits well with the social constructionist and social representation theories used for the research on cross-cultural perspectives on HIV/AIDS. Participants further defined the consequences of HIV/AIDS in terms of their reactions and relationships with infected and affected persons in terms of showing love or discrimination toward such people. The sexual construction of HIV/AIDS with promiscuous people in this study can be understood from the perspective of the low HIV/AIDS prevalence in Ghana compared to most Southern and Eastern African countries where HIV prevalence is high and HIV-positive persons are easily visible. In fact, some Ghanaians have never seen fully blown AIDS patients outside media and other abstract reportages. For as Antwi and Oppong (2006) argue, many Ghanaians till today have never encountered an HIV/AIDS patient before. What they know are the images from posters, billboards and other media sources shown through educational programs. Many people, therefore, see HIV/AIDS as an abstract disease and do not find themselves susceptible to it.

Additionally, because most Ghanaians have not encountered HIV/AIDS directly, they hold strange and fearful ideas about it with some associated misconceptions. Such misconceptions are, therefore, translated into stigma and discriminatory acts on infected and affected persons. The extreme stigma and discrimination associated with HIV/AIDS in Ghana tends to discourage most people from voluntary counseling and testing (VCT). Although some achievement have been chalked by the Ghana AIDS Commission with the reduction of HIV/AIDS prevalence to the current 0.8 %, there are still challenges, especially in the area of stigma reduction and discrimination. Education on stigma reduction and discrimination stand to suffer with a recent development (on 15 December, 2014) where one of the 'Heart to Heart' ambassadors[16] in the country revealed that she was not actually infected with HIV/AIDS although she has been parading herself over the years as an infected person for health promotion and stigma reduction reasons. This development has been taken very seriously by Ghanaians for public deception with possible negative repercussion on infected and affected persons. The ambassador explained her action for

[16] See http://ghanaaids.gov.gh/gac1/pubs/RESPONSE_TO_JOYCE_MENSAHS.pdf (Accessed 5/01/ 2015).

coming out publicly to deny her positive status as a result of the negative stigma and discrimination suffered by her two children in school and by the public. This situation poses great challenge for the country's stigma reduction efforts. Findings from the study also has policy implication, in the area of HIV/AIDS education and emphasis. Lastly, the chapter has revealed the essence of creative, child/youth sensitive methods, voice-centered and culturally sensitive methodology in research studies.

Acknowledgement I wish to thank the managers of the RECOUP studentship which enabled this study, as well as my supervisors, Prof. Madeleine Arnot and Prof. Colleen McLaughlin of the University of Cambridge, UK for their inputs.

References

Adomako-Ampofo, A. (2006). Intimate bargains: Sex workers and free women negotiate their sexual space. In C. Oppong, M. A. P. A. Oppong, & I. K. Odotei (Eds.), *Sex and gender in an era of AIDS: Ghana at the turn of the millennium* (pp. 137–168). Legon: Sub-Saharan Publishers.

Agadzi, V. K. (1989). *AIDS: The African perspective of the killer disease*. Accra: Ghana Universities Press.

Amuyunzu-Nyamongo, M., Tendo-Wambua, L., Babishangire, B., Nyagero, J., Yitbarek, N., Matasha, M., et al. (1999). Barriers to behaviour change as a response to STD including HIV/AIDS: The East African experience. In J. C. Caldwell, P. Caldwell, J. Anarfi, K. Awusabo-Asare, J. Ntozi, I. O. Orubuloye, et al. (Eds.), *Resistances to behavioural change to reduce HIV/AIDS infection in predominantly heterosexual epidemics in third world countries* (pp. 1–12). Canberra: Health Transition Centre.

Anarfi, J. K. (1999). Initiating behavioural change among street-involved youth: Findings from a youth clinic in Accra. In J. C. Caldwell, P. Caldwell, J. Anarfi, K. Awusabo-Asare, J. Ntozi, I. O. Orubuloye, et al. (Eds.), *Resistances to behavioural change to reduce HIV/AIDS infection in predominantly heterosexual epidemics in third world countries* (pp. 81–90). Canberra: Health Transition Centre.

Anning, A., & Ring, K. (2004). *Making sense of children's drawings*. Maidenhead: Open University Press.

Antwi, P. M., & Oppong, Y. P. A. (2006). Ghana's attempts at managing the HIV/AIDS epidemic: A review of efforts. In C. Oppong, M. A. P. A. Oppong, & I. K. Odotei (Eds.), *Sex and gender in an era of AIDS: Ghana at the turn of the millennium* (pp. 303–331). Legon: Sub-Saharan Publishers.

Assimeng, J. M. (1999). *Social structure of Ghana: A study of persistence and change*. Tema: Ghana Publishing Corporation.

Awusabo-Asare, K., Abane, A. M., Badasu, D. M., & Anarfi, J. K. (1999). 'All die be die': Obstacles to change in the face of HIV infection in Ghana. In J. C. Caldwell, P. Caldwell, J. Anarfi, K. Awusabo-Asare, J. Ntozi, I. O. Orubuloye, et al. (Eds.), *Resistances to behavioural change to reduce HIV/AIDS infection in predominantly heterosexual epidemics in third world countries* (pp. 125–132). Canberra: Health Transition Centre.

Badasu, D. (2004). Child care among ewe migrants in Accra: Cases of crisis. *Research Review Supplement, 16*, 17–28.

Berger, P., & Luckmann, T. (1991). *The social construction of reality*. London: Penguin Books.

Bhana, D. (2008). Beyond stigma? Young children's responses to HIV and AIDS. *Culture, Health & Sexuality, 10*(7), 725–738.

Boler, T., & Archer, D. (2008). *The politics of prevention: A global crisis in AIDS and education*. London: Actionaid, Pluto Press.

Bukuluki, P., Walakira, E., Sengendo, J., & Mugumya, F. (2006). Caught in the fear of pregnancy and HIV infection: A dilemma for youth in Jinja, Uganda. In A. Pertet (Ed.), *Re-thinking research and intervention approaches that aim at preventing HIV infection among the youth*. Nairobi: SOMA-Net, The Regal Press Kenya Ltd.

Burr, V. (2003). *Social constructionism* (2nd ed.). London: Routledge.

Caldwell, J. C., Orubuloye, I. O., & Caldwell, P. (1999). Obstacles to behavioural change to lessen the risk of HIV infection in the African AIDS epidemic: Nigerian research. In J. Caldwell, C. P. Caldwell, J. Anarfi, K. Awusabo-Asare, J. Ntozi, I. O. Orubuloye, et al. (Eds.), *Resistances to behavioural change to reduce HIV/AIDS infection in predominantly heterosexual epidemics in third world countries* (pp. 223–232). Canberra: Health Transition Centre.

Campbell, C. (2003). *'Letting them die': Why HIV/AIDS intervention programmes fail*. Bloomington: Indiana University Press.

Crentsil, P. (2007). *Death, ancestors and HIV/AIDS among the Akans of Ghana* (Research Series in Anthropology). Helsinki: Helsinki University Press.

De Waal, A. (2002). HIV/AIDS and young Africans. In A. De Waal & N. Argenti (Eds.), *Young Africa: Realising the rights of children and youth*. Trenton: Justice Africa -Africa World Press.

Dillabough, J., & Kennelly, J. (2010). *Lost youth in the global city: Class, culture and the urban imaginary*. New York: Routledge, Taylor and Francis Group.

Durkheim, E. (1893, 1960). *The division of labour in society*. (G. Simpson, Trans). New York: Free Press.

Ghana AIDS Commission/National AIDS Control Program. (2014). *HIV sentinel survey 2013 report*. Accra: Ghana Health Service, WHO, World Bank.

Gilligan, C. (1982). *In a different voice: Psychological theory and women's development*. Cambridge, MA: Harvard University Press.

Greene, S., & Hill, M. (2005). Researching children's experience: Methods and methodological issues. In S. Greene & D. Hogan (Eds.), *Researching children's experience: Approaches and method* (pp. 1–21). London: Sage.

Gupta, G. R. (2000). Gender, sexuality, and HIV/AIDS: The what, the why, and the how. *Canadian HIV/AIDS Policy Law Review, 5*(4), 86–93.

He, X. (n.d). *Construction and marginalisation of AIDS as a 'social virus' in China*. Available at http://www.wagnet.ox.ac.uk/eacs/abstracts/xhe.doc. Accessed 6 June 2013.

Hope, K. R., Sr. (Ed.). (1999). *AIDS and development in Africa: A social science perspective*. New York: The Haworth Press.

Kuffour, T. (2007). First Lady speaks against stigmatization in fight against AIDS, News item. *Ghana News Agency*, (25/05/2007). Available at http://www.modernghana.com/news-thread1/136548/4/. Accessed 24 Feb 2010.

Kunda, J. E. L. (2008). *'They have ears but cannot hear': Listening and talking as HIV prevention: A new approach to HIV and AIDS campaigns at three of the universities in KwaZulu Natal*. Unpublished PhD thesis, Faculty of Humanities, Development and Social Sciences, University of KwaZulu-Natal, Durban, South Africa.

Leach, F. (2006). Researching gender violence in schools: Methodological and ethical considerations. *World Development, 34*(6), 1129–1147.

Leclerc-Madlala, S. (2008). Age-disparate and intergenerational sex in Southern Africa: The dynamics of hypervulnerability. *AIDS, 22*(Suppl. 4), S17–S25.

Miles, M. B., & Huberman, A. M. (1994). *Qualitative data analysis: An expanded sourcebook* (2nd ed.). London: Sage.

Moscovici, S. (1963). Attitudes and opinions. *Annual Review of Psychology, 14*, 231–260.

MOWAC/UNICEF (Ministry of Women and Children's Affairs/UNICEF). (2009). *Children in Ghana*. Accra: UNICEF.

Nukunya, G. K. (1992). *Tradition and change in Ghana: An introduction to aociology*. Accra: Ghana Universities Press.

Oduro, G. Y. (2010). *Gender relations, sexuality and HIV/AIDS education: A study of Ghanaian youth cultures*. Unpublished PhD thesis, Faculty of Education, University of Cambridge, UK.
Oduro, G. Y., & Otsin, M. N. A. (2013). Perspectives on HIV/AIDS stigma and discrimination: voices of some Ghanaian young people in Ghana. *Sex Education: Sexuality, Society and Learning, 13*(2), 146–158.
Orubuloye, I. O., & Oguntimehin, F. (1999). Death is pre-ordained, it will come when due: Attitudes of men to death in the presence of AIDS in Nigeria. In J. C. Caldwell, P. Caldwell, J. Anarfi, K. Awusabo-Asare, J. Ntozi, I. O. Orubuloye, et al. (Eds.), *Resistances to behavioural change to reduce HIV/AIDS infection in predominantly heterosexual epidemics in third world countries* (pp. 101–112). Canberra: Health Transition Centre.
Osei-Hwedie, B. Z., & Osei-Hwedie, K. (1999). The social context of HIV/AIDS policy in Africa. In K. R. Hope Sr. (Ed.), *AIDS and development in Africa: A social science perspective* (pp. 121–133). New York: The Haworth Press.
Pattman, R., & Chege, F. (2003). *Finding our voices: Gendered and sexual identities and HIV/AIDS education*. Nairobi: UNICEF Eastern & Southern Africa Regional Office.
Radstake, M. (2000). *Secrecy and ambiguity: Home care for people living with HIV/AIDS in Ghana* (African studies centre research report 59/2000). Enchede: Print Partners Ipskamp B.V.
Rivers, K., & Aggleton, P. (1999). *Adolescent sexuality: Gender and the HIV epidemic*. UNDP Development Programme, HIV and Development Programme. Thomas Coram Research Unit, Institute of Education, University of London. Available at http://www.pwhce.ca/hivaids/scenario2/Gender_and_the_HIV_Epidemic.pdf. Accessed 27 Mar 2010.
Schwandt, T. A. (2000). Constructivist, interpretivist approaches to human inquiry. In N. K. Denzin & Y. S. Lincoln (Eds.), *Handbook of qualitative research* (pp. 118–137). Newbury Park: Sage.
Swartz, S. (2007). *The moral ecology of South Africa's township youth*. Unpublished PhD thesis, Faculty of Education, University of Cambridge, Cambridge.
Tonks, D. (1996). *Teaching AIDS*. New York: Routledge.
UNAIDS. (2013). *Report on global AIDS epidemic*. Geneva: UNAIDS. Available at http://www.unaids.org/en/datanalysis/knowyourepidemic. Accessed 8 Nov 2014.
UNFPA. (2009). *Preventing HIV/AIDS: Young people: The greatest hope for turning the tide*. Available at http://www.unfpa.org/hiv/people.htm. Accessed 3 Apr 2014.

Chapter 9
HIV/AIDS Knowledge and Risk of HIV/AIDS Among Youth in South Africa

Sylvia Niele and Pranee Liamputtong

Contents

S. Niele (✉)
Clinical Psychologist & Independent Researcher,
P O Box 633, Black Rock, VIC 3193, Australia
e-mail: sniele@ozemail.com.au

P. Liamputtong
School of Science and Health, Western Sydney University, Penrith 2751, NSW, Australia
e-mail: p.liamputtong@westernsydney.edu.au

P. Liamputtong (ed.), *Children and Young People Living with HIV/AIDS*,
Cross-Cultural Research in Health, Illness and Well-Being,
DOI 10.1007/978-3-319-29936-5_9

9.1 Introduction

Human Immunodeficiency Virus is a retrovirus that eventually causes Acquired Immunodeficiency Syndrome (AIDS), the stage in which there is a severe loss of the body's cellular immunity, and without antiretroviral (ARV) treatment, inevitable death. At the end of 2013, 35 million people globally were living with HIV with the greatest proportion (24.7 million) in Sub-Saharan Africa, with 67 % of men and 57 % of women living with HIV, not receiving antiretroviral therapy (UNAIDS 2014). An additional consideration is that defaulting on the ARV regimen, risks drug resistant strains of HIV being spread (Kallings 2008). Consequently those with HIV or AIDS experience considerable suffering with over 3000 people dying daily in Sub-Saharan Africa (UNAIDS 2014), and this affects the most productive in society, those aged 15–49 years, and the AIDS epidemic is the leading cause of death in South Africa (UNAIDS 2014) with an estimated 2.5 million South African children as at 2012 being orphaned by HIV/AIDS (UNICEF 2013).

HIV/AIDS continues to be perceived as a devastating and debilitating illness in developing countries, and South Africa has encountered additional risks affiliated with this disease. For example, HIV/AIDS is associated with increased risk of suicide in South Africa (Govender and Schlebusch 2012; Schlebusch and Govender 2012), and in KwaZulu-Natal, the region with the highest HIV/AIDS prevalence (UNGASS 2012), the occurrence of suicidal ideation in HIV-positive individuals was 25.4 % (Bertolote et al. 2009). Even pregnancy is not protective against suicidal thoughts (Rochat et al. 2013). Because HIV/AIDS continues to represent a serious threat to public health in South Africa, and particularly younger people, greater empirical understanding of the drivers of the epidemic is urgently needed.

9.2 Factors Undermining Prevention and Treatment of HIV/AIDS in South Africa

A number of factors have been proposed which may have hampered South Africa's response to the HIV/AIDS epidemic. The South African government has been widely criticized (Nattrass 2004) for initial denial of the link between HIV and AIDS, and an early ban on life-extending ARV treatment believing it to be toxic (Tomaselli 2009). This delay was estimated to have cost 330,000 lives (Abdool Karim et al. 2009) and may partially explain low uptake of ARV treatment (Adam and Johnson 2009).

Globally, proposed factors undermining HIV/AIDS prevention include a resistance to behavior change and beliefs regarding gender, sexuality, and culture (Coates et al. 2008). In South Africa, popular patriarchal notions of masculinity encourage men to have multiple wives and sexual partners, engage in frequent intercourse, emphasize procreation, and discourage sexual abstinence and condom use (Jordaan 2005; Simpson 2009), with women having little power to negotiate safe sex. In addition, extremely high rates of rape and violence, with one in three South African women reporting being raped in their lifetime (Moffett 2006) differentiates Western and South African cultures, and increases the risk of HIV transmission as condom use is unlikely.

Other pivotal practices which have been linked to HIV spread include transactional sex and the Virgin Myth. Transactional sex, where sex is exchanged for cash or material goods, is prevalent in South Africa. A cross-sectional study in Soweto found the practice was associated with violence, socio-economic disadvantage, and substance use, shaping women's behavior and their risk for HIV (Dunkle et al. 2004). A cluster randomized control trial in the Eastern Cape also found transactional sex increased young women's HIV risk (Jewkes et al. 2012). The Virgin Myth, where sexual intercourse with a young girl is believed to cure HIV/AIDS, is considered responsible for child rape increases and HIV spread amongst children in South Africa (Meel 2003; Ndlovu 2005). Structural inequities in South Africa have also been proposed to contribute towards, and exacerbate, HIV transmission by necessitating practices such as transactional sex (Jewkes et al. 2012) and with unemployment in South African townships estimated at 75 % (Stokes 2007), poverty, and transactional sex, may be increasing HIV risk. See also Chaps. 4, 7, and 15 in this volume.

9.3 Cultural Practices and HIV/AIDS

Few studies have explored the link between specific African cultural practices and HIV/AIDS. An anthropological study by Mchunu (2005) revealed that 'respect' in Zulu culture prohibited children discussing sexual matters with their parents. Mchunu also suggested that apartheid necessitated Zulu men to work in cities, and that the cultural practice of 'cleansing', sex with another woman to avoid bringing witchcraft back to their wives, may be proliferating the virus. Similar to Zulus, Xhosa culture is purported to consider HIV/AIDS a curse from the ancestors (Barr 2008). Circumcision is a common ritual in South Africa, usually amongst adolescents already sexually active, and may spread HIV if the same traditional knife is used (Peltzer et al. 2008). Consequently, numerous randomized control trials are promoting that earlier medical circumcision could reduce HIV transmission (Auvert et al. 2005; Bailey et al. 2007; Gray et al. 2007). If such factors are contributing to HIV spread, culturally sensitive HIV/AIDS interventions are needed (Teitelman et al. 2009), therefore more research exploring possible links between South African cultural beliefs and practices and HIV/AIDS is urgently required.

9.4 South African Street Youth and Risk for HIV/AIDS

A subgroup identified at particularly high risk for HIV/AIDS in South Africa are street youth who are generally aged between 11 and 17 years (Kruger and Richter 2003). The street youth population is considered to be increasing due to the familial impact of AIDS reducing the number of caregivers, and due to their homelessness, exact prevalence of street youth can only be estimated (Ward and Seager 2010). Based on a report by outreach workers in contact with street youth in Zimbabwe (Dube 1997), and a qualitative study with South African street youth (Richter and Swart-Kruger 1995), increased risks for contracting HIV have been suggested. These included, earlier sexual activity, engagement in consensual or survival sex, rare use or misconceptions regarding condom effectiveness, a high incidence of sexually transmitted diseases (STDs), and substance use. There also appears to be a lack of knowledge amongst street youth regarding HIV/AIDS and how it is spread (Bryan et al. 2006; Kruger and Richter 2003; Mufune 2000; Snell 2003) with a study of male street youth in Ethiopia suggesting day-to-day survival concerns were considered more pressing than the problem of HIV/AIDS (Tadele 2003). It is important to understand whether access to information and education regarding HIV/AIDS could play a significant role in addressing knowledge gaps and misconceptions amongst street youth.

9.5 The Study

The study on which this chapter is based investigated the knowledge, attitudes and cultural beliefs of South African street youth with respect to HIV/AIDS transmission, sequelae and treatments to address the significant current gaps in the literature. We utilized a qualitative semi-structured interview framework to: (1) ascertain current knowledge regarding HIV/AIDS in street youth in South Africa; (2) ascertain if participants consider HIV and AIDS to be linked; (3) ascertain cultural beliefs associated with HIV/AIDS; (4) further explore street youth attitudes towards HIV/AIDS; and (5) determine the part stigma plays in HIV/AIDS prevention and treatment behaviors. In addition, implications for HIV/AIDS prevention and treatment behaviors in South Africa were considered in respect of both the community generally and street youth in particular.

The final sample consisted of seven female and seven male street youth (n = 14) and one female and three male staff members (n = 4), aged 15–34 working or residing at Umthombo, a non-profit street youth shelter (See Results for details). An additional participant did not complete the entire interview, and his data was subsequently excluded from analysis.

The research was conducted at Umthombo, a South African non-government and fully registered non-profit organization that empowers street children towards leaving street life. Umthombo is situated in the central business district of Durban and provides meals, and ongoing or transient accommodation for 40–60 street youth ranging in age from 11 years to early 20s. At the time the research was undertaken, Umthombo employed 35 staff who were an amalgamation of trained former street children and social working professionals. Interviews occurred in early 2012.

Participants were recruited by staff announcing to street youth the opportunity to participate in research. To minimize feelings of coercion, potential participants were approached by an independent volunteer to ascertain interest and answer any questions. Eligibility criteria for participants included, being over 14 years of age (and for those 14 to less than 18 years, willingness to have an Umthombo staff member present during the interview), and sufficient English proficiency to communicate and understand exchanges when interviewed.

Semi-structured interviews, including ascertaining family of origin details using a genogram, and observation were conducted. Before interviews commenced all participants read, or had read to them, the Explanatory Statement and Consent Form. Questions pertaining to stigma were taken from The AIDS-Related Stigma Scale (Kalichman et al. 2005), the only reliable and valid stigma scale developed for Africa. It consisted of nine items asked as open questions to elicit greater depth of information. All other questions were developed based on the literature.

The interviews were opportunistic, taking place at a time and place convenient to the interviewee and would occur in various rooms at Umthombo based on availability. Measures were taken to ensure privacy with the interview being suspended when interruptions occurred. To facilitate confidentiality, all participants chose a pseudonym, used in place of their actual name in this report.

Interviewed staff members reported having been street youth themselves and/or having spent time as a child or adolescent in a shelter away from their family. Participant welfare was paramount and the researcher was sensitive to any distress or discomfort participants may have experienced, provided an option to not disclose information if this caused discomfort, reassured them regarding confidentiality and initiated interventions where necessary. Participants were invited to provide opinions or feedback, and street youth were encouraged to speak English as much as possible.

An Umthombo staff member was usually present during street youth interviews. Three staff members assisted including a social worker (one interview), shelter staffer (one interview) and youth worker/medical officer (seven interviews) and would also assist in translation as required. Due to the possibility of translator bias, it was decided to only include data directly provided, or confirmed by participants. One 17 year old female participant (pseudonym Latifa) refused to be interviewed with a staff member present because no staff members she trusted were available. Based on our assessment it was decided to conduct the interview without a staff member present.

Table 9.1 summarizes the demographic characteristics of all participants interviewed.

The mean ages for street youth and staff members were 17.6 and 29.5 years respectively. Of the remaining total sample (n = 18), 8 were female and 11 were male, with participants 15–19 participating in a focus group. Zulu was the

Table 9.1 Demographic characteristics of participants

Participant no.	Pseudonym	Age	Gender	Street youth or staff member	Culture	Parents still alive
1	Vavavoom	28	Male	Staff member	Xhosa	Father
2	James	34	Male	Staff member	Xhosa	Mother
3	Sindi	27	Female	Staff member	Sotho	None
4	Sbu	21	Male	Street youth	Zulu	Father[a]
5	Latifa	17	Female	Street youth	Zulu	Mother[a]
6	Mike	19	Male	Street youth	Zulu	None
7	Thabo	29	Male	Staff member	Xhosa	Mother
8	Friday[b]	14	Male	Street youth	Zulu	Mother
9	Sabelo	15	Male	Street youth	Zulu	Mother
10	Thamqasa	15	Male	Street youth	Zulu	Mother
11	Sboniso	17	Male	Street youth	Zulu	Mother/father
12	Sphiwe	19	Male	Street youth	Zulu	Father
13	Princess	16	Female	Street youth	Zulu	None
14	Brian	19	Male	Street youth	Zulu	Mother/father[a]
15	Rethabile	18	Female	Street youth	Zulu	Unknown
16	Olga	18	Female	Street youth	Zulu	Father
17	Sharon	18	Female	Street youth	Zulu	Mother/Father
18	Doris	18	Female	Street youth	Zulu	Father
19	Carol	17	Female	Street youth	Zulu	None

[a]Mortality status unknown as parent has been absent since participant was young

[b]Did not complete interview

predominant culture amongst street youth whilst most staff members were Xhosa. Only three participants indicated that both their parents were still alive, although one of these participants was unsure as their parent left when they were very young.

9.6 Knowledge About HIV/AIDS

This theme elicited general information regarding HIV/AIDS and where it was learnt. Knowledge pertaining to HIV transmission, prevention and testing, AIDS treatment, and positive outcomes as a result of this knowledge are also described.

9.6.1 General Knowledge About HIV/AIDS

Knowledge regarding HIV/AIDS varied across participants. Most knew about the virus and some had extensive knowledge (e.g., low CD4 count indicates AIDS, KwaZulu Natal has highest HIV rate in South Africa). Whilst some participants were able to differentiate between HIV and AIDS, many could not and used the terms interchangeably or considered them the same. Preferences regarding use of the term HIV or AIDS revealed that 55 % of participants preferred the term HIV, for 22 % it did not matter, 6 % did not know what HIV was, 6 % did not know what AIDS was, and 11 % knew neither about HIV or AIDS.

Participants acquired new information about HIV during interviews, particularly during the intervention, which confirmed knowledge gaps previously identified in the literature (Bryan et al. 2006; Eaton et al. 2003; Swart-Kruger and Richter 1997). For example, Sphiwe was unaware of the link between HIV and AIDS and how HIV undermines immunity, Princess did not know that HIV was a virus passed on through bodily fluids, and Brian did not realize people who are HIV-positive can look and feel well yet still be spreading HIV. All focus group participants were unaware that HIV was a small germ, subsequently becoming aware of the importance of condom use during the focus group. James was aware that an unborn baby could be protected from HIV but not the mother once she was infected. Sabelo did not know any intervention information, and both Sbu and Thamqasa were unaware of South Africa having the highest HIV/AIDS prevalence in the world, nor that HIV is spread primarily via heterosexual intercourse.

The difference between a street youth's awareness of HIV/AIDS, and their behaviour, was also salient. For example, Brian emphasized the importance of HIV testing yet later revealed: "I haven't checked it".

Sbu stated post intervention that he would use a condom in future but earlier in the interview had indicated that he already used them, as did Princess who said she would now use gloves and condoms but had also attested to their merits earlier. It is unclear whether these answers reflect a willingness to please, significant change, or an inability to translate increased knowledge into safer sexual practices (MacPhail and Campbell 2001; Marston and King 2006; Snell 2003).

Beliefs about level of infection in the community may also increase risk. Mike was aware of HIV and AIDS and that it was spread by not using a condom, but considered there was low prevalence in the community: "It's not in a lot of people". This may result in not practicing safe sex based on the belief that the chances of acquiring the virus are low.

9.6.2 How HIV/AIDS Knowledge Was First Acquired

Most participants learnt about HIV and AIDS during adolescence at school although some, (such as Princess) had ceased schooling after Year 8, and had consequently developed little knowledge. Other identified sources of knowledge regarding HIV/AIDS included doctors and nurses at clinics and hospitals, shelters, Xhosa initiation school, community outreach door to door, staff training at a hospital, and through outside organizations attending Umthombo such as on World AIDS Day.

Shelter staff rarely discussed HIV/AIDS with street youth. Sindi explained: "We prefer visitors because from us they [street youth] don't want to hear".

No exposure to external AIDS educators at the shelter, may explain why several street youth, such as Sabelo, did not know about HIV, AIDS or both. Shelter staff, such as James, believed that parents will need to begin discussing HIV/AIDS with their children, something that has not previously been common:

> But now the challenge is, we've got kids and they're growing. We also have to teach them about this thing. Our parents never taught us.

Traditions, such as parental respect in Zulu culture (Mchunu 2005), may explain why young people are unable to speak freely regarding issues that pertain to sex out of deference to adults. This affected interviews on several occasions and was overcome by asking impersonal questions ('they' rather than 'you'). The implication for HIV/AIDS is that if young people in South Africa are unable to discuss such matters with their parents, then their access to such knowledge is restricted to schools, which they no longer attend after becoming street youth. Therefore street youth or adolescents who do not attend school may have little or no access to HIV/AIDS information on the streets or in townships, apart from peers (Selikow et al. 2009).

9.6.3 Knowledge Related to Transmission

Participant knowledge regarding ways of contracting HIV/AIDS emphasized blood to blood transmission through, injury/violence, piercings, tattoos, intravenous drug use, injections, and heterosexual intercourse. Misinformation regarding HIV transmission methods included: penetration through fingernails, sweat, touch, just knowing someone, stepping on a rusty nail, sharing the same utensils, and kissing if gums were bleeding.

Regarding the question of whether a HIV-positive mother would transfer HIV to her baby, opinion and confidence of participants generally varied. The baby could become infected at birth or through breast milk, could remain naturally free of HIV or be protected through medication:

> The baby can be protected from that…I don't know how…the mother is not allowed to breast feed. (Vavavoom)

As procreation is an important expression of masculinity (Jordaan 2005; Simpson 2009) and most street youth are sexually active earlier (Kruger and Richter 2003; Swart-Kruger and Richter 1997), it seems that greater education for street youth regarding mother-to-child transmission (and the importance of testing and treatment) is warranted.

Information provided by some medical authorities may increase risk taking behavior among street youth. Sindi, when attending training about HIV/AIDS at a local hospital, was told that unless there was a cut during sexual intercourse, the partner cannot be infected. Proliferation of such information may justify unprotected sex, and incorrectly minimize estimation of risk. An emphasis on cuts may cause people to overlook possible transmission as a result of STDs or the micro tears that can occur during intercourse.

9.6.4 Knowledge Related to Prevention and Testing

Condom use, colloquially known as "condomise" was advocated by all participants that knew about HIV/AIDS although not all linked condom use with HIV/AIDS. Condoms were described as enabling "safe sex", "protecting you", "pieces of plastic", "prevent disease", and being used for contraception. Most knew that they were freely available from clinics and hospitals, and focus group participants also obtained condoms from the medical officer. This raises questions of whether condom use is practical for street youth who may have spontaneous or forced sexual encounters (Dube 1997; Lockhart 2008). Street youth have few possessions, clothes or places to store condoms on their person. However, most street youth knew about condoms and where to access them.

All staff interviewed voiced concerns regarding the reliability of free government provided condoms:

> They do protect you in a way, but not one hundred percent, cos [sic] they can break. (Thabo)

Others found that witnessing the suffering of friends with advanced AIDS, motivated prevention:

> The stage they are in, it's kind of bad…it makes someone to think twice… before you do things. (James)

Abstinence, marriage or monogamy was the only other form of prevention mentioned, mainly by staff. Whilst abstinence was supported in the focus group, another street youth, sharing her response to a nurse's abstinence recommendation, considered it unrealistic:

> As we're living…they know that people…they get married and sleep and get a child. (Latifa)

HIV/AIDS testing was advocated overall, with some participants considering it a fast way of confirming the HIV status of oneself or prospective partners, whilst others reported themselves or others being afraid to learn their status and subsequently avoiding being tested or waiting until symptoms occur:

> Other people they said no, if I get sick, then there's no cure for my sickness, then I check (Sindi)

Because Sindi considers men play a major part in the spread of HIV, she believes males should be targeted for prevention and testing education. This is also a perspective emerging in the literature (Betron et al. 2011; Jordaan 2005).

> I think they (men) are the ones who really, really, really need more education than other people…and they are the ones that don't want to go and check.

Some participants reported being tested when external educators accompanied by doctors visited and testing was also promoted prior to Xhosa initiation. Quarterly testing to ensure early detection was also recommended.

9.6.5 *Knowledge Related to Treatment*

Most participants who knew about ARVs, perceived them to be beneficial, and that they maintained a person's health and increased their life expectancy. Some ARV knowledge was sophisticated, such as ARV use being linked to one's CD4 count (number of helper T cells per cubic millimetre of blood):

> You have to find the CD4 count…to find out if they have to start the ARVs. (Sindi)

A healthy diet was considered an important aspect of HIV/AIDS treatment, particularly when taking ARVs. Special foods were recommended such as fruit, vegetables, and drinking water, whilst foods to be avoided included: junk food, onion, and oil. Some participants, such as Sboniso, believed that healthy food and exercise alone could stop the outward appearance of AIDS for up to 30 years:

> Let's say I got HIV positive when I was two years. I can even go and be thirty one years and tell my children that I have that, how long I've live with this virus.

Even staff with extensive HIV/AIDS knowledge, such as Thabo, believed that it would be possible to have the virus, live for an extended period of time and even have children if ARVs were adhered to:

> You must live for the next twenty to thirty years…you might still get kids, if you love children.

No participant indicated that ARVs or any other intervention could cure HIV/AIDS, with the exception of James citing that a baby who shares their mother's blood can be protected from HIV even if the mother is HIV-positive:

> I am sure there is a cure for HIV and AIDS. I don't know why them people they are not releasing it if it is there. How can you save the kid and you don't save the mother?

James attributed his beliefs to population control and apartheid in books he read about the origin of AIDS:

> They say, all over the world we are populated…so now people need to die because of this so that we can decrease them…In the beginning we were killing them but today they are killing themselves through sex.

AIDS and the implementation of Western scientific and medical interventions may inadvertently trigger recollections of apartheid oppression (Mbali 2004; Nattrass 2008). This was reflected in the data with repeated references to freedom, humanity and equal rights when discussing HIV stigmatization:

> They still a human being…we all mutually have equal freedom, irrespective of sickness. (Vavavoom)

A return to African traditions may attempt to offset perceptions of Western intervention (Maluleke 2012):

> African doctors will say they can cure AIDS but, for my understanding, there is no cure. (Sindi)

Our data showed knowledge regarding ARVs was mixed. Several participants made a consistent link between taking ARVs and the importance of eating healthy food, that ARVs control the proliferation of AIDS in the body, and that ARVs increase life expectancy. Others such as Thamqasa had not heard of ARVs, and Sboniso considered ARVs to be medication to treat TB, unaware of the link between AIDS and TB (Abdool Karim et al. 2009).

9.6.6 *Positive Outcomes of HIV/AIDS Knowledge*

Data highlighted how knowledge about HIV/AIDS was put into practice by the participants. Thamqasa volunteered that he promotes condom use amongst the other street youth: "I said to the other ones you have to use a condom". As an intern at Umthombo, and considering that staff generally to not discuss HIV/AIDS with street youth, Thamqasa plays a significant role in promoting safe sex amongst his peers. Sboniso's positive interaction with AIDS patients met through a shelter program was a normalising and stigma reducing experience: "They are friendly, kind, anything that you can think".

Others argued for promoting community spirit and reciprocity when coping with the realities of HIV/AIDS:

> You need to be friends with people, take care of people so that they can be able to take care of you…if you treat people like shit, then they will treat you like shit. (James)

A celebrity disclosing their HIV status via the media can play a powerful educative role, especially in negating stigma:

> There's a guy who used to play basketball back in the days cos I used to love basketball, Magic Johnson…from there I kind of changed my mind and said OK, even famous people you know can get this. It doesn't mean that because we are poor or because he or she is rich, they can't get this thing. It affects everyone. (Thabo)

Such disclosures humanise the condition, engender sympathy, and highlight that HIV/AIDS is an illness that does not discriminate.

9.7 Risk Factors Associated with HIV/AIDS

This theme elicited a number of discrete factors leading to street life which culminate in direct risks for acquiring HIV. Discrete factors were social and familial in nature, whilst direct risks were associated with street life and psychological issues.

9.7.1 Social and Familial Factors

For many street youth, a disintegration of the family unit has been a significant factor in choosing the streets where the risk for contracting HIV is high (Foster 2004; Grassly et al. 2004; Robbins et al. 2010; Ward and Seager 2010). Of the 13 participants who completed genograms, earlier death of family members was reported by all but 2 participants, some lost up to 4 members of their immediate family, 7 had suffered the death of one parent with another 3 orphaned. Additional deaths were reported by focus group members who did not complete genograms. Where mentioned, causes of death included undisclosed illness, suicide, shooting, stroke, HIV/AIDS or cancer. Most street youth had been exposed to the death of a family member at a young age, or witnessed their parent slowly dying, most due to AIDS. For some, the experience was particularly visceral:

> I was suffering too much when my mother was next to me and she was dying…then… my sister died, it was very bad. (Sphiwe)

Many street youth reported being neglected by family members who were dependent on alcohol. Abuse and maltreatment was frequently reported by participants. Examples included a female street youth molested by her grandfather, a male street youth raped and starved by his stepmother, adoption because of an auntie's mistreatment, being beaten by their 'granny', or abandonment by a parent. Some participants reported leaving for the streets as early as 8 years of age.

Fragmented families were frequently reported with several participants having little or no involvement from their fathers who often established new families elsewhere. This was highlighted in genograms where participants mentioned same aged siblings:

> My father was a policeman so he moved around a lot, so… he had girlfriends, in many places. (Thabo)

Mothers were usually responsible for bringing up children but the loss of either parent tended to exacerbate family fragmentation with children then staying with extended family. This is epitomized by Olga's story of her father denying her parentage: "He denied me when I was young…my mother…she kill herself".

Economic factors placed families under additional strain with street youth and staff citing unemployment, poverty, lack of food and poor living conditions (See Fig. 9.1) which likely aggravated family divisions and discrimination.

Latifa was taken by a social worker from her family and adopted despite having extended family because: "all of them got their own childrens…and…they are not working". In several cases, family conditions remained so dire that when returned to their homes, street youth immediately left for the streets.

Social changes such as increased freedom and rights were also considered to increase young people's exposure to HIV risk. Sindi highlighted government changes to the Children's Act in South Africa, now enabling children from 12 years

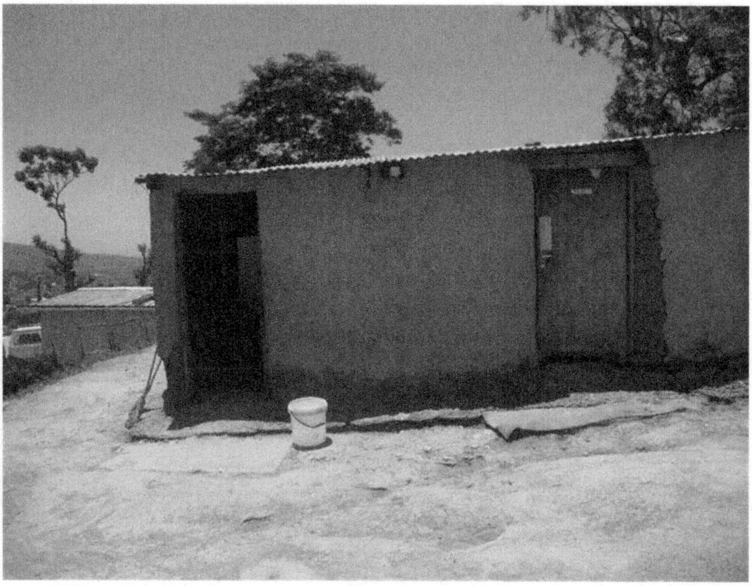

Fig. 9.1 Where street youth come from – a typical township home

to access contraception and abortion without parental consent, possibly leading young people to an earlier introduction to unprotected sex. Thamqasa agreed that street life also offered freedom in the form of "entertainment, disco, girls, unlimited hours" which played a significant role in his return to the streets.

Physical discipline of children both within the home and by the community is expected, but providing moral guidance and judgement can be difficult to differentiate from abuse.

> Sometimes they give you a speech…sometimes they beat you….if a child is not beaten down, I can tell you it is not respectful. (Sboniso)

In some cases, community justice can be taken to the extreme such as when Sboniso's family rejected him for his own protection:

> The reason for them to chase me out it's not that they doesn't like me…I did wrong in the community, the community when it beats you…it beats you to death. (Sboniso)

Although family fragmentation, abuse, and neglect motivated many participants to turn to the streets, others missed their friends, enjoyed having freedom or thought it would be fun compared to life at home. Other possible factors based on our observation included: conduct disorder; learning difficulties; trauma; grief; and other mental health issues.

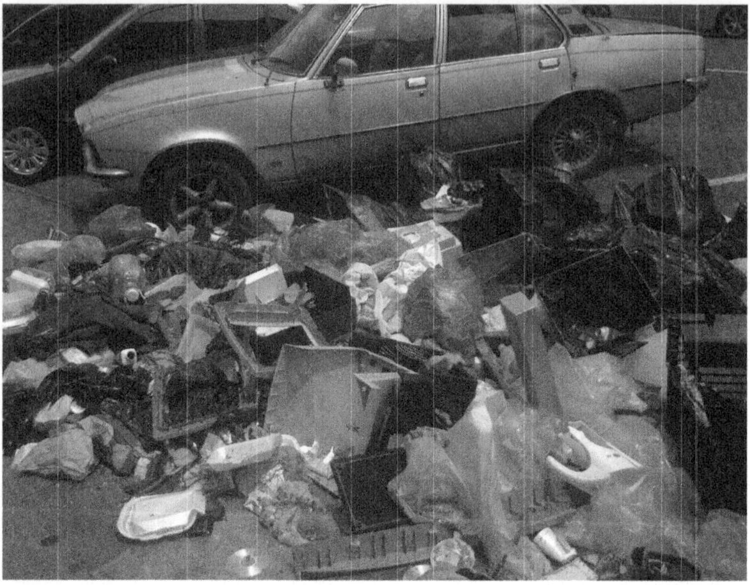

Fig. 9.2 A street in Durban close to the shelter

9.7.2 *Street Life*

All participants agreed that street life (See Fig. 9.2) was difficult and dangerous. To escape the stresses of street life, numerous participants indicated they had used (or continue to use) various substances including cigarettes, dagga (marijuana), glue sniffing, heroin and whoonga. This made them vulnerable to HIV through sexual exploitation whilst high, and the likelihood of taking greater risks when engaging in crime and violence to support their habit risking blood to blood transmission. Staff discussions revealed that whoonga consisted of marijuana, chlorine, rat poison and ARVs and was sprinkled on a cigarette and smoked, resulting in immediate addiction. Whoonga was reported to cause death in those with HIV and staff claimed people had deliberately become infected with HIV to access ARVs, on-selling them to drug dealers to fund their habit. This finding builds on what little is known about whoonga, also known as nyoape, in the literature which implicates the incorporation of ARVs into the drug (Moodley et al. 2012; TF Market Research 2011).

Princess and Latifa reported that female street youth smoked dagga inside the toilet at the shelter and Brian admitted previously using glue. Mike continues to use dagga but explained why he gave up whoonga:

> Whoonga…it's no good for me…I decided to quit it…because it makes you thin…it makes you steal a lot.

Others gave up one substance only to substitute it with another:

> I did smoke glue… I smoke it a lot…well I stop it and then I start smoking heroin. (Sbu)

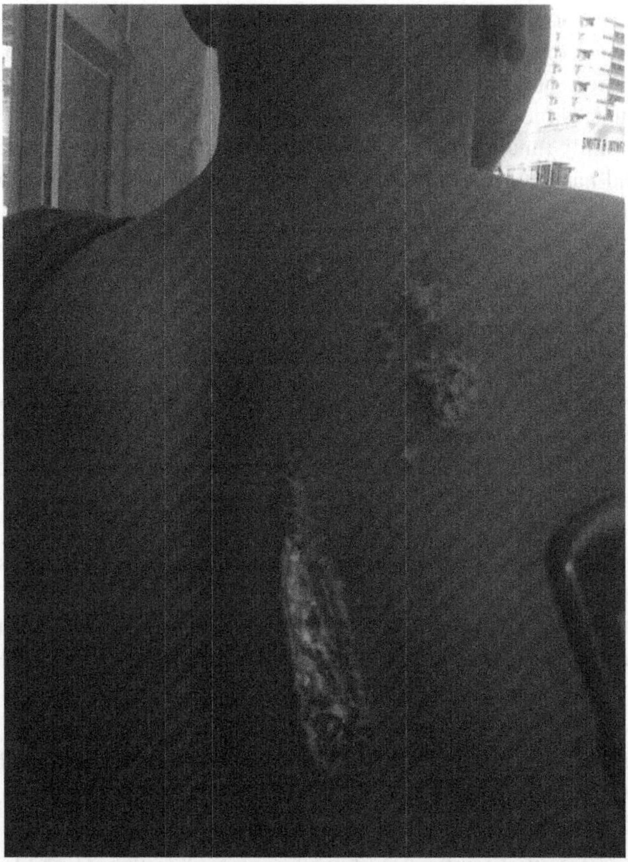

Fig. 9.3 Violence is a common risk on the streets – a street youth with infected stab wounds

Reliance on substances often lead to crime and made street youth vulnerable to exploitation, violence (See Fig. 9.3), prostitution, begging and subsequently HIV, with shelters offering only temporary refuge from the streets until street youth reached 18 years of age (Umthombo offered extended age accommodation). Thamqasa explained his involvement in crime before living at Umthombo:

> I was stealing too much, I was robbing people outside, stealing money, see now I am not doing that.

Participants described street youth engaging in violent behaviours such as hitting smaller children, carrying knives, threatening staff, accusations of child rape, and the researcher witnessed a volunteer being attacked with a knife.

Several participants reported police brutality during round-ups, describing being beaten, and even the use of pepper spray.

> I was sleeping and the Metro coming and they hit us and take us far away…with…pepper spray, yar. (Thamqasa)

For most participants, families are not a safe haven in South Africa with exposure to death and emotional and physical abuse often precipitating going to the streets. Street life offers ongoing vulnerability for acquiring HIV through substance use, violence, and crime with only shelters offering limited protection. Therefore, improving family functioning and homeless support are important aspects of reducing HIV and has been supported in previous research (Snell 2003; Swart-Kruger and Richter 1997).

9.7.3 Psychological Issues

Difficult family and socio-economic circumstances had a marked impact on street youth psychologically. Many participants cited reactions of being stressed, "sad" (depressed), whilst others cited boredom, loneliness, embarrassment and ostracism. Some had detached themselves socially and struggled with feelings of despair. When asked about the happiest time in his life, Sphiwe corroborated the translator's description: "He doesn't have it, been terrible (emphasised) abuse in his life".

Survival on the streets involved regular exposure to violence, likely to result in hypervigilance and aggressive responses to threat. James described a recent incident where a street youth at the shelter pulled a knife on him to which he responded violently:

> I was stabbed twice in my life, almost died…it was just my mind, it just went mad immediately…because he was coming straight to me…that's life on the street, so I've been there you know…because the minute you pull a knife on me, you want to kill me.

James' response not only reflects his childhood on the streets, but also how violence is a daily threat on the streets of Durban, thus increasing the risk of blood to blood HIV transmission.

'Living in the moment' represents a way of escaping from daily hardship and consequences. When asked why some people risk having unprotected sex, Sindi explained:

> Because there are a lot of things that happened…they lost interest in everything in life…they just want to enjoy themselves for that moment.

This suggests a sense of hopelessness about the future which is understandable in the context of risk factors such as unemployment, poverty, high rates of rape and violence and poor nutrition: all daily challenges for street youth and many South Africans. Consequently, enjoyment of immediate pleasures such as substances and sex may represent a welcome escape from daily survival struggles. Therefore, protecting against HIV, whose problematic symptoms manifest many years into the future, is unlikely to be a priority for street youth or South Africans struggling in cities or townships.

9.8 Discussion and Recommendations

The purpose of our research was to give street youth, one of the most disenfranchized groups in South Africa, a voice and ascertain their knowledge about, and vulnerability to acquiring, HIV/AIDS. The following summary of the main themes of our findings also has implications for addressing HIV/AIDS prevention and treatment across South Africa.

Knowledge regarding HIV/AIDS amongst street youth varied and numerous knowledge gaps were identified (e.g., that HIV is mainly spread through heterosexual intercourse), and many participants could not differentiate between HIV and AIDS. Beliefs regarding low prevalence are likely to increase risk, and exposure to outside educators in a shelter environment may increase knowledge about the virus. Cultural beliefs, such as not discussing sex in deference to adults, are likely to compromise HIV/AIDS knowledge acquisition. Misinformation regarding transmission, and preventative interventions such as abstinence and condoms, clashes with cultural beliefs such as the importance of procreation in expressing masculinity. HIV/AIDS stigma could lead to avoidance of HIV testing and men were identified as playing a major part in disease spread. ARVs were correctly linked by some to the need for a healthy diet and mistakenly as a treatment for TB. AIDS was also negatively linked to a Western interference and apartheid but numerous positives were also identified with HIV/AIDS understandings, such as increased compassion and sympathy, and the positive impact of celebrity disclosure, highlighted how the virus does not discriminate.

Discrete risk factors leading to street life and increased risk of acquiring HIV, included disintegration of the family unit through substance use, polygamy, death (often due to AIDS), and also through economic factors such as unemployment, and poverty, which could lead to neglect and abuse. Direct risks associated with street life, which is difficult and dangerous, often leads to 'self medication' via substance use. This results in increased vulnerability to sexual exploitation, crime, exposure to violence and consequently psychological issues such as depression, trauma related disorders and ultimately increased exposure to HIV transmission.

From a sexuality perspective, this study highlighted gender inequality and the need to empower women to be more active agents in negotiating safe sex, which cannot be done without the support of government regulated infrastructures such as police and courts to act against violence, crime and rape (Jewkes et al. 2009; Moffett 2006) which place women at risk for HIV infection. Prevention is further compromized and chances of transmission increased, when current interventions are contradicted by South African culture and beliefs such as polygamy, multiple partners, transaction sex and provider relationships, gender inequalities, and perceptions of masculinity which can drive unprotected intercourse and high rates of rape.

HIV/AIDS knowledge was inextricably linked with culture and beliefs. For example, outside educators could play a valuable and effective educative role in promoting accurate knowledge about HIV/AIDS but differences identified between what participants say and do in regarding HIV/AIDS practices indicates that other factors need to be identified that may mediate reluctance to take preventative action such as culture and beliefs about the disease. Data confirmed that suicide can occur in anticipation of a HIV/AIDS diagnosis, challenging recent findings (Govender and Schlebusch 2012; Schlebusch and Govender 2012) because suicide may not be solely linked to depression. Whilst medical circumcision is seen as a significant preventative intervention (Peltzer et al. 2008; Wilcken et al. 2010) this study progresses previous findings (Barr 2008) that practices such as using the same circumcision knife across initiates poses considerable risk irrespective of prior HIV testing and the importance of cultural consideration in developing interventions. Abstinence appears unrealistic in the South African context, and interventions need to reconcile cultural ideals, social reality and HIV risk in a sensitive and practical way, particularly if there is a resurgence of such traditions post-apartheid (Maluleke 2012).

In respect of treatment, whilst ARVs were viewed optimistically overall, efficacy and adherence can be compromized by HIV/AIDS stigma, structural inequities and inaccessibility to nutritious food. The poor uptake of ARVs generally (Adam and Johnson 2009) is exacerbated in the HIV-positive street youth population where attendance at a shelter risks transmission to others through violence, lack of knowledge, unprotected sex, and being kept unaware of their HIV status, whilst freedom to return to the streets negates ARV compliance and increases disease spread.

This chapter culminates in the following general recommendations (see Table 9.2) that address issues raised by the data. These are conditional upon being developed in consultation with health professionals and interest groups familiar with the diverse social and cultural traditions within South Africa to ensure appropriateness and maximize outcomes.

9.9 Conclusion

In this study we found that the links between HIV and AIDS for some street youth are unclear and HIV testing may only occur after developing AIDS symptoms. If this belief is widespread, HIV-positive people in South Africa may be undermining their health, limiting their life expectancy, and the effectiveness of ARVs, but most disturbingly, have been unwittingly spreading the virus for up to 10 years before becoming symptomatic. In the context of polygamy and culturally sanctioned multiple partner relationships, this could explain why the virus has spread so rapidly. Without intervention, the major factor likely to reduce the current HIV/AIDS prevalence figures in South Africa will be mortality. Halting the spread of HIV, in street youth in particular and South Africa in general, appears to be hampered by cultural and traditional norms and stigma and further compounded by a reluctance to use condoms which represent population control and have postcolonial/apartheid overtones. Whilst a biomedical approach is at the forefront of fighting this pandemic, it will need to collaboratively identify and incorporate culturally sensitive interventions or there will be no halting HIV's spread in South Africa.

Table 9.2 Recommendations regarding HIV/AIDS research and interventions for South Africa

No.	Recommendation
1.	Emphasize the link between HIV and AIDS and how HIV can be unwittingly spread for up to 10 years before AIDS symptoms become apparent
2.	More education for street youth, regarding mother to child transmission, and the importance of testing and treatment, is warranted
3.	Promotion of accurate knowledge is essential in reducing transmission and dispelling myths and misinformation
4.	Obstacles to prevention, testing and how to connect HIV to AIDS, especially targeting males, needs to be better understood as the risk of waiting until symptoms occur before testing can mean the virus is spread for many years prior to diagnosis and ARV efficacy and life expectancy is undermined
5.	Promoting the benefits of ARVs because of their ability to increase life expectancy and visibly improve health, could have an important impact against stigma which is often associated with outward appearance
6.	Further research into whoonga, or nyaope, to ascertain the veracity of reports about its ingredients, effects, dangers and the role of ARVs
7.	Consideration of media-based HIV/AIDS education campaigns headed by well-known public figures disclosing their HIV/AIDS status to counter stigma, acknowledge how cultural norms and gender inequity have contributed to the spread of HIV, and educational campaigns that address specific stigma beliefs, e.g., you cannot get HIVAIDS from touching someone, using the same crockery or cutlery
8.	Further implementation of the living positively intervention in South Africa as it reduces stigma, HIV re-infection, promotes self-care, medication adherence, and condom use
9.	Need for educational interventions that link HIV and AIDS, and early intervention for ARV treatment to extend life and combat beliefs that HIV/AIDS is a death sentence
10.	Criminal acts such as rape and violence against women need to be reported and prosecuted
11.	Use of education to dispel previous negative perceptions of AIDS death, when no treatment regime was available, by emphasizing that ARVs prolong life and its quality if taken as directed. A blanket campaign could instill hope for the future; reduce stigma, fear of testing and suicide
12.	Importance of educating and promoting the life extending benefits of ARVs to address the fearful recollection of the devastation of AIDS before ARVs became available. This may reduce suicidal ideation and completion
13.	Educational campaigns aimed at associating condoms with trust, rather than mistrust
14.	Incorporation of HIV prevention and intervention strategies that require community consultation and cooperation in practices such as traditional circumcision rituals and masculinity and procreation
15.	Encouragement of early ARV interventions and adherence and greater government intervention in addressing structural inequalities that compromize HIV/AIDS interventions
16.	Greater funding and implementation of HIV/AIDS educative interventions directed to street youth, who are at high-risk for HIV, via not-for-profit shelters who have direct contact with this population

References

Abdool Karim, S. S., Churchyard, G. J., Abdool Karim, Q., & Lawn, S. D. (2009). HIV infection and tuberculosis in South Africa: An urgent need to escalate the public health response. The Lancet, 374(9693), 921–933. doi:10.1016/s0140-6736(09)60916-8.

Adam, M. A., & Johnson, L. F. (2009). Estimation of adult antiretroviral treatment coverage in SouthAfrica. [Antiretroviral treatment; HIV/AIDS; Markov model]. South African Medical Journal, 99(9), 661–667.

Auvert, B., Taljaard, D., Lagarde, E., Sobngwi-Tambekou, J., Sitta, R., & Puren, A. (2005). Randomized, controlled intervention trial of male circumcision for reduction of HIV infection risk: The ANRS 1265 Trial. PLoS Medicine, 2, e298. doi:10.1371/journal.pmed.0020298.

Bailey, R. C., Moses, S., Parker, C. B., Agot, K., Maclean, I., Krieger, J. N., … Ndina-Achola, J. O. (2007). Male circumcision for HIV prevention in young men in Kisumu, Kenya: a randomised controlled trial. Lancet, 369, 643–656. doi:10.1016/S0140-6736(07)60312-2pmid:17321310.

Barr, B. K. (2008). The culture of AIDS in Xhosa society. Tennessee: University of Tennessee Honours Research Projects. Retrieved from http://trace.tennessee.edu/utk_chanhonoproj/1149.

Bertolote, J. M., Fleischmann, A., Leo, D., & Wasserman, D. (2009). Suicidal thoughts, suicide plans and attempts in the general population on different continents. In D. Wasserman & C. Wasserman (Eds.), Oxford textbook of suicidology and suicide prevention: A global perspective (pp. 99–104). Oxford: Oxford University Press.

Betron, M., Barker, G., Contreras, J. M., & Peacock, D. (2011). Men, masculinities and HIV/AIDS: Strategies for action: United Nations Development Programme (UNDP).

Bryan, A., Kagee, A., & Broaddus, M. R. (2006). Condom use among South African adolescents: Developing and testing theoretical models of intentions and behavior. AIDS Behavior, 10, 387–397. doi:10.1007/s10461-006-9087-5.

Coates, T. J., Richter, L., & Caceres, C. (2008). Behavioural strategies to reduce HIV transmission: How to make them work better. The Lancet, 372(9639), 669–684. http://dx.doi.org/10.1016/S0140-6736(08)60886-7.

Dube, L. (1997). AIDS-risk patterns and knowledge of the disease among street children in Harare, Zimbabwe. Journal of Social Development in Africa, 12(2), 61–73.

Dunkle, K. L., Jewkes, R. K., Brown, H. C., Gray, G. E., McIntryre, J. A., & Harlow, S. D. (2004). Transactional sex among women in Soweto, South Africa: Prevalence, risk factors and association with HIV infection. Social Science & Medicine, 59, 1581–1592.

Eaton, L., Flisher, A. J., & Aarø, L. E. (2003). Unsafe sexual behaviour in South African youth. Social Science & Medicine, 56(1), 149–165.

Foster, G. (2004). Safety nets for children affected by HIV/AIDS in southern Africa. In R. Pharoah (Ed.), A generation at risk? HIV/AIDS, vulnerable children and security in southern Africa (Vol. 109, pp. 65–92). Institute for Security Studies monograph series. Retrieved from http://www.iss.co.za/pubs/Monographs/No109/Chap4.htm 31 Mar 2011.

Govender, R. D., & Schlebusch, L. (2012). Hopelessness, depression and suicidal ideation in HIV-positive persons. South African Journal of Psychiatry, 18, 16–21.

Grassly, N. C., Lewis, J. J. C., Mahy, M., Walker, N., & Timaeus, I. M. (2004). Comparison of household-survey estimates with projections of mortality and orphan numbers in sub-Saharan Africa in the era of HIV/AIDS. Population Studies, 58, 201–217.

Gray, R. H., Kigozi, G., Serwadda, D., Makumbi, F., Watya, S., Nalugoda, F., … Wawer, M. J. (2007). Male circumcision for HIV prevention in men in Rakai, Uganda: A randomised trial. Lancet, 369(9562), 657–666.

Jewkes, R., Sikweyiya, Y., Morrell, R., & Dunkle, K. (2009). Understanding men's health and use of violence: Interface of rape and HIV in South Africa. Technical Report. Pretoria: Medical Research Council.

Jewkes, R., Dunkle, K., Nduna, M., & Jama Shai, N. (2012). Transactional sex and HIV incidence in a cohort of young women in the stepping stones trial. Journal of AIDS & Clinical Research, 3. doi:10.4172/2155-61131000158.

Jordaan, S. (2005). A gendered critique of the ABC prevention policy of the South African government concerning HIV/Aids: A case study of Northern KwaZulu-Natal. Unpublished dissertation. University of Johannesburg.

Kalichman, S. C., Simbayi, L. C., Jooste, S., Toefy, Y., Cain, D., Cherry, C., & Kagee, A. (2005). Development of a brief scale to measure AIDS-related stigma in South Africa. AIDS and Behavior, 9(2), 135–143. doi:10.1007/s10461-005-3895-x.

Kallings, L. O. (2008). The first postmodern pandemic: 25 years of HIV/AIDS. Journal of Internal Medicine, 263(3), 218–243. doi:10.1111/j.1365-2796.2007.01910.x.

Kruger, J. M., & Richter, L. M. (2003). South African street children at risk for AIDS? Children, Youth and Environments Spring, 13(1). Retrieved July, 25, from http://colorado.edu/journals/cye.

Lockhart, C. (2008). The life and death of a street boy in East Africa. Medical Anthropology Quarterly, 22(1), 94–115.

MacPhail, C., & Campbell, C. (2001). 'I think condoms are good but, aai, I hate those things': Condom use among adolescents and young people in a Southern African township. Social Science and Medicine, 52(11), 1613–1627.

Maluleke, M. J. (2012). Culture, tradition, custom, law and gender equality. Potchefstroom Electronic Law Journal, 15(1). Retrieved from http://ssrn.com/abstract=2045469.

Marston, C., & King, E. (2006). Factors that shape young people's sexual behaviour: A systematic review. [Article]. Lancet, 368(9547), 1581–1586. doi:10.1016/s0140-6736(06)69662-1.

Mbali, M. (2004). AIDS discourse and the South African state: Government denialism and post-apartheid AIDS policy making. Transformation, 54, 104–122.

Mchunu, M., R. (2005). Zulu fathers and their sons: Sexual taboos, respect and their relationship to the HIV/AIDS pandemic. Michigan: MPublishing. University of Michigan Library. Retrieved from http://quod.lib.umich.edu/p/passages/4761530.0010.013?rgn=main;view=fulltext.

Meel, B. L. (2003). The myth of child rape as a cure for HIV/AIDS in Transkei. Medicine, Science, and the Law, 43, 85–88.

Moffett, H. (2006). 'These women, they force us to rape them': Rape as a narrative of social control in post-apartheid South Africa. Journal of South African Studies, 32, 129–144.

Moodley, S. V., Matjila, M. J., & Moosa, M. Y. H. (2012). Epidemiology of substance use among secondary school learners in Atteridgeville, Gauteng. South African Journal of Psychiatry, 18, 2–9.

Mufune, P. (2000). Street youth in southern Africa. International Social Science Journal, 164, 233–243.

Nattrass, N. (2004). The moral economy of AIDS in South Africa. Cambridge: University Press.

Nattrass, N. (2008). AIDS and the scientific governance of medicine in post-apartheid South Africa. African Affairs, 107(427), 157–176. doi:10.1093/afraf/adm087.

Ndlovu, B. A. (2005). Perceptions of different subsets of African men and African traditional healers in the Durban Metropolitan area that sexual intercourse with young girl can cure HIV/AIDS. Unpublished master's thesis, Durban Institute of Technology, Durban, South Africa.

Peltzer, K., Nqeketo, A., Petros, G., & Kanta, X. (2008). Traditional circumcision during manhood initiation rituals in the Eastern Cape, South Africa: A pre-post intervention evaluation. BMC Public Health, 8(1), 64.

Richter, L. M., & Swart-Kruger, J. (1995). AIDS-risk among street children and youth: Implications for intervention. South African Journal of Psychology, 25, 31–38.

Robbins, C. L., Zapata, L., Kissin, D. M., Shevchenko, N., Yorick, R., Skipalska, H., … Hillis, S. D. (2010). Multicity HIV seroprevalence in street youth, Ukraine. International Journal of STD and AIDS, 21, 489–496.

Rochat, T., Bland, R., Tomlinson, M., & Stein, A. (2013). Suicide ideation, depression and HIV among pregnant women in rural South Africa. Health, 5, 650–661. doi:10.4236/health.2013.53A086.

Schlebusch, L., & Govender, R. D. (2012). Age, gender and suicidal ideation following voluntary HIV counseling and testing. International Journal of Environmental Research and Public Health, 9, 521–530.

Selikow, T. A., Ahmed, N., Flisher, A. J., Mathews, C., & Mukoma, W. (2009). I am not "umqwayito": A qualitative study of peer pressure and sexual risk behaviour among young adolescents in Cape Town, South Africa. Scandinavian Journal of Public Health, 2, 107–112.
Simpson, A. (2009). Boys to men in the shadow of AIDS: Masculinities and HIV risk in Zambia. London: Palgrave McMillan.
Snell, C. L. (2003). Help-seeking and risk-taking behavior among black street youth. Journal of Health and Social Policy, 16(1), 21–32.
Stokes, B. (2007). South Africa striving. National Journal, 39(5), 28–34.
Swart-Kruger, J., & Richter, L. M. (1997). AIDS-related knowledge, attitudes and behaviour among South African street youth: Reflections on power, sexuality and the autonomous self. Social Science & Medicine, 45(6), 957–966.
Tadele, G. (2003). Surviving on the streets: Sexuality and HIV/AIDS among male street youth in Dessie, Ethiopia. CODESRIA Bulletin, 2, 98–110.
Teitelman, A. M., Seloilwe, E. S., & Campbell, J. C. (2009). Voices from the frontlines: The epidemics of HIV/AIDS and violence among women and girls. Health Care for Women International, 30(3), 184–194. doi:10.1080/07399330902739239.
TF Market Research. (2011). South Africa pharmaceuticals and healthcare report Mar 01, 2011. New York: Business Monitor International Ltd.
Tomaselli, K. G. (2009). (Re)Mediatizing HIV/AIDS in South Africa. Cultural Studies ↔ Critical Methodologies, 9(4), 570–587. doi:10.1177/1532708609334101.
UNAIDS. (2014, July). The gap report. Retrieved from http://www.unaids.org/en/media/unaids/contentassets/documents/unaidspublication/2014/UNAIDS_Gap_report_en.pdf.
UNGASS. (2012). Global AIDS response progress report 2012: Republic of South Africa. South Africa: UNGASS.
UNICEF. (2013). Towards an AIDS-free generation – children and AIDS: Sixth stocktaking report, 2013.
Ward, C. L., & Seager, J. R. (2010). South African street children: A survey and recommendations for services. [Article]. Development Southern Africa, 27(1), 85–100. doi:10.1080/03768350903519374.
Wilcken, A., Keil, T., & Dick, B. (2010). Traditional male circumcision in eastern and southern Africa: A systematic review of prevalence and complications. Bulletin of the World Health Organization, 88, 907–914.

Chapter 10
"I Definitely Want Kids, But I Think the Risks Are Pretty High": Fertility Desires and Perinatal HIV Transmission Knowledge Among Adolescents and Young Adults with Perinatally-Acquired HIV

Cynthia D. Fair and Jamie Nicole Albright

Contents

10.1 Introduction

Perinatally-acquired HIV (PHIV) infection was first identified in 1983 (Rubinstein et al. 1983). Survival and health of children born with PHIV was poor until the discovery of antiretroviral treatment (ART) in 1992 when fewer infants were born to

C.D. Fair (✉)
Elon University, 100 Campus Drive CB 2337, Elon, NC 27244, USA
e-mail: cfair@elon.edu

J.N. Albright
Department of Psychology, University of Virginia,
102 Gilmer Hall, P.O. Box 400400, Charlottesville, VA 22904, USA
e-mail: jna2db@uva.edu

P. Liamputtong (ed.), *Children and Young People Living with HIV/AIDS*,
Cross-Cultural Research in Health, Illness and Well-Being,
DOI 10.1007/978-3-319-29936-5_10

HIV-positive mothers, and infected children and their mothers received life-extending treatment. The risk of mother-to-child transmission of HIV decreased from approximately 30 % in the mid-1980s to less than 1–2 % currently (Townsend et al. 2008) due, in part, to widespread HIV testing of pregnant women, and the use of preventative measures during pregnancy, delivery, and abstinence from breast-feeding (Fakoya et al. 2008). Although the mortality rate for childhood HIV infection was high in the late 1980s and early 1990s, there remains a surviving cohort of adolescents and young adults (AYA) living with PHIV in the United States and worldwide. In the United States, approximately 9100 individuals are living with PHIV (Centers for Disease Control and Prevention 2011). The demographics of AYA with PHIV reflect those of their mothers. Most are black/African American, of lower socioeconomic status, and experience high levels of psychosocial stressors (Frederick et al. 2000). Many AYA with PHIV have experienced substantial loss and turmoil in their lives, which complicate the developmental tasks of young adulthood.

The majority of AYA with PHIV have been engaged in medical care most of their lives. Health-related consequences of long-term survival of HIV are common. These include cognitive delays, poorer mental health status, physical limitations, co-morbidities, and complications related to extended exposure to ART (Mellins et al. 2009; Nozyce et al. 2006). The reality of the survival of AYA with PHIV, however, is that they must manage the same developmental tasks of young adulthood as their uninfected peers—including engaging in romantic and intimate relationships, establishing self-sufficiency, and pursuing a family of their own, all while dealing with a chronic, stigmatized illness (Erikson 1980; Ezeanolue et al. 2006; see also Chap. 4 in this volume).

10.2 Previous Literature

Little is known about perspectives of AYA with PHIV on reproductive decision-making (RDM) (Fair et al. 2013) although there is sufficient documentation of their engagement in intimate relationships, pregnancies, and participation in developmentally expected sexual behaviors (Ezeanolue et al. 2006; Wiener et al. 2007; Fair and Albright 2012). Research suggests that AYA with PHIV can have successful pregnancies, and most described in the literature have resulted in healthy postpartum outcomes and uninfected offspring (Phillips et al. 2011).

Although the perspectives of reproductive decision-making AYA with PHIV are not well understood, those of adults with HIV have been described (Williams et al. 1996; Bedimo-Rung and Clark 2005). Reproductive decision-making encompasses age at initiation and frequency of sexual intercourse, time spent in a sexual union, use of contraceptives, perceived health and socio-cultural influences. Such decision-making can be active or passive, and is characterized by varying levels of desire and intent to bear children (Hass 1974; Miller 1994; Gage 1998). Research suggests that age, health status, messages from partners or family, as well as religious and gender role orientation influence desires/intentions to have children among adult women (Sowell et al. 1999; Chen et al. 2001). Similarly, little is known about the fertility desires and intentions among adult men living with HIV (Sherr and Barry 2004). However, findings reported by Paiva and colleagues (2003) suggest that some men with HIV do want children.

The maturing population of AYA with PHIV are engaging in the same developmentally appropriate behavior of relationship and family formation as their uninfected peers. However, little is known about their childbearing intentions nor understanding of the risks of PHT. Further, the bulk of existing literature focuses exclusively on females. The study on which this chapter is based examines the fertility desires and intentions along with knowledge of PHT among AYA males and females living with PHIV.

10.3 Theoretical Framework

Miller et al.'s (2004) theoretical approach to understanding childbearing motivations, desires and intentions provides a framework for the current study. The Fertility Decision-Making Model, later known as the Traits-Desires-Intentions-Behavior (TDIB) Framework (Miler 1994; Miller et al.'s 2004) comprises a series of steps that ultimately influence reproductive behaviors. In short, traits are mental structures that guide behavior based upon biological characteristics and social experiences, including the biological impetus to have a child. Traits are activated into specific childbearing desires including number of children and the ideal time to have a child. Intentions are shaped by the context in which one lives, and this step in the fertility decision-making model most directly translates into what decisions one will ultimately make. Finally, the last step in the TDIB Framework is the behavior taken to either pursue or prevent conception.

The medical and cultural discourses around HIV are prominent features of the fertility decision-making processes of individuals living with HIV. While a biological drive to have children contributes to fertility desire, the social aspect of HIV stigma may reduce the likelihood that desire results in reproductive behavior, although this is historically-bound by fear of HIV transmission. During the 1980s and early 1990s, women with HIV were vilified as vectors of transmission and strongly encouraged to avoid having children due to the risk of PHT (Arras 1990). Reports of coerced sterilization and prejudicial treatment at the hands of medical providers are documented historically and presently in the literature (Sowell et al. 1999; Badell et al. 2012), underscoring the difficult context in which reproductive decisions were made by individuals living with HIV. Views on childbearing among those living with HIV have evolved over the course of the epidemic, although evidence suggests that in some countries, many patients still believe that their medical providers are not supportive of their desire to have children (Paiva et al. 2003; Gruskin et al. 2008). Still, the finding that the risk of PHT could be reduced from 25 to 30 % to less than 5 % radically altered the reproductive landscape for women

(Cooper and Charurat 2002). Today, the risk of PHT is less than 2 % and relatively few children are born with PHIV in high resource countries (Townsend et al. 2008). Further, clinicians and researchers have developed guidelines to support serodiscordant couples achieve childbearing goals, and large numbers of people living with HIV report a desire to have children in the future (Chen et al. 2001; Paiva et al. 2003; Matthews and Mukherjee 2009; Finocchario-Kessler et al. 2010). International reproductive health advocates affirm the right of those living with HIV to bear children and suggest risk reducing strategies designed to promote safe conception (Center for Reproductive Rights 2010). Adolescents and young adults living with PHIV navigate a different context than even those who acquired HIV as adults due to the nature of life-long management of the disease. Little is known about how researchers and clinicians should account for the unique experience of PHIV in their conceptualization of patient fertility decision-making.

10.4 The Study

During July 2011 through April 2012, AYA with PHIV were recruited using purposive sampling. Current or former patients of two pediatric clinics in the southeastern United States were referred to us by social workers at the clinic, who identified eligible participants. Eligible participants were over 14 years of age, free from cognitive impairments, and able to communicate in English. Interested participants were then referred to a member of the research team. A total of 42 AYA were invited to participate in the study. Two females and one male declined, and three males and one female could not be reached after initially agreeing to participate resulting in a final sample of 35 AYA. Elon University's Institutional Review Board (IRB) approved the study before recruitment began.

Upon consent from AYA or their guardians, semi-structured interviews were conducted by trained interviewers either in person or over the phone, based upon the participant's preference. Participants were provided a $25 gift card in compensation for their participation. Each interview was recorded and transcribed for later analysis.

The interview assessed levels of fertility desires and intentions as well as understanding of mother-to-child transmission and PHT preventative measures. In keeping with Miller et al.'s (2004) proposed fertility decision-making framework, interviewers elicited primary desires to have a child, medical knowledge of their ability to have a child, and their future intentions (including expected parity and anticipated age at the birth of their first or subsequent child). Interview questions were open-ended, and adapted from previous studies (Chen et al. 2001, Ezeanolue et al. 2006; Plotnick 2007; Finocchario-Kessler et al. 2010). Questions included:

Do you want/expect to have a child in the future? At what age?

Understanding of mother-to-child transmission was assessed as follows:

Do you know the risk of mother-to-child transmission? What would you estimate the risk to be?

To assess knowledge of preventative measures:

What steps, if any, would you take to prevent your baby and partner from contracting HIV if you were to have a child?

Demographic features and quantitative data were entered into SPSS for analysis.

Interviews were transcribed and then compared to the original recording to assure accuracy. Accuracy of PHT knowledge was coded as follows: 0 % underestimate, 1–2 % accurate, >3 % overestimate, and "I don't know" inaccurate (Finocchario-Kessler et al. 2010). The transcripts were entered into Atlas.ti 6.0, a qualitative data analysis software program. Answers to the open-ended question, "What steps, if any, would you would take to prevent your baby and partner from contracting HIV if you were to have a child?" were independently coded and counted upon consensus between the authors (Patton 1990).

10.5 Socio-Demographic Characteristics of the Participants

Thirty-five AYA with PHIV participated in the study. Demographic features of the sample are reflective of patients receiving care from the two recruitment sites. The mean age of participants was 20.7 (range 15–30 years). The majority of participants were African American (77.1 %) and female (65.7 %). See Table 10.1 for additional demographic details.

As Table 10.2 indicates, the majority (71.4 %) of participants were sexually experienced. Of those, only nine (36.0 %) reported using condoms during all sexual encounters. Many (69.6 %) used other forms of contraceptives, such as oral contraceptives, Depo-Provera, and Norplant. Eight (27.5 %) participants had ever experienced a pregnancy or gotten someone pregnant, and five (14.3 %) were current parents or pregnant at the time of the interview. Although not significant due to the small sample size, it is of note that all eight participants who had ever experienced a pregnancy reported that they did not have a biological mother who was currently living.

10.6 Fertility Desires and Intentions

Among participants, 31 (88.6 %) expressed a desire to have a child in the future, of whom 29 (93.5 %) intended to have a child. The average age at which participants desired to have a child was 27.1 years (range 19–33), and intended age of having a child was 27.0 years (range 20–35). The number of children desired and intended in the future were 2.4 children (range 1–6) and 1.9 children (range 0–4), respectively. Due to the high level of fertility desires and intentions, it was not possible to examine whether demographic or other features were positively associated with the desire or intent to have a child. See Table 10.3 for further details.

Table 10.1 Demographic features

Variable (n=35)	n (%)
Age	
Mean	20.7 years (15–30)
Females	23 (65.7)
Ethnicity	
Black/African American	27 (77.1)
White	3 (8.6)
Hispanic	2 (5.7)
Mixed race	3 (8.6)
Insurance	
Private insurance	12 (34.3)
Medicaid/ Ryan White	18 (51.4)
Uninsured	5 (14.3 %)
Taking HAART	31 (88.6 %)
HIV symptoms in past 6 months	5 (14.3 %)
AIDS diagnosis	9 (25.7 %)
Living situation	
Lives with parent	18 (51.4 %)
Lives independently	8 (25.7 %)
Lives with other relative	6 (17.1 %)
Lives with partner	2 (5.8 %)
Biological mother alive	15 (42.9)
Biological father alive	15 (42.9)
Education	2 (5.7 %)
Some HS	9 (25.7 %)
Currently in HS	5 (14.3 %)
HS graduate	16 (45.7 %)
Some college/vocational school	3 (8.6 %)
College/graduate degree	
Employed	19 (54.3 %)

Table 10.2 Relationship, sexual and reproductive features

Variable	n (%)
Ever sexually active	25 (71.4)
Using contraceptives (other than condoms) (females, n=23)	16 (69.6)
Condom use all the time (males and females, ever sexually active n=25)	9 (36.0)
Current relationship status	
Committed relationship	7 (20.0)
Uncommitted (not exclusive)	3 (8.6)
No relationship/single	25 (71.4)
Ever pregnant/gotten partner pregnant	8 (25.7)[a]
Currently caring for own child/pregnant at time of interview	5 (14.3)

[a]None had a biological mother who was currently living

Table 10.3 Desires/intentions: fertility, parity, and age

Variable	n (%)
Had live birth (all HIV-)/pregnant at time of interview	5 (14.3)
Desire to have child in the future:	31 (88.6)
# of desired children	Mean 2.4 children (range 1–6)
Desired 1 or 2 children	20 (64.5)
Ideal age to have desired child(ren)	Mean 27.1 years (range 19–33)
Intent to have child in the future (n=31):	29 (93.5)
# of intended children	Mean 1.9 children (range 1–4)
Intend 1 or 2 children	22 (75.9)
Ideal age to have intended child(ren)	Mean 27.0 years (range 20–35)

Table 10.4 Knowledge of perinatal HIV transmission

Variable	n (%)
Yes, I know the risk of a baby getting HIV from me/ my partner. (n=35)	21 (60.0)
Females (n=23)	11 (47.8)
Males (n=12)	10 (83.3)
Accurate report of PHT risk for total sample (n=35)	8 (22.8)
Females (n=23)	7 (30.4)
Males (n=12)	1 (8.3)
Mean reported PHT risk of those who offered a number (n=21)	32.5 (range 1–90 %)
Types of PHT knowledge errors (n=35)	
Overestimation of risk	13 (37.1)
"I don't know"	14 (40.0)

10.7 Knowledge of PHT

The mean perceived proportion of risk of PHT by the entire sample was 32.5 % (range 1–90 %). See Table 10.4 for more details. Only eight participants accurately reported the risk of PHT. All of the eight participants who accurately reported the risk of PHT had no children but wanted children in the future. All but one of the participants who accurately reported the risk of PHT were female, and had never been pregnant/gotten someone pregnant. However, these descriptive features were not statistically significant due to small sample sizes. Of note is the finding that 83.3 % of males reported knowing the risk of PHT, but only one (8.3 %) accurately reported the risk. Although the majority of participants did not accurately report the risk of PHT, 22 participants described the benefits of taking medicine for the prevention of PHT and/or the general benefit of "being healthy," 7 participants

Table 10.5 Working knowledge of PHT prevention steps

Preventative measure described	Age 14–18 (n=9)	Age 19–21 (n=14)	Age 22–30 (n=12)	Total sample (n=35)
General health/medications during pregnancy	3	9	10	22
C-section	3	2	2	7
Abstain from breastfeeding	3	4	1	8
Infant receives medications after birth	1	1	1	3
Sperm washing		1		

suggested that having a C-section reduced the risk of PHT, and 8 participants described the reduced risk of transmission associated with abstaining from breastfeeding. Gender, age, sexual experience and history of pregnancy did not appear to be associated with differences in knowledge about transmission prevention, although the small sample sizes limited the use of statistical analyses to test differences. Finally, the eight participants who were able to identify the correct proportion of transmission risk (1–2 %) did not identify more transmission prevention methods than those who did not know the precise risk of transmission (Table 10.5).

10.8 Case Studies

Below are four case studies that describe the complex factors that influence fertility desires among individuals with varying levels of knowledge about perinatal transmission.

Case Study 1: William

This case illustrates the possible effect of overestimating the risk of PHT on one's desire to have children. William is a single 21-year-old African American man who is uncertain about his desire to have children, and does not expect that he will have children in the future. He describes concerns about the complexities of protecting his partner from HIV during conception, and estimates the risk of transmission from mother to child to be "80 or 90 percent." However, he is aware of a few methods of preventing PHT, such as maintaining a low viral load, sperm washing and medications during pregnancy. William worries about infecting a child, and the implications of having a child as a person with HIV:

> [The] first thing would be making sure they didn't get it. So they wouldn't have to live with it like I had to. So that's the biggest thing, and after that I guess I would have to make sure to raise them in a way that makes them more I guess, understanding of it, than I guess a normal child, because eventually I'd want to tell them that, 'your father has it.'

Case Study 2: Rosa

The second case study focuses on the single parent of an uninfected 8 year-old child who also misunderstands the risk of PHT. Rosa is a 29 year-old woman whose Chilean born mother received a blood transfusion contaminated with HIV during childbirth. Rosa's mother died shortly afterwards and she was raised by her maternal aunt. She received excellent medical care throughout childhood and adolescence, but suffered from severe depression. She ultimately had to change schools due to the teasing she experienced once other children learned of her HIV status. At the age of 21, she became pregnant. Rosa's aunt initially asked her to move out upon hearing the news, but later agreed to let her return home. Her seronegative baby girl was delivered by C-section, a step she said was taken to reduce the risk of mother-to-child-transmission. The child's father was financially and emotionally unsupportive and is currently incarcerated. Rosa wishes to have additional children despite the fact that she estimates there is a 50 % chance future children will be born HIV-infected. According to her aunt, Rosa consistently becomes involved with men who treat her poorly. She refuses to end abusive relationships for fear of "being alone." Rosa reports that being a single parent is challenging but that her daughter is doing well in school. She hopes that her daughter completes high school and attends "so she's not like me, sitting at home doing nothing all day."

Case Study 3: Brianna

This case highlights the role that disclosure can play in someone's fertility desires and intentions. Brianna is a single 20-year-old African American woman who gave birth to an HIV-negative child at the age of 15. She explains that she felt unprepared for motherhood and decided on adoption after the birth. Brianna wants to have children in the future, but is most concerned with the requirement to disclose her HIV status to a sexual partner, and states that she would rather "go to a fertility bank." She did not know the risk of mother-to-child transmission, estimating it to be a 50 % chance of infection. She is aware of several preventative measures, including taking medication, having a C-section, and abstaining from breastfeeding, all of which she did during her previous pregnancy. Brianna explains that her desire for a child stems from the nature of the parent-child relationship: "You have somebody who loves you for you. Like, period. No matter your status, or whatever. They love you."

Case Study 4: Mark

The final case study provides insight into fertility desires that may originate from the wish to share a "good life" with another person. Twenty-year-old Mark is a biracial young man who was adopted as an infant by the nurse who cared for him after he was abandoned by his parents. Mark plans to pursue a career in the hospitality industry and intends to adopt two children once he has established a stable relationship. He is eager for his mother to become a grandmother and notes,

> I'm working overtime to find a guy so that I can have kids and I want to make sure she has grandchildren and she can have fun with them and enjoy them….I came from a really great family. I loved my childhood and I want to be able to provide that for another child and I think that I definitely want to share that with somebody.

Mark has a good understanding of the risk of mother-to-child-transmission noting that the chance is very low if the mother is on antiretroviral treatment and her viral load is undetectable.

10.9 Discussion

Fertility desires and intentions were considerably higher than documented in previous studies focused on adult women with HIV of reproductive age, and slightly higher than the few studies that have described fertility desires and intentions among youth with HIV (e.g., Ezeanolue et al. 2006). One study yielded similar rates of pregnancy desires among youth—ranging from 80 % among young females with behaviorally- and perinatally- acquired HIV, and 85 % among uninfected females (Finocchario-Kessler et al. 2012). The sample included in the current study solely consisted of AYA with PHIV. The mean age and age range of our cohort was slightly older at 20.7 years (range 15–30) compared to 19.9 years (15–24) in Finocchario-Kessler et al.'s (2012) sample; and whether the mean age of the 15 participants with PHIV in their study differed from their counterparts with BHIV was not reported. Older AYA may be more likely to desire children as they move toward the end of the developmental stage of establishing intimacy and on to the stage associated with establishing a family (Erikson 1980).

The finding that participants had low knowledge of PHT was consistent with recent studies that reported low knowledge of sexual risk factors among AYA with PHIV (Phillips et al. 2011; see also Chaps. 9 and 11 in this volume). Adult women with HIV also have low knowledge of PHT, which some researchers attribute to physician tendency to discourage pregnancy among adults with HIV (Craft et al. 2007). Findings from this study contradict previous research focused on adult women with HIV that indicates perceptions of high PHT risk lowers fertility desires and intentions (Sowell et al. 1999; Abiodun et al. 2007) and suggest that today, lack of knowledge does not influence childbearing desires or intentions. Still, low knowledge of PHT could adversely affect birth outcomes, and has significant implications for fertility outcomes and parenting as an individual living with PHIV.

Limited research has examined knowledge of PHT among adolescents with PHIV. Ezeanolue et al.'s (2006) study of sexual and reproductive health knowledge among adolescents with PHIV found that 56.1 % of participants perceived the risk of PHT as "high" or were unaware of the risk. However, it is unknown whether participants who described the risk of PHT as "low" were able to identify methods for prevention or the precise proportion of risk. In our study, participants were asked to identify or estimate a transmission risk percentage. Additionally, gender-specific responses were not reported. In the current study, all male participants believed they knew the risk of PHT, but only one of eight correctly identified the risk. Males and females alike reported high levels of fertility desires and intentions, which speaks to the relevance of education about perinatal transmission for both genders. Males with

HIV in serodiscordant couples who desire children face the risk of infecting their partner during attempts to conceive. Further, the risk to women and babies is compounded if infection occurs during pregnancy or postpartum if breastfeeding. In keeping with other researchers' recommendations, findings from our study suggest that providers should have broader discussions about PHT risk and prevention strategies regardless of the patient's gender (Matthews and Mukherjee 2009).

For the population of AYA living with PHIV, low knowledge of PHT may be attributable to age and extended involvement in exclusively pediatric care, as well as the public's tendency to discourage teenage pregnancies by focusing on contraception rather than family planning in young adulthood. That most participants overestimated the risk of PHT may appear in conflict with the levels of fertility desires and intentions reported by participants. Several factors in addition to the age of our sample may explain high rates of fertility desires and intentions, including demographic features and the unique aspects of living with PHIV. First, adolescence and young adulthood are characterized by a higher frequency of risk-taking behaviors and a sense of "invincibility" that may result in a disconnect between risk knowledge and risk taking (Cohn et al. 1995). The majority of our sample were female and black/African American. In the general U.S. population, rates of pregnancy are higher among black/African American women (Ventura and Curtin 2012). As evidenced by the reported insurance coverage (Medicaid/Ryan White) received by the majority of participants, many were of low socioeconomic status, which is similarly correlated with higher fertility rates among adolescents in the general population (Elfenbein and Felice 2003). However, due to the finding that nearly all participants desired children, any differences between the fertility desires and intentions of those groups with private insurance versus Medicaid/Ryan White could not be determined. In order to determine the predictive value of AYA reported fertility desires and intentions, longitudinal studies must be conducted to monitor childbirth rates and outcomes.

Second, the unique context in which individuals with PHIV enter young adulthood may offer further insight into our findings. It is relatively common for AYA living with PHIV to have experienced family disruption due to the loss of parent(s), siblings, or other family members to HIV, and some findings suggest that growing up in a "non-traditional" (e.g. single-parent, poor parent-child relationship) household increases fertility interests among the general population of AYA (Uhlenberg and Mueller 2003; Edin and Kefalas 2011). Although not significant in this study due to small sample sizes, parental loss may influence childbearing. All eight participants who had ever been pregnant or gotten someone pregnant did not have a living mother. The same was not true for the few fathers in our sample. Similar findings were produced by other research which indicated a relationship between maternal loss and a higher frequency of pregnancy among young women with PHIV, although the link was not statistically significant (Tepper et al. 2013). The anticipation of a shorter lifespan might influence the fertility desires and intentions of AYA with PHIV as they may not have been encouraged to consider aspects of future planning such as childbearing and career aspirations. As well, in circumstances of prolonged and intimate health supervision from parental figures and pediatric providers, childbearing may offer an alternative sense of attaining adulthood (Edin and Kefalas 2011).

Within the context of Miller et al.'s (2004) TDIB, it is possible that the biological and social experiences of growing up with HIV heightened childbearing motivations and, in turn, affected desires and intentions. The biological impetus to have a child could be influenced by living with a perinatally-transmitted illness, as well as experiences of maternal loss and family disruption. Early experiences of loss likely shape the development of attachment and nurturant schemas (Bowlby 1982). Further, despite progress, HIV is still a highly stigmatized illness (Nyblade et al. 2009) which may color the context in which AYA with PHIV make reproductive decisions.

Our findings must be considered in light of several limitations. The sample for the study included only 35 participants, all of whom were perinatally infected with HIV, so there is limited generalizability to AYA who acquired HIV behaviorally or through blood transfusion. Data were limited to self-report only, and all participants were engaged in medical care at the time of the interview. Knowledge of modes of PHT, the proportion of risk, and strategies for prevention were assessed using open-ended questions, which may not have captured all areas of AYA knowledge about the subject. The overwhelming majority of participants wanted and expected to have children, so it was not possible to determine what attributes or experiences might contribute to not desiring children. Our sample was recruited from two HIV clinics in the southeastern U.S., which may limit generalizability to other geographic locations.

10.10 Conclusion

In spite of the study limitations, findings highlight the importance of sexual and reproductive health education for AYA with PHIV. Such education must include discussion of fertility desires and intentions rather than simply focusing on pregnancy and transmission prevention as a means to heighten the effectiveness of harm reduction strategies. Although knowledge was not assessed in a questionnaire-format and may not reflect comprehensive and specific understanding of PHT, it is important to recognize that the open-ended nature of the questions allowed for the data to illustrate "working knowledge" of the topic; which is possibly the way in which AYA will make decisions regarding childbearing and prenatal care-seeking behaviors.

Further, those participants who were able to accurately identify the current risk of PHT did not describe a greater number of prevention strategies than those who did not know the risk of PHT. Comprehensive care should include education about specific prevention strategies which may translate into subsequent increased care-seeking behaviors. Anecdotal evidence provided by participants during interviews, made possible due to the semi-structured nature of the study, suggests that AYA with PHIV are interested in obtaining accurate information about PHT as well as general topics about pregnancy and childbearing, despite the prevalence of inability to identify aspects of PHT. Encouragingly, this may indicate that when fertility becomes a more immediate concern, AYA would take steps to access relevant information from medical providers or other resources.

The findings from this study are clinically important in that high fertility desires coupled with low knowledge of PHT risk might contribute to reduced health-seeking behaviors upon pregnancy. Despite the relatively young age of the sample, it is well-documented that higher fertility intentions at ages as young as 18 or 20 years are predictive of greater parity later in life, though less is known about whether this holds true for AYA with HIV (Schoen et al. 1999; Morgan and Rackin 2010). Discussing fertility desires and intentions offers providers an opportunity for anticipatory guidance about childbearing. Previous research indicates that adult women with HIV and other young adults with chronic illness want providers to initiate conversations regarding sexual and reproductive health (Finocchario-Kessler et al. 2010; Tuchman and Kalogiros 2010). The TDIB framework (Miller et al.'s 2004) offers providers a comprehensive view of reproductive behavior and the factors that influenced associated outcomes. That HIV did not appear to impede the desire-intention link for our sample is particularly important: findings suggest that Miller et al.'s (2004) TDIB theoretical framework, based on a "normative" population, is still useful to apply to this population; possibly even more than to their counterparts who acquired HIV later in life. A holistic perspective of sexual and reproductive health education in healthcare settings avoids a narrow approach focused solely on risk behaviors and supports the maturing cohort of AYA as they move forward into adulthood and possibly parenthood. Such an approach to sexual and reproductive health education for the aging population of AYA with PHIV has the potential to not only improve quality of life, but enhances public health efforts to reduce the spread of HIV and offer a model for comprehensive care for emerging populations of AYA with PHIV in developing countries.

Acknowledgements We would like express our deep gratitude to the young people who shared their stories with us. We would also like to thank the Elon University Faculty Research and Development Committee, the Lumen Prize, and the Elon College Fellows program for providing funding.

References

Abiodun, M., Ijaiya, M., & Aboyeji, P. (2007). Awareness and knowledge of mother-to-child transmission of HIV among pregnant women. *Journal of the National Medical Association, 99*(7), 758–763.

Arras, J. (1990). AIDS and reproductive decisions: Having children in fear and trembling. *The Milbank Quarterly, 68*(3), 353–382.

Badell, M. L., Lathrop, E., Haddad, L. B., Goedken, P., Nguyen, M. L., & Cwiak, C. A. (2012). Reproductive healthcare needs and desires in a cohort of HIV-positive women. *Infectious Diseases in Obstetrics and Gynecology, 2012*, Article ID 107878, 6 pages. doi:10.1155/2012/107878.

Bedimo-Rung, A., & Clark, A. (2005). Reproductive decision-making among HIV-Infected women. *Journal of the National Medical Association, 97*(10), 1403–1410.
Bowlby, J. (1982). Attachment and loss: Retrospect and prospect. *American Journal of Orthopsychiatry, 52*(4), 664–678.
Center for Reproductive Rights. (2010). Proceedings of the Ninth session of the UPR working group of the human rights council: *Report on the United States' compliance with its human rights obligations in the area of women's reproductive and sexual health.* United Nations Periodic Review.
Centers for Disease Control and Prevention. (2011). *Pediatric HIV surveillance 2011.* Retrieved May 30, 2014, from http://www.cdc.gov/hiv/topics/surveillance/resources/slides/pediatric/index.htm
Chen, J., Phillips, K., Kanouse, D., Collins, R., & Miu, A. (2001). Fertility desires and intentions of HIV-positive men and women. *Family Planning Perspectives, 33*(4), 144–152.
Cohn, L., Macfarlane, S., Yanez, C., & Imai, W. (1995). Risk-perception: Differences between adolescents and adults. *Health Psychology, 14*(3), 217–222.
Cooper, E., & Charurat, M. (2002). Combination antiretroviral strategies for the treatment of pregnant HIV-1-infected women and prevention of perinatal HIV-1 transmission. *Journal of AIDS, 5*, 484–494.
Craft, S., Delaney, R., Bautista, D., & Serovich, J. (2007). Pregnancy decisions among women with HIV. *AIDS and Behavior, 11*(6), 927–935.
Edin, K., & Kefalas, M. (2011). *Promises I can keep: Why poor women put motherhood before marriage*. Berkeley: University of California Press.
Elfenbein, D., & Felice, M. (2003). Adolescent pregnancy. *Pediatric Clinics of North America, 50*(4), 781–800.
Erikson, E. (1980). *Identity and the life cycle* (Reissue ed.). New York: W. W. Norton & Company.
Ezeanolue, E. E., Wodi, A. P., Patel, R., Dieudonne, A., & Oleske, J. M. (2006). Sexual behaviors and procreational intentions of adolescents and young adults with perinatally acquired human immunodeficiency virus infection: Experience of an urban tertiary center. *Journal of Adolescent Health, 38*(6), 719–725.
Fair, C., & Albright, J. (2012). "Don't tell him you have HIV unless he's 'he one'": Romantic relationships among adolescents and young adults with perinatal HIV infection. *AIDS Patient Care and STDs, 26*(12), 746–754.
Fair, C., Wiener, L., Zadeh, S., Albright, J., Mellins, C. A., Mancilla, M., Kapetnovic, S., et al. (2013). Reproductive health decision-making in perinatally HIV-infected adolescents and young adults. *Maternal and Child Health Journal, 17*(5), 797–808.
Fakoya, A., Lamba, H., Mackie, N., Nandwani, R., Brown, A., Bernard, E., … Gazzard, B. (2008). British HIV Association, BASHH and FSRH guidelines for the management of the sexual and reproductive health of people living with HIV infection 2008. *HIV Medicine, 9*(9), 681–720.
Finocchario-Kessler, S., Sweat, M. D., Dariotis, J. K., Trent, M. E., Kerrigan, D. L., Keller, J. M., & Anderson, J. R. (2010). Understanding high fertility desires and intentions among a sample of urban women living with HIV in the United States. *AIDS and Behavior, 14*(5), 1106–1114.
Finocchario-Kessler, S., Sweat, M. D., Dariotis, J. K., Anderson, J. R., Jennings, J. M., Keller, J. M., … Trent, M. (2012). Childbearing motivations, pregnancy desires, and perceived partner response to a pregnancy among urban female youth: Does HIV-infection status make a difference? *AIDS Care, 24*(1), 1–11.
Frederick, T., Thomas, P., Mascola, L., Hsu, H., Rakusan, T., Mapson, C., … Bertolli, J. (2000). Human immunodeficiency virus-infected adolescents: A descriptive study of older children in New York City, Los Angeles County, Massachusetts and Washington, DC. *Pediatric Infectious Disease Journal, 19*(6), 551–555.
Gage, A. J. (1998). Sexual activity and contraceptive use: The components of the decision making process. *Studies in Family Planning, 29*(2), 154–166.

Gruskin, S., Firestone, R., MacCarthy, S., & Ferguson, L. (2008). HIV and pregnancy intentions: Do services adequately respond to women's needs? *American Journal of Public Health, 98*(10), 1746–1750.

Hass, P. H. (1974). Wanted and unwanted pregnancies: A fertility decision-making model. *Journal of Social Issues, 30*(4), 125–165.

Matthews, L. T., & Mukherjee, J. S. (2009). Strategies for harm reduction among HIV-affected couples who want to conceive. *AIDS and Behavior, 13*(Suppl. 1), 5–11.

Mellins, C. A., Brackis-Cott, E., Leu, C.-S., Elkington, K. S., Dolezal, C., Wiznia, A., et al. (2009). Rates and types of psychiatric disorders in perinatally human immunodeficiency virus-infected youth and seroreverters. *Journal of Child Psychology and Psychiatry, and Allied Disciplines, 50*(9), 1131–1138.

Miller, W. B. (1994). Childbearing motivations, desires, and intentions: A theoretical framework. *Genetic, Social & General Psychology Monographs, 120*(2), 223–253.

Miller, W. B., Severy, L., & Pasta, D. (2004). A framework for modelling fertility motivation in couples. *Population Studies, 58*(2), 193–205.

Morgan, S., & Rackin, H. (2010). The correspondence between fertility intentions and behavior in the United States. *Population and Development Review, 36*(1), 91–118.

Nozyce, M., Lee, S., & Wiznia, A. (2006). A behavioral and cognitive profile of clinically stable HIV-infected children. *Pediatrics, 117*(3), 763–770.

Nyblade, L., Stangl, A., Weiss, E., & Ashburn, K. (2009). Combating HIV stigma in health care settings: What works? *Journal of the International AIDS Society, 12*(15), 1–7.

Paiva, V., Filipe, E. V., Santos, N., Lima, T. N., & Segurado, A. (2003). The right to love: The desire for parenthood among men living with HIV. *Reproductive Health Matters, 11*(22), 91–100.

Patton, M. (1990). *Qualitative evaluation and research methods* (2nd ed.). Thousand Oaks: Sage Publications.

Phillips, U., Rosenberg, M., & Dobroszycki, J. (2011). Pregnancy in women with perinatally acquired HIV-infection: Outcomes and challenges. *AIDS Care, 23*(9), 1076–1082.

Plotnick, R. D. (2007). Adolescent expectations and desires about marriage and parenthood. *Journal of Adolescence, 30*(6), 943–963.

Rubinstein, A., Sicklick, M., & Gupta, A. (1983). Acquired immunodeficiency with reversed T4/T8 ratios in infants born to promiscuous and drug-addicted mothers. *Journal of the American Medical Association, 17*(249), 2350–2356.

Schoen, R., Astone, N., Kim, Y., Nathanson, C., & Fields, J. (1999). Do fertility intentions affect fertility behavior? *Journal of Marriage and the Family, 16*(3), 790–799.

Sherr, L., & Barry, N. (2004). Fatherhood and HIV-positive heterosexual men. *HIV Medicine, 5*(4), 258–263.

Sowell, R., Phillips, K., & Misener, T. (1999). HIV-infected women and motivation to add children to their families. *Journal of Family Nursing, 5*(3), 316–331.

Tepper, V., Kriebs, J., Lovelace, S., & Nair, P. (2013). *The next generation: Perinatally infected adolescents and their reproductive health*. In 19th international AIDS conference: Abstract no. WEAC0103. Retrieved August 18, 2014, from http://ias2015.org/Abstracts/A200746172.aspx

Townsend, C. L., Cortina-Borja, M., Peckham, C. S., de Ruiter, A., Lyall, H., & Tookey, P. A. (2008). Low rates of mother-to-child transmission of HIV following effective pregnancy interventions in the United Kingdom and Ireland, 2000–2006. *AIDS, 22*(8), 973–981.

Tuchman, L., & Kalogiros, I. (2010). Reproductive knowledge and preferences of adolescents and adults with cystic fibrosis: A web-based assessment. *International Journal of Sexual Health, 22*, 72–83.

Uhlenberg, P., & Mueller, M. (2003). Family context and individual well-being. In J. T. Mortimer & M. J. Shanahan (Eds.), *Handbook of the life course* (pp. 123–148). New York: Springer.

Ventura, S., & Curtin, S. (2012). Estimated pregnancy rates and rates of pregnancy outcomes for the United States, 1990–2008. *National Vital Statistics Report, 60*(7), 1–21.

Wiener, L., Battles, H., & Wood, L. (2007). A longitudinal study of adolescents with perinatally or transfusion acquired HIV infection: Sexual knowledge, risk reduction self-efficacy and sexual behavior. *AIDS and Behavior, 11*(3), 471–478.

Williams, H., Watkins, C., & Risby, J. (1996). Reproductive decision-making and determinants of contraceptive use in HIV-infected women. *Clinical Obstetrics and Gynecology, 39*(2), 333–343.

Chapter 11
Men Who Have Sex with Men (MSM) in Accra, Ghana and Lome, Togo: Sexual History and HIV Risk Behavior

Ami Moore and Adobea Owusu

Contents

11.1 Introduction

An estimated 24.7 million of the world's population were infected with HIV in 2013 (WHO 2014). Africa is recognized as the epicenter for the HIV/AIDS pandemic as it contributes 70 % of the world's HIV/AIDS infections. It has 90 % of children orphaned from the disease as well as a very high proportion of the AIDS-related morbidity and mortality. This calls for urgent action among at-risk and the vulnerable populations infected and affected by HIV/AIDS (UNAIDS 2011; Okonofua 2012).

A. Moore (✉)
University of North Texas, 1401 Eufemia Dr, Denton, TX 76207, USA
e-mail: Ami.Moore@unt.edu

A. Owusu
ISSER (Institute of Statistical, Social and Economic Research), University of Ghana, LG 74, Legon, Accra, Ghana
e-mail: gaowusu@ug.edu.gh

P. Liamputtong (ed.), *Children and Young People Living with HIV/AIDS*,
Cross-Cultural Research in Health, Illness and Well-Being,
DOI 10.1007/978-3-319-29936-5_11

One of such groups all over the world, and in Africa particularly, is men who have sex with men (MSM) (Muraguri et al. 2012a, b; Okonofua 2012). Both HIV/AIDS control programs in Ghana and Togo list MSM as an important risk group for HIV infection (Ghana AIDS Commission (GAC) and UNAIDS 2012). Although initially heterosexual sex was the main source of HIV infection in Africa (John 1988; Okonofua 2012), a trend is evolving where same-sex sexual relationships are contributing an unprecedented proportion of the HIV infection in Africa as a whole (Smith et al. 2009; Okonofua 2012). For example, the UNAIDS (2010a, b) has recorded 10 to about 15 % HIV prevalence among MSM in Ghana and Togo, while 20–50 % has been reported in Abidjan, Cote D'Ivoire, Central Nigeria and Dakar in Senegal.

Ghana, with an estimated population of 25.9 million people, had a 1.5 % HIV prevalence in the general population in both 2010 and 2011. In 2013, a national HIV prevalence of 1.3 % was reported (GAC 2014). The HIV incidence for 2010 was 12,890, and 7812 in 2013; with 224,488 prevalence in 2013. Deaths attributed to AIDS in 2010 were 16,319 and 10,074 in 2013. The number of children who were living with HIV in 2010 was 32,329, and 34,557 (15 %) in 2013 (GAC 2014). The age group most affected by HIV is people aged 15–24 (GAC 2011; National AIDS Control Program (NACP), Ghana Health Service (GHS), and Ministry of Health (MOH) 2012). Additionally, findings from a "Ghana Men's Study" in 2011 reported that 17.5 % of MSM were HIV-positive (GAC and UNAIDS 2012: 61). Thus, although HIV/AIDS is generally on a downward trend in Ghana, it still constitutes a great health and socio-economic problem in Ghana (United National Development Program (UNDP) Ghana 2007).

In Togo, with a population of 7,351,374 million (The World Factbook 2014), estimates in 2012 of people living with HIV/AIDS was 128,100, with a prevalence rate of 2.9 % in persons aged 15–49 years, and with an estimated 110,000 adults (15 years and above) living with the pandemic. Also, the number of infected children (0–17 years) was 17,000. Deaths due to AIDS stood at 7158 in 2010, with 90,000 estimated AIDS orphans. New infections during 2010 were 4835. Data also show that compared to females aged 15–49 years, males within the same age group had a much higher sexual risk behavior. Additionally, a study of HIV prevalence among MSM reported 19.6 % of seropositive status (GARPR Togo 2014).

Given the high HIV prevalence rates in MSM in both Ghana and Togo, studying the sexual history and risky sexual behavior of MSM is important for both policy and health intervention. Not until recently, MSM in Africa were given no recognition when it came to the fight against HIV/AIDS for several reasons (Muraguri et al. 2012a, b; Okonofua 2012). Talking about sex and sexual expression in African settings is a near-taboo, even in the era of HIV/AIDS (Owusu et al. 2013; Yankah 2004). Also, some people question the existence of homosexuality among African men especially, as it is believed to be counter-cultural. In fact, the existence of same-sex sexual relationships in Africa in general has until very recently been denied or shrouded in mystery (Dankwa 2009; Essien and Aderinto 2009; Owusu et al. 2013). Furthermore, ethnographic studies on sexual behavior by Africans are rare (Epprecht 2008). Some scholars also believe that denial of the existence of MSM in Africa, cultural, moral and religious rejection of MSM, social stigmatization, and/or criminalization of MSM are some of the reasons for the reluctance of authorities to adequately tackle the sexual health needs of MSM (McKenna 1996). Our chapter therefore contributes immensely to the discourse of risky sexual behavior that African MSM exhibit which may put them and their sexual partners at risk of sexually transmitted infections, including HIV. Beyond this academic exercise, our study has the potential of contributing to policy debates and actions, as well as health interventions for MSM in Ghana and Togo (Okonofua 2012).

11.2 The Phenomenon of MSM in Africa

It has been documented that same-sex sexual expression among men is universal across cultures and societies (Epprecht 2004, 2008; Muraguri et al. 2012a, b). Yet, in the immediate past, and even currently, the phenomenon of MSM has been met with passiveness and denial in most African societies, with the idea that MSM is either non-existent or a foreign practice (Dankwa 2009; Legrand et al. 2010; Okonofua 2012; Owusu et al. 2013). This is in spite of the fact that a number of anthropological accounts have emerged recently, indicating that same-sex relationships, including MSM behaviors and identities, have always existed in African societies (Rupp 1999). In fact, currently in Africa, more people are consenting to same-sex sexual relationships than it was before (Okonofua 2012). Owusu et al. (2013) reported that same-sex sexual practices in Africa have followed a trend where such behaviors were openly practiced in the past, without stigmatization. But, they probably were put at the backdoor during the colonial era particularly with the advent of Christianity and Islam across the continent in the past two centuries or so. Currently, they are gradually coming into the open but with intense stigmatization, requiring several attempts to manage one's same-sex sexual behavior with indirections and verbal discretions (Gaudio 1998; Dankwa 2009; Owusu et al. 2013). In Ghana for instance, Owusu et al. (2013) indicated that MSM relationships are greatly frowned upon, perceived to be distant from mainstream Ghanaian society, and thought of as a socio-cultural deviation, a bad omen, demonic act, and an abnormality which deserves punishment, including criminalization and banishment from communities. However, there are accounts of MSM sexual practices in literally all African countries. For instance, Attipoe (2004), Dankwa (2009), and Essien and Aderinto (2009) document the existence of MSMs in Ghana; the same observation has been made in Togo (CNLS-IST and UNAIDS 2012; GARP Togo 2012).

Additionally, accounts of MSM have come from Epprecht (2008) and Gaudio (2009) in even northern Nigeria where Islam is said to be more strictly practiced. Other accounts of MSM practices have been made in Senegal (Niang et al. 2003; Wade et al. 2005; Geibel et al. 2010), Botswana (Baral et al. 2009), Lesotho (Baral et al. 2011) and several other parts of sub-Saharan Africa (Epprecht 2004; Muraguri et al. 2012a, b; Okonofua 2012). These accounts call for the need to open the Pandora box regarding MSM sexual behavior in Africa. While it has been established that MSM behavior is nearly universal, it is difficult to estimate the prevalence of male same-sex sexual behavior, particularly in Africa where MSM behavior is highly stigmatized (Muraguri et al. 2012a, b; Okonofua 2012). Estimates of the MSM population in Africa based on limited information in places such as South Africa and Tanzania is pegged at 2 % life time MSM activity on the continent (Caceres et al. 2008; Muraguri et al. 2012a, b).

11.3 MSM as a High Risk Group for HIV/AIDS in Africa

MSM are of particular importance when it comes to HIV/AIDS. Several studies have concluded that MSM constitute a high risk group for HIV infection in Africa and worldwide (Smith et al. 2009; Beyrer et al. 2010a, b; Legrand et al. 2010; McDaid and Hart 2010; Millett et al. 2012; Muraguri et al. 2012a, b). This makes paying attention to their risky sexual behaviors important. The UNAIDS (2006) reported that a 5–10 % of the global HIV burden is contributed by MSM. However, the extent of the burden varies from country to country and different regions in the world. In regions with generalized HIV epidemic, such as in Eastern and Southern Africa, MSM have higher HIV infection rates than the general population (Smith et al. 2009; Beyrer et al. 2010a, b; McDaid and Hart 2010; Muraguri et al. 2012a, b; GAC 2012; Okonofua 2012). Beyrer et al. (2010a, b) estimated 3.8 times likelihood of higher HIV infection among MSM in Africa, compared to men within the reproductive age in the general populations. More specifically, Muraguri et al. (2012a, b) reported 50 % HIV prevalence rates among MSM in Abidjan, Cote D'Ivoire; 49.5 % in Johannesburg, South Africa; 37.6 % in the Federal Capital Territory, Nigeria; 24.5 % in Mombasa, Kenya; 21.4 % in Blantyre and Lilongwe, Malawi; 21.8 % in Dakar, Senegal; 19.7 % in Gaborone, Botswana; 18.2 % in Nairobi, Kenya and 15.8 % in Lagos, Nigeria.

Furthermore, McDaid and Hart (2010) reported a range of 8 % HIV prevalence in Sudan to 34 % in Cape Town, South Africa, among MSM. The only known HIV incidence rate among MSM, reported in Mombasa and Nairobi, in Kenya, cited 6.8 per 100 person-years (Muraguri et al. 2012a, b). Similarly, Millett et al. (2012) indicated that diasporan African MSM had as much as 15 times higher likelihood of being HIV-positive compared with the general populations in the countries in which they live, and also they were 8.5 times more likely to be infected by HIV than black male populations. Although these rates need to be treated with caution because some of the studies did not use representative sampling (McDaid and Hart 2010; Muraguri et al. 2012a, b), they still give an indication of rather high rates of HIV among MSM in Africa. Importantly, MSM groups suffer other STIs as well (Muraguri et al. 2012a, b).

11.4 Risk Behaviors That Put MSM at a Higher Risk of HIV

Evidence strongly suggests that MSM in Africa engage in risky sexual behavior. MSM engage in both insertive and receptive anal sex (McDaid and Hart 2010; Muraguri et al. 2012a, b). Some African MSM consider anal sex not to expose one to the risk of HIV transmission, possibly leading to active pursuit of such behavior (Geibel et al. 2008; Kalamar et al. 2011; Muraguri et al. 2012a, b). However, as noted by McDaid and Hart (2010: 312), "receptive unprotected anal intercourse (UAI) remains the behavior with the greatest risk of HIV transmission". Also, MSMs may not use condoms during anal sex (barebacking) or use it inconsistently (McDaid and Hart 2010; Muraguri et al. 2012a, b). In fact, studies have shown that the use of condom rates vary from 9 % over the past 1 month in Ugunja, Zanzibar in 2007 (Dahoma et al. 2011) to 80 % over the past 2 months in Pretoria (Tun et al. 2012). Additionally, Muraguri et al. (2012a, b) documented consistent use of condoms during MSM sexual encounters from a minimal 7 % (in Kano, Nigeria, in 2010) to 63 % (in Kampala, Uganda in 2004), over the past 6 months (Kajubi et al. 2008; Federal Ministry of Health (FMOH) 2011). In Togo, in 2010, for example, condom use at last intercourse with a man was about 48 % (*CNLS-IST* and UNAIDS 2012). Additionally, MSM may use condom less often with their main sexual partners (Sullivan et al. 2009).

Several reasons account for inconsistent condom use among MSM. These include desire for sexual pleasure and adventure, trust for partner, fulfilling a transactional obligation, having casual/unplanned/unintended sex, inadequate self-efficacy for condom use, inadequate information about self- and/or partner's serostatus (Carballo-Diéguez 1989; Sullivan et al. 2009; Kalamar et al. 2011). Even when they use condoms, it is known that MSM in Africa usually use lubricants such as petroleum products, baby oils and other lotions during anal sex (Onyango-Ouma et al. 2005; Baral et al. 2009; FMOH 2011; Muraguri et al. 2012a, b). The use of these products typically lead to breakage of the condoms (Geibel et al. 2008; Muraguri et al. 2012a, b), rendering their use ineffective with possible implications for HIV transmission from an infected partner to an uninfected one. MSM in Africa use such lubricants because of a lack of knowledge about the impact of such lubricants on latex condoms, difficulty finding water based lubricants, high cost of condoms, and inappropriate packaging of the condoms (Moreau et al. 2007).

Also, MSM in general are noted to have greater frequency of sexual acts (McDaid and Hart 2010), and they also have high rates of multiple sexual partners (Niang et al. 2003; McDaid and Hart 2010; FMOH 2011; Kalamar et al. 2011; Muraguri et al. 2012a, b). The number of reported male sexual partners over a relatively short time for some MSM is rather high. For instance, in Mombasa, Kenya, 74 % of MSM reported multiple male sexual partners in the past 7 days in 2006, while 63 % of them reported multiple male sexual partners over the same time frame in 2008 (Geibel et al. 2012). In Kisumu, Kenya, as many as 92 % of MSM studied reported multiple male sexual partners in the past 12 months in 2010 (Plenty et al. 2011).

A study of MSM in Malawi, Namibia and Botswana found that 15 % of them reported having at least five male sexual partners in the past 6 months, with a mean of 3.2 male sexual partners over that time frame. Additionally, 54 % of the sample reported having both male and female sexual partners in the past 6 months (Baral et al. 2009).

Yet another risky sexual behavior among African MSM is payment for sex or sex work (Muraguri et al. 2012a, b). According to Muraguri et al. (2012a, b), a range of 6–74 % of MSM in Africa who had been studied over various time frames reported having engaged in anal sex with other MSM after having paid for it or engaged in it as sex work for pay. For instance, 87 % of MSM in Mombasa in 2006 had either paid for sex or were sex workers in the past 7 days. In 2008, 81 % of MSM interviewed in Mombasa over the same time frame (past 7 days) reported either paying for sex or being a sex worker (Geibel et al. 2012). Similarly, 67 % of MSM recruited in Kisumu in 2010 using random sampling reported commercial sex work or having paid for sex in the past 2 months. Also, 64 % of MSM interviewed in Kano, Nigeria, in 2010 using random sampling had ever paid for sex or engaged in commercial sex work with other men in the past 6 months, and 59 % of MSM interviewed in Ugunja (Zanzibar), Tanzania, using random sampling in 2007 had also paid for sex or undertaken commercial sex work in their lifetime experience as MSM (Dahoma et al. 2011). It is noteworthy to mention that 50 % of the MSM who reported engaging in transactional sexual intercourse with other MSM in Abidjan in 2007–2008 reported being HIV positive (Vuylsteke et al. 2012).

In some instances, substance use and abuse has also been blamed for the lack of and/or inconsistent use of condoms among MSM in Africa. The use and abuse of alcohol has been reported in some studies (Lane et al. 2008; Luchters et al. 2011). Other studies have reported limited drug use (Sanders et al. 2007; Lane et al. 2008; Muraguri et al. 2012a, b). In their study on MSM and HIV transmission in general, McDaid and Hart (2010: 312) documented an association between drug use, risky sexual behavior and HIV acquisition and transmission. However, injecting drug use risk behavior is reportedly not common among African MSM (Sanders et al. 2007; Lane et al. 2008; Muraguri et al. 2012a, b).

Quite unique to Africa, MSM in this region have a preponderance to be bisexual, and often, these relationships are concurrent with both other MSM and also wives or other women with whom they have long term sexual relationships (Epprecht 2008; Kalamar et al. 2011; Muraguri et al. 2012a, b; Owusu et al. 2013). This implies that MSM in Africa also contribute to heterosexual transmission of HIV (GAC and UNAIDS 2012; Muraguri et al. 2012a, b). MSM in Africa's usual bisexual behavior is typically to conceal their true sexual orientation (Beyrer et al. 2010a, b; Broz et al. 2011; Kalamar et al. 2011; Muraguri et al. 2012a, b). Bisexual behavior has also been report among MSM in other countries such as Thailand, though (McDaid and Hart 2010). (See also Chap. 12 for MSM in China).

11.5 The Study

Human sexuality is a complex phenomenon that is influenced by biology, psychology, culture, religion and law (DeLamater and Sill 2005; Shapiro and Ray 2007). The psychological and cultural influences of sexuality are basically about the way sex is viewed, what is desired, what is expected, and intensity of sexual desire. Psychological as well as cultural factors are socially constructed and hence vary from one society to another. Through language, different labels are used to praise or denigrate any sexual behavior deemed socially acceptable or inappropriate (Brickell 2006). Homosexuality being highly stigmatized in Africa in general, and in both Ghana and Togo in particular, we wanted to understand how our participants became MSM and their sexual histories. Specifically, we asked our study participants about their first sexual activity with a man, their age at this first sexual encounter, the circumstances under which it occurred, and their relationship with the male partner. We also examined risky sexual behavior that these MSM exhibited.

We conducted a cross-sectional survey and interviews among 60 MSM in Accra, Ghana and Lome, Togo. Participants were recruited via a convenience sampling from October 2012 to July 2013. We have established working relationships in both cities. We contacted a director of the only HIV center that caters to the needs of MSM in Lome, Togo, explained the purpose of the study to him and asked him to help recruit potential participants. In Ghana, we contacted an MSM program manager who was himself an MSM, explained the purpose of the study to this person and asked him to help recruit potential participants. They then talked to the MSM and those who agreed to participate were interviewed by the first author. To be included, one must be at least 18 years old and an MSM. The study protocol was approved by the University of North Texas Institutional Review Board. A consent form was signed by each participant prior to both survey and interview. Interviews lasted 50 min on average. The data were transcribed verbatim. The present chapter presents the findings of the interviews that focused on the sexual histories and risky sexual behaviors of our study participants.

The interview data were analyzed manually, using the successive approximation method (Wolfer 2007) in combination with the approach of grounded theory. First, through open coding, recurrent concepts were generated. Second, through axial coding, we created relationships within the concepts. We identified two ways through which first sexual encounter happened – planned and unplanned, and three types of risky sexual behavior: exchange sex for a valued resource, inconsistent use of condoms, and having multiple sexual partners.

The mean age of the participants was about 22 years. They had a mean of about 11 years of education. They were all single, but about 7 % had children. The mean age at which they had their first sexual intercourse was 14 years. The mean number of the people they had had sex with in their lifetime was 22. Also, in the past 6 months prior to the study, the MSM had sex with a mean number of eight people. They were mostly HIV-negative (about 82 %). Seventeen percent reported they had ever had a sexually transmitted infection, and about 32 % had ever exchanged sex

Table 11.1 Demographic characteristics of the MSM (N=60)

	Mean	Percent
Age	22.33	
Age at 1st sex	14.20	
Number of years of education	11.33	
Number of life time sexual partners	22.57	
Number of people had sex with past 6 months	8.19	
Number of people had sex with past 3 months	4.68	
HIV serotatus		
Negative		81.7
Positive		6.7
Do not know		11.7
Had children		
Yes		6.7
No		93.3
Had sex with women		
Yes		21.67
No		78.33
Had ever had sexually transmitted disease		
Yes		17
No		83
Had ever sold sex		
Yes		31.6
No		68.4
Consistently use condoms		
Yes		28.8
No		65.4
Currently employed or in school		
Employed		48.3
School		40
Unemployed		11.7

for money or a valuable resource. While 48 % were employed, 40 % were still attending school, and almost 12 % were unemployed. Additionally, participants exhibited some risky sexual behavior: exchange sex for a valued resource, having multiple sexual partners, and inconsistent use of condoms (Table 11.1).

11.6 Sexual Histories

Mostly, our participants had their very first sexual encounter with a male (78 %). However, their first homosexual experience happened with males who were family members, classmates, friends, neighbors, people met online, and teachers (Table 11.2).

Table 11.2 Relationship with first male sexual partner

Relationship	Number	Percent (%)
Family member	10	17
Classmate	19	32
Friend	15	25
Neighbor	12	20
Teacher	2	3
Men met online	2	3
Total	60	100

While having sex with a male classmate was the most cited first homosexual experience, the least was with a male teacher or with a male person met on the internet. Also, some of the respondents who had sex with their male classmates had the experience in a boarding school. While in some of the cases, the participants planned and initiated the encounter, in other cases, it was the partner that planned and initiated the act. However, in other cases, sexual activity was not planned, but it just happened.

Mike, who had his first homosexual sexual encounter at age 15, explained how this activity happened in the following case where the male classmate had planned this encounter.

> It happened with a classmate. He invited me over to his place. When I arrived, we began to talk and then he turned on a pornographic video and asked me if we could have sex. I did not refuse and we had it. After that encounter, then I began to have sex with an uncle who was 28 years old. I then met other guys afterward and continue on having sex with men.

Another respondent, Kwame, who had his first homosexual encounter at age 12, described the circumstance as follows:

> I am a bit effeminate, you know. So, this male friend used to tease me all the time. One day we were watching a movie at his house, and there was a love scene. So I asked him if we can have sex and he did not refuse. So, that is how it happened.

For almost all of our participants, their first homosexual experience began prior to their becoming young adults (before they turned 20 years old). However, three of the participants had had their first homosexual experience in their twenties. Such was the case of Alfred, a 27 year old father of two. He told us:

> My homosexual life began when I was in training to become a tailor. I was 21 and there was a classmate who invited me to homosexual evening get-to-together. I met one guy there who courted me and afterward we went to his house and had sex.

11.7 Risky Sexual Behavior

We identified three types of risky sexual behavior among our study participants: exchange sex for a valued resource, having multiple sexual partners, and inconsistent use of condoms. Several reasons were given for these risky sexual activities.

11.7.1 Exchange Sex for Valued Resources

Participants exchanged sex for mainly financial reasons. Some had older married men who provided them with foods and paid for their school fees and other amenities. Steven simply stated: "when I am hungry, I go out with men who can give me money to buy food". While Steven's reason shows that some of the participants would trade sex for basic needs to survive, it seems like this is a relatively pervasive issue among some of the young men who do not have traditional means (education and skills) to gainfully support themselves. In fact, our participants also discussed how some of the young men who were supposedly not MSM but were using their bodies to secure finances or any valuable resources by sleeping with other men. They said these men were 'situational' or 'occasional' MSM. In fact, Ohene described this phenomenon in great detail:

> … Sometimes, the men can make about 3000CFA (about 6USD) or less. Sometimes, the male partners will just buy them a meal and a drink. Others become MSM in order to steal from people. They come to your place of residence and sleep with you. Afterwards, they steal something from you. I witnessed such a case when I was with my friend one day. That day, I was very sick and my friend asked me to stay with him at his place instead of leaving me alone at my place. His roommate brought a guy home with him. I then left the bedroom and sat in the living room. Then after they had sex, the guy came to the living room and grabbed something. Then he left. After a while, the roommate came out looking for his cell phone. He asked me if I saw the phone. I told him that the guy that left grabbed something of the table before he left but I did not look to see what he took. The phone was later recovered from the guy. … You know, there are many young men today who just love sex and will sleep with you. Some claim to be heterosexual but they come to you and ask you to make love to them. They claim not to be able to sleep with a man (insertive sex), so they accept a receptive sex and then ask for money or steal something from you afterward. They will accept a receptive sex to get whatever necessities they need.

Others slept with a man as a sign of gratitude for helping them. Thomas, a 25-year old MSM who identified himself as homosexual because he had never slept with a female, noted:

> I was in need of money and called this guy to see if I could come and see him at home. I knew that if I go to his house, we will make love and he would give me some money. He is a 40-year old man who is a bit well-off. … I sleep with him whenever I get something valuable from him.

Some participants had a project that had to be financed but did not have the funds for it. Thus, they would sell sex in order to obtain the necessary funds. Often, these young MSM would look for foreign men as the rumor was that they usually pay good money. This was Eric's situation, a 20-year old barber. He confided:

> I needed money to open my shop. Then a friend told me that there are some European men who want to have sex for money. When I went to see these guys, I noticed that they were not white but black (Nigerians and Cameroonians). These guys wanted me to be in a pornographic video that they were making. I refused and then they gave me 25,000 CFA (about $50) and asked me not to tell anyone.

Another respondent, Edem, remarked:

> It was in the month of April this year (2014) when a friend of mine called me and informed me that there were two gay foreign men (Egyptians) who wanted two men. We went to meet them and we went to Aneho (a town about 30 miles from Lome, the Capital city of Togo). In the evening of our second stay, they paid each of us 30,000 CFA (about $60).

11.7.2 Having Multiple Sexual Partners

Some of our participants had multiple sexual partners in order to make ends meet as indicated earlier. They traded sex for money or food for example. However, others had multiple partners, especially females, to conceal their homosexual orientation. For instance, Tom, an 18-year old MSM, who was caught when he was 15 years old having sex with another male and was severely beaten by his parents noted the following:

> Whenever my parents asked me if I still continue that lifestyle (having sex with men), I tell them no. I even found a girlfriend and bring her to my house to prove them (parents) that I am now straight.

11.7.3 Inconsistent Use of Condoms

Different reasons were given for not consistently using condoms. Some participants believed that since antiretroviral drugs are relatively readily available, they would be able to use them in case they became infected. They did not fear HIV, but they were cautious about having sex with men that they considered violent or too aggressive in bed. Sam told us:

> I do not like condoms, yes, I do not like condoms at all. I never use condoms when I know my partner. I am more cautious about having my buttom tear up. I am careful about the men that I sleep with in that regard.

When asked why having his bottom tear up more important than getting HIV, he responded:

> If I ever get HIV, I will take drugs for it. But if I have my buttom torn up, I will need someone to care for me. However, I do not have anybody who will do that.

Other MSM wanted their partners to ejaculate faster especially in cases of receptive sex. Partners ejaculate faster when condom is not used.

> The life of MSM is difficult especially you may meet some men who would not want to come. Hence, they would stay in you for a long time. This is very uncomfortable. So I do not use condoms with such men as it helps them to come quicker. (Senam)

Intense, uncontrollable urge prior to anal sex was another common reason shared by our participants. A few MSM reported that they could not control their sexual desire and use condom prior to anal intercourse. Kokou revealed: "At times, the feelings that one has for the other guy is too intense and one is unable to get a condom and use it. The sexual urge is just too intense".

11.8 Conclusion

In this study, we examined the sexual history and risky sexual behavior among MSM in both Accra, Ghana and Lome, Togo. Our findings show that the first homosexual activity that our study participants experienced were with mainly classmates, especially in boarding schools, friends, neighbors, and family members. Also, the MSM in both countries exhibited risky sexual behavior that put them and their sexual partners at risk for HIV and other sexually transmitted infections. Additionally, while some of our findings, especially the reasons for exhibiting risky sexual behavior, concur with previous studies, our study also found that some of the MSM did not use condoms because they wanted their partner to quickly ejaculate as they were uncomfortable during sexual activities when they were the passive partners. While we do not know why this was the case, some of the MSM explained that some men could be wild and will not take into consideration that anal sex is not the same as vaginal sex. However, this may also stem from abuses that these men encounter as they trade sex for valued resources.

A few policy recommendations are warranted. First, we believe that policymakers and stakeholders should come up with programs to train and/or educate these young men. With education and skills, they will not feel obligated to trade sex for valued resources. Second, it is important for authorities to recognize that the sexual risk behavior of MSM is partly facilitated by a climate of difficult structural barriers which are social, political and legal (Smith et al. 2009; Kalamar et al. 2011; Muraguri et al. 2012a, b; Okonofua 2012). These barriers include the strong stigma and discrimination African societies attach to MSM behavior (Smith et al. 2009; Legrand et al. 2010; GAC 2012; Muraguri et al. 2012a, b; Okonofua 2012; Owusu et al. 2013) and also for HIV and AIDS (Onyango-Ouma et al. 2005; Moreau et al. 2007; Muraguri et al. 2012a, b; Tenkorang and Owusu 2013). In fact, Muraguri et al. (2012a, b) noted that MSM sexual behavior and expression is illegal in 31 African countries, and in four countries, MSM sexual behavior can attract death penalty. Both the Ghanaian and Togolese National AIDS Control programs' reports cite criminalization of same sex sexual activities and stigma and discrimination as current challenges (GAC and UNAIDS 2012; CNLS-IST and UNAIDS 2012).

References

Attipoe, D. (2004). *Revealing the pandora box or playing the ostrich? A situational appraisal of men having sex with men in the Accra Metropolitan area and its environs – Ghana*. Unpublished. Accra, Ghana: West Africa Project to Combat HIV/AIDS and STI (WAPCAS).

Baral, S., Trapence, G., Motimedi, F., Umar, E., Lipinge, S., Dausab, F., et al. (2009). HIV prevalence, risks of HIV infection, and human rights among men who have sex with men (MSM) in Malawi, Namibia and Botswana. *PLoS ONE, 4*(3), e4997. 1–8.

Baral, S., Adams, D., Lebona, J., Kaibe, B., Letsie, P., Tshehlo, R., et al. (2011). A cross-sectional assessment of population demographics. HIV risks and human rights context among men who have sex with men in Lesotho. *Journal of International AIDS Society, 14*(36), 1–9.

Beyrer, C., Baral, S. D., Walker, D., Wirtz, A. L., Johns, B., & Sifakis, F. (2010a). The expanding epidemics of HIV type 1 among men who have sex with men in low and middle-income countries: Diversity and consistency. *Epidemiology Reviews, 32*(1), 137–151.

Beyrer, C., Trapence, G., Motimedi, F., Umar, E., Lipinge, S., Dausab, F., et al. (2010b). Bisexual concurrency, bisexual partnerships, and HIV among Southern African men who have sex with men. *Sexually Transmitted Infections, 86*(4), 323–327.

Brickell, C. (2006). The sociological construction of gender and sexuality. *The Sociological Review, 54*(1), 87–113.

Broz, D., Okal, J., Tun, W., Sheehy, M., Mutua, M., Muraguri, N., et al. (2011). *High levels of bisexual behaviors among men who have sex with men in Nairobi, Kenya*. 6th IAS conference on HIV pathogenesis, Treatment and prevention, Rome, Italy, July 17–20. Abstract no MOLBPEO46.

Caceres, C., Konda, K., Segura, E., & Lyerla, R. (2008). Epidemiology of male same-sex behavior and associated health indicators in low- and medium-income countries: 2003–2007 estimates. *Sexually Transmitted Infections, 84*(Suppl. 1), i49–i56.

Carballo-Diéguez, A. (1989). Hispanic culture, gay male culture, and AIDS: Counseling implications. *Journal of Counseling & Development, 68*(1), 26–30.

Conseil National de Lutte Contre le SIDA et les IST &UNAIDS. (2012). *Rapport de progres sur la riposte au SIDA au Togo (GARP) 2012*. http://www.unaids.org/en/regionscountries/countries/togo/. Accessed 25 Oct 2013.

Dahoma, M., Johnston, L. G., Holman, A., Miller, L. A., Mussa, M., Othman, A., et al. (2011). HIV and related risk behavior among men who have sex with men in Zanzibar, Tanzania: Results of a behavioral surveillance survey. *AIDS and Behavior, 15*(1), 186–192.

Dankwa, S. O. (2009). 'It's a silent trade': Female same-sex intimacies in Post-Colonial Ghana. *Nordic Journal of Feminist and Gender Research, 17*, 192–205.

DeLamater, J. D., & Sill, M. (2005). Sexual desire in later life. *The Journal of Sex Research, 42*, 138–149.

Epprecht, M. (2004). *Hungochani: A history of a dissident sexuality in Southern Africa*. Montreal: McGill-Queen's University Press.

Epprecht, M. (2008). *Hungochani: A history of a dissident sexuality in Southern Africa*. Montreal: McGill-Queen's University Press.

Essien, K., & Aderinto, S. (2009). Cutting the head of the roaring monster: Homosexuality and repression in Africa. *African Study Monographs, 30*, 121–135.

Federal Ministry of Health (FMOH). (2011). *HIV integrated biological and behavioral surveillance survey (IBBSS) 2010*. Abuja: FMOH.

GARPR (2014). *Raport de progres sur la riposte au VIH et au SIDA au Togo*. Retrieved from http://www.unaids.org/sites/default/files/en/dataanalysis/knowyourresponse/countryprogressreports/2014countries/TGO_narrative_report_2014.pdf

Gaudio, R. P. (1998). Male lesbians and other queer notions in Hausa. In S. O. Murray & W. Roscoe (Eds.), *Boy-wives and female husbands: Studies of African homosexualities* (pp. 115–128). New York: St. Martin's Press.

Gaudio, R. P. (2009). *Allah made us: Sexual outlaws in an Islamic African City*. Malden: Wiley-Blackwell.

Geibel, S., Luchters, S., King'ola, N., Esu-Williams, E., Rinyiru, A., & Tun, W. (2008). Factors associated with self-reported unprotected anal sex among male sex workers in Mombasa, Kenya. *Sexually Transmitted Disease Infections, 35*(8), 746–752.

Geibel, S., Tun, W., Tapsoba, P., & Kellerman, S. (2010). HIV vulnerability of men who have sex with men in developing countries: Horizons studies, 2001–2008. *Public Health Report, 125*, 316–324.

Geibel, S., King'ola, N., Temmerman, M., & Luchters, S. (2012). The impact of peer outreach on HIV knowledge and prevention behaviours of male sex workers in Mombasa, Kenya. *Sexually Transmitted Diseases, 35*(8), 746–752.

Ghana AIDS Commission. (2011). *AIDS country progress report for January 2009 – December, 2010*. Accra: GAC.

Ghana AIDS Commission. (2012). *Ghana country AIDS progress report for January 2011 – December 2011*. Accra: GAC.

Ghana AIDS Commission. (2014). *Summary of the 2013 HIV sentinel survey report*. http://ghanaids.gov.gh/gac1/aids_info.php. Accessed 23 Oct 2014.

Ghana AIDS Commission and UNAIDS. (2012). *Ghana country AIDS progress report (January 2010 – December 2011)*. Submitted March 2012. http://www.unaids.org/en/dataanalysis/knowyourresponse/countryprogressreports/2012countries/ce_GH_Narrative_Report[1].pdf. Access 25 Oct 2013.

John, A. M. (1988). *A model of HIV-1 transmission dynamics and of the demographic impact of HIV-1 infection in developing countries. Paper 0018. Food Research Institute*. Stanford: Standford University. May.

Kajubi, P., Kamya, M. R., Raymond, H. R., Chen, S., Rutherford, G. W., Mandel, J. S., et al. (2008). Gay and bisexual men in Kampala, Uganda. *AIDS and Behavior, 12*(3), 492–504.

Kalamar, M., Maharaj, P., & Gresh, A. (2011). HIV prevention interventions targeting men having sex with men in Africa: Field experiences from Cameroon. *Culture, Health & Sexuality, 13*(10), 1135–1149.

Lane, T., Shade, S. B., McIntyre, J., & Morin, S. F. (2008). Alcohol and sexual risk behavior among men who have sex with men in South African township communities. *AIDS and Behavior, 12*(Suppl. 4), S78–S85.

Legrand, A., Yomb, Y., Bourrelly, M., Lorente, N., & NKom, A. (2010). MSM law in francophone Africa and the fight against AIDS: The hypocrisy of certain countries. *HIV AIDS Policy Law Review, 14*(3), 13–17.

Luchters, S., Geibel, S., Syengo, M., Lango, D., King'ola, N., Temmerman, M., et al. (2011). Use of AUDIT, and measures of drinking frequency and patterns to detect associations between alcohol and sexual behavior in male sex workers in Kenya. *BMC Public Health, 11*(384), 1–8.

McDaid, L. M., & Hart, G. (2010). Sexual risk behavior for transmission of HIV in men who have sex with men: Recent findings and potential interventions. *Current Opinion in HIV and AIDS, 5*, 311–315.

McKenna, N. (1996). *On the margins: Men who have sex with men and HIV in developing countries*. London: Panos Institute.

Millett, G. A., Jeffries, W. L., Peterson, J. L., Malebranche, D. J., Lane, T., Flores, S. A., et al. (2012). HIV in men who have sex with men. Common roots: A contextual review of HIV epidemics in black men who have sex with men across the African diaspora. *Lancet, 380*, 411–423.

Moreau, A., Tapsoba, P., Ly, A., Niang, C. I., & Diop, A. K. (2007). *Implementing STI/HIV prevention and care interventions for men who have sex with men in Senegal, Horizons Research Summary*. Washington, DC: Population Council.

Muraguri, N., Temmerman, M., & Geibel, S. (2012a). A decade of research involving men who have sex with men in sub-Saharan Africa: Current knowledge and future directions. *Journal of Social Aspects of HIV/AIDS, 9*(3), 137–147.

Muraguri, N., Tun, W., Okal, J., Broz, D., Raymond, H. F., Kellogg, T., et al. (2012b). *Burden of HIV and sexual behaviour among men who have sex with men and male sex workers in Nairobi, Kenya*. XIX international AIDS conference, Washington, DC, July 23. Abstract no MOPE301.

NationalAIDS/STI Control Programme, Ghana Health Service, Ministry of Health. (2012). *2011 HIV sentinel survey report*. Accra: NACP, GHS and MOH.

Niang, C. I., Tapsoba, P., Weiss, E., Diagne, M., Niang, Y., Moreau, A. M., et al. (2003). 'It's raining stones': Stigma, violence and HIV vulnerability among men who have sex with men in Dakar, Senegal. *Culture, Health & Sexuality, 5*(6), 499–512.

Okonofua, F. (2012). Same sex relationships and HIV/AIDS in Africa: Need for research and programmatic focus. *African Journal of Reproductive Health, 16*(4), 9–12.

Onyango-Ouma, W., Birungi, H., & Geibel, S. (2005). *Understanding the HIV/STI risks and prevention needs of men who have sex with men in Nairobi, Kenya*. Washington, DC: Population Council.

Owusu, A. Y., Anarfi, J. K., & Tenkorang, E. Y. (2013). Attitudes and views on same-sex sexual behavior in Ghana. *Global Advanced Research Journal of Social Science (GARJSS), 2*(8), 176–186.

Plenty, A., Bailey, R., Geibel, S., & Adinya-Achola, J. O. (2011). *Men's health study: Preliminary findings of a respondent-driven sampling study of MSM in Kisumu. University of Nairobi* STD/HIV Collaborative Group 2011 Annual Review Meeting, Nairobi. 22 January.

Rupp, L. J. (1999). *A desired past: A history of same-sex love in America*. Chicago: University of Chicago Press.

Sanders, E. J., Graham, S. M., Okuku, H. S., van der Elst, E. M., Muhaari, A., Davies, A., et al. (2007). HIV-1 infection in high risk MSM in Mombasa, Kenya. *AIDS, 21*(18), 2513–2520.

Shapiro, K., & Ray, S. (2007). Sexual health for people living with HIV. *Reproductive Health Matters, 15*(29 Suppl.), 67–92.

Smith, A. D., Tapsoba, P., Peshu, N., Sanders, E. J., & Jaffe, H. W. (2009). Men who have sex with men and HIV/AIDS in sub-Saharan Africa. *The Lancet, 374*(9687), 416–422.

Sullivan, P. S., Salazar, L., Buchbinder, S., & Sanchez, T. H. (2009). Estimating the proportion of HIV transmission from main sex partners among men who have sex with men in five US cities. *AIDS, 23*, 1153–1162.

Tenkorang, E. Y., & Owusu, A. (2013). Examining HIV-related stigma and discrimination in Ghana: What are the major contributors? *Sexual health, 10*(3). doi:10.1071/SH12153

The World Factbook. (2014). Africa: Togo. https://www.cia.gov/library/publications/the-world-factbook/geos/to.html. Accessed on 26 Jan 2015.

Tun, W., Kellerman, S., Maimane, S., Fipaza, Z., Sheehy, M., Vu, L., et al. (2012). HIV-related conspiracy beliefs and its relationships with HIV testing and unprotected sex among men who have sex with men in Tshwane (Pretoria), South Africa. *AIDS Care, 24*(4), 459–467.

UNAIDS. (2006). *2006 Report on the Global AIDS Epidemic*. Available at http://data.unaids.org/pub/report/2006/2006_gr_en.pdf. Accessed 22 Sep 2012.

UNAIDS. (2010a). *United nations general assembly special session on HIV/AIDS 09: Monitoring the declaration of commitment on HIV/AIDS. Guidelines on construction on core indicators, 2010 reporting*. Geneva: UNAIDS.

UNAIDS. (2010b). *UNAIDS report on the global AIDS epidemic 2010*. Geneva: UNAIDS.

UNAIDS. (2011). *World AIDS day report*. Geneva: UNAIDS.

United National Development Program (UNDP) Ghana (2007). *Ghana Human development Report, 2007: Towards a more inclusive society*. Accra/Ghana: UNDP, Ghana Office.

Vuylsteke, B., Semde, G., Sika, L., Crucitti, T., Ettiegne Traore, V., Buve, A., et al. (2012). High prevalence of HIV and sexually transmitted infections among male sex workers in Abidjan, Cote d'Ivoire: Need for services tailored to their needs. *Sexually Transmitted Infections, 88*(4), 288–293.

Wade, A. S., Kane, C. T., Diallo, P. A., Diop, A. K., Gueye, K., Mboup, S., et al. (2005). HIV infection and STIs among MSM in Senegal. *AIDS, 19*(18), 2133–2140.

Wolfer, L. (2007). *Real research: Conducting and evaluating research in the social sciences.* Boston: Allyn and Bacon.

World Health Organization. (2014). *HIV/AIDS: Fact sheet N°360.* www.who.int/mediacentre/factsheets/fs360/en. Accessed 19 Jan 2015.

Yankah, K. (2004). Narrative in times of crisis: AIDS stories in Ghana. *Journal of Folklore Research, 41*, 181–198.

Chapter 12
Mental Health Problems and Associated Socio-Ecological Factors Among HIV-Positive Young Migrant Men Who Have Sex with Men in China

Haochu (Howard) Li, Joseph T.F. Lau, Eleanor Holroyd, and Xiaoming Li

Contents

H.(H). Li (✉)
UNC Project-China, Institute for Global Health and Infectious Diseases, University of North Carolina at Chapel Hill, Chapel Hill, NC, USA

School of Public Health, Shandong University, Jinan, Shandong Province, China
e-mail: haochuli@med.unc.edu; hcli@alumni.cuhk.net

J.T.F. Lau
Jockey Club School of Public Health and Primary Care, The Chinese University of Hong Kong, Hong Kong SAR, China
e-mail: jlau@cuhk.edu.hk

E. Holroyd
School of Clinical Sciences, Auckland University of Technology, 90 Akoranga Drive, Northcote, Auckland
e-mail: eleanor.holroyd@aut.ac.nz

X. Li
Department of Health Promotion, Education, and Behavior, Arnold School of Public Health, 915 Greene Street, Room 408, Columbia, SC 29208, USA
e-mail: xiaoming@mailbox.sc.edu

P. Liamputtong (ed.), *Children and Young People Living with HIV/AIDS*, Cross-Cultural Research in Health, Illness and Well-Being,
DOI 10.1007/978-3-319-29936-5_12

12.1 Introduction

As compared to heterosexual populations, gay, lesbian and bisexual (LGB) populations have a higher prevalence of mental health problems such as depression, anxiety, substance use and suicidal ideation (Cochran et al. 2007; Hirshfielda et al. 2008; Chae and Ayala 2010). The elevated risks may be caused by institutional and interpersonal forms of stigma, discrimination and prejudice, instances of verbal and physical violence and harassment (Huebner et al. 2004; Chae and Yoshikawa 2008; see also Chaps. 1, 11, 13, and 18 in this volume).

For people living with HIV/AIDS (PLWH), the prevalence of depression reported in international studies ranges from 22 to 71 % (Savetsky et al. 2001; Campos et al. 2008). Moreover, PLWH commonly experience negative life experiences such as traumatic events, mental illnesses, lack of trust in the health care system, and stigma (Whetten et al. 2008). Amongst HIV-positive men who have sex with men (MSM), high prevalence of depression (58.1 %) and anxiety (38.2 %) have been reported (Berg et al. 2004). Anxiety symptoms were found to be associated with contextual factors of homelessness, recent experience of HIV symptoms, injection drug use, and lifetime sexual abuse (Semple et al. 2011). Poor mental health status increases the risk of sexual transmission of HIV (O'Cleirigh et al. 2010; Semple et al. 2011). It has been reported that about one third of PLWH who are aware of their HIV status continue to engage in HIV-related risk behaviors, and mental health is one of the important associated factors (Fisher et al. 2010). Improvement of mental health status among PLWH is hence an essential mean to contain the spread of HIV infection (Cournos et al. 2005).

In China, high prevalence of mental health problems among PLWH, including depression and suicidal ideation, have been reported (Lau et al. 2010). Associated risk factors included inaccessibility to antiretroviral treatment (ART), poor physical functioning, perceived discrimination from relatives and friends, low level of resilience (Yu et al. 2009), low self-acceptance, poor social support and negative life events (Chen et al. 2004), and stress related to HIV/AIDS (Wang et al. 2005). However, these epidemiological and behavioral studies provided limited knowledge and exemplification of how mental health problems (i.e. depression symptoms and anxiety) are embedded in its socio-ecological contexts.

HIV-positive MSM in China constitute a vulnerable and important population as they are facing stressors and have to adapt to their HIV status, which may affect the entire course of the disease. Depression is highly prevalent among persons who have been newly diagnosed with HIV (67 % screened positive for depression) (Bhatia et al. 2011). To date, however, very limited qualitative studies have investigated potential causes of mental health problems among PLWH, including HIV-positive MSM. The underestimation of subjective experience limited contextual and insightful explanations of mental health problems among PLWH.

12.2 Theoretical Framework

To better understand the full range of factors associated with mental health, we advocate the use of the socio-ecological model that integrates both cultural and structural factors to provide an alternative to more individualistic behavioral research paradigms (Parker 2001). A qualitative approach guided by the socio-ecological model can embed the specific mental health problems, such as depression and anxiety, in multi-level and multi-dimensional psychosocial and structural contexts. Medical anthropologists argue that disease is not only a natural object, which cannot be separated from human consciousness, and humans can experience the external material world only through their cultural frames (Good 1994; Baeret al. 2003). Ecological models are powerful when a specific behavior is exemplifying both cultural values and beliefs as well as shaped by structural constraints in the environment (Sallis et al. 2008). A socio-ecological approach to understanding mental health problems among HIV-positive MSM requires an exploration of the comprehensive social cultural context (McLeroy et al. 1988; Baer et al. 2003; Poundstoneet al. 2004).

A socio-ecological model (McLeroy et al. 1988), which examines both individual and social environmental factors influencing behavior as an outcome of interest in multiple levels and multiple dimensions, was therefore adapted in the current study to guide the data collection and analysis. Before formal study, pilot work (e.g. interviewing five HIV-positive MSM and discussing with five healthcare workers and volunteers) were conducted to refine the model in the context of Shenzhen. We then explored key factors, such as affective and cognitive factors and subsistence in individual level, partners, social support, and intimacy in interpersonal level, and cultural concept of face, filial piety, taboos, stigma and discrimination in the community and family level. Understanding the social ecological context of mental health problems will provide insight of how to provide effective mental health care to this group of men and therefore facilitate positive prevention.

12.3 The Study

The current study was conducted in Shenzhen, China. In 2010, Shenzhen had a population of 13.1 million and over 80 % of the population were internal migrants, locally known as the "domestic floating population" (Shenzhen City Government General Office 2011). It was estimated that there were 100,000–200,000 MSM living in Shenzhen (Xie et al. 2010). In-depth interviews and repeated in-depth interviews were conducted in Shenzhen from January to September 2010, in collaboration with a local non-government organization (NGO). The NGO worked closely with

Table 12.1 Summary of the characteristics of participants (HIV-positive young MSM)

Characteristics	$N=19$
Occupations	
Office	3
Service/seller	3
Technician	1
Laborer	2
Sex worker	7
Jobless	3
Education	
College	5
High/technological school	9
Secondary school	5
Income (per month)	
More than 6000	1
3000–6000	5
Less than 3000	10
No income	3
Sexual identity	
Homosexual	15
Bisexual	3
Heterosexual	1

the Shenzhen Centre for Disease Prevention and Control (CDC) to provide HIV/AIDS prevention services to MSM and was well connected to some grass root groups of the PLWH. A life profile approach was used to focus on individual life narratives that provide background and context to an individual's contemporary community life (McCance et al. 2001). The interview guide mainly included: after the HIV diagnosis, how do you feel and what do you think? What do you do to response to it or adjust yourself? How do others react to you? And how do you handle their reactions?

We used purposive sampling to recruit participants from diverse background characteristics (Table 12.1). Eligibility criteria included participants who were 18 years of age or older, diagnosed as HIV-positive, identified as a man who has sex with men, and willing and able to provide written informed consent. In total, 45 eligible participants took part in in-depth interviews. All participants were internal migrants. In this chapter, we include only 19 young participants who aged from 18 to 25.

The collaborating NGO approached potential participants through their contacts and networks according to our purposive sampling scheme. Participants had explained that refusal would not affect their right to use services and they were further informed that the content of the discussion was to be audio recorded. Written informed consent was obtained. Each man was assured of data confidentiality, use of pseudonyms, safe storage of the data and the right to withdraw at any time without being questioned. The second interviews were conducted 3 months after the initial interview. Before starting the second interview in each case, translated verbatim in the initial interview was read through first and emerging themes, missing points from the interview guide, or incomplete information in the initial interview were emphasized and explored in the second interview. Each interview lasted from 1.5 to 2 h and was conducted in a private room in the NGO's office. Participants were given RMB 200 (about USD 30) in cash for the first interview and an extra RMB 300 (about USD 50) for the second interview to compensate their time. The first author also conducted participant observations in venues of men who have sex with men, NGO offices, and local health care settings and took field note. From these contacts 12 men accepted the first author's engagement in their daily life, such as visiting their homes or work places, and hanging out with them and their friends. Ethics approval was granted by the Ethics Committee in the Chinese University of Hong Kong.

The tape-recorded interviews were transcribed verbatim into Chinese immediately at the completion of each interview. The first author translated the transcripts into English, and the co-authors cross-checked the accuracy and completeness of the translation. We employed thematic content analysis (Green and Thorogood 2009) concurrently with data collection in order to capture emerging themes. In subsequent bi-week meetings, we discussed areas of emerging importance and reached agreement on a set of preliminary codes. The later in-depth analysis first involved preliminary reading of all the transcripts, noting initial reactions and assigning preliminary thematic codes. Symptoms of major depression and anxiety disorder were identified from the narratives. Such symptoms were coded with the assistance of a senior psychiatrist with a specialist background in HIV and MSM issues. Related psycho-social and cultural factors emerging from participants' reflections on their mental health problems were also coded, using the aforementioned socio-ecological model as a guiding framework. We grouped informative quotes relevant to the themes together and then synthesized them. We further refined the thematic structures based on collective discussion.

12.4 Depressive and Anxiety Symptoms

Most newly diagnosed HIV-positive MSM (14/19) reported depressive symptoms (e.g., fatigue, hopelessness and despair); almost half (8/19) experienced anxiety symptoms (e.g. catastrophizing, anxiety and avoidance), whilst about one third (6/19) experienced both types of symptoms. Examples of quotations potentially reflecting relevant symptoms are summarized in Table 12.2.

Table 12.2 Examples of quotations reflecting symptoms of depression and anxiety

Depressive symptoms	Representative quotes
Fatigue (tired/weary)	"I was very 'tui fei' (颓废grey and dispirited) at the beginning and totally in a 'wei mi' (萎靡 weary) situation…'shen xin pi bei' (身心疲惫 a state of emotional and physical exhaustion/burnout)"
Hopelessness/despair	"When I was just diagnosed positive, my psychological situation was very bad. I felt the heavens were falling down. Everything became unimportant…In the first 1 or 2 weeks, I felt despair, and had nightmares every night. Once I fell asleep I had nightmares. I then woke up and felt I was dying soon"
	"When I had the diagnostic report, I was numb and lost feeling in my whole body, so giddy. A lot of things went into my mind. I felt my life was over and I felt despair, very sad, and my future looked bleak"
Anxiety symptoms	**Representative quotes**
Catastrophizing	"Many times I feel there is something extra in my body, and I resist it in my mind. I really want to get rid of it, but I can't… (I think I will) die in a terrible way, looks not like human nor ghosts"
Anxiety and avoidance	"Now I don't want to attend any activities organized by non-infectors' organizations. Even though others don't know that I am an infector, I have some thinking in my mind. I see others so happy, and then I will be in low spirits and feel stressed"

12.5 Social-Ecological Factors Associated with Mental Health

We explain in the following sections that in support of the aforementioned socio-ecological model, many newly diagnosed HIV-positive MSM experienced various types of stressors related to individual, interpersonal, and socio-cultural conditions.

12.5.1 Individual-Level Cognitive and Affective Factors

12.5.1.1 Internalized HIV Stigma

Some participants developed internalized HIV stigma and reported strong self-stigmatization. They regarded themselves as being toxic, inferior, evil, shameful, a virus bringing bad luck, or a "monster". Internalized HIV stigma stimulated negative emotions and further exacerbated their self-reported poor mental health. Expressions from participants Wu and Lv are presented below:

> It's a kind of punishment. Heaven (god) is really punishing me. I remember when my father passed away, I did not go back home to '*shou si*' (death-watch which is the role of a son at his father's funeral)…I am now HIV-positive and I am very toxic. I feel I am inferior to others and I feel I am evil. Only those dubious characters would get this rubbish disease. (Wu)

> It's very taboo, and infectors are seriously looked down upon and treated as a virus, like a monster (which is regarded as bringing with bad luck). In my life, I know they slandered and disgusted HIV infectors. (Lv)

12.5.1.2 Internalized Homophobia

Participants developed negative perceptions about themselves in relation to their experience of HIV infection, such as feeling dirty, promiscuous, and being punished, such testimonies further stimulated a spoiled identity of being a *tongzhi* (gay or bisexual men), especially a HIV-positive one. Feng remarked:

> I am not very accustomed to the men-men relationships …sometimes feel very good, but sometimes feel very uncomfortable … I do not like those men who are so feminine … I believe in Buddha, but Buddhism does not support *tongzhi* (gay) … They think *tongzhi* is not correct, instead *tongzhi* is sexual misconduct.

According to Miao:

> Feminine *tongzhi* are strongly urged not to join [a QQ group for general HIV-positive people]. Only normal men can join this group. I feel I am quite feminine. … I suspect that normal men would feel disgusting against *tongzhi*.

12.5.1.3 Perceptions of ART and Side-Effects

Some participants were taking ART and suffering from side-effects, such as vomiting, skin rashes and stomach ache. They wondered whether these medicines were really good. These problems became stressors that made them low spirited, in grief, indignant and wishing to give up. Ge provided his experiences as the following:

> What I worry most is complicating diseases and the side effect of ART. When I was hospitalized, I thought of death. This disease made me suffer too much. I could not eat, got serious fever over 40 degree. At that moment, I suffered too much and wanted to give up treatment. I would rather die.

12.5.1.4 Perceived Constraints to a Meaningful Future

Some participants worried that working too hard would reduce their CD4 count and therefore further deteriorate their immune system. HIV prohibited them from working hard and therefore made them feel disabled and worthless, which decreased their confidence and self-esteem. Hei told us that:

> After taking part in this activity, I saw others were very happy, and I became more downhearted and felt more stressed. I admired how others would not get infected and they still have a long way to go and can fulfil a lot of things. But I cannot work as hard as them to fulfil my dream since I get too tired and my body doesn't allow that. I therefore became especially afflicted.

12.5.1.5 Frightening Images of HIV/AIDS

The terrible images of AIDS as portrayed in the media made some participants scared or anxious. These images were shared within HIV-positive groups, or presented in the media and on the Internet. Star remarked:

> Anyone who has common knowledge realize that once getting infected…I don't want my families to see I die in such a terrible way, looks not like human nor ghosts.

12.5.2 Individual-Level Factors Related to Subsistence

12.5.2.1 Financial Burden

No participant reported paying for antiretroviral treatment (ART), since they were covered by "Four Free and One Care" services. However, high spending on health care and medication, including general medical costs or specific spending on HIV (e.g. treating complications and the side-effects of ART), and household-bounded conditions for access to free ART made participants feel stressed. Qin elaborated:

> I do not feel safe, because I just come to Shenzhen without a penny, I am in debt and owe nearly four thousand … my wages are very low, a thousand RMB a month. … Probably because of the money, I am in a very low mood and feel very oppressed. I have to think about the future. I heard from some patients that to address medication allergies cost one thousand RMB in hospital one day, and then two weeks to ten thousand. My company has not yet arranged my social security. For me, it is very insecure in future.

12.5.2.2 Difficulties in Employment and Poor Working Conditions

Some participants were fired or demoted in their workplace after their HIV-positive status was disclosed to others. HIV constrained some participants from working hard, and limited them in their job seeking. Deterioration of the participants' economic status as a migrant worker created a downward cycle of poverty and potentially increased propensity for ill mental health. These adversities made some participants felt angry, that they were unfairly treated, upset, gloomy, depressed and stressed. Hei who was infected with HIV and hepatitis B. said: "I cannot pass the body check…I can only work in small workshops or small factories where only employ around ten to twenty workers, since they do not require employees to take body check." Another participant, Fang, provided his testimony as following:

> After getting HIV infectionn, I can not continue working at bars. Because I am afraid my body cannot bear it. Working at bars need to stay up late. I want to change my job, but do not know what to change. …I have been jobless for three months.

12.5.3 Interpersonal Factors

12.5.3.1 Difficulties in Finding Partners

Participants reported difficulty in finding a lover or stable partner in MSM circles and HIV made them even more difficult to look for partners. Some participants became worried about being refused and hurt again or transmitting HIV to their partner(s). Hei provided his view as following:

> I feel it is really difficult to look for a partner. …Even in the circle of HIV-positive people, the people like me who are lowly educated, lack of training in working skills or technologies and low income are difficult to look for someone.

Han too remarked that:

> I have many one night stand. In my impression, I think those people did not want to find a stable partner, because they felt they were so privilege or strongly that they did not need to look for a stable partner. They wanted to look for more sexual partners.

12.5.3.2 Self-Isolation and Reduced Social Support

The diagnosis of being HIV-positive narrowed some participants' social network, and restricted their sources of social support. Feelings of boredom, loneliness, low spirit, and being afraid were testified to have been experienced. Wu told us that:

> When we were on the way to the hospital, he said we would face difficulties together and gave me a lot of promises. I was so innocent. After I told him my seropositivity, he said that we should not meet again. …I used to go to some parties. But a lot of people in the parties cursed me that how dare you come to have fun after getting AIDS and whether you want to play or harm others.

Ge also said that:

> My brothers were so scared, not to mention my Dad. I was hospitalized three times, but my Dad never gave me a phone, not to mention giving me money. That's to say they gave me up.

12.5.3.3 Conflict of Intimacy and Safer Sex

Participants presented their needs for intimacy and sex. When they met partners with unknown HIV status, however, having sex and developing intimacy frightened them. Non-disclosure or fear of disclosure created anxiety, and the dilemma between casual and regular relationships resulted in mental conflicts as the participants did not know whether they should maintain casual sex or instead to build up regular relationships with others.

> When two lovers are ramping up the feelings, we actually need very harmonious sexual life. We want to make love very actively. If we are very comfortable in sex, we feel great happiness. But because of a condom, we feel being barred by something. …If he does not feel good (he does not want to use condoms), I will feel losing something as well. …Emotional attachment also needs to be sublimed by having good sex. (Qin)

12.5.4 Socio-cultural Factors in Community and Family

12.5.4.1 Losing "face" of Oneself and One's Family

In Chinese cultural context, "*lian*" (脸 face) is about integrity of one's moral character and reputation (Hu 1944). It is related to property (embedding with the cultural stigmatization of avoiding poverty), marriage (embedding a stigma against single adults who do not fulfil family obligations), and moral judgments against PLWH (embedding a stigma against those people who became infected through culturally immoral ways, such as multiple sex partners, homosexual activities, commercial sex and taking drugs). This Chinese cultural factor of "*lian*" (脸 face) made some participants worried or anxious. Zhou told us that:

> I haven't been home for nine years. Honestly speaking, I feel I am so dirty…my uncle is very serious about the issue of face…I am afraid relatives in my home know about (his homosexuality and HIV-positive) …I am really afraid to go back to hometown.

12.5.4.2 Significance of Filial Piety

HIV infection made some participants feel sorry for their parents. In Chinese culture, children are expected to take care of aged parents, which is an important component of filial piety. If one dies before one's parents, he/she cannot fulfil filial piety. Therefore, some participants felt very impiety when they thought they may die before their parents.

> When I think of my parents and relatives, I feel very uncomfortable. Once I think of them, my tear would come down. I feel very sorry for them. I thought if I really die, I am sorry for them. (Sun)

Not getting married and having children to maintain the family bloodline is another very serious deviation from filial piety, as illustrated by a Chinese saying: "*bu xiao you san, wu hou wei da*" (不孝有三,无后为大), meaning that "without male offspring is the worst form of impiety."

> I am the only child of my family. …If I die …If there is no hope, no continuity of life, my family and parents will collapse. I don't know how they can accept this reality. It is really too cruel for them. (Ren)

12.5.4.3 Taboos and Prohibitions in Open Discussion of HIV/AIDS and Sexuality

It is a cultural restriction for open and in-depth discussion of being homosexual and HIV-positive, which prohibited participants from developing sound psychological adjustments. Some participants could talk to someone, such as their close friends, boyfriends, and family, but the communication was likely to be partial. They could not openly and fully talk about sex, love and HIV/AIDS. Hei disclosed his condition to his mother, but they did not have an in-depth conversation. Hei said: "I really got annoyed and didn't want to talk to others."

12.5.4.4 Social Stigma and Discrimination Against PLWH

Some participants experienced social stigma and discrimination after disclosing their HIV status to others. They were humiliated, isolated, gossiped about, extorted for money, refused health services or judged morally on the basis of how they got infected. Moreover, there were stigma and discrimination among PLWH. Hei told us that:

> Some people abused me after I disclosed my condition to them on the QQ group. ...They scolded me '*shen jing bing*' (madness), 'don't transmit (HIV) to others', 'I don't want to talk to you', etc. They used lot of abusive terms to humiliate me.

Sun too remarked that:

> Even within HIV-positive groups, there is stigmatization/discrimination. I can feel this. In the first meeting, if he/she was infected through receiving blood, he/she would give you a strange look. ...Since many homosexual men got infected, an infected man is usually regarded as gay. If he is straight, he would be regarded as having gone whoring. If it is a girl, she would be usually regarded as a prostitute. Actually this thinking is a kind of background discrimination.

12.6 Conclusion

After being diagnosed as HIV-positive, the participants encountered new stressors, such as frightening images toward HIV/AIDS, perceptions on ART and side-effects, conflict of intimacy and safer sex, stigma and constraints due to the disease, making them feel disabled and worthless (see also Chaps. 2, 3, 4, 6, 9, 14, and 18 in this volume). On top of these emerging stressors, pre-existing stressors became more serious as a result of their HIV-positive status. These pre-existing stressors included social adversities faced by migrants, social suffering as MSM, cultural trauma, stigma and discriminations.

Social adversities in migrants' lives have been widely reported (Li et al. 2007; Wong et al. 2008). In China, the Hukou system (the household registration system) contributed to the experience of marginalization of rural migrant workers in urban cities, since it determines social welfare and medical benefits (Wong et al. 2007). Migrant status contributes to poor mental health (Wong et al. 2008), obsession, compulsion, and phobia (Shen et al. 1998), and difficulties in interpersonal relationship (Wong 2008). Very few (less than 1 %) migrants had received any professional help for depression or anxiety (Li et al. 2007). In the current study, all participants were internal migrants, making it difficult for them to access social security, health care insurance and free ART in Shenzhen. Most of them migrated to Shenzhen from poor areas and shouldered an obligation to support their family at the hometown. Failure to do so would put them in a stigmatized and shameful situation. Some participants encountered unstable jobs and financial difficulties. Their HIV-positive status aggregated the situation tremendously in multiple dimensions (e.g., poorer health, heavier financial burden, job instability, narrower social networks and less social support) and appeared to further exacerbate downward social mobility and life stressors. Governmental inter-departmental co-ordinations are hence important and may be lacking in China and many other places. HIV prevention policy efforts targeting HIV-positive MSM need to involve departments in charge of internal migration, welfare and mental health services. We suggest a joint force to improve the situation, such as removing the household-based boundaries of access to social welfare and health care, integrating prevention, treatment, care and mental health services, including health psychologists and social workers into the team.

MSM generally could only express their social and sexual needs in some MSM venues or circles, hiding their sexual identity in the mainstream heterosexual society. In Shenzhen, 52.6 % of MSM were not in a steady or spousal relationship (Behringer 2008). In our study, many MSM expressed unmet needs for love and stable partnership. It seems that wealth, appearance and sexual sensations are more important than care and spirituality in relationships in the local MSM subculture. It would even more difficult for HIV-positive MSM to establish significant personal relationships, since it involved issues of disclosure, self-confidence, fear of rejection, and conflict of intimacy and safer sex. These HIV-positive MSM had diminished support networks but increased burdens. They testified to having to hide not only their sexual orientation but also their seropositivity and not only from the mainstream heterosexual society but also from MSM communities. The MSM communities in general may show stigma to HIV-positive MSM, making disclosure to other MSM equally difficult. Their social spaces hence almost disappeared. Therefore, these HIV-positive MSM generated even more negative attitudes both towards themselves and the MSM communities, such as more serious internalized homophobia, potentially creating a vicious cycle involving feelings of inferiority, guilt, mistrust and even hatred, informing a spoiled identity (Goffman 1963), which would further deteriorate their self-esteem and destroy their confidence in MSM circles. It is hence important to build up vital communities for HIV-positive MSM and connect them to diverse supportive groups. The rise of social media provides a good opportunity to build up virtual communities which is a good potential source of social support (Lewis et al. 2011; see also Chap. 18 in this volume).

Many MSM in China (18.25–33.5 %) are in married heterosexual relationships (Lau et al. 2008), and the majority of the MSM (64 %) older than 39 years had been married (Choi et al. 2003). Many participants planned to get married with a woman before being diagnosed as HIV-positive. The HIV-positive diagnosis confronted their life picture of fulfilling cultural competency and success, such as marrying to a woman and having children to maintain family bloodlines, which are deeply and culturally internalized (Li et al. 2010), and therefore put them in the midst of "cultural trauma" (Alexander 2004), elaborating the adverse and dysfunctional effects on MSM caused by the HIV diagnosis. Moreover, these HIV-positive MSM cannot fulfill their family obligation of maintaining "*lian*" (face), and exercising filial piety. In the Chinese context, *lian* (face, moral position) and *mianzi* (face as self-affirming social status) are key moral resources (Kleinman and Kleinman 1997). The destruction of this moral capital (Bourdieu 1984) would enhance the negative impact of the cultural trauma, creating negative life attitudes such as loss of life meaning and self-esteem, contributing to poor mental health among HIV-positive MSM. Such stressors are mostly related to the family. But there is currently no supportive services provided to family members of the HIV-positive MSM, which is possibly the most stable and significant source of support, if available. Interventions to support disclosure of one's HIV status to his family members are also warranted.

HIV/AIDS stigma exists within the gay community and has a negative effect on the mental health of HIV-positive MSM (Courtenay-Quirk et al. 2006; see also Chaps. 11, 13, and 18 in this volume). The current study presented enacted, perceived and internalized stigma (self stigma) (Goffman 1963; Steward et al. 2008). Enacted stigma was felt by the MSM interviewed with their seropositivity being disclosed to others, including humiliation, isolation, gossip, extortion for money and refusal to use services. Most HIV-positive MSM did not disclose their seropositivity publicly but they were still affected by perceived stigma, which is associated with a marked decrease in the likelihood of a resilient outcome (Fleming and Ledogar 2008). Some participants showed internalized stigma (self-stigma), regarding themselves as being toxic, dirty, inferior, shameful and bringing bad luck to others. Moreover, layered stigma (Henkel et al. 2008) exerts a strong force on these migrant HIV-positive MSM, as stigma results from multiple sources: sexual orientation, route of infection, "*mei su zhi*" (low quality/ poor distinction, including low education and having a rural background), and poverty. However, very few efforts have been made to remove stigma against HIV-positive MSM among MSM communities. Interventions of counseling for empowerment, training of communications with significant others, strengthening self esteem, and building healthy life styles are important.

In this regard, some basic psycho-social and cultural factors not directly related to HIV exercised strong influence over these HIV-positive MSM's mental health, corroborating with the results of other studies (Rogers et al. 2003; Mao et al. 2009). In line with the argument that HIV risk in the MSM population is embedded in multiple co-occurring public health problems (a syndemic) (USCDC 2008; Safren et al. 2010), the current study informed that both the pre-existing and emerging stressors related to adverse psycho-social and cultural conditions interacted with each other to result in poor mental health status of HIV-positive MSM. These men hence experienced complicated and synthesized traumatic experiences. We theorize that HIV/AIDS is a trigger that amplifies pre-existing stress and conflicts that are deeply embedded at different socio-ecological levels among migrant MSM.

There are limitations in this study. First, the use of a digital recorder may have prohibited some participants to openly talk about their negative views. Second, the nature of qualitative research meant that the sample size was small and sampling was limited to social networks of participants and local MSM/PLWH groups who collaborated with us. We failed to recruit those participants who had not contacted health care workers or volunteers. Third, although an interview guide was provided, in order to be mindful of the cultural context of discussing sensitive information, the first author concurrently analyzed themes, and hence, not all participants received the exactly same series of questions in the same order.

Despite these limitations, this study fills up the knowledge gap of potential causes of mental health problems among HIV-positive MSM. The study informs that HIV-positive MSM encounter significant mental health problems, and the causes of these problems are multiple and socio-ecological. We found potential influences of socio-ecological factors at individual, interpersonal, and socio-cultural levels, constituting a syndemic and possibly a vicious cycle between pre-existing adversities and emerging stressors due to the HIV diagnosis. It is very likely that the joint effects of these conditions are interactively rather than additive. This study implicates that the mental health problems faced by HIV-positive MSM are more complicated than it seems. It is not only to provide counseling on HIV-related problems that would be able to relieve the prevalent and serious mental health problems among HIV-positive MSM. HIV care services need to use the socio-ecological framework to address pre-existing problems including adverse conditions of migrants, societal acceptance of HIV-positive MSM, creation of social space, and self-empowerment. Policy makers and healthcare providers need to be aware of the multiple causes and syndemic nature of mental health problems among HIV-positive MSM as well as the consequences of such problems, and to put a priority to review current policies so as to create a better socio-ecological environment to alleviate the problems. One of the emphases is to integrate user-friendly mental health services into current HIV/AIDS prevention and intervention campaigns. A stronger effort to improve the overall conditions faced by HIV-positive MSM is greatly warranted.

Acknowledgements This research obtained funding from the Center for Health Behaviors Research of the Jockey Club School of Public Health and Primary Care (JCSPHPC), The Chinese University of Hong Kong (CUHK), a postgraduate study grant in JCSPHPC, and the Global Scholarship Programme for Research Excellence – CNOOC Grants 2010–2011 in CUHK. Authors wish to thank all participants who shared their life histories and experiences, Shenzhen 258 Rainbow Workgroup and Shenzhen CDC who helped significantly in the fieldwork and access to the populations. Dr. Conall O'Cleirigh from Harvard Medical School provided significant assistance in coding depression and anxiety symptoms.

References

Alexander, J. C. (2004). Toward a theory of cultural trauma. In J. C. Alexender, R. Eyerman, B. Giesen, N. J. Smelser, & P. Sztompka (Eds.), *Cultural trauma and collective identity* (pp. 1–30). Berkeley: University of California Press.

Baer, H. A., Singer, M., & Susser, I. (Eds.). (2003). *Medical anthropology and the world system*. Westport: Praeger.

Behringer, K. (2008). HIV/AIDS prevention: Factors affecting risky sexual behaviors among MSM in Shenzhen, China. UCHC Graduate School masters theses 2003–2010. Paper 144. Retrieved from http://digitalcommons.uconn.edu/uchcgs_masters/144.

Berg, M. B., Mimiaga, M., & Safren, S. A. (2004). Mental health concerns of HIV-infected gay and bisexual men seeking mental health services: An observational study. *AIDS Patient Care and STDs, 18*(11), 635–643.

Bhatia, R., Hartman, C., Kallen, M. A., Graham, J., & Giordano, T. P. (2011). Persons newly diagnosed with HIV infection are at high risk for depression and poor linkage to care: Results from the steps study. *AIDS and Behavior, 15*, 1161–1170.

Bourdieu, P. (1984). *Distinction: A social critique of the judgement of taste* (Trans: Nice, R.). Cambridge, MA: Harvard University Press.

Campos, L. N., Guimaraes, M. D., & Remien, R. H. (2008). Anxiety and depression symptoms as risk factors for non-adherence to antiretroviral therapy in Brazil. *AIDS and Behavior, 14*, 289–299.

Chae, D. H., & Ayala, G. (2010). Sexual orientation and sexual behavior among Latino and Asian Americans: Implications for unfair treatment and psychological distress. *Journal of Sex Research, 47*(5), 451–459.

Chae, D. H., & Yoshikawa, H. (2008). Perceived group devaluation, depression, and HIV-risk behavior among Asian gay men. *Health Psychology, 27*(2), 140–148.

Chen, Q., Zhou, Z., Wen, Y., Lu, W., Huang, G., & Jia, M. (2004). Effects of mental health and psychosocial factors in individuals with HIV/AIDS. *Chinese Mental Health Journal, 18*, 850–853. Retrieved from http://en.cnki.com.cn/Article_en/CJFDTOTAL-ZXWS200412008.htm.

Choi, K. H., Liu, H., Guo, Y., Han, L., Mandel, J. S., & Rutherford, G. W. (2003). Emerging HIV-1 epidemic in China in men who have sex with men. *Lancet, 361*, 2125–2126.

Cochran, S. D., Mays, V. M., Ortega, A. N., Alegria, M., & Takeuchi, D. (2007). Mental health and substance use disorders among Latino and Asian American lesbian, gay, and bisexual adults. *Journal of Consulting and Clinical Psychology, 75*(5), 785–794.

Cournos, F., McKinnon, K., & Wainberg, M. (2005). What can mental health interventions contribute to the global struggle against HIV/AIDS? *World Psychiatry, 4*(3), 135–141.

Courtenay-Quirk, C., Wolitski, R. G., Parsons, J. T., & Gomez, C. A. (2006). Is HIV/AIDS stigma dividing the gay community? Perceptions of HIV-positive men who have sex with men. *AIDS Education and Prevention, 18*(1), 56–67.

Fisher, J. D., Smith, L. R., & Lenz, E. M. (2010). Secondary prevention of HIV in the United States: Past, current, and future perspectives. *Journal of Acquired Immune Deficiency Syndromes, 55*(2), s106–s115.

Fleming, J., & Ledogar, R. J. (2008). Resilience, an evolving concept: A review of literature relevant to aboriginal research. *Pimatisiwin, 6*(2), 7–23.

Goffman, E. (1963). *Stigma—notes on the management of spoiled identity*. New York: Simon and Schuster/Touchstone Books.

Good, B. (1994). *Medicine, rationality, and experience—an anthropological perspective*. Cambridge: Cambridge University Press.

Green, J., & Thorogood, N. (2009). *Qualitative methods for health research* (2nd ed.). London: Sage.

Henkel, K. E., Brown, K., & Kalichman, S. C. (2008). AIDS-related stigma in individuals with other stigmatized identities in the USA: A review of layered stigmas. *Social and Personality Psychology Compass, 2*(4), 1586–1599.

Hirshfielda, S., Wolitskib, R. J., Chiassona, M. A., Remienc, R. H., Humberstonea, M., & Wong, T. (2008). Screening for depressive symptoms in an online sample of men who have sex with men. *AIDS Care, 20*(8), 904–910.

Hu, H. C. (1944). The Chinese concepts of "face". *American Anthropologist, 46*(1), 45–64.

Huebner, D. M., Rebchook, G. M., & Kegeles, S. M. (2004). Experiences of harassment, discrimination, and physical violence among young gay and bisexual men. *American Journal of Public Health, 94*, 1200–1203.

Kleinman, A., & Kleinman, J. (1997). Moral transformations of health and suffering in Chinese society. In A. M. Brandt & P. Rozin (Eds.), *Morality and health* (pp. 101–118). New Yourk: Routledge.

Lau, J. T. F., Wang, M., Wong, H. N., Tsui, H. Y., Jia, M., Cheng, F., Zhang, Y., Su, X., & Wang, N. (2008). Prevalence of bisexual behaviors among men who have sex with men (MSM) in China and associations between condom use in MSM and heterosexual behaviors. *Sexually Transmitted Diseases, 35*(4), 406–413.

Lau, J. T. F., Yu, X. N., Mak, W. W. S., Cheng, Y. M., Lv, Y. H., & Zhang, J. X. (2010). Suicidal ideation among HIV+ former blood and/or plasma donors in rural China. *AIDS Care, 22*(8), 946–954.

Lewis, M. A., Uhrig, J. D., Ayala, G., & Stryker, J. (2011). Reaching men who have sex with men for HIV prevention message with new media: Recommendations from an expert consultation. *Annals of the Forum for Collaborative HIV Research, 13*(3), 11–18.

Li, L., Wang, H. M., Ye, X. J., Jiang, M. M., Lou, Q. Y., & Hesketh, T. (2007). The mental health status of Chinese rural-urban migrant workers: Comparison with permanent urban and rural dwellers. *Social Psychiatry and Psychiatric Epidemiology, 42*(9), 716–722.

Li, H. C., Holroyd, E., & Lau, J. T. F. (2010). Negotiating homosexual identities: The experiences of men who have sex with men in Guangzhou. *Culture, Health & Sexuality, 12*(4), 401–414.

Mao, L., Kidd, M., Rogers, G., Andrews, G., Newman, C. E., Booth, A., Saltman, D. C., & Kippax, S. C. (2009). Social factors associated with major depression disorder in homosexually active, gay men attending general practices in urban Australia. *Australian and New Zealand Journal of Public Health, 33*(1), 88–86.

McCance, T. V., McKenna, H. P., & Boore, J. R. P. (2001). Exploring caring using narrative methodology: An analysis of the approach. *Journal of Advanced Nursing, 33*(3), 350–356.

McLeroy, K. R., Bibeau, D., Steckler, A., & Glanz, K. (1988). An ecological perspective on health promotion programs. *Health Education and Behavior, 15*(4), 351–377.

O'Cleirigh, C., Mimiaga, M., Safren, S. A., Stall, R., & Mayer, K. H. (2010). Synergistic effects of psychosocial and substance use problems on increased sexual transmission risk among HIV-infected men who have sex with men. XVIII International AIDS Conference, Vienna [abstract WEPE0515].

Parker, R. (2001). Sexuality, culture, and power in HIV/AIDS research. *Annual Review of Anthropology, 30*, 163–179.

Poundstone, K. E., Strathdee, S. A., & Celentano, D. D. (2004). The social epidemiology of human immunodeficiency virus/acquired immunodeficiency syndrome. *Epidemiological Reviews, 26*, 22–35. doi:10.1093/epirev/mxh005.

Rogers, G., Curry, M., Oddy, J., Pratt, N., Beilby, J., & Wilkinson, D. (2003). Depressive disorders and unprotected casual anal sex among Australian homosexually active men in primary care. *HIV Medicine, 4*(3), 271–275.

Safren, S. A., Traeger, L., Skeer, M. R., O'Cleirigh, C., Meade, C. S., Covahey, C., & Mayer, K. H. (2010). Testing a social-cognitive model of HIV transmission risk behavior in HIV-infected MSM with and without depression. *Health Psychology, 29*(2), 215–221.

Sallis, J. F., Owen, N., & Fisher, E. B. (2008). Ecological models of health behavior. In K. Glanz, B. K. Rimer, & K. Viswanath (Eds.), *Health behavior and health education: Theory, research, and practice* (4th ed., pp. 465–485). San Francisco: Jossey-Bass.

Savetsky, J. B., Sullivan, L. M., Clarke, J., Stein, M. D., & Samet, J. H. (2001). Evolution of depressive symptoms in human immunodeficiency virus-infected patients entering primary care. *Journal of Nervous & Mental Disease, 189*(2), 76–83.

Semple, S. J., Strathdee, S. A., Zians, J., McQuaid, J., & Patterson, T. L. (2011). Psychosocial and behavioral correlates of anxiety symptoms in a sample of HIV-positive, methamphetamine-using men who have sex with men. *AIDS Care, 23*(5), 628–637.

Shen, Q., Lu, Y. W., Hu, C. Y., Deng, X. M., Gao, H., Huang, X. Q., & Niu, E. H. (1998). A preliminary study of the mental health of young migrant workers in Shenzhen. *Psychiatry and Clinical Neurosciences, 52*(suppl), 370–373.

Shenzhen City Government General Office. (2011, September 14). *Shenzhen Shi Renkou Fazhan "shi er wu" Guihua [the 12th Five years Shenzhen City population development plan]*. Retrieved from http://www.sz.gov.cn/zfgb/2011/gb758/201110/t20111012_1738467.htm.

Steward, W., Herek, G., Ramakrishna, J., Bharatd, S., Chandye, S., Wrubelf, J., & Ekstranda, M. L. (2008). HIV-related stigma: Adapting a theoretical framework for use in India. *Social Science and Medicine, 67*(8), 1225–1235.

USCDC/Centers for Disease Control and Prevention. (2008). *Syndemic prevention network: Spotlight on syndemics*. Atlanta: Centers for Disease Control. Web page. Retrieved from http://www.cdc.gov/syndemics/.

Wang, J., Lin, X., Wu, H., & Qu, W. (2005). The mood state of paid blood donors with HIV and its relation to stress and cognitive appraisal. *Acta Psychologica Sinica, 37*, 106–112.

Whetten, K., Reif, S., Whetten, R., & Murphy-McMillan, L. K. (2008). Trauma, mental health, distrust, and stigma among HIV-positive persons: Implications for effective care. *Psychosomatic Medicine, 70*, 531–538.

Wong, D. F. K. (2008). Differential impacts of stressful life events and social support on the mental health of mainland Chinese immigrant and local youth in Hong Kong: A resilience perspective. *British Journal of Social Work, 38*, 236–252.

Wong, D. F. K., Li, C. Y., & Song, H. X. (2007). Rural migrant workers in urban China: Living a marginalized life. *International Journal of Social Welfare, 16*, 32–40.

Wong, D. F. K., He, X. S., Leung, G., Lau, Y., & Chang, Y. L. (2008). Mental health of migrant workers in China: Prevalence and correlates. *Social Psychiatry and Psychiatric Epidemiology, 43*, 483–489.

Xie, W., Chen, L., Cai, W., Liu, G., Zhao, J., & Tan, J. (2010). Estimation of the population size of men who have sex with men in Shenzhen in 2010. *Chinese Journal of AIDS & STDs, 17*(4), 414–415. Retrieved from http://www.cqvip.com/qk/90479a/201104/39201795.html.

Yu, X. N., Lau, J. T. F., Mak, W. W. S., Cheng, Y. M., Lv, Y. H., & Zhang, J. X. (2009). Risk and protective factors in association with mental health problems among people living with HIV who were former plasma/blood donors in rural China. *AIDS Care, 21*(5), 645–654.

Chapter 13
Young LGBT People, and HIV/AIDS Risks: A Metasynthesis

Pattaraporn Moolchaem and Pranee Liamputtong

Contents

P. Moolchaem (✉)
Department of Public Health, School of Psychology and Public Health, College of Science, Health, and Engineering, La Trobe University,
Bundoora Campus, Melbourne, VIC 3086, Australia
e-mail: becki.pm@gmail.com

P. Liamputtong
School of Science and Health, Western Sydney University, Penrith 2751, NSW, Australia
e-mail: p.liamputtong@westernsydney.edu.au

P. Liamputtong (ed.), *Children and Young People Living with HIV/AIDS*,
Cross-Cultural Research in Health, Illness and Well-Being,
DOI 10.1007/978-3-319-29936-5_13

13.1 Introduction

Lesbian, gay, bisexual, and transgender (LGBT) people form a gender minority group who are vulnerable to HIV infection, and the young age population among this group have a heighten vulnerability (Centers for Disease Control and Prevention 2014; Friedman et al. 2003; Wilson et al. 2010). Of this gender minority population, young men who have sex with men (MSM) have been at increased risk for HIV infection. This can be seen from previous epidemic studies that the HIV prevalence and estimated incidence among this group remain high (Balaji et al. 2013; Centers for Disease Control and Prevention 2005). Although few data are available on HIV prevalence and risk among young lesbian and bisexual women, previous reports have also shown that this young group of lesbian and bisexual women are at risk for HIV infection (Friedman et al. 2003; Lemp et al. 1995).

It has been suggested from previous studies that the lifestyles of young LGBT people place them at risk for HIV infection (Bockting 2009; Centers for Disease Control and Prevention 2014; Khan et al. 2009; Kwong-Lai Poon and Trung-Thu Ho 2002; Moolchaem et al. 2015). According to Centers for Disease Control and Prevention (2014), LGBT youth have experienced violence in their daily lives. This violence can include verbal and physical behaviors that result in stress experienced by LGBT youth, driving them to depression, substance use, and sexual risk behaviors. This place them at risk for HIV infection (Centers for Disease Control and Prevention 2014; Moolchaem et al. 2015). Experiencing rejections, discriminations, exclusions, and loneliness from peers, family, and society also tend to lead young LGBT people to HIV-related risk behaviors. For instance, Yadegarfard et al. (2014) quantitatively examined health outcomes among Thai male-to-female transgender adolescents and found that family rejection, social isolation, and loneliness were predictors of depression, suicidal ideation, and sexual risk behavior which may put them at risk for HIV infection.

In order to better understand the increase of HIV prevalence among young LGBT people, researchers have also conducted qualitative studies exploring the perspectives of young LGBT individuals in different cultures to better understand what place LGBT youth at risk for HIV infection, and the complexity of HIV risk, prevention, and needs. Timm et al. (2013), for example, investigated sexually transmitted infection and HIV risk among young black women who have sex with women. They found that lack of adult supervision, alcohol use, and unacceptance of homosexual relationship from heteronormative society drove them to sexual risk behavior such as practicing unsafe sex which resulted in the increased risk of HIV infection. Similarly, the work of Flores Iii et al. (2011) revealed the factors that contributed to infection among young MSM who were newly diagnosed with HIV infection. The factors that these young MSM reported included self-awareness which they believed they were not at risk for HIV infection despite engaging in high-risk behaviors (Flores Iii et al. 2011). Flores Iii et al. (2011) also elaborated that bullying, sexual abuse, personal sexual behaviors, and the lack of relevant education were contributing factors of their HIV infection.

Young LGBT individuals participating in existing qualitative studies did not only reveal their perspectives about HIV risk factors, but also articulated their perceptions on HIV-related issues, strategies they used to prevent themselves from acquiring the infection, obstacles to and needs for HIV prevention. Young LGBT individuals' perceptions on the issues related to HIV infection included risk behaviors and awareness, condom use and sexual partners, health care providers and services (Farrell 2006; Flores Iii et al. 2011; Ginsburg et al. 2002; Magee et al. 2012). For strategies used to prevent themselves from getting HIV prevention, LGBT youth expressed that seeking HIV-related and sexual health information, safe sex negotiation and practice with partners, learning from peers or partners, access to sensitive and nonjudgmental health care services, and participating HIV prevention program were used to enhance their HIV-related health (DeHaan et al. 2013; Eisenberg et al. 2011; Ginsburg et al. 2002; Kubicek et al. 2010; Kwong-Lai Poon and Trung-Thu Ho 2002). The obstacles to and the needs for HIV prevention revealed that young LGBT found supports from family and social group were unavailable or insufficient for them (Flores Iii et al. 2011; Kwong-Lai Poon and Trung-Thu Ho 2002). They expressed their needs for interesting and appropriate HIV prevention programs (Flores Iii et al. 2011; Kwong-Lai Poon and Trung-Thu Ho 2002).

In order to better understand the complexity of HIV infection and prevention among LGBT youth as well as to seek better solution for this public health problem, a number of qualitative papers related to HIV risk of LGBT youth, HIV-related health enhancing strategies including its obstacles and their needs in regards to these HIV issues has been conducted. We are interested in reviewing, integrating, and synthesizing those qualitative findings in order to reach a clearer picture of the perceptions of HIV risk among LGBT youth, health strategies that they used to prevent themselves from having infection, and obstacles to and needs for HIV prevention and health enhancing strategies. In order to reach our goal, we adopted an approach used to analyze, synthesize, and interpret qualitative findings, called 'metasynthesis' which will allow us to achieve an integrative interpretation of those findings.

13.2 Synthesizing Qualitative Research: A Metasynthesis

'Metasynthesis' refers to an approach used to analyze, synthesize, and interpret findings from qualitative studies (Major and Sevin-Baden 2010). It is both interpretive creation and analytic processes by mean of "the findings of studies are aggregated, summarized, or otherwise put together" (Barroso et al. 2003: 154). Sandelowski and Barroso (2003: 227) suggest that "qualitative metasynthesis is a form of systematic review or integration of qualitative research findings in a target domain that are themselves interpretive syntheses of data, including phenomenologies, ethnographies, grounded theories, and other integrated and coherent descriptions or explanations of phenomena, events, or cases". The goal of metasynthesis is to reach an integrative interpretation of results which is more substantive than those findings from individual study, resulting in greater understanding and development of new or modified theory (Bondas et al. 2013). Thus, metasynthesis is a method used to systematically review, analyze, and synthesize qualitative studies in a field of interest in order to achieve deeper understanding, possibly leading to the development or creation of a new body of knowledge.

The development of metasynthesis began with the work of Noblit and Hare (1988), called meta-ethnography which refers to the method of systematic comparison, involving the translation of studies into each other to create new meanings. Then, the methods of metasynthesis have been developed by scholars in different fields and given different name having the key characteristic of each method (Bondas et al. 2013). Paterson et al. (2001), for example, developed 'meta-study' to conduct metasynthesis in nursing sciences, having its philosophical foundation rooted in a constructivist orientation. This method comprises three component of the analysis process: meta data-analysis, meta-method, and meta-theory, followed by synthesis (Paterson et al. 2001). Sandelowski and Barroso (2003) then further developed 'metasummary' to synthesize the results from qualitative studies through effect sizes. Similarly, 'thematic synthesis' has been created by Thomas and Harden (2008) to synthesize qualitative research in systematic review. Thematic synthesis involves three stages including coding of text line-by-line, developing descriptive themes, and generating analytical themes (Thomas and Harden 2008).

Due to the increase numbers of qualitative studies, metasynthesis is one of the significant approaches used to develop knowledge in area of interests. Bondas et al. (2013) suggest that metasynthesis not only has a potential to present condensed knowledge in the area of interest, and strengthen research-base care in the field, it also make knowledge accessible and easier to use in evidence-based health care. In other words, metasynthesis is designed to facilitate the development of knowledge (Thorne et al. 2004). However, validity of conducting a metasynthesis needs to be ensured in order to achieve the goal of this synthesis approach; otherwise, it may be instead critical literature review and a replication of descriptive findings from original studies (Bondas et al. 2013; Thorne et al. 2004).

There are different processes to conduct a metasynthesis, depending on its concepts developed by different scholars. In this chapter, we only present the method of meta-ethnography proposed by Noblit and Hare (1988) and thematic synthesis developed by Thomas and Harden (2008) as we have adopted these two approaches to conducting this metasynthesis. According to Noblit and Hare (1988), there are seven steps to conduct metasynthesis. It consists of getting started which involves identifying an area of interest for conducting a meta-synthesis, deciding what is relevant to the initial interest, reading the studies, determining how studies are related, translating the studies into one another, synthesizing translation, and expressing the synthesis (Noblit and Hare 1988). Similarly, Thomas and Harden (2008) propose the method of synthesizing qualitative studies, called a thematic synthesis. This method focuses on the use of thematic analysis to develop new themes from original studies. It takes three stages of the synthesis, including coding text line by line, developing descriptive themes, and generating analytical themes. We are presenting how we adopted these two approaches to conducting our meta-synthesis in the next section.

13.3 Conducting a Metasynthesis

This chapter is a part of our metasynthesis project investigating perceived risk for HIV infection, HIV-related health enhancing strategies, and needs for HIV preventions among young LGBT people emerging adulthood. We adopted the seven phases of the meta-ethnographic approach of Noblit and Hare (1988) and the thematic synthesis proposed by Thomas and Harden (2008) to conduct our metasynthesis. The meta-ethnographic approach is used to identify an area of interest for conducting a meta synthesis, to determine what is relevant to the initial interest, including defining the focus of the synthesis, to systematically search and retrieve relevant studies, and then to appraise the resulting studies. Then, we used the methods of thematic synthesis to synthesize qualitative findings and develop the new themes from included studies.

13.3.1 Identify an Area of Interest

As a result of the rapidly rising numbers of qualitative studies from different disciplinary perspectives in health and social sciences conducted to understand HIV risks and health enhance strategies among young LGBT people emerging adulthood, we are interested in exploring the perceptions of HIV risk, what HIV-related risk behaviors that young LGBT individuals have engaged in, and what HIV-related health enhancing strategies they used to enhance their health including its obstacles and their needs in regards to this issue, by integrating and synthesizing findings from those qualitative studies. In this paper, we are discussing only the findings of perceived risk for HIV infection of LGBT youth.

13.3.2 Inclusion and Exclusion Criteria

To be considered for inclusion in this metasynthesis, the study needed to meet the following criteria: (1) must be related to young LGBT's HIV risks and HIV-related health enhancing strategies, (2) the participants in the included studies must be LGBT individuals having age between 13 and 29 years (3) utilised a qualitative methodology or a combination of qualitative and quantitative methods, (4) had sufficiently detailed information on themes and concepts as part of their results, and (5) was published in English. Studies with various perspectives or participants (young LGBT people/LGBT people, young LGBT people/health care providers, and others) are included if the various results specific to young LGBT participants could be separated from those of other respondents. Reviews and editorial articles were excluded, as were Masters' theses and dissertations, as it would be difficult to retrieve a whole thesis.

13.3.3 Search Strategy and Retrieving Studies

Computerized searches of relevant databases were conducted between November 2012 and September 2013, including CINAHL, PsycINFO, SocINDEX, Science Direct, LGBT Life, Medline, ProQuest Social Sciences, Google Scholar, and La Trobe University digital library databases. Key search words included 'young/youth/adolescent/teen LGBT OR lesbian/gay/bisexual/transgender/men who have sex with men/women who have sex with women/homosexual/gender minority AND HIV/AIDS/health/risk. We applied the Boolean operators AND/OR in combination with MeSH (medical subject heading) and free text terms. Additionally, we conducted a manual search of key journals (Journal of LGBT youth, International Journal of Transgenderism, and Journal of Homosexuality). The initial number of literature 'hits' (a total of all key search words in nine databases) was 9947 papers. All titles and abstracts were then screened by the first author and confirmed by the second, and our exclusion criteria were used to initially filter out papers that were irrelevant and/or did not meet the criteria. Duplicate papers were also sorted out in this stage using bibliography management software – Endnote X7. As a result, 9476 papers were excluded and 471 were considered potentially eligible. After scanning the full texts of the remaining articles, 51 papers were considered eligible, and 420 excluded, based on our inclusion criteria. After re-reading the full text of these 51 studies, one article were an HIV prevention program evaluation using statistical test, two articles were considered to consist of a combined group of participants (LGBT and non-LGBT), thus precluding separation of results, and thus, these were also excluded. Although 18 papers investigated the issues about LGBT individuals' self-destructive behaviors, sexuality, and health care access, the research purposes, questions, and/or findings have no relation to HIV infection; thus, it did not meet our inclusion criteria and, therefore, these were also excluded. This resulted in 30 eligible papers. From hand-searching of these 30 eligible articles, we found an additional article that met our inclusion criteria but it was a duplicate of one that has already been included. Therefore, 30 eligible papers have been remained and were the final included articles (see Table 13.1).

Table 13.1 Characteristics of the included studies

No.	Author	Year	Purpose of study	Research design	Participants	Age of participants	Number of participants	Place of study	Methods of data collection	Methods of data analysis
1	DeHaan, S., et al.	2013	To investigate the interplay between online and offline explorations of multiple dimensions of sexual health, which include sexually transmitted infections, sexual identities, romantic relationships, and sexual behaviors	Mixed methods	LGBT	16–24	32	USA	Individual Semi-structured interviews An ordinal scale item Open-ended discussions	Coding and generating themes using Ethno notes mixed method analysis program
2	Eisenberg, A., et al.	2011	To explore the use of internet as a dating tool and sexual behavior of young gay men	Qualitative study	Gay men	18–24	34	USA	Phone semi-structured interviews	Thematic analysis using Nvivo software to manage data
3	Farrell, K.P.	2006	To explore how undergraduate gay men make sense of HIV and its representation in a fictional TV storyline	Qualitative study	Gay men	18–24	16	USA	Focus group discussions	Coding and developing themes
4	Flores, D.D., Blake, B.J., & Sowell, R.L.	2011	To investigate the factors that may have contributed to each young gay man's recent HIV diagnosis and to elicit his perspectives on the design and efficacy of existing HIV prevention programs	Qualitative Study	Gay men	18–24	10	USA	Individual semi-structured interviews	Thematic content analysis

(continued)

Table 13.1 (continued)

No.	Author	Year	Purpose of study	Research design	Participants	Age of participants	Number of participants	Place of study	Methods of data collection	Methods of data analysis
5	Ginsburg, K.R., et al.	2002	To investigate factors that sexual minority youth believe make them feel safe in health care settings	Mixed methods	LGBTQ	14–23	215 (41 in focus groups)	USA	Focus group discussions	Statistical analysis for quantitative data
									Survey using 5 point Likert scale questionnaire	Qualitative data was presented to supplement quantitative data (no qualitative dada analysis mentioned)
6	Hall, N.M. & Applewhite, S.	2013	To investigate the relationship between masculine ideology, adherence to norms, and HIV prevention among young Black heterosexual and gay men on the campus of a historically Black college/university	Mixed methods	Black Gay men and heterosexual men	18–24	35 (Gay men 12 out of 35)	USA	Focus group discussions	Coding and identifying themes using Atlas.ti 6.2 software
				(only qualitative findings were presented in this study)					Individual interviews	
7	Kubicek, K., et al.	2010	To examine how and where young men who have sex with men receive relevant information on sexual health/behavior	Mix methods	MSM	18–24	58 (a total of 526 of mixed method project)	USA	Semi-structured interviews	Grounded theory (A constant comparative), using Atlas.ti software
				(only qualitative findings were presented in this study)						
8	Kubicek, K., et al.	2012	To investigate the use of Photovoice in the adaptation process of an evidence-based intervention (Adult Identity Mentoring) to make it developmentally and culturally appropriate HIV prevention interventions for African American young MSM	Qualitative study	African American MSM	18–24	36	N/A	Photovoice methods	Grounded theory (A constant comparative)

9	Kwong-Lai Poon, M., & Trung-Thu Ho, P.	2002	To examine cultural and social barriers that may increase HIV risk among gay, lesbian, and bisexual Asian youth	Qualitative study	Asian LGB	17–24	15	Canada	Individual interviews Focus group discussions	Coding and identifying themes
10	Lemos, D., Hosek, S.G., & Bell, M.	2015	To investigate perceptions of HIV risk behaviors and how HIV prevention services can be tailored to be culturally appropriate and effective for the House Ball community	Qualitative study	Black MSM	17–24	21	USA	Focus group discussion	Coding and identifying themes
11	Lyons, T., Johnson, A.K., & Garofalo, R.	2013	To describe syndemic factors that young MSMs have engaged which related to their HIV infection, and explore these factors that be used to strengthen HIV prevention program	Qualitative study	MSM	18–24	21	N/A	Semi-structured interviews	Constant comparative method
12	Magee, J.C., et al.	2012	To investigate the positive and negative aspects of Internet use for sexual health information among LGBT youth	Mixed methods	LGBT	16–24	32	USA	Semi-structured interviews	Constant comparative method, using EthnoNotes, a mixed method analysis program
13	McClelland, A., et al.	2012	To examine the ways in which social and environmental conditions influence vulnerability to adverse sexual health outcomes for young LGBT people with intellectual disabilities	Qualitative study (community-based approach)	LGBT youth with intellectual disabilities	17–26	10	Canada	Semi-structured interviews Focus group discussion	Coding and identifying themes using Nvivo software program

(continued)

Table 13.1 (continued)

No.	Author	Year	Purpose of study	Research design	Participants	Age of participants	Number of participants	Place of study	Methods of data collection	Methods of data analysis
14	McDermott, E., Roen, K., & Scourfield, J.	2008	To investigate the connections between sexual identities and self-destructive behaviors in young people	Qualitative study	LGBT	16–25	27	UK	Interviews Focus group discussions	Foucauldian discourse analysis
15	Middelthon, A.L. & Aggleton, P.	2001	To examine the influence of habitual signs governing interpersonal relations and to explore young men's capacity to self-reflect upon situations they have practiced unsafe sex, as well as those in which they may be vulnerable to such actions	Qualitative study	Gay men	17–22	20	Norway	Repeated in-depth interviews	Thematic analysis (not clearly specified in the paper)
16	Moeller et al.	2013	To examine how young gay and bisexual men make decisions about and experience their sexual behaviors	Qualitative study (Discovery-Based Research)	Gay and Bisexual men	18–27	10	USA	Discovery-based interviews (Open-ended questions; Method of Psychological Inquiry)	Listening Guide Method (3 steps of listening and synthesizing the stories told by participants)
17	Mustanski, B., Lyons, T., & Garcia, S.C.	2011	To investigate internet-related behaviors among young MSM that positively and negatively impact their sexual health	Mixed-methods	Gay men	18–24	16 (Total of 329 of mixed method project)	Not mention in the study	Interview	Constant comparison method Atlas.ti was used to manage the data

18	Mutchler, M.G.	2000a	To illustrate a community empowerment HIV prevention project considered to significantly reduce rate of unprotected anal sex among young gay males	Qualitative study (Ethnography)	Gay men and bisexual men	19–30	25	USA	Individually formal semi-structured interviews Informal interviews Participant observations	Closely to grounded theory
19	Mutchler, M.G.	2000b	To examine the sexual stories of young gay men in the era of AIDS and investigate how interpersonal dynamics, social contexts, and masculinities shape and constrain their sexual experiences	Qualitative study	Gay men	18–24	30	USA	Individual interviews	Thematic analysis (not clearly specified in the paper)
20	Mutchler, M.G., et al.	2013	To investigate the effectiveness of peer ethnography to gain insider views on substance use and sex among a diverse range of high-risk substance- using Black and Latino young men who have sex with men.	Qualitative study (Peer Ethnography)	MSM and Bisexual men	21–24	9 (peer ethnographers) 150 (young msm & bisexual men observed)	USA	Field notes from participant observations	A modified grounded theory and analytical induction approach
21	Pachankis, J.E. et al.	2013	To explore young gay and bisexual men's views of HIV prevention; experiences with former HIV prevention project; and attitudes towards online HIV prevention pro- grams, specifically a program to be delivered via the instant messaging (IM) feature of Facebook	Qualitative study	Gay and bisexual men	18–29 (young and emerging adulthood)	13	USA	Focus group discussions and individual interviews	Generating themes from data derived from focus groups and interviews

(continued)

Table 13.1 (continued)

No.	Author	Year	Purpose of study	Research design	Participants	Age of participants	Number of participants	Place of study	Methods of data collection	Methods of data analysis
22	Pingel, E.S. et al.	2013	To examine young gay men's use of the internet as a dating tool and their sexual behavior in order to reach a greater understanding of the opportunities for HIV prevention and health promotion among this population	Qualitative study	Gay men	18–24	34	USA	Semi-structured in-depth phone interviews	Thematic analysis
23	Scourfield, J., Roen, K., & McDermott, L.	2008	To investigate the cultural context of youth suicide and more specifically any connections between sexual identity and self-destructive behavior	Qualitative study	LGBT	16–25	69	UK	Focus group discussions Individual Interviews	Thematic analysis
24	Seal, D. W. et al.	2000	To explore elicit the recommendations from young MSM concerning the kinds of HIV prevention programs that would best meet their needs and would address risk issues they believed are critical	Qualitative study	MSM	16–25	72	USA	Ethnographic observations Semi-structured individual interviews	Coding and qualitatively generating themes

25	Singh, A.K., Sharma Mahendra, V., & Verma, R.	2008	To investigate the levels and range of sexual practices and attitudes of the homosexually active male youth by comparing them with their peers who reported heterosexual experiences.	Mixed method	Homosexual men	15–24	55	India	Individual interviews	Coding and generating themes
									Questionnaires	Statistical test for quantitative data
26	Stevens, R., Bernadini, S., & Jemmott, J. B.	2013	To explore the sexual behaviors of gay and transgender African American young people as embedded within the unique social and structural environments affecting this population	Qualitative study	African American gay men and transgender youth	18–24	54	USA	Focus groups	Grounded theory coding method
27	Timm, T.M. et al.	2013	To examine young black lesbian women's consensual sexual debut experiences with both males and females	Qualitative study	Black lesbian women	16–24	14	USA	Semi-structured interviews	Qualitative case, and cross-case analysis using cross-case matrices
28	Travers, R., & Paoletti, D	1999	To investigate how lesbian, gay, and bisexual youth who were HIV positive thought and felt about their situations and to identify the services they required or sought out	Qualitative study	LGB youth	17–25	32	Canada	In-depth semi-structured interviews	Thematic analysis

(continued)

Table 13.1 (continued)

No.	Author	Year	Purpose of study	Research design	Participants	Age of participants	Number of participants	Place of study	Methods of data collection	Methods of data analysis
29	Voisin, D.R. et al.	2013	To identify sources of HIV prevention information and barriers to adopting protective behaviors among young African American men who have sex with men	Qualitative study	African American MSM	18–24	10	USA	Focus group discussions	Coding and identifying themes
30	Wilson, E.C. et al.	2012	To explore HIV risk in transgender female youth	Qualitative study (Subsample of participants in mixed method project)	Transgender female youth	16–24	21	USA	Individual in-depth interviews	A phenomenological exploratory approach

L lesbian, *G* gay, *B* bisexual, *T* transgender, *Q* questioning, *MSM* men who have sex with men, *N/A* not available (not mention in the study)

13.3.4 Quality Appraisal

We read and reread the 30 included studies individually, in order to be familiar with them and to identify their main concepts, key metaphors, and/or themes. The first author extracted the data from the 30 selected studies to summarize their main concepts, with sample quotations, describing the methodology of each, including its research purposes, participants, fieldwork, data collection methods, data analysis, and information on methodological rigor. All were then evaluated for quality, using the quality assessment checklist, for qualitative studies, of the Critical Appraisal Skills Programme (CASP), developed as a tool to appraise evidence (particularly in health and social care) for their trustworthiness and value (Critical Appraisal Skill Programme 1993).

CASP consists of 10 questions assessing qualitative studies with no rating scores, with two authors reading each individually and assessing it according to the CASP questions. In the present case, however, we adopted a three-point rating system developed by Duggleby et al. (2010) to determine quality scores. According to the Duggleby's rating system, a rating point is given to each article for each of the CASP's eight questions (from question number 3 to 10). Duggleby and colleague also determined the range of score for weak, moderate, and strong. A weak score is a value of one point, for articles having little to no justification or explanation for a particular issue; a moderate score is a value of two points for articles discussing an issue but not elaborating on it, and a strong score is three points, for articles with extensive justification for and explanation of the issue at hand (Duggleby et al. 2010). Thus, the quality scores for each article ranged from 8 to 24, based on Duggleby's rating system. According to Moolchaem et al. (2015), the quality scores were then categorized in three levels based on Duggleby's rating system, including weak score of 8–15, a moderate one from 16 to 23, and a strong one of 24. We discussed results of this quality appraisal, but no studies were excluded based on the CASP score.

13.3.5 Analysis and Synthesis

In this metasynthesis, we adopted three stages of the thematic synthesis proposed by Thomas and Harden (2008). Stage one and two include coding texts and developing descriptive themes. In these two stages, we coded the texts from the findings of included studies according to meanings and contents within the framework of our research questions. We then developed the descriptive themes by grouping those new codes (see Table 13.2). The third stage involves generating analytical themes which can be equivalent to the development of the 'third order interpretations in meta-ethnography (Thomas and Harden 2008). We used metaphors and concepts we had identified from the original studies to discuss, compared and determined how they were related; resulting in forming the model illustrating what are HIV

Table 13.2 Themes emerged from included studies

Overarching themes	Number of sources	Number of coded references	First-order themes	Second-order themes
Exposure to high risk behaviors, unsafe sexual environment, experiences and activities	24	113	Having early sexual experiences, having high risk lifestyles and behaviors (drugs and alcohol use, engaging in clubs or party in which drugs and sex are involved), finding sex partner online, having unprotected sex, homeless, having multiple sex partners, having unsafe sexual and mental environments, engaging in sex work, experiencing sexual abuse, unhealthy sexual acts and desire.	Exposure to HIV risk resulted from two factors including intrinsic (characteristic of this age group) and extrinsic factor (related to the environment); internet make the possibility to easily find sex partners and engage in unhealthy sex, unsafe and unhealthy environment may create the possibility to expose to HIV risk; Sexual desire in young people may lead to the experiments of sexual experiences which may be the unhealthy experiences.
Perceptions of, attitudes to, and awareness of sexuality, HIV risk and prevention	17	45	Unawareness of HIV risk, the belief of not being at risk for HIV infection, women who have sex with woman believed AIDS was a "gay disease", perceiving low risk of contracting STIs/HIV, perceiving young people were not at risk for HIV infection, negative attitudes on condom use, intentional and accidental inconsistent/non-condom use, unwanted HIV screening, not interest in HIV prevention program.	Sexual abuse experiences impacted the perceptions of sexuality, and risk behaviors; The discrepancy between perceived risk for HIV and actual risky behaviors put LGBT youth at risk for HIV infection; Beliefs and norms impacted the ways that participants thought about communication, relationships with others, and the types of risky and preventative practices they engaged in

Psychosocial factors influencing HIV risk	16	54	Facing stigma, homophobia and discrimination, low self-esteem due to nonconforming gender identity, lack of parent supports, and lack of self-control, confusion/stress of non-conforming gender identity leading to seeking self through sexual experimentations/coping mechanism, resulting in risk behaviors.	Negative lived experiences resulted from unaccepted gender identity by society may lead LGBT youth to risk behaviors; stigma influenced attitude, decision to test for HIV, gender role expectations, and sexual scripts of young people which place LGBT youth at risk for HIV infection; The confusion/stigma of gender identity and gender disclosure may lead to psychological stress resulting in risk behaviors; experiencing psychological distress resulted from nonconforming gender identity, homophobia, discriminations, and social exclusions led LGBT youth to unhealthy coping mechanism resulting in risk behaviors; not disclosing sexuality to parents and feeling embarrassing to come to parents for same-sex sexual education information resulted in the lack of parent support.
Lack of relevant and appropriate skills, knowledge, resources, and HIV prevention program	13	40	Lack of HIV/STI education, lack of appropriate and relevant education relating to sexuality, lack of appropriate and interesting HIV prevention programs, HIV information and sources are not interesting, lack of negotiating skills (safe sex), miscommunication relation to sexual intercourse leading to unsafe sex, lack of ability to deal with the sexual situation leading to unsafe sex despite of having HIV/SIT educations.	Contents of information/educations as well as the methods providing educations regarding HIV and sexuality were not interesting and relevant to young LGBT, in term of age, gender identity, and culture; LGBT youth did not participate or interest in HIV education/preventive programs due to perceiving themselves invulnerable to HIV; the lack of skills regarding HIV prevention resulted from inexperienced, young age, and lacking of adult supervisions/supports; Schools and parents played important roles in providing appropriate and relevant HIV/sexuality educations; Gaps in sexual knowledge at the time of their sexual debut led young participants to engage in high-risk sexual activities.

(continued)

Table 13.2 (continued)

Overarching themes	Number of sources	Number of coded references	First-order themes	Second-order themes
Intimacy and HIV risk	12	29	Having unprotected sex with partners because of the trust feelings, the desire of satisfying partners, and the desire to feel more intimacy; having relationship with older partner or a partner having more power, which may lead to unsafe sexual intercourse.	Unbalanced power dynamics within the relationship (older/younger, financial dependence) may create the situation of unhealthy sexual intercourse; Partners are one of important sources that young participants learned about sex through actual experimentation; The confidence and trust in partners as well as the desire to experience sexual pleasure and satisfy partners may place young LGBT at vulnerability for HIV risk; Making decision to engage in safe sex/ unsafe sex with partners depended on participants' HIV knowledge, awareness regarding HIV risk, perception of a threat, the motivation to stay HIV-negative, and senses of self-efficacy.
Limited to HIV test and health care access	4	5	Avoiding HIV test due to fear (fear of being positive, stigma, and the impact on the future); ignoring HIV test due to perceiving not at risk/ low risk for HIV; ignoring or refusing HIV screening due to being aware of engaging in risk behaviors and anticipating HIV-positive test; apathy toward self-care; fear of being judged by health care providers; feeling of uncomfortable and unsafe to discuss about sexual orientation and sexuality issues with health care providers; concern about privacy, confidentiality, and infection control of health care settings when made decision to utilize health care services.	Stigma (non-conforming gender identity, and anticipated HIV-positive test) prevented LGBT youth from getting HIV test and utilizing health care services; The attitudes of participants towards health care providers (knowledge, competency, sensitivity, perceptions, and interpersonal skills, regarding sexuality, sexual orientation, and HIV issues) and health care settings (privacy, confidentiality, infection control, and safe) were the factor whether to access health care settings and get HIV test or not.
Total	30 (repeated sources excluded)	286		

Notes. The first-order themes reflect the perspective and understanding of participants of included studies. The second-order themes represent the primary authors' interpretations of participants' understandings

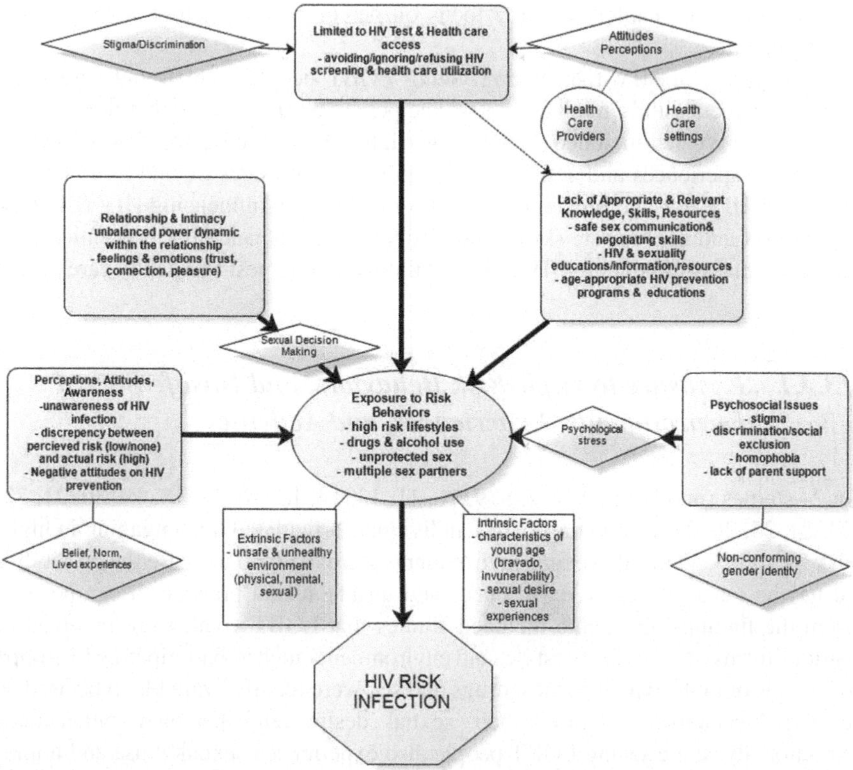

Fig. 13.1 Conceptual model of HIV risk among young LGBT young people

risks among young LGBT people, strategies they used to enhance their HIV-related health, and their HIV prevention needs (see Fig. 13.1). Nvivo, a qualitative data management software, was used to manage all stages including coding texts, generating themes, comparing concepts, and illustrating the models of perceived risk for HIV infection among young LGBT population.

13.4 HIV Risk Among Young LGBT People

There were approximately 999 young LGBT people participating in qualitative research projects, conducted and published during 1999–2015 included in this metasynthesis. The locations where most of the included studies conducted their research were in western countries, mostly in the USA. The most commonly adopted method for collecting data was individual in-depth interviews and thematic analysis method was commonly used for data analysis (the characteristics of original studies were illustrated in Table 13.1). Six majors themes emerged from these original studies. In these chapter, we only focus on perceived risk factors among LGBT young people.

Perceptions of HIV risk among young LGBT people were found across the included papers (study number 1–30). The perceived risk factors that these young population revealed included: exposure to high-risk behaviors, unsafe sexual environment, experiences and activities; perceptions of, attitudes to, and awareness of sexuality, HIV risk and prevention; psychosocial factors influencing HIV risk; lack of relevant and appropriate skills, knowledge, resources, and HIV prevention program; intimacy influencing HIV risk; and limited to HIV test and health care access

13.4.1 Exposure to High-Risk Behaviors, and Unsafe Sexual Environments, Experiences, and Activities

In 24 studies (number 1, 2, 4, 7, 8, 9, 10, 11, 13, 14, 15, 16, 17, 18, 19, 20, 21, 22, 23, 24, 25, 26, 27, 30), young LGBT individuals articulated that engaging in high-risk lifestyle, and unsafe sexual environments were likely to increase the possibility of having negative sexual experiences and unsafe sexual practice. It can be seen from the findings across the included studies that LGBT youth were involved in various forms of high risk lifestyle, and environments such as participating in groups of friends or clubs where parties, drugs and sex were readily available to be used as coping mechanism or fulfil their sexual desire, and personal satisfaction. Additionally, some young LGBT people also experienced sexual abuse and homelessness. These high-risk lifestyles and negative lived experiences tended to lead them to risky behaviors including drugs and alcohol abuse, and prostitution which would place them to risk of unprotected sexual intercourse. One young gay man said:

> It's about the drugs: it's about the party, sex – like rock and roll when you come out to it. Depending upon the group of people you hang around, you get into certain things. When I came out I was with the right people and didn't get into all these parties – sex parties. (Stevens et al. 2013: 1152)

Another one added:

> Of course we know marijuana is going to relax your body, and I think the least you're going to be thinking of is having safer sex. But that age, it loosened me up. It relaxed me, and I didn't really care about anything else. (Lyons et al. 2013: 373)

Sexual desire also contributed to young LGBT people's exposure to sexual experiences and activities. Sexual desire drove them to 'sexual curiosity and experiment'. Consequently, LGBT youth would seek partners via both online and offline methods. Seeking sexual partners online mostly included dating or hook up websites while the offline ones tended to be some public locations such as public parks and toilets. As a result, the possibility of engaging in sexual activities were increased which were likely to lead young people to have multiple sex partners as well as unsafe sexual practice.

13.4.2 Perceptions of, Attitudes to, and Awareness of Sexuality, HIV Risk and Prevention

LGBT youth's sexuality and perceived HIV risk, prevention, and risk awareness were unfolded through 17 studies (number 2, 3, 4, 6, 8,9,10, 12, 13, 15, 17, 19, 24, 26, 28, 29, and 30). These young people revealed that according to social attitudes towards sex, it was embarrassing to talk about this issue which resulted in preventing them seeking information about sex. This might put LGBT you at risk for unsafe sexual practice.

Regarding perceived HIV risk and self-awareness, some believed that HIV infection was not a significant issue in their life despite knowing that HIV was not curable. This tended to be because they perceived that, for them, HIV risk-taking was inevitable. However, some young LGBT people thought that although HIV infection was not curable, antiviral medication was sufficiently effective to deal with this disease. One expressed:

> Some people don't think it is a risk and think it's overrated, since AZT is so effective, you don't see it close to home anymore. (Stevens et al. 2013: 1154)

As a result of perceiving unimportance of HIV infection and the effectiveness of its treatments, they did overlook or not pay much attention to HIV-related information and prevention, which significantly placed them at risk for HIV infection.

Lack of HIV risk awareness was another cause that drove young LGBT people to HIV risk infection. It has been revealed through this metasynthesis that some young participants were not aware that HIV infection would happen to them despite engaging in high-risk behaviors. In other words, these young people did not believe that they were at risk for HIV infection. One lesbian expressed that "HIV only happen to older gay men" (Travers and Paoletti 1999, p. 274). Similarly, a young gay man remarked:

> Young people have this mentality that I'm gonna live forever and nothing can really affect me and if it happens to somebody else it's fine, but it'll never happen to me. (Flores Iii et al. 2011, p. 379)

Nevertheless, there were young LGBT individuals who were aware that they were at risk for HIV infection but had fear about the knowledge of being HIV-positive. Because of this, this group of people did not acknowledge their HIV risk and avoided having HIV test. Therefore, it was clear that young LGBT people being unaware their HIV risk had been placed at risk for transmitted HIV infection.

13.4.3 Psychosocial Factors Influencing HIV Risk

Not surprisingly, psychosocial issues had also been articulated that it was one of the significant factors placing young LGBT at risk for HIV infection. It can be seen from 15 included studies (number 1,6, 7, 8, 9, 10, 11, 14, 21, 24, 26, 27, 28, 29, and

30) that young LGBT people experienced various forms of homophobia, stigma, discriminations, and social exclusions including the lack of parent and social supports. This had resulted in low self-esteem and psychological distress that drove young people to risky behaviors such as drugs and alcohol abuse, prostitution, and engaging in an unsafe sexual environment and unprotected sex. As reflected in the study of Kwong-Lai Poon and Trung-Thu Ho (2002), LGBT youth had to deal with emotional stresses, and these drove those who lack positive coping mechanisms to use substances. Although this could ease some of their stress, it created awkward feelings about intimacy with a same-sex partner. Not only this, to gain a sense of social connection and to validate their sexual identity, many of these young gendered minority sought anonymous sexual encounters, which may increase their risk for HIV infection (Kwong-Lai Poon and Trung-Thu Ho 2002).

13.4.4 Lack of Relevant and Appropriate Skills, Knowledge, Resources, and HIV Prevention Program

Through 13 studies (number 2, 4, 7, 9, 10, 11, 15, 16, 17, 26, 28, 29, and 30), it was evident that the lack of relevant skills, knowledge, resources, and HIV prevention program forced young LGBT to risk for HIV infection. For instance, lack of skills for safe sex negotiation and miscommunication had brought these young LGBT people to the possibility of engaging in risk behaviors. As we could see from a young male account:

> I assumed that we were going to use a condom, first of all. And I think I said that he initiated it. And he – and I was going to bottom. So, he – I said, "Do you have something?" And he said, "Sure." And then he went away, and he came back. But he – and he put something on. But it was not a condom. It was a cock ring. And so, I was – I should have been a lot more upset and said to stop, but I was just like, "OK, whatever," and went along with it which is not good at all…but that's what happened. (Eisenberg et al. 2011: 9)

Another male participant also remarked that:

> My first few partners, for instance, I never asked them (their HIV and STD status) because I don't know …I just felt um …hm…I didn't know how to. (Kwong-Lai Poon and Trung-Thu Ho 2002: 53)

Insufficient sexual education and HIV-related knowledge, resources, and prevention programs were also the reasons why these young people were at risk for HIV infection. The youth articulated that information learnt from school was not relevant and interesting to them. For example, it was too conservative and sexualities of the gendered minority group were not often included in the lessons or school discussions. Also, available HIV resources were not appropriate designs for their age and hence did not catch their attentions. One participant said that "they (school) didn't talk about gay sex at all" (Kubicek et al. 2010: 247). Another agreed, saying that "it was all hetero and had nothing to do with what I was interested in, I just ignored it" (Flores Iii et al. 2011: 380). Another example was that sexual educations in school were based on a heterosexual context and only when homosexual sex was brought up. According to young men (in school), it was "just that", and "it was wrong" (Kubicek et al. 2010: 248). Similarly, for HIV prevention program, the LGBT participants felt that some programs or campaigns lack age and cultural appropriateness. For example, the participants articulated in Kwong-Lai Poon and Trung-Thu Ho (2002)'s work that safer sex campaign lacked Asian representation.

As a consequence of the lack of relevant information and resources, knowledge as well as campaigns of sexuality and HIV-related issues of young LGBT people may be insufficient to deal with the transmission of HIV. As presented in the study of Kubicek et al. (2010), some participants believed that the pain and bleeding they were experiencing was "normal" and so did not feel they could or should say anything to their partner. Thus, insufficient relevant skills and knowledge place young LGBT persons at high risk of HIV infection. Nevertheless, it was interesting that although some young LGBT people were well educated in the relevant issues, they confessed that their education had nothing to do with self-control when they were in real situations in which unprotected sex intercourse was convinced. The example of this was reflected by one young male medical student who elaborated that:

> I feel like, yea, I have all this medical knowledge and, you know, maybe, in other people's eyes, might be held to a higher standard, but I feel like I'm just another person out there, you know. So, I mean, we all make mistakes, I think. I've done my best to behave responsibly, um. I can't say I have 100 % of the time. But, um, again I think a lot of that comes down to just, you know, substance use and not necessarily making the decisions you would sober. I mean, I don't use drugs but I certainly have gotten myself into situations when I've been drunk that has been-I've done things that I wouldn't do sober, so. Um, I think we all, like I said, make mistakes. But, I mean, safe sex is something that, certainly on paper and most often in practice I would advocate, so. I do, I've tried to make that a reality. (Moeller et al. 2013: 781)

13.4.5 Intimacy Influencing HIV Risk

Eleven included studies revealed that another the risk factor that put young LGBT people at risk for HIV infection was an intimacy or relationship that somehow highly influenced HIV risk behaviors (study number 4, 7, 8, 10, 11, 15, 16, 22, 26, 27, and 30). Many young LGBT people engaged in unprotected with their partners, both casual and steady ones. According to this metasynthesis, we summarized that there were two situations in which LGBT people were put into risk behaviors. Firstly, personal attributes or behaviors of LGBT youth themselves that created the situations of engaging in practicing unsafe sex. That is the physical attributes that were considered attractive allowing LGBT youth having more chances to meet more partners. In other words, they had more possibilities of engaging in unsafe sexual activities. In addition, the willingness and intention of practicing unsafe sex of LGBT youth also were articulated. Many young people mentioned that because they wanted to retain their relationship with a partner, especially the one they felt emotionally connected with, they did not want protected sex to be a barrier of trust, and sexual satisfaction in the relationship. One youth remarked: "When you're in love and care about that person at the end of the day you're willing to do anything for that person" (Lemos et al. 2015: 74). Another agreed, stating that "I don't need a condom. I trust him so, I was kinda, like, yeah whatever" (Flores Iii et al. 2011: 380).

The second situation that put young LGBT individuals at risk for HIV infection was that the partners of LGBT youth created the possibility of unsafe sex. This tended to happen when the partner was older or was an influential person who has more power over the youth. One respondent said that "being 'in debt' might make me at risk. It is easy to give a bit more than your partner. It is good not to be 'in debt', but it is painful not to be able to reciprocate" (Middelthon and Aggleton 2001: 520). Young LGBT people also did articulate how they felt with their older partner; they saw older people were the source of money as well as taking them (young men) under their wings (Stevens et al. 2013).

Not only having more power over young LGBT persons, some partners of the LGBT youth also persuaded these young participants to have unprotected sex, using 'sweet conversation' and genuine intimacy as the convincing tools. This can be seen from the explanation of one man that "he is vulnerable to a partner who can 'sweet talk me' and I'll do whatever you want" (Moeller et al. 2013: 783). Therefore, young LGBT people were forced into risk for HIV infection through unhealthy intimacy.

13.4.6 Limited to HIV Test and Health Care Access

Although only two included studies did mention about limited to HIV test and health care access driving LGBT youth to risk for HIV infection (study number 5 and 28), these issues were significantly impact on their HIV-related health. These young participants explained that offending behaviors of health care providers, non-sensitive and non-confidential health care services prevented them from utilizing health care services including HIV test. They also shared that they were assumed they were at greater risk for HIV infection. One participant stated: "Are you (participant) going to get HIV tested? Don't think that just because somebody's gay that that means they have to have HIV … Don't place labels on people" (Ginsburg et al. 2002: 413). This was likely to impact on LGBT youth's satisfaction and attitudes towards health care that would result in non-returning for health care including screened HIV status.

Not just only clinician characteristics and health care service issues that prevented those young LGBT population from health care and HIV screening, but mental issues also played an important role in seeking health care and HIV test. That is LGBT youth avoided utilizing health care because they feared that once they were screened for HIV infection and the testing result was positive, their HIV status would be disclosed and judged by peers and family. This was reflected in an HIV-positive youth's statement, saying that "I didn't see a doctor and I didn't get medical treatment right away, I pretended like I wasn't positive and I was afraid of how my friends would be" (Travers and Paoletti 1999: 275). Consequently, this greatly affected their health status and in return, other LGBT youth were also at risk for acquiring HIV virus.

13.5 Discussion and Conclusion

This metasynthesis, using the meta-ethnography method of Noblit and Hare (1988), has systematically analyzed and synthesized the findings from 30 qualitative studies related to HIV risk of young LGBT people. Based on the themes emerged from this metasynthesis, exposure to high-risk behaviors, and unsafe sexual environments, experiences, and activities play the negative role of placing young LGBT at greater risk for HIV infection. Taking risk from this exposure seems to be associated with their marginalized gender identity and the nature of their young age. Curiosity and attempts to experience new things in life are what young people tend to do despite the fact they have to take some risk. Flores Iii et al. (2011) have suggested in their study that young gay men utilized available resources to find out their gender identity and fulfil their sexual desire, resulting in becoming sexually active. Pachankis et al. (2013) have also revealed in their study that early sexual and substance use experiences potentially influence on subsequent risk behavior patterns of these young people. Singh et al. (2008) also suggested that the reasons why some young gendered minority people engage in various risk behaviors were to assert their manhood because they felt they did not meet their gender role expectations.

Psychosocial factors consisting of stigma, low self-esteem, discriminations, social exclusions, and psychological distress are also the significant HIV risk infection. Social exclusion, as defined by the Social Exclusion Knowledge Network (SEKN) (2008), is a condition that individuals or groups are assumed to be excluded from the systems and relationships of society, by dynamic and multi-dimensional processes driven by unequal power relationships. According to Fish (2010), the social exclusion concept can be used to describe the exclusion of and discrimination against the gender minority group of people, who have been placed within the boundary of homosexuality and seen as sinners. It can be seen from the existing studies that lifestyles of LGBT people are perceived as deviant. Consequently, they are considered as a moral underclass and excluded from social institutions, including being excluded from the rights associated with citizenship (de Lind van Wijngaarden et al. 2012; Khan et al. 2009; Moolchaem et al. 2015; Ocha 2013). These exclusions can be situated within the three paradigms of social exclusion proposed by Silver (1994), which consist of solidarity, specialization, and monopoly. In the solidarity paradigm, exclusion occurs when the social bond between the individual and society breaks down. This paradigm focuses on a relationship between groups based on cultural or moral boundaries. With young LGBT individuals who transgress the gender norm, the bond between them and the mainstream society has broken down. This has resulted in the rejections that LGBT people face due to their gender identity. Moolchaem et al. (2015) suggested that psychosocial distress and social exclusion drive the gendered minority group of people to risk behaviors and greatly affected their health and well-being.

Our synthesis can be conceptualized as presented in Fig. 13.1.

We contend that this metasynthesis provides a clear account of perceived risk for HIV infection among young LGBT people. Our findings can be used as an evidence to create an evidence-based practice of sensitive care and HIV prevention programs in order to reach the goal of decreasing HIV prevalence and incidence among this high-risk group.

References

Balaji, A. B., Bowles, K. E., Le, B. C., Paz-Bailey, G., Oster, A. M., & Group, f. t. N. S. (2013). High HIV incidence and prevalence and associated factors among young MSM, 2008. *AIDS, 27*(2), 269–278. doi:10.1097/QAD.0b013e32835ad489.

Barroso, J., Gollop, C. J., Sandelowski, M., Meynell, J., Pearce, P. F., & Collins, L. J. (2003). The challenges of searching for and retrieving qualitative studies. *Western Journal of Nursing Research, 25*(2), 153–178. doi:10.1177/0193945902250034.

Bockting, W. O. (2009). Transforming the paradigm of transgender health: A field in transition. *Sexual and Relationship Therapy, 24*(2), 103–107.

Bondas, T., Hall, E. O. C., & Wikberg, A. (2013). Metasynthesis in health care research. In P. Liamputtong (Ed.), *Research methods in health: Foundations for evidence-based practice* (2nd ed., pp. 280–294). Melbourne: Oxford University Press.

Centers for Disease Control and Prevention. (2005). HIV prevalence, unrecognized infection, and HIV testing among men who have sex with men – five US cities, June 2004–April 2005. *MMWR Morbidity and Mortality Weekly Report, 54*(24), 597.

Centers for Disease Control and Prevention. (2014). *Lesbian, gay, bisexual, and transgender health*. Retrieved June, 20, 2015, from http://www.cdc.gov/lgbthealth/youth.htm.

Critical Appraisal Skill Programme. (1993). Critical appraisal skills programme: Making sense of evidence. Retrieved from www.casp-uk.net. Retrieved Dec, 26, 2013, from www.casp-uk.net.

de Lind van Wijngaarden, J. W., Schunter, B. T., & Iqbal, Q. (2012). Sexual abuse, social stigma and HIV vulnerability among young feminised men in Lahore and Karachi, Pakistan. *Culture, Health & Sexuality, 15*(1), 73–84. doi:10.1080/13691058.2012.743186.

DeHaan, S., Kuper, L. E., Magee, J. C., Bigelow, L., & Mustanski, B. S. (2013). The interplay between online and offline explorations of identity, relationships, and sex: A mixed-methods study with LGBT youth. *Journal of Sex Research, 50*(5), 421–434. doi:10.1080/00224499.2012.661489.

Duggleby, W., Holtslander, L., Kylma, J., Duncan, V., Hammond, C., & Williams, A. (2010). Metasynthesis of the hope experience of family caregivers of persons with chronic illness. *Qualitative Health Research, 20*(2), 148–158. doi:10.1177/1049732309358329.

Eisenberg, A., Bauermeister, J. A., Pingel, E., Johns, M. M., & Santana, M. L. (2011). Achieving safety: Safer sex, communication, and desire among young gay men. *Journal of Adolescent Research, 26*(5), 645–669. doi:10.1177/0743558411402342.

Farrell, K. P. (2006). HIV on TV: Conversations with young gay men. *Sexualities, 9*(2), 193–213. Retrieved from http://search.ebscohost.com/login.aspx?direct=true&db=qth&AN=20549605&site=ehost-live.

Fish, J. (2010). Conceptualising social exclusion and lesbian, gay, bisexual, and transgender people: The implications for promoting equity in nursing policy and practice. *Journal of Research in Nursing, 15*(4), 303–312. doi:10.1177/1744987110364691.

Flores Iii, D. D., Blake, B. J., & Sowell, R. L. (2011). "Get Them While They're Young": Reflections of young gay men newly diagnosed with HIV infection. *Journal of the Association of Nurses in AIDS Care, 22*(5), 376–387. http://dx.doi.org/10.1016/j.jana.2011.01.001.

Friedman, S. R., Ompad, D. C., Maslow, C., Young, R., Case, P., Hudson, S. M., … Garfein, R. S. (2003). HIV prevalence, risk behaviors, and high-risk sexual and injection networks among young women injectors who have sex with women. *American Journal of Public Health, 93*(6), 902–906. Retrieved from http://www.ncbi.nlm.nih.gov/pmc/articles/PMC1447865/.

Ginsburg, K. R., Winn, R. J., Rudy, B. J., Crawford, J., Zhao, H., & Schwarz, D. F. (2002). How to reach sexual minority youth in the health care setting: The teens offer guidance. *Journal of Adolescent Health, 31*(5), 407–416. http://dx.doi.org/10.1016/S1054-139X(02)00419-6.

Hall, N. M., & Applewhite, S. (2013). Masculine ideology, norms, and HIV prevention among young black men. *Journal of HIV/AIDS & Social Services, 12*(3/4), 384–403. doi:10.1080/15381501.2013.781974.

Khan, S. I., Hussain, M. I., Parveen, S., Bhuiyan, M. I., Gourab, G., Sarker, G. F., … Sikder, J. (2009). Living on the extreme margin: Social exclusion of the transgender population (hijra) in Bangladesh. *Journal of Health Population and Nutrition, 27*(4), 441–451.

Kubicek, K., Beyer, W. J., Weiss, G., Iverson, E., & Kipke, M. D. (2010). In the dark: Young men's stories of sexual initiation in the absence of relevant sexual health information. *Health Education & Behavior, 37*(2), 243–263. Retrieved from http://0-heb.sagepub.com.alpha2.latrobe.edu.au/content/37/2/243.full.pdf.

Kubicek, K., Beyer, W., Weiss, G., & Kipke, M. D. (2012). Photovoice as a tool to adapt an HIV prevention intervention for African american young men who have sex with men. *Health Promotion Practice, 13*(4), 535–543. doi:10.1177/1524839910387131.

Kwong-Lai Poon, M., & Trung-Thu Ho, P. (2002). A qualitative analysis of cultural and social vulnerabilities to HIV infection among gay, lesbian, and bisexual Asian youth. *Journal of Gay & Lesbian Social Services, 14*(3), 43–78. Retrieved from http://0-search.proquest.com.alpha2.latrobe.edu.au/docview/61532809?accountid=12001, http://CM8EK7ZY3D.search.serialssolutions.com/?ctx_ver=Z39.88-2004&ctx_enc=info:ofi/enc:UTF-8&rfr_id=info:sid/ProQ%3Asocialservicesshell&rft_val_fmt=info:ofi/fmt:kev:mtx:journal&rft.genre=unknown&rft.jtitle=Journal+of+Gay+%26+Lesbian+Social+Services&rft.atitle=A+Qualitative+Analysis+of+Cultural+and+Social+Vulnerabilities+to+HIV+Infection+among+Gay%2C+Lesbian%2C+and+Bisexual+Asian+Youth&rft.au=Kwong-Lai+Poon%2C+Maurice%3B+Trung-Thu+Ho%2C+Peter&rft.aulast=Kwong-Lai+Poon&rft.aufirst=Maurice&rft.date=2002-01-01&rft.volume=14&rft.issue=3&rft.spage=43&rft.isbn=&rft.btitle=&rft.title=Journal+of+Gay+%26+Lesbian+Social+Services&rft.issn=10538720, http://0-www.tandfonline.com.alpha2.latrobe.edu.au/doi/pdf/10.1300/J041v14n03_03

Lemos, D., Hosek, S. G., & Bell, M. (2015). Reconciling reality with fantasy: Exploration of the sociocultural factors influencing HIV transmission among black young men who have sex with men (BYMSM) within the house ball community: A Chicago study. *Journal of Gay & Lesbian Social Services, 27*(1), 64–85. doi:10.1080/10538720.2015.988837.

Lemp, G. F., Jones, M., Kellogg, T. A., Nieri, G. N., Anderson, L., Withum, D., & Katz, M. (1995). HIV seroprevalence and risk behaviors among lesbians and bisexual women in San Francisco and Berkeley, California. *American Journal of Public Health, 85*(11), 1549–1552. doi:10.2105/AJPH.85.11.1549.

Lyons, T., Johnson, A. K., & Garofalo, R. (2013). "What Could Have Been Different": A qualitative study of syndemic theory and HIV prevention among young men who have sex with men. *Journal of HIV/AIDS & Social Services, 12*(3–4), 368–383. doi:10.1080/15381501.2013.816211.

Magee, J. C., Bigelow, L., DeHaan, S., & Mustanski, B. S. (2012). Sexual health information seeking online: A mixed-methods study among lesbian, gay, bisexual, and transgender young people. *Health Education & Behavior, 39*(3), 276–289. Retrieved from http://0-search.proquest.com.alpha2.latrobe.edu.au/docview/1312424713?accountid=12001, http://CM8EK7ZY3D.

search.serialssolutions.com/?ctx_ver=Z39.88-2004&ctx_enc=info:ofi/enc:UTF-8&rfr_id=info:sid/ProQ%3Aericshell&rft_val_fmt=info:ofi/fmt:kev:mtx:journal&rft.genre=unknown&rft.jtitle=Health+Education+%26+Behavior&rft.atitle=Sexual+Health+Information+Seeking+Online%3A+A+Mixed-Methods+Study+among+Lesbian%2C+Gay%2C+Bisexual%2C+and+Transgender+Young+People&rft.au=Magee%2C+Joshua+C.%3B+Bigelow%2C+Louisa%3B+DeHaan%2C+Samantha%3B+Mustanski%2C+Brian+S.&rft.aulast=Magee&rft.aufirst=Joshua&rft.date=2012-06-01&rft.volume=39&rft.issue=3&rft.spage=276&rft.isbn=&rft.btitle=&rft.title=Health+Education+%26+Behavior&rft.issn=10901981, http://0-heb.sagepub.com.alpha2.latrobe.edu.au/content/39/3/276.full.pdf

Major, C. H., & Sevin-Baden, M. (2010). *An introduction to qualitative research synthesis: Managing the information explosion in social science research*. New York: Routledge.

McClelland, A., Flicker, S., Nepveux, D., Nixon, S., Vo, T., Wilson, C., … Proudfoot, D. (2012). Seeking safer sexual spaces: Queer and trans young people labeled with intellectual disabilities and the paradoxical risks of restriction. *Journal of Homosexuality, 59*(6), 808–819. doi:10.1080/00918369.2012.694760.

McDermott, E., Roen, K., & Scourfield, J. (2008). Avoiding shame: Young LGBT people, homophobia and self-destructive behaviours. *Culture, Health & Sexuality, 10*(8), 815–829. doi:10.1080/13691050802380974.

Middelthon, A. L., & Aggleton, P. (2001). Reflection and dialogue for HIV prevention among young gay men. *Aids care, 13*(4), 515–526.

Moeller, R. W., Halkitis, P. N., Pollock, J. A., Siconolfi, D. E., & Barton, S. (2013). When the emotions really started kicking in, which ended up being a problem: Sex, HIV, and emotions among young gay and bisexual men. *Journal of Homosexuality, 60*(5), 773–795. doi:10.1080/00918369.2013.773825.

Moolchaem, P., Liamputtong, P., O'Halloran, P., & Muhamad, R. (2015). The lived experiences of transgender persons: A meta-synthesis. *Journal of Gay & Lesbian Social Services, 27*(2), 143–171. doi:10.1080/10538720.2015.1021983.

Mustanski, B., Lyons, T., & Garcia, S. C. (2011). Internet use and sexual health of young men who have sex with men: A mixed-methods study. *Archives of Sexual Behavior, 40*(2), 289–300. doi:10.1007/s10508-009-9596-1.

Mutchler, M. G. (2000a). Making space for safer sex. *AIDS Education and Prevention, 12*(1), 1–14. Retrieved from http://0-search.proquest.com.alpha2.latrobe.edu.au/docview/198002769?accountid=12001, http://CM8EK7ZY3D.search.serialssolutions.com/?ctx_ver=Z39.88-2004&ctx_enc=info:ofi/enc:UTF-8&rfr_id=info:sid/ProQ%3Acriminaljusticeperiodicalsshell&rft_val_fmt=info:ofi/fmt:kev:mtx:journal&rft.genre=article&rft.jtitle=AIDS+Education+and+Prevention&rft.atitle=Making+space+for+safer+sex&rft.au=Mutchler%2C+Matt+G&rft.aulast=Mutchler&rft.aufirst=Matt&rft.date=2000-02-01&rft.volume=12&rft.issue=1&rft.spage=1&rft.isbn=&rft.btitle=&rft.title=AIDS+Education+and+Prevention&rft.issn=08999546, http://media.proquest.com/media/pq/classic/doc/51975850/fmt/pi/rep/NONE?hl=&cit%3Aauth=Mutchler%2C+Matt+G&cit%3Atitle=Making+space+for+safer+sex&cit%3Apub=AIDS+Education+and+Prevention&cit%3Avol=12&cit%3Aiss=1&cit%3Apg=1&cit%3Adate=Feb+2000&ic=true&cit%3Aprod=ProQuest+Central&_a=ChgyMDE0MDIxOTAxMjU0NTczOTo5NDQ5NTASBjEwMjEzNxoKT05FX1NFQVJDSCINMTMxLjE3Mi4zNi40NSoFMzI2MDQyCTE5ODAwMjc2OToNRG9jdW1lbnRJbWFnZUIBMFIGT25saW5lWgJGVGIDUEZUagoyMDAwLzAyLzAxcgoyMDAwLzAyLzI5egCCATJQLTEwMDcwMjUtMTIwMDEtQ1VTVE9NRVItMTAwMDAwMzkvMTAwMDAxNDctMTEyOTY5OZIBBk9ubGluZcoBB0VuZE5vdGXSARJTY2hvbGFybHkgSm91cm5hbHOaAgdQcmVQYWlkqgIoT1M6RU1TLVBkZkRvY1ZpZXdCYXNlLWdldE11ZGlhVXJsRm9ySXRlbbICALoCAMoCD0FydGljbGV8RmVhdHVyZQ%3D%3D&_s=Z%2BjxEsdubR36tIFabj2%2FokZalP0%3D

Mutchler, M. G. (2000b). Young gay men's stories in the states: Scripts, sex, and safety in the time of AIDS. *Sexualities, 3*(1), 31. Retrieved from http://search.ebscohost.com/login.aspx?direct=true&db=qth&AN=5435374&site=ehost-live

Mutchler, M. G., McKay, T., McDavitt, B., & Gordon, K. K. (2013). Using peer ethnography to address health disparities among young urban Black and Latino men who have sex with men. *American Journal of Public Health, 103*(5), 849–852. doi:10.2105/AJPH.2012.300988.

Noblit, G. W., & Hare, R. D. (1988). *Meta-ethnography: Synthesizing qualitative studies*. Newbury Park: Sage.

Ocha, W. (2013). Rethinking gender: Negotiating future queer rights in Thailand. *Gender, Technology and Development, 17*(1), 79–104. doi:10.1177/0971852412472125.

Pachankis, J., Lelutiu-Weinberger, C., Golub, S., & Parsons, J. (2013). Developing an online health intervention for young gay and bisexual men. *AIDS and Behavior, 17*(9), 2986–2998. doi:10.1007/s10461-013-0499-8.

Paterson, B. L., Thorne, S. E., Canam, C., & Jillings, C. (2001). *Meta-study of qualitative health research*. Thousand Oaks: SAGE Publications.

Pingel, E. S., Bauermeister, J. A., Johns, M. M., Eisenberg, A., & Leslie-Santana, M. (2013). "A Safe Way to Explore": Reframing risk on the internet amidst young gay men's search for identity. *Journal of Adolescent Research, 28*(4), 453–478. http://dx.doi.org/10.1177/0743558412470985.

Sandelowski, M., & Barroso, J. (2003). Creating metasummaries of qualitative findings. *Nursing Research, 52*(4), 226–233.

Scourfield, J., Roen, K., & McDermott, L. (2008). Lesbian, gay, bisexual and transgender young people's experiences of distress: Resilience, ambivalence and self-destructive behaviour. *Health & Social Care in the Community, 16*(3), 329–336. http://dx.doi.org/10.1111/j.1365-2524.2008.00769.x.

Seal, D. W., Kelly, J., Bloom, F., Stevenson, L., Coley, B., Broyles, L., & Team, T. M. C. O. W. C. P. R. (2000). HIV prevention with young men who have sex with men: What young men themselves say is needed. *AIDS care, 12*(1), 5–26. Retrieved from http://www.tandfonline.com/doi/pdf/10.1080/09540120047431

Silver, H. (1994). Social Exclusion and Social Solidarity: Three Paradigms. *International Labour Review, 133*(5–6), 531–578. http://www.ilo.org/public/english/revue/index.htm

Singh, A. K., Mahendra, V. S., & Verma, R. (2008). Exploring context and dynamics of homosexual experiences among rural youth in India. *Journal of LGBT Health Research, 4*(2/3), 89–101. doi:10.1080/15574090902913719.

Social Exclusion Knowledge Network. (2008). *Understanding and tackling social exclusion: Final report to the WHO Commission on Social Determinants of Health From the Social Exclusion Knowledge Network*. Retrieved from http://www.who.int/social_determinants/publications/socialexclusion/en/index.html

Stevens, R., Bernadini, S., & Jemmott, J. B. (2013). Social environment and sexual risk-taking among gay and transgender African American youth. *Culture, Health & Sexuality, 15*(10), 1148–1161. doi:10.1080/13691058.2013.809608.

Thomas, J., & Harden, A. (2008). Methods for the thematic synthesis of qualitative research in systematic reviews. *BMC Medical Research Methodology, 8*(1), 45. Retrieved from http://www.biomedcentral.com/1471-2288/8/45.

Thorne, S., Jensen, L., Kearney, M. H., Noblit, G., & Sandelowski, M. (2004). Qualitative metasynthesis: Reflections on methodological orientation and ideological agenda. *Qualitative Health Research, 14*(10), 1342–1365. doi:10.1177/1049732304269888.

Timm, T. M., Reed, S. J., Miller, R. L., & Valenti, M. T. (2013). Sexual debut of young black women who have sex with women: Implications for STI/HIV risk. *Youth & Society, 45*(2), 167–183. doi:10.1177/0044118x11409445.

Travers, R., & Paoletti, D. (1999). Responding to the support needs of HIV positive lesbian, gay and bisexual youth. *Canadian Journal of Human Sexuality, 8*(4), 271–283. Retrieved from http://search.ebscohost.com/login.aspx?direct=true&db=cin20&AN=2000068402&site=ehost-live, http://0-media.proquest.com.alpha2.latrobe.edu.au/media/pq/classic/doc/60613987/fmt/pi/rep/NONE?hl=&cit%3Aauth=Travers%2C+Robb%3BPaoletti%2C+Dino&cit%3Atitle=Responding+to+the+support+needs+of+HIV+positive+lesbian%2C+gay+and+bisexual

+youth&cit%3Apub=The+Canadian+Journal+of+Human+Sexuality&cit%3Avol=8&cit%3Aiss=4&cit%3Apg=271&cit%3Adate=Winter+1999&ic=true&cit%3Aprod=ProQuest+Central&_a=ChgyMDE0MDIxOTAxMjYwMTY1ODozNTU1OTASBjEwMjEzNxoKT05FX1NFQVJDSCINMTMxLjE3Mi4zNi4yNCoFMzM0MDAyCTIyMDc3MDAyMToNRG9jdW1lbnRJbWFnZUIBMFIGT25saW5lWgJGVGIDUEZUagoxOTk5LzAxLzAxcgoxOTk5LzAzLzMxegCCATJQLTEwMDcxMDYtMTIwMDEtQ1VTVE9NRVItMTAwMDAwMzkvMTAwMDAxNjAtMTEyOTc4MpIBBk9ubGluZcoBB0VuZE5vdGXSARJTY2hvbGFybHkgSm91cm5hbHOaAgdQcmVQYWlkqgIoT1M6RU1TLVBkZkRvY1ZpZXdCYXNlLWdldE11ZGlhVXJsRm9ySXRlbbICALoCAMoCD0FydGljbGV8RmVhdHVyZQ%3D%3D&_s=gq7TyJLojXFRF1G5O0nWx46080E%3D

Voisin, D. R., Bird, J. D. P., Shiu, C. -S., & Krieger, C. (2013). 'It's crazy being a Black, gay youth.' Getting information about HIV prevention: A pilot study. *Journal of Adolescence, 36*(1), 111–119. Retrieved from http://0-search.proquest.com.alpha2.latrobe.edu.au/docview/1347782681?accountid=12001, http://CM8EK7ZY3D.search.serialssolutions.com/?ctx_ver=Z39.88-2004&ctx_enc=info:ofi/enc:UTF-8&rfr_id=info:sid/ProQ%3Asocabsshell&rft_val_fmt=info:ofi/fmt:kev:mtx:journal&rft.genre=unknown&rft.jtitle=Journal+of+Adolescence&rft.atitle=%26%2339%3BIt%26%2339%3Bs+crazy+being+a+Black%2C+gay+youth.%26%2339%3B+Getting+information+about+HIV+prevention%3A+A+pilot+study&rft.au=Voisin%2C+Dexter+R%3B+Bird%2C+Jason+D.P.%3B+Shiu%2C+Cheng-Shi%3B+Krieger%2C+Cathy&rft.aulast=Voisin&rft.aufirst=Dexter&rft.date=2013-02-01&rft.volume=36&rft.issue=1&rft.spage=111&rft.isbn=&rft.btitle=&rft.title=Journal+of+Adolescence&rft.issn=01401971, http://ac.els-cdn.com/S0140197112001601/1-s2.0-S0140197112001601-main.pdf?_tid=764d0054-96bc-11e3-a9fc-00000aab0f6c&acdnat=1392522373_e392ba6bf4925830929829994fe9a5a1

Wilson, C. M., Wright, P. F., Safrit, J. T., & Rudy, B. (2010). Epidemiology of HIV infection and risk in adolescents and youth. *Journal of Acquired Immune Deficiency Syndromes (1999), 54*(Suppl 1), S5–S6. doi:10.1097/QAI.0b013e3181e243a1.

Wilson, E. C., Iverson, E., Garofalo, R., & Belzer, M. (2012). Parental support and condom use among transgender female youth. *JANAC: Journal of the Association of Nurses in AIDS Care, 23*(4), 306–317. doi:10.1016/j.jana.2011.09.001.

Yadegarfard, M., Meinhold-Bergmann, M. E., & Ho, R. (2014). Family rejection, social isolation, and loneliness as predictors of negative health outcomes (depression, suicidal ideation, and sexual risk behavior) among Thai male-to-female transgender adolescents. *Journal of LGBT Youth, 11*(4), 347–363. doi:10.1080/19361653.2014.910483.

Part III
Children, Young People, Health Care, Interventions and Policies

Chapter 14
Protecting HIV-Positive Children in Jamaica: Exploring Policy, Practice and Institutional Responses

Paul Miller and Stephen Wallder

Contents

P. Miller (✉)
Department of Education, Brunel University, London, UK
e-mail: paul.miller@brunel.ac.uk

S. Wallder
Faculty of Education & Liberal Studies, University of Technology, Jamaica, Kingston, Jamaica
e-mail: stephen.wallder@utech.edu.jm

P. Liamputtong (ed.), *Children and Young People Living with HIV/AIDS*, Cross-Cultural Research in Health, Illness and Well-Being,
DOI 10.1007/978-3-319-29936-5_14

14.1 Introduction

Perhaps not many individuals could conceive that the HIV/AIDS pandemic could well be one of earth's worst weapons of mass destruction, endangering young and old alike. Its spread has had a severe impact on many of the worlds' poorest and most under resourced peoples. Consequently, Jamaica, like other countries across the world, must continue to combat ignorance, denial, stigma and discrimination which are themselves potent agents contributing to the spread of HIV/AIDS.

George Alleyne, a former medicine professor at the University of the West Indies and a former Director of the Pan American Health Organization (PAHO), in a speech to the Jamaican parliament in 2002 suggested the HIV epidemic "requires appropriate policies and a legal framework so that organising against AIDS is supported, and the corrosive impact of discrimination countered, including that against those groups and individuals in society who are most vulnerable to AIDS" (Kelly 2003: 21). Alleyne also advocated for the Caribbean to be free from a cycle of mental slavery which he argued was fuelling homophobia and discrimination against persons perceived as living a lifestyle of which others in society did not or do not approve.

At a Regional Meeting of Ministers of Education in Latin America and the Caribbean in 2002, it was discussed that education is integral to the fight against HIV and AIDS, and that the disease will not be overcome without the full involvement of the education sector. For example, the education ministers present at the meeting acknowledged that more could be done through the education of teachers and students to prevent the spread of HIV. They also affirmed the need to provide support and care to affected and infected educators and learners, and they recognized that creative measures were required to limit the impact of the epidemic on the region's education sector (UNESCO 2002).

Health and education demand serious investment since each has to do with the trajectory of humans. Freedom from disease is closely related to freedom from ignorance and both can lead to other freedoms. All three conditions – disease, ignorance and hunger – promote poverty, and their alleviation and eradication underpins a nation's development agenda. National development, therefore, makes more sense when human beings, in terms of their health and well-being, their education and aspirations, are placed at the heart of the process of development. When this is done, good health, a widely recognized indicator of the quality of life and a positive measure of social capital, takes on new meaning.

But education must not be only for the young. Kelly and Bain cites McCaw-Binns as suggesting that "the control of the major chronic diseases will require renewed health promotion efforts at community level to bring about the lifestyle changes needed to reduce the risks associated with the development of HIV" (Kelly 2003: 23). In other words, education at all ages is necessary to clarify myths and allay fears associated with HIV/AIDS. Linking policy leadership to educational leadership and the potential for change through combining them, Miller asserts that, "...if sound leadership at the policy level is a seed of development, then sound leadership of educational institutions and at the classroom level is arguably a flower of development (Miller 2012: 9).

In the Caribbean, the spread of HIV is second only to that occurring in southern Africa; and within the Caribbean region itself, Jamaica has the second highest rate of HIV-positive persons, behind Hispaniola (UNAIDS 2010a). The social and economic implications are extensive since the disease threatens to deprive the entire region of much of its youth who are, put simply, tomorrow's generation. In the Introduction of Kelly's book, former University of the West Indies Vice Chancellor, Professor Rex Nettleford argued, "the HIV/AIDS pandemic is to this generation of Caribbean people what tuberculosis was to the generation of the 50s–60s" (Kelly 2003: 24).

Although new HIV infections in Jamaica have declined by 25 % in the last decade (UNAIDS 2014), children and young people in Jamaica are at risk of losing their lives due to the spread of the disease among young men, young women of child-bearing age, and children born to mothers with the virus. Consequently, and in addition, Jamaica must do all it can to not replicate the tragedy of some southern African countries where tens of thousands of children are orphaned and are left to raise themselves; up from 0.2 % of all children in 1980 to 3.2 % in 2010 (Avert 2012).

14.2 Conceptual Framework

14.2.1 International Legal Context

Human rights concerns of the HIV/AIDS epidemic cover the full range of civil, political, economic, social and cultural rights. There is only limited discussion about human rights and HIV in the Caribbean (Chill News 2011). Nevertheless, customary international law and international legal treaties, signed by Jamaica, underpin the basis of the international law of human rights. The International Covenant on Economic, Social and Cultural Rights (1966); the International Covenant on Civil and Political Rights (1966); the Convention on the Elimination of all forms of Discrimination against Women and the Convention on the Rights of the Child (1989) are all examples.

The treaties of the International Labour Organization (ILO) on issues such as workplace discrimination are also important, as are general comments of UN treaty committees, resolutions of the Commission on Human Rights, and the International Guidelines on HIV/AIDS and Human Rights. The Office of the High Commissioner on Human Rights (OCHR 2002) outlines the following human rights relevant to HIV and AIDS.

- The right to non-discrimination, equal protection and equality before the law
- The right to life
- The right to the highest attainable standard of physical and mental health
- The right to freedom of expression

- The right to freedom of movement
- The right to seek and enjoy asylum
- The right to privacy
- The right to freedom of opinion and expression and the right to freely receive and impart information
- The right to freedom of association
- The right to work
- The right to marry and found a family
- The right to equal access to education
- The right to an adequate standard of living
- The right to social security, assistance and welfare
- The right to share in scientific advancements and its benefits
- The right to participate in public and cultural life
- The right to be free from torture and cruel, inhuman or degrading treatment or punishment (OCHR 1998; OCHR/UNAIDS 2002)

International law recognizes that some rights, such as those relating to universal education or health care, must necessarily be achieved progressively in developing countries such as Jamaica. However, even among these rights, are 'core obligations' (such as essential primary health care, basic housing and education) which should be met immediately. In all cases, State parties should take deliberate, tangible and targeted steps towards fulfilling these obligations. Where appropriate legislation does not exist, States parties are expected to adopt legislation to ensure services are provided without discrimination of any kind (United Nations CESCR 1990).

14.2.2 Inclusion, Participation and Non-Discrimination

A key principle that has come from decades of responding to HIV/AIDS is that people living with and affected by HIV/AIDS are at the center of a human rights approach. Referred to as the 'GIPA Principle', the Greater Involvement of People Living with HIV/AIDS (GIPA), this principle supports the non-discrimination agenda and underlines the importance of participation by all persons infected or affected by HIV/AIDS as set out in the pyramid of involvement (UNAIDS 1999).

Discrimination leads to fear, denial, apathy, and isolation. By limiting or preventing the participation of people who are infected and affected by HIV/AIDS, discrimination retards public health prevention and care efforts. Respecting and enforcing human rights are essential to securing meaningful inclusion and effective participation. As suggested by the United Nations, "an environment in which human rights are respected ensures that vulnerability to HIV/AIDS is reduced" (United Nations 1998: 5). Additionally, as has been suggested by the Canadian International Development Agency (CIDA), a human rights approach to HIV/AIDS is both objective (safeguarding human dignity) and goals orientated (providing an enabling environment). In other words, both *processes* (such as, participation, transparency, accountability), and *substantive elements* (such as, the protection of the vulnerable – especially women and children, and protection from discrimination) must be seen to be in sync (United Nations 1998).

14.3 HIV and AIDS in the Caribbean

The AIDS epidemic in the Caribbean is believed to have started in 1981 when the first cases of AIDS were recorded in Haiti. However, retrospective analysis of patients affected by Kaposi's sarcoma has shown that the first cases of AIDS were documented in 1979 (UNAIDS 2010a, b). Cases of AIDS had also been documented among Haitians living in the United States at that time (Gilbert et al. 2007). In 1982, cases were reported in Jamaica and Bermuda (Caribbean Epidemiology Centre 2004) and, by 1987, all Caribbean countries had reported at least one case. By 2001 there were an estimated 210, 000 people living with HIV/AIDS (PLHIV) and, in 2013, UNAIDS estimated this number had increased to circa 250,000 (UNAIDS 2013) 16,000 of these children.

The largest number of people living with the virus is on the island of Hispaniola, where the combined number of PLHIV in Haiti and the Dominican Republic is 182,000 (Avert 2014). This accounts for approximately 70 % of all PLHIV in the Caribbean. In the English-speaking Caribbean, Jamaica has the largest number of individuals living with HIV, at an estimated 30,265 (Ministry of Health 2014). However, the data on adult HIV prevalence offers a different perspective (UNAIDS 2010a, b). The Bahamas (3 %) has the highest adult HIV prevalence, followed by Suriname (2.4 %) and Haiti (2.2 %). Although there is some variation in terms of those persons living with HIV in the Caribbean, it is to be understood that nine of the ten larger countries have generalized epidemics, with prevalence of over 1 % among the adult population.[1] However, it should be noted that increased access to antiretroviral treatment (ART) has led to a decrease in the mortality associated with AIDS (UNAIDS 2013).

Since 2001, there has been a 40 % decline in AIDS-related mortality in the Caribbean. Furthermore, the most pronounced decline in new cases of HIV infections since 2001 (49 %) has occurred in the Caribbean (UNAIDS 2013). This level of decline is noticeable among children and young people also and is believed to be the result of scaled-up HIV prevention services, which saw, between 2001 and 2012, a 52 % decline in new HIV infections among children and young people (UNAIDS 2013).

[1]With the exception of Cuba, Bahamas, Barbados, Belize, Dominican Republic, Guyana, Haiti, Jamaica, Suriname, Trinidad and Tobago each have HIV prevalence rates over 1 %.

14.4 HIV/AIDS in Jamaica

Jamaica currently has no law that criminalizes the transmission of HIV. UNAIDS estimates that as at 2012, 30,265 persons or approximately 1.7 % of the Jamaican adult population is HIV-infected and that almost two thirds of HIV-infected persons are unaware of their status. Higher HIV prevalence has been recorded in such vulnerable groups as sex workers (4.2 %), men who have sex with men (MSM) (32.9 %), individuals with other sexually transmitted infections (3.6 %), homeless persons/drug users (8.2 %), and prison inmates (2.5 %). Between 1982 and 2011, 29,069 persons were reported with HIV in Jamaica and the cumulative number of reported AIDS deaths was 8498. Circa 79 % of all reported AIDS cases in Jamaica are in the 20–49 year old age group, and 90 % of reported AIDS cases are individuals between 20 and 60 years old. In 2006, the number of newly reported AIDS cases in young girls aged 15–24 was twice as high compared with boys in the same age group. More HIV-positive men are reported in the age group 20–60 compared with women in that age group, although this gap is continuing to narrow. All 14 parishes in Jamaica are affected by the HIV epidemic though urban parishes have higher numbers of HIV-positive individuals (Ministry of Health 2011).

Despite vigorous national efforts, the HIV/AIDS epidemic continues to spread in Jamaica. Of the estimated 30,265 people in Jamaica living with HIV close to 10 % are children under 18, and 20 % are aged 20–29 years. This suggests many may have been infected during their adolescent years.

Efforts to prevent mother-to-child transmission (PMTCT) in the public services have resulted in significant reductions in the mother-to-child transmission rate, from 25 % in 2002 to fewer than 5 % in 2008 and less than 1 % currently (Ministry of Health 2011). Eighty four percent of HIV-positive pregnant women in Jamaica now receive antiretroviral medication, and more than 90 % of infants born to HIV-positive mothers receive ARV treatment. According to UNICEF (2015), Jamaica has made significant progress in treating more HIV-positive children.

However, increased knowledge about HIV among Jamaican children and young people, due largely to targeted interventions in schools and communities, is yet to bring significant results in terms of reducing risky sexual behavior. According to the Youth Risk and Resiliency Behaviour Survey conducted among 4320 sexually active children (aged 10–14) and young people (aged 15–24), 76 % of males and 21.4 % of females reported being involved in multiple partner relationships. In addition, 23 % of males and 43.5 % of females did not use a condom during their last sexual encounter. Transactional sexual relationships have emerged as a serious cause for concern among young people, with 39 % reporting they have either given or received money or gifts in exchange for sex. Almost 13 % of the young people (aged 15–24) reported they have been forced to have sex, whilst 14 % admitted to forcing someone else to have sex with them.

14.5 Government Intervention in Jamaica

Jamaica's response to the HIV epidemic is outlined in the HIV/AIDS/STI National Strategic Plan (JHANSP) (Ministry of Health 2002). This plan acknowledges the seriousness of the HIV epidemic and its negative consequences for national development. HIV and AIDS are key government priorities and alleviating the effects of stigma and discrimination is among a range of policy issues the government seeks to tackle. The goals of the JHANSP are to build an effective multi-sectoral response to HIV and AIDS; mitigate the socio-economic and health effects of HIV and AIDS; decrease individual vulnerability to HIV infection; reduce the transmission of HIV infection; and improve care, support and treatment services of PLHAs.

The education ministry's response is part of a national multi-sectoral approach aimed at reducing individual vulnerability to HIV infection through the revised Health and Family Life Education [HFLE] curriculum. The HFLE curriculum is part of the Behaviour Change Intervention and Communication (BCIC) initiative that promotes the ministry's HIV and AIDS policy. This was reinforced in the Ministry of Education's work plan as set out in the Jamaica HIV/AIDS/STI National Strategic Plan (JHANSP) that aims to, inter alia:

- produce appropriate teaching and learning materials to generate awareness;
- provide training for teachers in order to develop competence in the delivery of the HIV/AIDS/STI education program including the development of peer educators;
- increase awareness by the Ministry's personnel and stakeholders of the need for greater responsibility for adopting programs and workplace policies relating to HIV/AIDS/STI.

In addition to the generalized JHANSP and the BCIC initiatives, there has also been the "Hold on, Hold Off" program delivered by Regional Health Authorities since 2008; the "Sex Ed, Best Said" program delivered by Jamaica Youth Advocacy Network [JYAN], 2009; a revision, in 2008, of the Health and Family Life Education curriculum that embeds HIV and AIDS issues in the education system (in 2011, some 87 % of schools were delivering HFLE to 418,517 students); the Ministry of Education/Secondary Schools Council 2008 anti-discrimination campaign called "Yes I Can Support Someone Living with HIV"; and the 2009 "Children First" and "Safe Kids", projects aimed specifically at primary school children aged 9–12 which promotes personal safety and well-being. We should note that a number of these initiatives are *donor* funded (and initiated) and at times their objectives seem to overlap one another.

In addition partnership between both the government and non-government sectors have enriched the response with policies and programs derived from supranational bodies, such as those instigated through the ILO (International Labour Organisation 2002). At the local level, the Jamaica Employers Federation in collaboration with both the ILO and the Ministry of Health initiated a Workplace Education Programme. This initiative not only sensitized the core labor force but assisted in driving policy nationally, firstly for a National Workplace Policy for HIV/AIDS, to be followed by its incorporation into the forthcoming Occupational Safety and Health Act. Currently, over 200 companies are in *voluntary compliance* with the policy, of which 58 have been visited by the Ministry of Labour and Social Security. Furthermore, since 2008 the Jamaica Employers Federation has published and distributed a handbook to its members and beyond so as to sensitize employers and employees to information regarding HIV/AIDS and its related impact in the workplace (Jamaica Employers Federation 2008).

14.6 The Study

The findings presented in this chapter were gathered during two phases. The first phase was conducted between June 2011 and August 2011. The second phase, a continuation study, was conducted between October and December 2014. Both phases sought to gather data in reference to the effectiveness of national policy and institutional responses in seeking to protect HIV-positive children in Jamaica. Additionally, the second phase was undertaken to examine the extent to which phase one findings, completed 3 years earlier, were still the case. Participants in the study were selected through a combination of deterministic and snowball sampling and representatives of relevant actors within including education, health, employment federation and industry. The content of this study was thus gathered through face to face interviewing, focus groups and documentary analysis.

The main research questions in phase one were: "To what extent does the HIV-positive and AIDS status of children in Jamaica impact their learning/schooling experience?" "How have these impacts been identified and assessed by education and health care professionals?" The main question in phase two was: "To what extent, are HIV-positive children and young people in Jamaica adequately protected by existing legal, policy and other frameworks?" Phase one included three HIV-positive young persons, one health care worker, one manager of services at a facility for HIV-positive homeless children and young people, two officials from the ministry of education and two officials from the ministry of health. Phase two data collection included a senior official from a worker lobby group, two officials from the ministry of health and an HIV-positive young person. Phase one had two males and eight females whereas phase two had two females and two males.

The findings from this study are presented in three sections below: Jamaica's legislative framework; Jamaica's policy framework; and Jamaica's policy-practice frameworks.

14.7 Jamaica's Legislative Framework

There is no specific legislation addressing a range of HIV and AIDS related issues in Jamaica. However, national legislations relevant to a study on the schooling experiences of HIV-positive children and young people are identified below (for a more detailed list, see Appendix A).

The Education Act 1980
A number of parts of the Act may assist in protecting school children affected by HIV/AIDS, significantly though it enshrines rights for both the administration and the child as regard to when for health reasons a student may be excluded from school, but must not be deprived of the opportunity to complete schooling.

Public Health Act 2003
No distinction is made between HIV/AIDS and any other notifiable disease thereby *normalizing* its status (and thus that of its sufferers) as one of a number of life threatening conditions.

The Childcare and Protection Act 2004
The Act, worded as such, whilst protecting a child's rights, ensures the mandatory nature of formal schooling.

14.8 Jamaica's Policy Framework

Jamaica has in place several policies regarding the management of HIV and AIDS in society. These have benefited from several sector-based policies including:

National Policy on Children (MoH 1997)
This policy supports the rights of children so as to enable them to reach their full potential, mentally, physically and emotionally, whilst also protecting those most vulnerable.

National HIV/AIDS Policy (MoH 2005)
Principally aimed at preventing new HIV infections and strongly aligned to the International Labour Organisation's (ILO) "10 Guiding Principles" (International Labour Organisation 2001).

National Policy for the Management of HIV/AIDS in Schools (MoE 2004, Revised 2010)
This important policy is centered on the UNGASS Declaration of Commitment on HIV and AIDS, the Millennium Development Goals, the Dakar Framework for Action for "Education for All", the ICPD Programme of Action, the Vienna Declaration of Human Rights. It aims to assure the rights of children to access to

and participation in education. Further, for both students and school staff it propagates open access, equity and the inviolability of one's human rights.

14.9 Policy: Practice Environments

14.9.1 Policy Awareness

Those interviewed during the course of the study displayed a well formed knowledge of much of the legislation relating to the country's response to HIV/AIDS, whether it be in regard to education, health (including services), the workplace and thus had a clear understanding of how, in all its facets, it should act to ensure that in all aspects of an individual's human rights, the law should *seamlessly* protect. The multi-sectoral approach was one that all recognized as a strong and important component of the overarching country response to the epidemic, notably this topic drew much comment and criticism in relation to the perceived (some with actual experiences of) effectiveness of the parties to this approach.

Policy particularly relevant to this study included the National Policy for the Management of HIV/AIDS in Schools (2004, revised 2010). The 2004 policy has eight tenets. The revised policy has nine tenets. The newly introduced tenet is about access or referral of students to reproductive health services. The policy speaks to reducing new incidents of HIV/AIDS among school-aged children; management of the disease for those infected with it; confidentiality and the right to access education and work regardless of one's status; responsibility of the education ministry to provide prevention education programs. The policy also addresses non-discrimination and universal precautions to be employed in schools. Expressly, this new tenet should further protect children whilst within the school system in their *day to day* experiences; thus recognizing the need for policy to seriously drive real protection at the practice level?

14.9.2 Stigma and Discrimination

Evidence of stigma and discrimination is reported anecdotally by many within the education sector, particularly in the secondary sector. However, due to fear, very little or no reporting occurs. As reported by Miller et al. (2011), many individuals working in schools will admit *off the record* to being aware of instances of stigma and discrimination against children at school, but feel unwilling or unable to report this due to socio-cultural pressures and for fear of repercussions. Many of those involved in this study cited instances of such child abuse that they were aware of, ranging from name calling, alienation, segregation through to sexual and physical abuse being experienced by children with (or labelled as) HIV-positive. These instances occurring in school, in the family and in the local and wider community and normally recounted with no *happy ending*!

Oftentimes people are uneducated about HIV/AIDS stated one education officer, this statement furthered by one health ministry official who cited a "lack of (correct) information" [in the public domain] which "breeds fear and ignorance" and which is underpinned by a strong anti-homosexual culture manifested in the music, especially among secondary school pupils. The "High level of stigma and poor level of understanding of the issues and a clear disconnect between: medics, teachers, researchers and parents" stated one state agency researcher is surely furthering stigma and discrimination.

Compared to the aforementioned, one education ministry policy official was quick to point out that stigma may often be 'self-inflicted' a position seemingly indexed by a health ministry Human Rights Officer who explained that many individuals in society saw those persons who are HIV-positive as having a form of 'Judgment on themselves'.

Reluctance thus to act *on the ground* utilizing appropriate policy seems apparent and thus the formation of the National HIV Related Discrimination Reporting and Redress System (NHDRRS) is a positive one, so as to drive interventions and address such incidences. However, its effectiveness is dependent upon its reporting, appropriate staffing and physical and financial resources. In 2011, it received a total of 19 cases of discrimination, noticeably the number of complaints has reduced from 2008 to date by 62 % (Ministry of Health 2011). One commentator expressing the view that "this is not due to reduced incidences of stigma and discrimination, it's because redress has *no teeth*." Thus, whilst reporting is limited, it remains a serious problem.

14.9.3 Promoting Inclusion

One education ministry official reported successfully delivering workshops to principals and to close to 1000 staff (all categories) working in schools. In collaboration with the Ministry of Health and assistance from persons infected with the HIV/AIDS virus and civil society organizations, a number of sensitization campaigns have also been staged in the nation's schools. In her view, "When HIV-positive individuals can contribute to intervention plans, this provides a definite benefit to both students and staff". In our view, this also underlines the fundamental principle of GIPA which asserts the involvement of persons with HIV/AIDS.

Inclusion efforts at both the strategic and operational levels are also actively driven by the Ministry of Education. The education ministry official pointed to national policy, "Every child can learn; every child must learn", arguing that the ministry has a role to play in supporting children at school no matter their health, socio-economic or other conditions. The regulatory role played by the ministry is underlined by Section 31 of the Education Act which stipulates that if a child's illness does not [directly] affect the wider school population they should not be denied entry.

At the operational level, the Ministry of Education provides a range of sensitization and public awareness engagements for teachers, the school community and parents, aimed at countering popular myths associated with HIV and AIDS. The introduction of Health and Family Lifestyle Education (HFLE) curriculum in all schools is also a part of this process of sensitization. Furthermore, the Ministry of Health provides social workers who work in Regional Health Authorities and schools to provide psychosocial support for children affected by HIV and AIDS.

The education ministry also operates a Safety and Security Programme which is now being implemented across the country. In addition to the already 164 participating schools, in September, 2014 implementation began in a further 595 primary schools (Jamaica Information Service 2014) backed by a Ministry of Education led – Behaviour Modification Programme. In addition to these, safety and security policy guidelines are in place in schools, underpinning Critical Incident Management Plans that have established procedures for handling a wide range of issues such as contact sports and bullying.

14.10 Evaluation of Policy, Practice and Institutional Responses

Having a range of policy and programs in place to support the treatment and care of HIV-positive children and young people is important. This shows good leadership and a degree of forward thinking by leaders at different levels. However, regardless of the range of policies and/or programs in place, effective change will only come about when leaders at all levels apply and enforce the policies – whether already in place or newly created.

At the moment, the monitoring of national policy implementation is by regional education officers, one of whom pointed to gaps in the current arrangements: "[T]o have better monitoring of the policies and interventions, it is important that the parents, students and entire school population be involved." Once more this requires leadership; and leadership of a kind that follows through. Monitoring of what goes on in schools is undertaken by the Health Promotion Officers appointed by the education ministry to monitor such intervention as the delivery of and response to the HFLE curriculum. Health Promotion Officers also engage in "follow up" activities with school principals and students affected or infected with HIV. In addition to these processes, principals provide regular updates to the education ministry's Guidance and Counselling Unit.

There are obvious challenges in terms of the appropriateness of the level and type of response provided to HIV-positive students. Pointing to a mismatch, one participant suggested, (an educational ministry official) HIV-positive persons need to do more to help themselves. Although it is not immediately clear what is meant by this, one could argue that effective self-leadership is a crucial component in enabling an infected child or young person to exercise restraint when jeered or mocked, or simply to turn their 'misfortune' into a lesson for others. But these can only occur in an environment where tolerance is promoted and where discrimination is frowned upon, such that notions of HIV being 'self-inflicted' and/or that HIV-positive individuals have called down a form of 'Judgment on themselves' are isolated from everyday thinking.

There is ample evidence that the government and related agencies have done and are doing much to safeguard HIV-positive children in Jamaica through a range of policy and practice based initiatives. It is also apparent that those who support HIV-positive children, on a day to day basis, have done much to protect and safeguard them. In both cases, these sets of actions are found to be consistent with the Jamaica's Child Care and Protection Act and a number of international legal instruments including the Convention and the Rights of the Child and guidelines from the Office of the High Commissioner on Human Rights. Nevertheless, the current system of monitoring appears to be fragmented and disjointed. In 2011, Miller quoted one participant in his original study as saying the monitoring of associated HIV policies will be overseen by the National Education Inspectorate. There is no evidence of this being done. Furthermore, there is no indication that there is a coherent approach to monitoring the implementation of policies and procedures nor is there a consistent plan that can be deployed across the island in all schools, context aside. Once more this calls for leadership that connects the dots; that reduces waste and does not duplicate efforts; and that publicize and use success stories as capacity building artefacts. For example, as a developing country, Jamaica is reliant upon donor funds from international entities that are often tied to specific donor targets. In pursuit of such financial assistance, there may be, at times, several concurrent initiatives, contributing to what appears a fragmented approach in the implementation and monitoring of cross-sectoral campaigns and initiatives.

14.11 Conclusion

Our conclusion is, despite the impressive list of local and international legislations and policies, and despite some evidence of good practice, there remains, in some cases, a clear mismatch between what the law and/or policies demand versus what is actually done. To achieve greater coherence between intent and outcomes, we also propose the implementation of fewer, deeper and more meaningful initiatives rather than the current practice of having several initiatives running at any one time – without unequivocal evidence of their effectiveness. For this to be achieved, however, there needs to be an interlocking of leadership energy and activities at national, regional and local levels, demanding that all efforts contribute to national development through robust accountability mechanisms in the implementation and monitoring of activities and initiatives aimed at safeguarding and protecting HIV-positive young persons.

Appendix A

Legislative and Policy Environments

The table below indicates specific legal and policy references as appropriate within each legislative Act or Policy as per section 14.7/14.8

Legislation/policy	Details of supporting applicable sections
The Education Act 1980:	Exclusions for health reasons:
	31.1 A student shall be excluded from attending a public educational institution during any period in which he is known to be suffering from a communicable disease or infestation
	31.3 Arrangements may be made to enable students who have been suspended, or excluded from school for pregnancy or other health reasons, to sit important examinations in connection with the completion of their education
Public Health Act 2003:	2.1 In this Act, unless the context otherwise requires – "communicable (or notifiable) disease" means any disease due to a specific infectious agent or its toxic products, which arises through transmission of that agent or its products from an infected person to another, or from animal to a susceptible person either directly or indirectly…
	Both HIV and AIDs are considered Class 1 Notifiable Diseases
The Childcare and Protection Act 2004:	2.2 Where there is a reference in this Act to the best interests of a child, the factors to be taken into account in determining the child's best interests shall include the:
	(a) Safety of the child;
	(b) Child's physical and emotional needs and level of development
National Policy on Children (Ministry of Health 1997)	(a) To ensure the right of every child to life and the attainment of the highest standard of health for children
	(b) To guarantee protection from all forms of maltreatment and special care for the disabled children and children without families
	(c) To ensure protection from interference with privacy
	(d) To recognize children as whole human beings having an inalienable right to participate in society's affairs within their intellectual and emotional capacities
	(e) To ensure special care, education and training for all children with disabilities to enable them to reach their fullest potential
	(f) To facilitate the involvement of children in all aspects of Civil Society in keeping with the child's evolving capacity
National HIV/AIDS Policy (Ministry of Health 2005)	2.1 The principle focus of the national response is the prevention of new HIV infections; the treatment, care, and support of those infected or affected by HIV/AIDS; mitigation of the impact of the epidemic; strengthening of the enabling environment including legislative changes and the reduction of HIV/AIDS related stigma and discrimination

(continued)

Legislation/policy	Details of supporting applicable sections
National Policy for the Management of HIV/AIDS in Schools (Ministry of Education 2004, (revised 2010)	(a) Access to Education: Every child has the right to education. No student shall be denied access to education on the basis of his or her actual or perceived HIV status
	(b) Access to Information: All Ministry of Education staff and students have the right to relevant and factual HIV and AIDS information and behavior change communication that is appropriate to their age, developmental level, gender, culture, language and context
	(c) Participation: The meaningful involvement of people living with and affected by HIV and AIDS and most vulnerable groups, including youth, in the design, implementation, monitoring and evaluation of the response to achieve stated outcomes
	(d) Equity: All responses to HIV and AIDS should ensure that no student or staff will be denied access to prevention, knowledge, skills and services or treatment, care and support services on the basis of their real or perceived HIV status, gender, age, disability, religious or other beliefs, socio-economic status, geographical location, level of literacy, capacity to understand the nature of HIV/AIDS and how it is prevented and treated or vulnerability to exposure. This includes orphans, wards of the state, street and working children, out of school youth and children living with disabilities
	(e) Promotion and protection of human rights: an important aspect of the response to the epidemic requires that the rights to equality before the law and freedom from discrimination are respected, protected and fulfilled. Discriminatory practices create and sustain conditions leading to vulnerability to HIV infection and to inadequate treatment, care and support as well as access to preventive services. Promotion and protection of human rights ensures that there is no discrimination based on race, class, gender, sex, sexual orientation, religious or cultural beliefs
	(f) Political Leadership and Commitment: Strong political leadership and commitment at all levels of Education is essential for a sustained and effective response to HIV and AIDS

References

Avert, C. (2012). *HIV/AIDS statistics.* Available at: http://www.avert.org/Caribbean-hiv-aids-statistics.htm

Caribbean Epidemiology Centre. (2004). *Status and trends. analysis of the Caribbean HIV/AIDS Epidemic* 1982–2002. Available at http://caribbean.scielo.org/scielo.php?script=sci_arttext&pid=S0043-31442009000200006

Chill News. (2011, January) *Education: The best weapon to combat HIV/AIDS stigma.* Issue 12, University of the West Indies (UWI) Cave Hill. Available at: ssuu.com/uwicavehill/docs/chill_12_17sm

Gilbert, M. T. P., Rambaut, A., Wlasiuk, G., Spira, T. J., Pitchenik, A. E., & Worobey, M. (2007). The emergence of HIV/AIDS in the Americas and beyond. *Proceedings of the National*

Academy of Sciences of the United States of America – PNAS, 104(47), 18566–18570. doi:10.1073/pnas.0705329104.
International Labour Organisation. (2001). *ILO principles on HIV/AIDS and the world of work.* 92-2-112562-9[ISBN] ILO 2001.
International Labour Organisation. (2002, May 17). Code of practice on HIV/AIDS and the world of work and the platform for action on HIV/AIDS and the world of work, signed in Barbados, 17th May, 2002.
Jamaica Employers Federation. (2008). *HIV/AIDS; what every employer should know!* Jamaica: Jamaica Employers Federation.
Jamaica Information Service. (2014, February 5). Safe schools policy will be implemented in 595 schools. Available at http://www.jis.gov.jm
Kelly, J. in cooperation with Bain, B. (2003). UNESCO/IEEP. *Education and HIV/AIDS in the Caribbean*. International Institute for Educational Planning/UNESCO 7–9 rue Eugène-Delacroix, 75116 Paris.
Miller, P., Kelly, K., & Spawls, N. (2011). Human rights as safeguarding: The schooling experiences of HIV+ children in Jamaica. *Education, Knowledge and Economy, 5*(3), 135–135.
Miller. P. (2012, December). The changing nature of educational leadership: 'Educational Leadership in the Caribbean & Beyond' (Editorial). *Journal of the University College of the Cayman Islands, Special Issue, 6*, 9–12.
Ministry of Education Youth & Culture (2004) National Policy for HIV/AIDS Management in Schools, Kingston, Jamaica. Available at: http://www.ilo.org/wcmsp5/groups/public/---ed_protect/---protrav/---ilo_aids/documents/legaldocument/wcms_132638.pdf
Ministry of Health. (2002). *HIV/AIDS/STI national strategic plan 2002–2006*. Jamaica: MoH Available at http://www.nhpjamaica.org/informationCentre/publications/reports
Ministry of Health. (2011). *National HIV/STI programme: Annual report*. Jamaica: MoH. Available at http://www.nhpjamaica.org/informationCentre/publications/reports
Ministry of Health/UNAIDS. (2014, September). *Spending Assessment* – Jamaica, Sept 2014. Available at http://www.unaids.org/sites/default/files/en/dataanalysis/knowyourresponse/countryprogressreports/2014countries/JAM_narrative_report_2014.pdf
OCHR. (1998). *HIV/AIDS and human rights: International guidelines*. Geneva: UNAIDS and Office of the High Commissioner for Human Rights. HR/PUB/98/1.
OCHR/UNAIDS. (2002). *HIV/AIDS and human rights: International guidelines – Revised guideline 6*. Geneva: UNAIDS and Office of the High Commissioner for Human Rights.
UN Committee on Economic, Social and Cultural Rights (CESCR). (1990, December 14). *General comment no. 3: The nature of states parties' obligations (Art. 2, Para. 1, of the Covenant)*, 14 Dec 1990, E/1991/23. Available at: http://www.refworld.org/docid/4538838e10.html
UNAIDS. (1999). *From principle to practice: Greater involvement of people living with or affected by HIV/AIDS (GIPA)*. Geneva: UNAIDS. www.unaids.org.
UNAIDS. (2010). *Global report: UNAIDS report on the global AIDS epidemic*. Geneva: UNAIDS. Available at http://www.unaids.org/sites/default/files/media_asset/20101123_globalreport_en_1.pdf
UNAIDS. (2010). *The status of HIV in the Caribbean*. Geneva: UNAIDS. Available at http://hiv.health.gov.tt/site_media/media/filer_public/2013/01/21/2010_status_of_hiv_in_the_caribbean_-_unaids.pdf
UNAIDS. (2013). *Global report: UNAIDS report on the global AIDS epidemic*. Geneva: UNAIDS. Available at http://www.unaids.org/sites/default/files/media_asset/UNAIDS_Global_Report_2013_en_1.pdf
UNESCO. (2002, November). *First inter governmental meeting of the regional education project for Latin America and the Caribbean*. Havana, Cuba, 14th–16th November 2002.
UNICEF. (2015). *Jamaica: Children and HIV/AIDS*. Available at http://www.unicef.org/jamaica/hiv_aids.html
United Nations. (1998). *HIV/AIDS and human rights: International guidelines*. New York: United Nations.

Chapter 15
HIV Prevention for Adolescent Women in Africa: Structural Driver Interventions

Catherine MacPhail and Audrey Pettifor

Contents

15.1 Introduction

Advances in HIV treatment have been phenomenal over the past two decades but prevention remains a significant challenge, particularly in less developed countries where HIV is most prevalent. Young women in sub-Saharan Africa (SSA) remain one of the most significantly HIV affected groups globally. Recent estimates from UNICEF suggest that 41 % of all infections globally are among young people aged 15–24 years. Young people in southern and eastern Africa comprise slightly more than half of these infections (Gibbs et al. 2012). In such generalized epidemic

C. MacPhail (✉)
School of Health, University of New England, Armidale, NSW, Australia, 2351
e-mail: cmacphai@une.edu.au

A. Pettifor
Gillings School of Public Health, University of North Carolina – Chapel Hill, Chapel Hill, NC, USA
e-mail: apettif@email.unc.edu

P. Liamputtong (ed.), *Children and Young People Living with HIV/AIDS*, Cross-Cultural Research in Health, Illness and Well-Being,
DOI 10.1007/978-3-319-29936-5_15

settings, it is young women who particularly bear the brunt of HIV infections. In SSA, young women have HIV infection rates that are two to eight times as high as those of young men the same age (Laga et al. 2001), and account for 31 % of all new infections and 72 % of prevalent infections (UNICEF 2011). In Africa, HIV remains a specifically female disease: women are most at risk of infection and the impact of HIV rests most heavily on women through their provision of much of the palliative care and household duties required in families affected by HIV. Maternal death as a result of HIV is common: in South Africa and Botswana, 41.4 % and 23.5 % of maternal deaths respectively are attributable to HIV (World Health Organization 2013). For countries in SSA, managing HIV infection generally requires a specific focus on young women (see Table 15.1).

Along with increasing recognition of biological mechanisms heightening young women's vulnerability (Quinn and Overbaugh 2005), social and cultural issues impact most strongly on women's vulnerability to HIV (see Chap. 7 in this volume). Particularly in sub-Saharan African adolescent populations, it makes sense to look beyond individual-level behavior. Evidence has shown that measures of sexual risk behaviors among young people living in countries with high HIV prevalence are no higher, and are frequently lower, than those of young people in living countries with limited HIV epidemics among heterosexual youth (Pettifor et al. 2011). It is the social relations and economic realities of African women's lives and their unequal access to assets, social power and vulnerability to violence that contribute to women's substantial representation in HIV prevalence statistics. Inequalities in social relations mean that, for young women, adopting individual-level behavioral change to protect themselves from HIV is challenging and might place them at risk of violence and poverty. Women's unequal access to power makes requesting a partner to use condoms or test for HIV, or disclosing one's own HIV status a potentially dangerous undertaking (MacPhail and Campbell 2001; Medley et al. 2004; Hoffman et al. 2006). Compounding this risk are the additional barriers of inadequate access to youth-friendly sexual and reproductive health and HIV services.

In this chapter, we will examine the importance of structural factors in understanding HIV vulnerability with specific focus on young women in SSA. After considering the evidence for the impact of structural factors on women's HIV vulnerability, we will examine structural interventions and, specifically, focus on interventions currently proven to work with young women in sub-Saharan African settings or currently being evaluated. Finally, we will examine some of the concerns with structural approaches to HIV prevention and challenges with moving recognition of such factors from scientific evidence to policy change and implementation for this population.

15.2 Changing Face of Interventions for HIV Prevention: Individual to Structural

Over 30 years into the HIV epidemic and with massive resources having been directed to HIV prevention, there is limited evidence that individual-level behavior change interventions are impacting on new HIV infections. Indeed, HIV prevention

Table 15.1 Prevalence of HIV in 15–24 year olds in sub-Saharan African countries, 2012 (Adapted from UNAIDS 2013, p. A34–39)

Country	Female estimate	Male estimate
Sub-Saharan Africa total	*2.5 (2.3–3.0)*[a]	*1.2 (0.9–1.6)*
Angola	1.2 (0.9–1.5)	0.6 (0.4–0.9)
Benin	0.4 (0.3–0.5)	0.2 (0.2–0.3)
Botswana	6.7 (5.8–8.4)	3.7 (2.3–5.5)
Burkina Faso	0.5 (0.4–0.6)	0.4 (0.3–0.5)
Burundi	0.6 (0.4–0.8)	0.4 (0.3–0.6)
Cameroon	1.8 (1.6–2.3)	1.0 (0.6–1.4)
Cape Verde	<0.1 (<0.1–0.2)	<0.1 (<0.1–0.1)
Central African Republic	–	–
Chad	1.1 (0.8–1.5)	0.6 (0.4–0.9)
Comoros	–	–
Congo	1.3 (1.1–1.6)	0.8 (0.6–1.1)
Côte d'Ivoire	1.2 (1.0–1.6)	0.7 (0.5–1.0)
Democratic Republic of the Congo	0.8 (0.7–1.0)	0.4 (0.3–0.6)
Equatorial Guinea	3.1 (1.6–5.5)	1.6 (0.7–3.1)
Eritrea	0.2 (0.1–0.3)	0.2 (0.1–0.3)
Ethiopia	0.5 (0.3–0.6)	0.3 (0.2–0.3)
Gabon	1.6 (1.1–2.6)	0.4 (0.2–0.4)
Gambia	0.5 (0.3–0.8)	0.2 (0.1–0.5)
Ghana	0.5 (0.4–0.6)	0.3 (0.2–0.4)
Guinea	0.8 (0.6–1.1)	0.4 (0.2–0.6)
Guinea-Bissau	1.7 (1.1–2.6)	0.9 (0.5–1.5)
Kenya	3.6 (3.0–4.6)	1.8 (1.5–2.3)
Lesotho	10.7 (9.4–13.0)	5.8 (3.8–8.4)
Liberia	0.1 (<0.1–0.2)	0.1 (<0.1–0.1)
Madagascar	0.3 (0.2–0.4)	0.3 (0.2–0.4)
Malawi	4.5 (4.0–5.4)	2,7 (2.0–3.7)
Mali	0.3 (0.2–0.5)	0.2 (<0.1–0.3)
Mauritania	0.2 (0.1–0.4)	0.1 (<0.1–0.2)
Mauritius	0.3 (0.2–0.3)	0.3 (0.2–0.5)
Mozambique	6.6 (5.7–8.1)	2.8 (2.1–3.8)
Namibia	4.1 (3.2–5.5)	2.2 (1.4–3.4)
Niger	0.1 (<0.1–0.2)	<0.1 (<0.1–0.1)
Nigeria	1.3 (1.1–1.6)	0.7 (0.4–1.0)
Rwanda	1.3 (1.2–1.6)	1.0 (0.8–1.2)
Sao Tome and Principe	0.4 (0.3–0.7)	0.3 (0.1–0.6)
Senegal	0.3 (0.2–0.4)	0.1 (<0.1–0.2)
Sierra Leone	1.0 (0.6–1.7)	0.3 (0.1–0.5)
South Africa	13.9 (12.9–16.8)	3.9 (2.5–5.7)
South Sudan	1.2 (0.7–2.0)	0.6 (0.3–1.2)
Swaziland	20.0 (17.2–24.5)	10.3 (6.7–14.7)

(continued)

Table 15.1 (continued)

Country	Female estimate	Male estimate
Togo	0.9 (0.7–1.3)	0.5 (0.3–0.8)
Uganda	4.0 (3.4–4.9)	2.3 (1.6–3.2)
United Republic of Tanzania	3.6 (3.1–4.6)	1.8 (1.3–2.6)
Zambia	4.6 (4.1–5.6)	3.5 (2.5–4.9)
Zimbabwe	6.3 (5.6–7.5)	3.9 (2.9–5.2)

[a]Brackets indicate lower and upper estimates

interventions based on behavior change have rarely had large-scale impact through being taken to scale, despite best efforts to make use of known theories of behavior change. This has been true for programs directed at young people and most other at-risk populations globally. Historically, the focus of HIV prevention has been on the individual, specifically concentrated on increasing knowledge about HIV transmission, increasing preventative behaviors and reducing stigma towards those already infected. While both knowledge and attitudes have shown to be successfully changed across a range of interventions in SSA (Ross 2010), almost no interventions have shown significant changes in behavior, and even fewer have demonstrated change in biological outcomes, such as the incidence of HIV or other sexually transmitted diseases (Cowan and Pettifor 2009). As an example, Wight et al. (2012) examined why the school-based intervention *MEMA kwa Vijana*, effectively implemented in Tanzania from 1998 to 2002, showed improved sexual health knowledge, more desirable attitudes, fewer reported sexual partners and improved condom use, yet there were no changes in HIV, HSV-2 or pregnancy. They note that a range of structural barriers to effective change operate in Tanzanian society: economic, social status, cultural and gender. For women and girls, individual-level behavior change messages just do not reflect the realities of their lives or effect change to broader social issues, such as gender inequalities, that limit young women's ability to act on prevention messaging (Kim and Watts 2005). Increasingly, it is being recognized that effective HIV prevention interventions require a multi-level focus: some attention to individual-level factors, but also addressing structural or contextual factors in a way that places HIV centrally in development.

Criticism of individual-level behavior change interventions has focused on these interventions' lack of focus on structural factors or contexts which both shape and constrain individual agency (Tawil et al. 1995; Phillips and Pirkle 2011). Individual actions or practices are shaped by a range of factors impacting social life such as norms, values, networks, structures and institutions. In many situations, these elements, which constitute the fabric of social life, create and maintain inequalities between groups in regards to a range of elements, including health (Auerbach et al. 2011). It has been suggested that this focus on structural drivers of HIV risk is not new. Waldo and Coates (2000) note the social determinants of HIV risk in their ecological model, which dates from the late 1990s. UNAIDS defines social drivers of HIV as "the social and structural factors, such as poverty, gender inequality, and humans rights violations, that are not easily measured, that increase people's vulnerability to HIV infection" (UNAIDS 2007).

While these factors are generally discussed with regard to risk of HIV acquisition, they might also limit people's ability to engage in care and to prevent onward transmission of disease once HIV infected.

There is currently no standard definition of the structural drivers of HIV (Auerbach et al. 2011), with terminology and emphasis differing according to disciplinary focus (Parker et al. 2000). What is agreed is that HIV vulnerability is linked to social, political, environment and economic factors (Gupta et al. 2008), and can be predominately viewed as stemming from gender inequalities and poverty. Definitions of structural drivers have variously also included violence, education, transactional sex and legal discrimination. But in this chapter, we focus specifically on gender inequalities and poverty.

In 2008, The Lancet published a series devoted to promoting understanding of HIV prevention in which structural approaches to HIV were specifically highlighted. This literature noted that while structural drivers of HIV impact on men and women, their sway over women is more substantial. They also drew attention to the fact that structural factors associated with HIV risk are both deeply entrenched and challenging to alter; being broad in scope and escaping easy definition. Structural factors have largely been ignored by both health and HIV-specific policies, both because they are 'upstream', and therefore, difficult to implement, and because many changes at a structural level are viewed as falling outside of a health scope of work (Gupta et al. 2008). Structural drivers do not have a simple, linear causative relationship with HIV risk; they differ by context and change over time. Indeed, there is increasing recognition that there might be a range of contributing casual factors that may modify or amplify one another. Further, they do not operate independently of one another, and interact with behavioral and psychological actions (at an individual-level).

There have been differing attempts to classify structural drivers of HIV risk (see Fig. 15.1). Sweat and Denison (1995) proposed a classification system that described influence at a number of levels ranging from the individual up to the superstructure (national cultural identity), while Barnett and Whiteside (2002) assessed structural factors based on their distance from risk. Proximal factors would, therefore, have short, relatively simple causal pathways, while distal factors would be more complicated and less likely to have straight-forward causal relationships. Thus, the complexity of structural factors makes understanding the mechanisms through which structural drivers lead to HIV infection challenging, and also suggests that intervening on any one factor will not be sufficient to have a meaningful impact on the epidemic.

During the mid- to late-2000s, a number of policy developments reemphasized the importance of HIV prevention, despite advances in treatment. These policies focused specifically on the need to address structural drivers, emphasizing the importance of HIV prevention as a human rights issue, and the need to pay attention to gender equality. A movement to ensure universal access to HIV prevention, treatment, care and support saw numerous countries pledge more focused, ethically sound and contextually relevant HIV prevention efforts. Significantly, the signatories to this agreement "committed to overcoming structural barriers to effective HIV

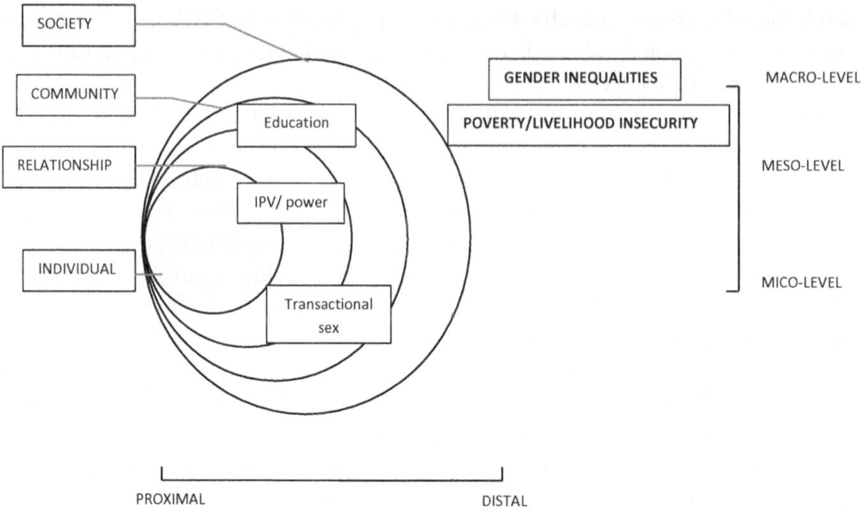

Fig. 15.1 Structural drivers of young women's HIV vulnerability in sub-Saharan Africa

prevention – including harmful social, political, legal and economic conditions that individuals alone cannot change" (Hankins and de Zalduondo 2010: S72). Strong political commitment and leadership was recognized as being crucial to success in HIV prevention (Coates et al. 2008; see also Chaps. 14 and 16 in this volume).

Focusing on structural drivers of HIV demands that we develop and examine new ways of evaluating interventions that aim to act on these factors. Documentation of context is key to understanding how and why success varies. Process is vital and the mechanisms by which change is promoted or not must be documented. Measurement of process requires that assessment is conducted along the hypothesized causal pathway. There are, however, challenges to evaluating structural interventions: they do not always conform to standard biomedical measures in which evidence is assessed according to a strict study design hierarchy (Bonnell et al. 2006). Auerbach et al. (2011) note that it is precisely the 'noise' of context, usually excluded in biomedical study designs that should be inherent in evaluation of structural interventions.

Intervention on structural factors, particularly those that are distal to HIV outcomes, and therefore, more complicated, may change other structural risks or create new ones. There have been concerns about unintended negative consequences of structural interventions. For example, that microfinance programs for women might increase intimate partner violence (IPV) if not implemented in conjunction with parallel changes to gender norms. Findings from programs such as Stepping Stones[1]

[1] Stepping Stones is a training package in gender, HIV, communication and relationship skills. The intervention uses participatory learning methods for community-based group activities. The program was originally developed in Uganda during the mid-1990s but has now been adapted and used in a range of countries. See http://www.Steppingstonesfeedback.org.

where young women reported increased transactional sex after participation, show that such fears of unintended changes are plausible. The potential for unintended negative consequences has been particularly highlighted for urban youth. Given the vulnerability of young urban populations, particular attention will need to be paid to this issue as structural interventions for these populations are developed.

15.3 What Is the Evidence? Associations Between Structural Drivers and Young Women's HIV Risk

There is mounting evidence of the role of structural drivers in HIV risk; evidence that particularly locates young women as central to the HIV epidemic and at particular risk. Two major conceptualizations of structural driver risk have been postulated. The first, driven by public health theory and a concern with causal determinants of ill health and the second more focused within the social sciences (Parkhurst 2013). An overview of associations between structural factors and HIV vulnerability suggest that three major categories of risk have been identified: relating to economic under-development and poverty; mobility and; gender inequalities (Parker et al. 2000).

Certainly, among young women in SSA, gender inequalities and poverty/livelihood insecurity lie at the heart of their increased HIV vulnerability. Although sometimes viewed as structural drivers themselves, mechanisms of young women's vulnerability such as intimate partner violence (IPV), transactional sex and poor education are pathways through which these structural drivers impact on individual vulnerability. Among young women, attempts to disengage structural drivers from one another are challenging, given that the pathways through which young women's vulnerability is increased are often related to both the key structural drivers identified here (Masanjala 2007). Indeed, it has been noted that "poverty and gender inequalities operate cyclically: the myriad manifestations of poverty – insufficient income, restrictions in educational attainment and access to labor markets, and minimized decision-making autonomy – are fueled by inequities in gender-based norms and values and thus reinforce women's lower social and economic status" (Krishnan et al. 2008: 101).

15.3.1 Gender Inequalities

Persistent inequalities in allocation of power, status and privilege are outcomes of gender norms in society in which appropriate roles and behaviors are allocated according to gender. Gender inequalities are damaging for men and women, but women are particularly vulnerable when norms dictate submissiveness and sexual ignorance, and where multiple sexual partners, unprotected sex and male power over women are viewed as legitimate expressions of masculinity (MacPhail and

Campbell 2001; MacPhail 2003; Naidoo et al. 2014; see also Chap. 7 in this volume). Over the past decade increasing attention has been paid to the role that gender inequalities play in HIV risk for women, specifically in southern and eastern Africa, as well as parts of Asia (Gupta et al. 2011). Gender inequalities are specifically evident in the association between gender power and sexual risk behaviors and the role of IPV in HIV risk.

The relationship between power and HIV vulnerability has been extensively explored among minority women in the United States, but less information is available about young women in SSA. A study of young women in the Eastern Cape of South Africa found a relationship between low relationship power and HIV incidence (Jewkes et al. 2010), and a nationally-representative survey of 15–24 year old South Africans found that low relationship control was associated with inconsistent condom use and forced sex with most recent sexual partner (although not HIV prevalence) (Pettifor et al. 2004). Evidence from adult women in Botswana has demonstrated similar relationships between control and condom use (Greig and Koopman 2003) and more empowered Ghanaian women were more likely to use contraception (Crissman et al. 2012).

A more substantial body of literature (particularly from South Africa) provides increasing evidence of the link between IPV and risk for HIV infection (Dunkle et al. 2004, 2006; Jewkes et al. 2006, 2010). Maman et al. (2000) have noted three key ways in which violence might increase women's risk of HIV infection. First, women may be at increased risk through coercive sex from already infected men. Second, women may fear violence as a consequence of suggesting HIV prevention behaviors such as using a condom or getting tested for HIV. Finally, a past experience of sexual or physical violence might be associated with increased HIV risk behaviors such as early age at first sex, multiple partners and unprotected sex at a later stage in a woman's life. Further research has shown that even subtle forms of IPV are associated with increased HIV risk. A study conducted among women attending antenatal services in South Africa, showed that women in relationships with men characterized as controlling were at increased risk of HIV through an increased likelihood that their male partner would himself be HIV-positive and subject his partner to sexual risk behaviors (Dunkle et al. 2004).

15.3.2 Poverty and Limited Livelihood Opportunities

There is increasing evidence of an intersection between poverty and gender in the African context, suggesting that women are likely to be economically subordinate to men and that gendered responses to poverty and inequality drive women to risky sexual practices (Masanjala 2007). Secondary school completion rates are low for young women in SSA (<40 %) and young people make up 40 % of the unemployed globally, with young women being significantly less likely to be employed than young men. In South Africa, almost 50 % of young people are unemployed; with Black women in rural areas disproportionately affected (Lam et al. 2010). These unemployment figures are among the highest in the world. Among young women, livelihood insecurity has been found to be associated with early age of first sex, coerced sex, transactional sex and reduced ability to negotiate and practice safe sex behaviors (Hardee et al. 2014).

Analysis of Demographic Health Surveillance data shows that South African women's HIV risk is increased through poverty, likely through an increased financial dependence on their partners (Tladi 2006). However, this has been contradicted by other researchers. More recent research has indicated that wealth inequalities rather than poverty are the main drivers of HIV vulnerability (Fox 2012). A study in three communities in the Western Cape of South Africa found that there was an association between poverty-related stressors and HIV risk (Kalichman et al. 2006) and poverty in urban Cameroon has been linked to a range of sexual risk behaviors for young men and women (Rwenge 2003). Mounting evidence from South Africa shows the converse; that there are reduced sexual risk behaviors in young women whose families have access to social support such as the Child Support Grant (CSG). While provision of the CSG (approximately USD25) is intended for poverty alleviation among the poorest members of South African society rather than sexual health promotion, evidence from a study in two rural and two urban areas has found that young women in families receiving the CSG had a lower incidence of both transactional sex and age-disparate sex (partners more than 5 years older). Receipt of the CSG did not, however, appear to impact on having unprotected sex, multiple partners or sex associated with alcohol and drug use (Cluver et al. 2013). While our understanding of the relationships between poverty, wealth and HIV vulnerability may still be murky, identifying context-specific risk is needed to understand how poverty or wealth may drive HIV infection so that prevention initiatives can be tailored to local context (Parkhurst 2010).

15.3.3 Education and School Attendance as a Key Pathway for Young Women

A range of evidence from SSA shows that for countries with generalized HIV epidemics, vulnerability to HIV is reduced by school attendance and educational attainment (Jukes et al. 2008). For example, a study of young people in KwaZulu-Natal province of South Africa found that increased education among young women significantly reduced their risk of having had sex in the past 12 months (Kaufman et al. 2004). It appears that this relationship exists for both educational attainment and school attendance, although we still do not completely understand the mechanisms by which protection is conferred. There is some evidence that it is the smaller sexual networks of students that offers protection from HIV infection (Hargreaves et al. 2008), but also speculation that school attendance delays marriage and childbearing for young women, increases socioeconomic status and has socio-cognitive impacts that lead to greater self-efficacy towards HIV prevention.

Data from Masaka District in Uganda have shown that over time reduction in HIV risk has been most pronounced among the most educated individuals: the greatest reduction being among young women with secondary school education (de Walque et al. 2005). Similar findings have been noted from Zambia, although this association was not significant for young rural women (Michelo et al. 2006). Pettifor et al. (2008) documented a fourfold increase in HIV risk for young women reporting only one sexual partner who had not completed high school. This finding is mirrored by research from other countries in the sub-Saharan region. However, we still know very little about the mechanisms through which education serves to reduce young women's vulnerability to HIV. Might this be through increasing self-efficacy to practice individual-level safer sex behaviors? Possibly through providing young women with increased employment opportunities associated with better education and therefore reduced economic reliance on sexual partners? Or might remaining within the confines of a school environment limit the social and sexual networks that young women are exposed to and thereby limit their risk of HIV acquisition? The impact of number of years of education obtained versus currently being in school may serve to limit risk of HIV infection at different times in the life-course and through different channels.

Despite recognition that education is beneficial for young women, there are a range of barriers to school attendance for young women in SSA including poverty and gender inequality. Cost remains a major barrier to school attendance for many young people in SSA. Policy changes have promoted free schooling (e.g. removing schools fees) to reduce economic barriers, but other barriers remain: costs of transport, uniforms and food; policy or social exclusions during pregnancy and; inadequate facilities for menstruating girls (Grant and Hallman 2008; Sommer 2010). Gender inequality can result in a perceived lack of value for girls' education and school completion, particularly in contexts where the costs of school attendance, either direct or indirect, are high.

15.4 Developing Structural Interventions

Structural interventions ameliorate the influence of social inequalities on people's health and allow them to manage the risks in their environment (Seely et al. 2012). There are two key elements to the development of structural interventions to reduce HIV risk and vulnerability. First, a vital element to developing successful interventions is identification of the casual pathways through which such factors impact on risk. It is too simplistic to say that particular social-structural factors do or do not lead to HIV – rather, we should consider *how*, in *what* circumstances and for *whom* particular combinations of factors contribute to vulnerability. Thus, interventions to address structural drivers need to be locally informed and contextually relevant. There is consensus that interventions should be grounded in and guided by theoretical frameworks accepted in the social sciences that ensure hypothesized causal pathways are 'sociologically plausible' for the populations targeted for intervention

(Krishnan et al. 2008; Auerbach et al. 2011). Second, interventions require a clear idea of the level at which they hope to impact. Given that interventions to challenge structural drivers can include strategies from the mico- to macro-level (as previously discussed), different information might be needed to operationalize distinct interventions within appropriate timeframes and outcomes (Auerbach et al. 2011).

The Aids2031 Social Drivers Working Group (Auerbach et al. 2011) identified key steps in the *process* of making decisions about structural interventions: (1) identify the target populations and/or locations for intervention; (2) identify the key behavioral patterns and drivers of behavioral patterns for the target population; (3) choose level of structural intervention; (4) describe planned and potential changes and outcomes; (5) design the intervention; (6) implement, monitor, evaluate and feedback. Within this process, interventions need not always be designed from scratch, but should be chosen based on evidence from other locations and the hypothesis that similar factors are at work in the intervention community. Within this suggested process, Auerbach et al. (2011) have described six main types of structural interventions, implemented individually or in combination: (i) policy-legal changes, (ii) increasing environmental enablers, (iii) shifting harmful social norms, (iv) catalyzing social and political change, (v) empowerment of communities and groups and, (vi) economic empowerment. Within these potential avenues of change, the proximal or distal location of structural factors will impact on the success of interventions. Interventions addressing proximal factors are likely to be easier to implement but their impact might be smaller and less enduring that more difficult-to-implement distal interventions (Parkhurst 2013).

The recognition that social change is central to future success in HIV prevention has pushed the acceptance of forms of evidence outside of traditional biomedical paradigms. Thus, the need to focus on context and to address broad social structures suggests that qualitative methodologies located in the social sciences might offer appropriate methodologies for designing and understanding mechanisms through which structural interventions effect change (Sanson-Fisher et al. 2007; Auerbach et al. 2011).

15.5 Current Structural Interventions for Young Women in Sub-Saharan Africa

Increasing recognition of the structural drivers of HIV risk is being translated into intervention programs. A range of programs are being implemented by sub-Saharan African governments and with local and international researchers. Importantly, many interventions also include program evaluations which will allow for a better understanding of what works and how. A full systematic review is beyond the scope of this chapter. However in a review of social and structural approaches to HIV prevention for women and girls, Hardee et al. (2014) noted that successful interventions have been undertaken across six domains: transforming gender norms;

addressing violence; transforming legal norms; promoting employment; advancing education; and reducing stigma and discrimination. In the Hardee et al. review, intervention success was rated according to depth, breadth and strength of evidence (Hardee et al. 2014), although few were evaluated with HIV or sexual and reproductive health outcomes. Of structural interventions deemed successful, all but transforming legal norms have shown some success in adolescent female populations. However, impact on stigma and discrimination has been focused predominately in Asia and will not be discussed here further. Current structural interventions have a strong focus on community mobilization but there are other methods, such as training on HIV, violence and gender for individuals, communities and providers, being used. For young women, there has been a particular interest in the use of social protection as HIV mitigation, through payment of conditional or unconditional grants that are generally tied to education in some form. Among young women, few policy change approaches have been implemented to date (Hardee et al. 2014).

15.5.1 Transforming Gender Inequalities

Evaluations of interventions among young women in Africa show that gender-awareness training, peer and partner discussions and community-based education about changing gender norms appear offer effective pathways to transforming gender norms. Mass media campaigns and programs to change norms around multiple partners also show promise (Hardee et al. 2014). In South Africa, a 50-h participatory program to build knowledge, communications skills and to stimulate critical reflection among young people aged 15–26 years showed mixed results. Positive behavior change was reported largely by young men: there were reductions in partner numbers, transactional sex, IPV and misuse of alcohol and drugs. Young women did not report positive behavior change, and indeed transactional sex appeared to increase in the initial 12-month period after the intervention. There was no impact on HIV incidence, although HSV-2 incidence was reduced by 33 % (Jewkes et al. 2008). In Tanzania, a community-based program to reduce violence and HIV has also shown limited success. While the program did improve attitudes towards IPV, there was no impact on IPV behaviors (Maman and Mbwambo 2007). A further community mobilization intervention targeting IPV in Uganda included young women from age 18 years and found that the intervention reduced experiences of both physical and sexual IPV among women in the previous 12 months (Abramsky et al. 2014). This intervention is now being replicated in other African countries.

Across Africa, Sonke Gender Justice is involved in community-based participatory work to challenge existing gender norms. The 'One Man Can' campaign uses a rights-based approach to reducing violence against women and work towards HIV reduction in men and women. Impact assessment of the program in three South African provinces has demonstrated promising trends in reducing male violence and challenging hegemonic masculinities (Dworkin et al. 2013). The program was recently adapted based on a model of community mobilization and is currently being evaluated using a community randomized trial in South Africa to determine the impact on negative gender norms, IPV and HIV risk behaviors among men and women 18–25 years of age (Lippman et al. 2013). Other programs with a focus on intimate partner violence made use of micro-finance as the vehicle for engaging women and are reported in the next section.

15.5.2 Impacting on Limited Livelihood Opportunities

Explicitly noting the realities of women's risk and vulnerability and the need for multi-faceted interventions addressing multiple structural drivers, a further review has focused specifically on the intersection between combating gender inequalities and enhancing livelihood security for young people in Africa (Gibbs et al. 2012). This review grouped interventions into three main categories, including: (i) combination microfinance and gender empowerment interventions; (ii) interventions for greater support of young women in education; and (iii) combination gender empowerment and financial literacy interventions.

Microfinance initiatives might be viewed as poverty alleviation, but also serve to impact on women's empowerment. Thus, evaluations of microfinance programs targeted at poverty reduction among women have also led to women's increased control of sexual and reproductive health decision-making within families, through increased acceptance and uptake of contraceptives (Kim and Watts 2005). A microfinance program for adult women in South Africa showed significant reductions in IPV for participating women as well as challenges to gender inequitable views (Pronyk et al. 2006). Particularly among younger participants, the intervention also generated higher levels of HIV communication, increased use of HIV testing and reduced unprotected sex (Pronyk et al. 2008). Attempts to focus micro-finance programs specifically on young women have not shown successful outcomes to date. In Zimbabwe, the SHAZ! program targeted young women aged 16–19 years with micro-grants and training in financial literacy (Dunbar et al. 2010). Unpublished results showed that while the program demonstrated changes in inequitable gender norms and a reduction in physical and sexual violence, these changes were not significantly different to changes in the control group. Other livelihood programs for youth have found similar challenges. In Congo, maintaining engagement with an income generation program for young people was limited: only a quarter remained engaged after an initial 3-month period. However, 4 years later there were reductions in unprotected sex with a new sex partner in those still engaged in income-generating activities. Behavior change was believed to be the result of income, increased sense of control and autonomy, new skills and having activities to engage young people's time. Migration for income generation, however, served to increase risk (Boungou Bazika 2007). The results of these interventions emphasize the role of context on the potential for structural interventions to have impact on specific populations in certain places.

The *Siyakha Nentsha* program in KwaZulu-Natal, South Africa focused on financial training, rather than the provision of actual cash, and did not note changes in young women's sexual behaviors (Hallman and Roca 2011). Likewise, the SUUBI Research Program in Uganda did not document changes in attitudes towards sexual risk taking among young women after ensuring access to child savings accounts and providing training on asset building and financial planning. There were, however, improved attitudes documented among young men (Ssewamala et al. 2010). Additional intervention studies in Zambia and urban South Africa are currently underway. These interventions will attempt to address livelihoods, gender relations and access to health care for young people.

In addition to these specifically focused HIV prevention programs, an increasing number of African countries are introducing social protection programs modelled on those that have existed in Latin America for decades. While most programs have poverty alleviation as their main aim, there is escalating interest in the impact that such programs might have on sexual health and HIV risk for young people, intended or unintended. There is growing evidence from evaluations of national programs that social protection interventions are efficacious in reducing sexual risk behaviors and/or HIV risk. An evaluation of the Government of Kenya's Cash Transfer for Orphans and Vulnerable Children program showed a reduction in the likelihood of sexual debut among adolescents aged 15–25 years of 31 % (Handa et al. 2014). Other sexual behaviors remained unchanged despite receipt of the grant, and the impact on sexual debut was stronger for women than it was for men. Similarly, evaluation of recipients of the South African Child Support Grant has shown that young women have reduced incidence and prevalence of both transactional sex and age-disparate sex when receiving the grant (Cluver et al. 2013). The addition of 'care' (psychological support) offered further protection for young women, and interestingly, halved young men's risk behaviors (Cluver et al. 2014).

Otherwise, it has also been common for interventions targeting young women in Africa to focus on the combination of poverty alleviation and promoting school attendance or increased education. A widely cited study of cash transfers in Malawi showed that providing young women and their families with small monthly transfers was effective in reducing pregnancy, early marriage, sexual activity and risky sexual behavior. Young women receiving the transfer were also more likely to be enrolled in school (Baird et al. 2010). A year and a half after the program was initiated, HIV prevalence among young women receiving the cash transfers was 60 % lower than in young women who did not receive the cash (Baird et al. 2012). This study compared both a conditional and unconditional cash transfer. Similar results in both arms suggest that it was poverty alleviation rather than education that promoted behavior change for these young women; specifically through a reduction in transactional sex. Thus providing young women with access to their own money may be instrumental in alleviating their dependence on male partners and engaging in sexual behaviors they might otherwise avoid.

Few other education interventions have documented success through measuring biological outcomes. However, other education-focused interventions for young women in Kenya and Zimbabwe have shown impact on increasing school attendance, delaying sexual debut, reducing teen marriage and pregnancy (Duflo et al. 2006; Cho et al. 2011; Hallfors et al. 2011). Other intervention programs promoting school attendance (largely through financial assistance) are underway in Mpumalanga and KwaZulu-Natal, South Africa, but have not yet generated results (MacPhail et al. 2013). Intervening in education currently appears to be one of the pathways through which structural drivers can be addressed with promising outcomes, and there are suggestions that all programs might need to include some element of increasing access to schooling to have impact (Gibbs et al. 2012).

15.5.3 Other Structural Interventions

Many African countries have policies that reflect the broader gender norms in which women's rights are given less credence than men's. In particular, women's lack of legal rights associated with their subordination to men increases their HIV risk; limiting women's options for leaving abusive relationships in which their HIV risk is increased and reducing their legal recourse in situations where they are abandoned, potentially due to HIV status. While some small-scale interventions, such as Kenyan programs to ensure property and inheritance rights show promise, none are currently focused specifically on young women (Hardee et al. 2014). In the African context, where early marriage is common, such interventions might assist young women nonetheless.

15.6 Conclusions

Given the pervasive impact of gender inequalities on women's HIV vulnerability and its integration with other structural drivers of women's risk, addressing gender inequalities is key to future responses to HIV in Africa (and elsewhere). Specifically, addressing gender inequalities should be built into comprehensive national approaches to HIV prevention and management. This would be achieved through ensuring a legal environment in which the rights of women are protected and *upheld in practice*, engaging communities in change and including women affected by HIV in the development of gender-sensitive strategies (Gupta et al. 2011). Of vital importance is the need for structural drivers of HIV to be viewed and treated as a core component of all responses to HIV. This includes new enthusiasms for the ability of treatment as prevention to make a significant impact on new HIV infections (Seely et al. 2012). This is noteworthy given that many of the structural factors currently determined to impact of HIV risk will also be instrumental in facilitating differential access and uptake of treatment. Interventions to reduce of Gender Based Violence (GBV) and increase the livelihoods of young women are key to a combination prevention approach.

Just as behavioral interventions have failed through not taking broader contextual factors into account, structural interventions might have limited success if they fail to acknowledge that multiple structural factors are at play in any given situation. Thus, interventions to mitigate HIV vulnerability cannot focus narrowly on a single structural driver without understanding when and how it interacts with other drivers. While this need to focus on the complexities of intertwined structural factors may pose challenges for implementation and evaluation; it may facilitate financing of expensive development-orientated large-scale social protection programs. Cofinancing is likely to be important in the implementation of structural interventions and evaluation of cost benefits should be assessed across health and development sectors (Remme et al. 2014).

Structural interventions for HIV prevention have not yet been adopted as a component of large-scale initiatives at the country level; largely because there is a small pool of evidence-based strategies from which to choose (Auerbach et al. 2011). Significantly, if we are to work towards structural interventions for HIV prevention, we need to ensure that such interventions are adequately evaluated. Many programs are community-based and implemented at the grassroots level, therefore do not necessarily including evaluation experts. The inclusion of an evaluation team with skills to measure social, economic, political and cultural factors is vital to ensure that a body of evidence is developed to direct future work (Gupta et al. 2008). Our experience of changing associations with risk through the HIV epidemic, such as with income and education, suggest that we need to continually assess and evaluate the contributory role of different structural factors as the epidemic evolves.

References

Abramsky, T., Devries, K., Kiss, L., Nakuti, J., Kyegombe, N., Starmann, E., et al. (2014). Findings from the SASA! study: A cluster randomized controlled trial to assess the impact of a community mobilization intervention to prevent violence against women and reduce HIV risk in Kampala, Uganda. *BMC Medicine, 12*(1), 122. doi:http://dx.doi.10.1186/s12916.

Auerbach, J., Parkhurst, J., & Cáceres, C. F. (2011). Addressing social drivers of HIV/AIDS for the long-term response: Conceptual and methodological considerations. *Global Public Health, 6*(supp 3), s293–s309.

Baird, S., Chirwa, E., McIntosh, C., & Özler, B. (2010). The short-term impacts of a schooling conditional cash transfer program on the sexual behavior of young women. *Health Economics, 19*(S1), 55–68.

Baird, S. J., Garfein, R. S., McIntosh, C., & Özler, B. (2012). Effect of a cash transfer programme for schooling on prevalence of HIV and herpes simplex type 2 in Malawi: A cluster randomised trial. *The Lancet, 379*(9823), 1320–1329.

Barnett, T., & Whiteside, A. (2002). *AIDS in the twenty-first century: Disease and globalisation.* Basingstoke: Palgrave Macmillan.

Bonnell, C., Hargreaves, J., Strange, V., Pronyk, P., & Porter, J. (2006). Should structural interventions be evaluated using RCTs? The case of HIV prevention. *Social Science & Medicine, 63*, 1135–1142.

Boungou Bazika, J. (2007). Effectiveness of small scale income generating activities in reducing risk of HIV in youth in the Republic of Congo. *AIDS Care, 19*(Suppl 1), s23–s24.

Cho, H., Hallfors, D. D., Mbai, I., Itindi, J., Milimo, B. W., Halpern, C. T., & Iritani, B. J. (2011). Keeping adolescent orphans in school to prevent human immunodeficiency virus infection: Evidence from a randomized controlled trial in Kenya. *Journal of Adolescent Health, 48*(5), 523–526.

Cluver, L., Boyes, M., Orkin, M., Prantelic, M., Molwena, T., & Sherr, L. (2013). Child-focused state cash transfers and adolescent risk of HIV infection in South Africa: A propensity-score-matched case-control study. *Lancet Global Health, 1*(6), e362–e370.

Cluver, L., Orkin, M., Boyes, M., & Sherr, L. (2014). Cash plus care: Social protection cumulatively mitigates HIV-risk behaviour among adolescents in South Africa. *AIDS, 28*(Suppl 3), s389–s397.

Coates, T., Richter, R., & Cáceres, C. F. (2008). Behavioural strategies to reduce HIV transmission: How to make them work better. *The Lancet, 372*(9639), 669–683.

Cowan, F., & Pettifor, A. (2009). HIV in adolescents in sub-Saharan Africa. *Current Opinion in HIV and AIDS, 4*(4), 288–293.

Crissman, H., Adanu, R., & Harlow, S. D. (2012). Women's sexual empowerment and contraceptive use in Ghana. *Studies in Family Planning, 43*(3), 201–2012.

de Walque, D., Nakiyingi-Miiro, J., Busingye, J., & Whitworth, J. A. (2005). Changing association between schooling levels and HIV-1 infection over 11 years in a rural population cohort in south-west Uganda. *Tropical Medicine and International Health, 10*(10), 993–1001.

Duflo, E., Pascaline, D., Kremer, M., & Sinei, S. (2006). *Education and HIV/AIDS prevention: Evidence from a randomized evaluation in Western Kenya*. Washington, DC: World Bank.

Dunbar, M. S., Maternowska, M. C., Kang, M. J., Laver, S. M., Mudekunye-Mahaka, I., & Padian, N. S. (2010). Findings from SHAZ!: A feasibility study of a microcredit and life-skills HIV prevention intervention to reduce risk among adolescent female orphans in Zimbabwe. *Journal of Prevention & Intervention in the Community, 38*(2), 147–161.

Dunkle, K. L., Jewkes, R. K., Brown, H. C., Gray, G. E., McIntyre, J. A., & Harlow, S. D. (2004). Gender-based violence, relationship power, and risk of HIV infection in women attending antenatal clinics in South Africa. *The Lancet, 363*(9419), 1415–1421.

Dunkle, K. L., Jewkes, R. K., Nduna, M., Levin, J., Jama, N., Khuzwayo, N., Koss, M. P., & Duvvury, N. (2006). Perpetration of partner violence and HIV risk behaviour among young men in the rural Eastern Cape, South Africa. *AIDS, 20*(16), 2107–2114 2110.1097/2101.aids.0000247582.0000200826.0000247552.

Dworkin, S. L., Hatcher, A. M., Colvin, C., & Peacock, D. (2013). Impact of a gender-transformative HIV and antiviolence program on gender ideologies and masculinities in two rural, South African communities. *Men and Masculinities, 16*(2), 181–202.

Fox, A. (2012). The HIV-poverty thesis re-examined: Poverty, wealth or inequality as a social determinant of HIV infection in sub-Saharan Africa? *Journal of Biosocial Science, 44*(4), 459–480.

Gibbs, A., Willan, S., Misselhorn, A., & Mangoma, J. (2012). Combined structural interventions for gender inequality and livelihood security: A critical review of the evidence from southern and eastern Africa and the implications for young people. *Journal of the International AIDS Society, 15*, 17362. doi:http://dx.doi.org/10.7448/IAS.15.3.17362.

Grant, M. J., & Hallman, K. K. (2008). Pregnancy-related school dropout and prior school performance in KwaZulu-Natal, South Africa. *Studies in Family Planning, 39*(4), 369–382.

Greig, F., & Koopman, A. (2003). Multilevel analysis of women's empowerment and HIV prevention: Qualitative survey results from a preliminary study in Botswana. *AIDS and Behavior, 7*(2), 195–208.

Gupta, G.R., Parkhurst, J., Ogden, J. A., Aggleton, P., & Mahal, A. (2008). HIV prevention 4: Structural approaches to HIV prevention. *The Lancet, 372*(9640), 764–775.

Gupta, G.R., Ogden, J., & Warner, A. (2011). Moving forward on women's gender -related HIV vulnerability: The good news, the bad news and what to do about it. *Global Public Health, 6*(Suppl 3), s370–s382.

Hallfors, D. P., Cho, H. P., Rusakaniko, S., Iritani, B., Mapfumo, J., & Halpern, C. (2011). Supporting adolescent orphan girls to stay in school as HIV risk prevention: Evidence from a randomized controlled trial in Zimbabwe. *American Journal of Public Health, 101*(6), 1082–1088.

Hallman, K., & Roca, E. (2011). *Siyakha Nentsha: Building economic, health, and social capabilities among highly vulnerable adolescents in KwaZulu-Natal, South Africa*. Washington, DC: Population Council.

Handa, S., Tucker Halpern, C., Pettifor, A., & Thirumurthy, H. (2014). The government of Kenya's cash tranfer program reduces the risk of sexual debut among young people age 15–25. *PLoS One, 9*(1), e85473.

Hankins, C., & de Zalduondo, B. (2010). Combination prevention: A deeper understanding of effective HIV prevention. *AIDS, 24*(suppl 4), s70–s80.

Hardee, K., Gay, J., Croce-Galis, M., & Peltz, A. (2014). Strengthening the enabling environment for women and girls: What is the evidence in social and structural approaches in the HIV response? *Journal of the International AIDS Society, 17*, 18619. doi:http://dx.doi.org/10.7448/IAS.17.1.18619.

Hargreaves, J., Morison, L., Kim, J. C., Bonell, C. P., Porter, J. D. H., Watts, C., et al. (2008). The association between school attendance, HIV infection and sexual behaviour among young people in rural South Africa. *Journal of Epidemiology and Community Health, 62*, 113–119.

Hoffman, S., O'Sullivan, L. F., Harrison, A., Dolezal, C., & Monroe-Wise, A. (2006). HIV risk behaviors and the context of sexual coercion in young adults' sexual interactions: Results from a diary study in rural South Africa. *Sexually Transmitted Diseases, 33*(1), 52–58.

Jewkes, R., Dunkle, K., Nduna, M., Levin, J., Khuzwayo, N., Koss, M., Puren, A., & Duvvury, N. (2006). Factors associated with HIV sero-status in young rural South African women: Connections between intimate partner violence and HIV. *International Journal of Epidemiology, 35*(6), 1461–1468.

Jewkes, R., Nduna, M., Levin, J., Jama, N., Dunkle, K., Puren, A., & Duvvury, N. (2008). Impact of stepping stones on incidence of HIV and HSV-2 and sexual behaviour in rural South Africa: Cluster randomised controlled trial. *BMJ [British Medical Journal], 337*(7666), 391–395.

Jewkes, R., Dunkle, K., Nduna, M., & Shai, N. (2010). Intimate partner violence, relationship power inequality, and incidence of HIV infection in young women in South Africa. *Lancet, 376*(9734), 41–48.

Jukes, M., Simmons, S., & Bundy, D. (2008). Education and vulnerability: The role of schools in protecting young women and girls from HIV in southern Africa. *AIDS, 22*(suppl 4), s41–s56.

Kalichman, S. C., Simbayi, L. C., Kagee, A., Toefy, Y., Jooste, S., Cain, D., & Chauncey, C. (2006). Associations of poverty, substance use, and HIV transmission risk behaviors in three South African communities. *Social Science & Medicine, 62*(7), 1641–1649.

Kaufman, C. E., Clark, S., Manzini, N., & May, J. (2004). Communities, opportunities, and adolescents' sexual behavior in KwaZulu-Natal, South Africa. *Studies in Family Planning, 35*(4), 261–274.

Kim, J., & Watts, C. (2005). Gaining a foothold: Tackling poverty, gender inequality, and HIV in Africa. *British Medical Journal, 331*(7519), 769–772.

Krishnan, S., Dunbar, M. S., Minnis, A. M., Medlin, C. A., Gerdts, C. E., & Padian, N. S. (2008). Poverty, gender inequities, and women's risk of human immunodeficiency virus/AIDS. *Annals of the New York Academy of Sciences, 1136*(1), 101–110.

Laga, M., Schwärtlander, B., Pisanai, E., Sow, P. S., & Caraël, M. (2001). To stem HIV in Africa, prevent transmission to young women. *AIDS, 15*(7), 931–934.

Lam, D., Leibbrandt, M., & Mlatsheni, C. (2010). Education and youth unemployment in South Africa. In R. Kanbur & J. Svejnar (Eds.), *Labour markets and economic development* (pp. 90–109). Oxon: Routledge.

Lippman, S., Maman, S., MacPhail, C., Twine, R., Peacock, D., Kahn, K., & Pettifor, A. (2013). Conceptualizing community mobilization for HIV prevention: Implications for HIV prevention programming in the African context. *PLoS One, 9*(10), e78208.

MacPhail, C. (2003). Challenging dominant norms of masculinity for HIV prevention. *African Journal of AIDS Research, 2*(2), 141–149.

MacPhail, C., & Campbell, C. (2001). 'I think condoms are good, but aai, I hate those things': Condom use among adolescents and young people in a southern African township. *Social Science and Medicine, 52*, 1613–1627.

MacPhail, C., Adato, M., Kahn, K., Selin, A., Twine, R., Khoza, S., Rosenberg, M., Nguyen, N., et al. (2013). Acceptability and feasibility of cash transfers for HIV prevention among adolescent South African women. *AIDS and Behavior, 17*(7), 2301–2312.

Maman, S., & Mbwambo, J. (2007). Evaluation of a community-based HIV and violence prevention intervention targeting young men in Dar es Salaam, Tanzania. *Horizons Final Report.* Washington, DC: Population Council.

Maman, S., Campbell, J. C., Sweat, M. D., & Gielen, A. C. (2000). The intersections of HIV and violence: directions for future research and interventions. *Social Science & Medicine, 50*(4), 459–478.

Masanjala, W. (2007). The poverty-HIV/AIDS nexus in Africa: A livelihood approach. *Social Science & Medicine, 64*(5), 1032–1041.

Medley, A., Garcia-Moreno, C., McGill, S., & Maman, S. (2004). Rates, barriers and outcomes of HIV serostatus disclosure among women in developing countries: Implications for prevention of mother-to-child transmission programmes. *Bulletin of the World Health Organization, 82*(4), 299–307.

Michelo, C., Sandoy, I., & Fylkesnes, K. (2006). Marked HIV prevalence declines in higher educated young people: Evidence from population-based surveys (1995–2003) in Zambia. *AIDS, 20*, 1031–1036.

Naidoo, P., Chirinda, W., Mchunu, G., Swartz, S., & Anderson, J. (2014). Social and structural factors associated with vulnerability to HIV infection among young adults in South Africa. *Psychology, Health and Medicine*. doi:http://dx.doi.org/10.1080/13548506.2014.936883

Parker, R., Easton, D., & Klein, C. H. (2000). Structural barriers and facilitators in HIV prevention: A review of international research. *AIDS, 14*(Suppl 1), s22–s32.

Parkhurst, J. (2010). Understanding the correlations between wealth, poverty and human immunodeficiency virus infection in African countries. *Bulletin of the World Health Organization, 88*(7), 519–526.

Parkhurst, J. (2013). Structural drivers, interventions, and approaches for prevention of sexually transmitted HIV in general populations: Definitions and an operational approach. Structural approaches to HIV prevention. In *Position Paper Series*. Arlington.

Pettifor, A., Measham, D., Rees, H., & Padian, N. (2004). Sexual power and HIV risk, South Africa. *Emerging Infectious Diseases, 10*(11), 1996–2004.

Pettifor, A., Levandowski, B., MacPhail, C., Padian, N., Cohen, M. S., & Rees, H. V. (2008). Keep them in school: The importance of education as a protective factor against HIV infection among young South African women. *International Journal of Epidemiology, 37*(6), 1266–1273.

Pettifor, A., Levandowski, B., MacPhail, C., Miller, W. C., Tabor, J., Ford, C., Stein, C. R., Rees, H., et al. (2011). A tale of two counties: Rethinking sexual risk for HIV among young people in South Africa and the United States. *Journal of Adolescent Health, 49*, 237–243.

Phillips, A., & Pirkle, C. (2011). Moving beyond behaviour: Advancing HIV risk prevention epistomologies and interventions (A report on the state of the literature). *Global Public Health: An International Journal for Research, Policy and Practice, 6*, 577–592.

Pronyk, P. M., Hargreaves, J. R., Kim, J., Morison, L. A., Phetla, G., Watts, C., Busza, J., & Porter, J. D. (2006). Effect of a structural intervention for the prevention of intimate-partner violence and HIV in rural South Africa: A cluster randomised trial. *The Lancet, 368*(9551), 1973–1983.

Pronyk, P., Kim, J., Abramsky, T., Phetla, G., Hargreaves, J., Morison, L. A., Watts, C., Busza, J., et al. (2008). A combined microfinance and training intervention can reduce HIV risk behaviour in young female participants. *AIDS, 22*(13), 1659–1665.

Quinn, T. C., & Overbaugh, J. (2005). HIV/AIDS in women: An expanding epidemic. *Science, 308*(5728), 1582+.

Remme, M., Vassall, A., Lutz, B., Luna, J., & Watts, C. (2014). Financing structural interventions: Going beyond HIV-only value for money assessments. *AIDS, 28*(3), 425–434.

Ross, D. (2010). Behavioural interventions to reduce HIV risk: What works? *AIDS, 24*, s4–s14.

Rwenge, M. (2003). Poverty and sexual risk behaviour among young people in Bamenda, Cameroon. *African Population Studies, 18*(2), 91–104.

Sanson-Fisher, R., Bonevski, B., Green, L., & D'Este, C. (2007). Limitations of the randomised controlled trial in evaluating population-based health interventions. *American Journal of Preventative Medicine, 33*(2), 155–161.

Seely, J., Watts, C., Kippax, S., Russell, S., Heise, L., & Whiteside, A. (2012). Addressing the structural drivers of HIV: A luxury or necessity for programmes? *Journal of the International AIDS Society, 15*(suppl 1), 17397.

Sommer, M. (2010). Where the education system and women's bodies collide: The social and health impact of girls' experiences of menstruation and schooling in Tanzania. *Journal of Adolescence, 33*(4), 521–529.

Ssewamala, F. M., Han, P., Neilands, T. B., Ismayilova, L., & Sperber, E. (2010). Effect of economic assets on sexual risk-taking intentions among orphaned adolescents in Uganda. *American Journal of Public Health, 100*(3), 483–488.

Sweat, M., & Denison, J. (1995). Reducing HIV incidence in developing countries with structural and environmental interventions. *AIDS, 9*(Suppl A), s251–s257.

Tawil, O., Verster, A., & O'Reilly, K. R. (1995). Enabling approaches for HIV/AIDS prevention: Can we modify the environment and minimiza the risk? *AIDS, 9*, 1299–1306.

Tladi, L. (2006). Poverty and HIV/AIDS in South Africa: An empirical contribution. *SAHARA, 3*(1), 369–381.

UNAIDS. (2007). *Practical guidelines for intensifying HIV prevention: Towards universal access*. Geneva: UNAIDS.

UNAIDS. (2013). *Global report: UNAIDS report on the global AIDS epidemic 2013*. Geneva: UNAIDS.

UNICEF. (2011). *Opportunity in crisis: Preventing HIV from early adolescence to young adulthood*. Geneva: UNICEF.

Waldo, C., & Coates, T. (2000). Multiple levels of analysis and intervention in HIV prevention science: Exemplars and directions for new research. *AIDS, 14*(Suppl 2), s18–s26.

Wight, D., Plummer, M., Ross, D. A., & Changalucha, J. (2012). The need to promote behaviour change at the cultural level: One factor explaining the limited impact of the *MEMA kwa Vijaana* adolescent sexual health intervention in rural Tanzania. A process evaluation. *BMC Public Health, 12*, 788.

World Health Organization. (2013). *Trends in maternal mortality 1990 to 2013*. Geneva: World Health Organization.

Chapter 16
In Search of Entrepreneurs, Children and HIV/AIDS in Cameroon: A Marginalized Issue?

Larissa Kojoué

Contents

16.1 Introduction

Political sciences have the potential to make a unique contribution to the study of and response to the epidemic, oriented as they are to the explanation of decision-making actors, institutions, ideas and processes (Paxton 2012). Because the political aspects of the epidemic can not be ignored, our paper is a contribution to the understanding of actors, ideas and processes that shape the present and the future of children facing HIV/AIDS epidemic in Cameroon.

The objectives of the fight against HIV/AIDS can only be reached if the reduction of inequalities with regard to the epidemic is taken into consideration (Piot 2010). Among the populations most vulnerable to the epidemic and its consequences are children under the age of 15. Ninety percent of the children most affected by

L. Kojoué (✉)
Research associate, LAM/Bordeaux,
MEOS/Montréal, Québec, Canada
e-mail: Larissa.kojoue@hotmail.fr

P. Liamputtong (ed.), *Children and Young People Living with HIV/AIDS*,
Cross-Cultural Research in Health, Illness and Well-Being,
DOI 10.1007/978-3-319-29936-5_16

HIV/AIDS are found in Africa (UNAIDS 2013; see also Chaps. 2 and 9 in this volume). This significantly undermines social and economic development of countries, which are permanently affected (UNAIDS et al. 2004; UNICEF 2006, 2013). Cameroon is one of the countries where 90 % of people live with limited or no access to antiretroviral treatment (ONUSIDA 2013). While children represent about 10 % of the 550,000 people living with HIV (PLWHIV), pediatric antiretroviral treatment coverage represents less than 5 %. The mother-to-child transmission of HIV (MTCT) is still the main mode of infection for persons under the age of 15. Besides fighting against AIDS programs, only 2 % of public expenditure in 2012 is devoted to orphans and other children made vulnerable by AIDS (OVC or HIV/AIDS-infected/affected children) (GTC-CNLS 2012). In the context of generalized epidemics where HIV prevalence is 4.3 %, the real importance given to children in HIV/AIDS public policies is of concern. Other related questions include: who are the stakeholders involved in the management of medical and what are the social consequences of children getting infected? What are the terms of their interventions? Can we attribute the lack of visibility of this issue to the weakness of local actors or unfavorable global economic conditions?

Based on actions carried out for children less than 15 years confronting HIV/AIDS, this chapter examines social mobilization and its impact on care and support for HIV/AIDS infected and affected children in Cameroon. A study of the context that led to the inclusion of this issue on the national agenda, as well as measures implemented since early 2000s, suggest that besides the weakness of local public policies entrepreneurs and their intervention capacities, care to children confronting HIV/AIDS raises issues that go beyond medical and social aspects which concern the social determinants of health, well-being and protection of all children (see also Chaps. 2, 3, and 14 in this volume).

16.2 Agenda Setting as an Indicator of Power Relations

Putting a question on agenda is one of the fundamental steps of public action. It refers to the process by which a problem is set to be examined by the State. It is important to identify why the State is particularly interested in certain problems at a given moment rather than others. According to available literature, agenda setting is the result of a dynamic and interactive process (Cobb and Elder 1972; Kingdon 1984; Stone 1989; Garraud 1990; Hassenteufel 2010). This process takes into account several factors. Some factors are related to the capacity of stakeholders (politicians, experts, social groups, and so on) to have their problem considered by public authorities. These are public policies entrepreneurs (Kingdon 1984), moral entrepreneurs (Becker 1985) or committed entrepreneurs (Cobb and Elder 1972). Other factors are related to the inherent characteristics or intrinsic properties of the problem (incidence, severity, scope), or more precisely how it is presented (a crisis, a scandal, an affair). Some structural and circumstantial factors related to the political context (change of government) and economic (budget) are also factors influencing agenda setting.

According to Jacques Lagroye (2003, 2006), the emergence of a problem in the public arena is the result of a process of collective mobilization and action. All problems do not have the same ability to access the public and the State, and this ability depends on factors more often related to the characteristics of stakeholders involved in these moments than on the problems themselves. Moreover, despite the severity of the HIV epidemic in sub-Saharan Africa and despite knowledge on its dramatic consequences on the health, the well-being and the future of children, I argue that the idea of taking care of children under 15 years (in ways programs have been defined) was not self-imposed in the Cameroonian political agenda. I will show that it is precisely the combined action of some actors that led to various support programs (that we shall develop in the next section). In the same vein, the low interest for this problem at the operational level is indicative of the weakness of the actors involved in the definition of public policies relating to AIDS in Cameroon. This weakness in actors contrasts with the image of the entrepreneur developed by political sociology.

Although the contexts and stakeholders to which the concepts of entrepreneurs have been applied vary, the dominant approach in political sociology assigns to the entrepreneur, a disruptive and transformative role, and even a modifier of social order (Eisenstadt 1980; Fligstein 2001; Lagroye 2003; Hassenteufel 2010; Bergeron et al. 2011). Public policies entrepreneurs are indeed stakeholders who have the ability to influence and control public action, from its definition to its implementation. These actors play an active role in providing guidelines to a problem, and thereby showing how to solve it (Muller 2000). Entrepreneurs of public policies or committed entrepreneurs differ from other social actors in their leadership abilities, their desire to satisfy their interests by transforming the existing orders rather than reproducing them (Bergeron et al. 2011).

In the Cameroonian context, this theoretical framework raises several issues: Could non-State actors in the fight against AIDS be described as entrepreneurs or leaders? How are they involved in the development and implementation of AIDS public policies? Do they have the opportunity and the capacity to intervene in State action? With agenda setting analysis, it will be possible to see what importance is given to children's health and social care in HIV/AIDS policies; and also, what are the conditions for a sustainable continuation of this problem among government's priorities.

16.3 Children and HIV/AIDS in Cameroon (OVC): Agenda Setting Conditions and Challenges

The term OVC, for orphans and other vulnerable children due to HIV/AIDS, appeared in the early 2000s (Hunter and Williamson 2000). While until the late 1990s, the predominant picture of the impact of HIV on children were AIDS orphans, taking into account the vulnerability criterion will lead to the institutionalization of the orphans and other vulnerable children due to HIV/AIDS category. This term refers to all children who in one way or the other suffer the consequences of the epidemic: children living with HIV, children exposed to HIV, children living in households affected by AIDS, children who lost one or both parent due to AIDS, and so on (see also Chaps. 2 and 3 in this volume). The argument that guides this classification is that OVC are more exposed than their peers to some problems: education, healthcare, nutrition, loneliness, and so forth. Medical criterion goes along with social and psychological criterion (UNICEF 2006). Despite the ambivalence in this category being criticized for the non-operational nature of the concept of vulnerability under AIDS[1] (Singhal et al. 2003; Skinner et al. 2004; Gillespie et al. 2005; Williamson 2008), governments of countries most affected by AIDS are invited to take measures targeting OVC in their national response. This chapter is based on three national programs of care and support to OVC.

Program 1 The first government program to support OVC was introduced in Cameroon in 2004. This was a pilot program jointly supported by UNICEF, the French Cooperation and the Ministry of Social Affairs (Minas). It is the bi-multi OVC program (bilateral and multilateral cooperation) covering a period of 36 months. The program included provision of social, nutritional, medical and academic support to 10,000 children identified as AIDS OVC. Initially limited to three pilot sites (three urban councils of medium density), this project will then be scaled-up nationwide.

Program 2 Due to substantial funding from the Global Fund, Cameroon government will develop a National Support Program for OVC (NSP-OVC) modeled on the bi-multi project. For an initial term of 5 years (2006–2010), NSP-OVC is the first national program of social pediatrics for children under 18 years in Cameroon. 180,000 OVC will be identified as having special needs for support. The program's goal was to support 75 % of the targeted children from 2006 to 2010. To implement this program, the government relied on about 50 local associations. Some of the associations were incompetent. One of the leaders of this program explained:

> The first part of the program was a real mess (…). The Minas sent social workers in all partner associations of the program. Some of them had no office space to work. Some associations were not motivated by the desire to help, but by the means allocated for work.

Two years later (2008), and barely 70,000 OVC (i.e. barely 25 % of the target) having received support, the program stopped abruptly. Government authorities indicated that the project was suspended and not stopped. They were expecting it to start over before the end of the National Strategic Plan (NSP) to fight AIDS and STIs from 2011 to 2015 and funding from Round 10 of the Global Fund. This focus

[1] In the context of generalized poverty, irrespective of HIV/AIDS, almost all children are exposed to the same risks, though at varying levels. For example, the fact of being an orphan because of AIDS does not automatically make a child vulnerable if he is taken care of by the extended family where his needs can be met. On the other hand, a child who lost his parents due to another illness can be extremely vulnerable if he is taken care of by a poor family or if he lives in the street.

on subsidies from the Global Fund brings to light the extreme dependence of national policies on foreign funding. The suspension of NSP-OVC did not raise many reactions from care providers, possibly because UNICEF launched another program for OVC that drawn their attention.

Program 3 As part of its global campaign "Unite for children, Unite against AIDS," UNICEF identified four priorities (known as the 4P): Preventing mother-to-child transmission (PMTCT), Providing treatment for children, Preventing new infections among adolescents and youths, and Protecting and supporting OVC. These four priorities serve as a framework for the implementation of cooperation programs to fight against HIV and AIDS. Hinted in the bi-multi project, it is from 2008, with the signing of a cooperation program for 2008–2012 with the Cameroonian government that all 4P components were activated. *Children, HIV and AIDS* (CHA) is a UNICEF program, which serves as the last framework of action for OVC in Cameroon. Although it is a national program, it covers only few cities by region, and every activity is almost entirely funded by UNICEF. With the CHA program, for the first time, the management of pediatric HIV infection was considered as part of priority support programs for OVC.[2] Since 2000, as part of PMTCT programs, free access to treatment has been established for infected children born from HIV-positive mothers. Inspite of this, it was only in 2008 that its visibility was enhanced. Thus, despite the measures targeting children HIV-infected, few associations were aware of the HIV status of children in their care, let alone that of their parent. This confirms the difficulty in operationalizing the concept of vulnerability in a context like Cameroon (country with limited resources).

Be it the bi-multi program or the NSP-OVC or CHA program, though all of them fall within HIV and AIDS policies, in practice, the HIV criterion was not really taken into account. Statistics on HIV-infected children or AIDS orphans are particularly imprecise. Given the context of fragility of most children, HIV infection (for parents or children) was not decisive as a selection criterion. It was quickly abandoned, considered as not contributing or contributing very little to the children's vulnerability rate (Femba 2007; CNLS 2008). These three programs show that the situation of children facing AIDS appears to be receiving particular attention in the global agenda of the fight against HIV/AIDS. In fact, what is noticed is the systematic presence of an international body behind each Cameroonian initiative (UNICEF, French Cooperation, Global Fund). Till date, there is no internal program led by the Cameroon government and not carried out by foreign actors. Can we then conclude to the marginality of this issue on the agenda of national stakeholders?

[2]The delay in pediatric care provision of the infection maybe justified by poor knowledge of the HIV infection in children, the existence of unqualified or poorly trained staff (and also unmotivated), early pediatric diagnosis challenges, insufficiency, and even lack of antiretroviral formulae adapted to children (Kojoué 2013).

16.4 A Plural Marginality Fuelled by the Weakness of Local Stakeholders and the Political Context

The conditions for the emergence and implementation of support programs for OVC in the fight against HIV/AIDS policies in Cameroon show that these programs are the product of institutional and international offers rather than as a result of formal requests. This confirms the idea of a "dissonant model" about Cameroonians AIDS public Policies (Eboko and Kerouedan 1999; Eboko 2002). Particularly in Cameroon, public action precedes requests, or even exists without specific requests (although needs are real). Thus, it is with the three programs described above. These programs were designed and developed without the participation of local (and key) actors: associations, local political leaders and local NGOs. The latter were only involved at the end of the process, which is the execution of the program. Moreover, even after the arbitrary suspension of NSP-OVC in which they were officially engaged for 5 years, no specific reaction of protest or complaint was recorded. Support to OVC, therefore, appears as a priority at global level, but not at national level, and this may be due to the inertia of local agents.

16.4.1 An Assisting Role and Not an Entrepreneur's Role: About Cameroonian Associations Supporting OVC

The setting up of local associations for collective action in Cameroon experienced fewer constraints than that related to freedom of the press, trade unions or political parties. With the liberalization of the political life in 1990 and in 1996, freedom of assembly took an unprecedented scale in the early 2000s; period during which the HIV epidemic became essential as a health issue, a challenge for development, international security, human rights and governance, and civil society highly participated in the fight against HIV/AIDS (Eboko and Mandjem 2010; Eboko et al. 2011; Kojoué 2013). With increased means of fight granted to States by international institutions such as the Global Fund and PEPFAR,[3] the Cameroonian associations witnessed a significant peak between 2002 and 2007. According to the National Committee on AIDS, there has been an increase of over 300 % in 5 years (Kojoué 2013). Today, there are about 500 associations to fight against HIV/AIDS, only in the country's big city centers (GTC-CNLS 2013).

Before the implementation of NSP-OVC in 2006, very few associations had included the component "Children and HIV/AIDS" in their programs. Open calls for tenders addressed by the Government and UNICEF led most entities to get involved. The NSP-OVC, as well as the bi-multi or CHA program, could certainly rely on a dynamic civil society engaged in the fight against HIV and AIDS. Yet this movement proved to be not only far away from concerns relating to children and

[3] PEPFAR is the President's Emergency Plan for AIDS Relief. It is a U.S. Government initiative created in 2003.

AIDS, but also somehow not committed for the improvement of social determinants of HIV infection. In fact, it is widely accepted that social inequalities are the main cause of inequalities in health. The social environment where people are born, live, grow, work and age (the social determinants of health), refers to policy choices expressed in the form of social justice (Moleux et al. 2011).

This calls for the following observation: the participatory nature of non-State organizations to national AIDS policies is a fact. This free participation in public action is not, however, accompanied by an advocacy action on the social determinants of health, nor on a real participation in the deliberations and final choices. Few associations involved in the fight against HIV/AIDS have the intellectual, social and economic capital to emerge as key actors in decision-making. Apart from some leading associations connected to international stakeholders, the institutionalization of OVC care providers remains low. Three main factors explain this low mobilization and the inability of local actors to stand as public policy entrepreneurs: an institutional weakness, an authoritarian political environment and the non-confrontational nature of the issue "Children and HIV/AIDS" (a non political issue).

Different actors with whom we conducted our survey in Cameroon show signs of extreme dependence vis-à-vis the State and vis-à-vis foreign partners. Reciprocity of interests between the State (who need the participation of civil society) and organizations fighting against HIV/AIDS (who need both resources and support from the State) vis-à-vis international partners has strengthened relations of mutual dependence. Thus, when there are no funded projects underway, all association activities are paused, and their staff is inactive. There is clear absence of consistent advocacy and monitoring of the issues surrounding AIDS, particularly issues related to children less than 15 years.

In addition to this institutional weakness of Cameroonian associations, the private, social and non-controversial nature of the issue of children and HIV/AIDS may explain the OVC marginality. In many interviews, two arguments regularly came up: the social and private arguments, and the argument presenting HIV/AIDS as a health imperative. These two arguments are used to prevent any increase in generalization or politicization. Whether health professionals, NGOs or local associations, the biggest challenge in pediatric and social care for HIV-infected or affected children is primarily its environment, not the organizational and functional structure of national strategies[4] : These speeches show how private the OVC issue is seen.

> Taking care of children is very difficult and it mostly depends on the state of the family. Children are usually from poor families who sometimes do not have any information. It is a family issue. (An NGO leader)
>
> The difficulty is that they are children and they are entirely dependent on parents, grandparents, guardians, and extended family, in short, adults. Most of them stay in their families and still HIV/AIDS is a taboo, nobody wants to talk about it in public. (A doctor)

[4]This means that there is too little criticism concerning budgets (even if there is criticism concerning funds management), neither on the legitimacy of roles nor on the accountability of political authorities.

The second argument that makes AIDS a health imperative suggests that it is a medical issue and decisions related are taken by professionals and are not to be argued. This means that all decisions regarding the fight against HIV/AIDS pertain to a class of experts that exclude laypersons. Local stakeholders in the fight against HIV/AIDS, therefore, exclude themselves from decisions spheres. Doing so, they are finally losing all ability to access the political arena, institutionalized space within which all negotiations and formal decisions are taken (Jobert and Muller 1987).

One factor, which probably explains why few actors dare to consider, is that taking care of OVC as a political issue, as well as other HIV/AIDS-related issues as PMTCT and access to care for men having sex with men (MSM) is probably a habitus, a long tradition of subordination to State power (Bourdieu 2000). Indeed, habitus lies in a gradual incorporation of social structures, patterns of thoughts and social practice adjusted to social positions. React by habitus is reacting spontaneously, without any calculation or express intention (Bourdieu 2000). In other words, the social, economic and political environment in which Cameroonian stakeholders operate pushes them to react spontaneously on the side of the HIV/AIDS victims, without seeking the culprits or criticizing the capabilities and ways in which political authorities deal with the problem. This habitus of avoidance of politics and conflict maintain political neutrality, which not only strengthens the dominant position of the central government, but also marginalizes the cause for which they act collectively.

16.4.2 A Political Environment Not Particularly Favorable to Public Policies Entrepreneurship

It was with Paul Biya's accession to power in 1982 that the Cameroonian society witnessed some liberalization of the political space. President Biya is described as a liberal reformer in comparison to his predecessor Ahmadou Ahidjo, autocratic and backward looking (Bayart 1985; Bigombé Logo and Menthong 1996; Sindjoun and Courade 1996). This opening-up paved way for political debates and led to the public emergence of strengthened non-State social dynamics, as is the case with the fight against HIV/AIDS. These dynamics are, however, closely related to State power that partially regulates their existence through its ability to control and sanction.

Despite the evolution of the Cameroonian legal framework regarding freedom of the press, freedom of assembly in associations and political parties and to hold meetings,[5] the political openness of Cameroonian public action remains controlled

[5]Law of 19 December 1990 on the rights and freedoms of association, Freedom of the press and Freedom of assembly puts an end to close to 25 years of bans on freedom to publicly express political opinion contrary to that of the Unique party. Revised in 1996, this law extends even to collective and individual Cameroonian actors. This explains increase in the number of associations and NGOs will significantly increase and the dynamics of global mobilization against HIV/AIDS.

(Sindjoun 1996; Pommerolle 2008). The social and medical management of HIV infection in children demonstrates the constant centrality of the State and its institutions, as well as the weaknesses of decentralized actors. In fact, the concern for State control is permanent. This is the case with the National Committee to fight against HIV/AIDS, Malaria and Tuberculosis, which was established to coordinate the national response to HIV/AIDS (Country Coordinating Mechanism). These committees bring together all stakeholders involved in fighting AIDS: Government actors, financial partners, international actors, NGOs and local private associations or religious groups. Although this committee has many members who do not belong to State departments, its primary strategic positions are made by the Ministry of Public Health (the chair and the secretariat). This makes the government to be both judge and jury in the process of collective deliberations (Moulin 2004).

Including non-State actors in the political fight against HIV/AIDS is a dual meaning strategy for political and administrative authorities. They acquire some legitimacy among patients living with HIV/AIDS and increase their credibility vis-à-vis their international partners (Kojoué 2013). The constant centrality of State power is also explained by Cameroon tensed economic environment since the succession of structural adjustment plans that deeply undermined its ability to deliver public services (health, education, agriculture, and so on) since the early 1990s. The scarcity of public resources and new governance requirements required from States with limited resources by the World Bank or the International Monetary Fund put them in competition with the leadership of new stakeholders who are increasingly numerous. In this context, civil society therefore has several reasons to be wary of financial sanctions (no more subsidies), civil sanctions (closure and seizure of premises) or criminal sanctions (fines, trials and convictions). Those who dare to publicly oppose State power run the risk of being severely punished. This is the case of the leader of Positive Generation a Non-governmental association who has been fighting against AIDS since the early 2000s. This leader admits to have been taken to court so many times for disturbing public order and threatening the security of the State because his organization, has repeatedly organized public demonstrations to advocate for the rights of PLWHIV. The relatively confined management of public action for OVC, therefore, reflects a quest for strong State control, a quest that never dropped with the democratization of health policies.

16.5 Conclusion

Non-state stakeholders can play an important role in the political dynamics to fight AIDS in Cameroon, but only if they become involved politically. However, most of them exclude themselves from the political debate, and thereby, give a free rein to government officials to set up priorities and lead their implementation. This is what is revealed by the analysis of OVC national policies in Cameroon.

Several factors explain the non-politicization of civil society and AIDS-related actors. These factors are mostly related to the inability of civil society actors to disrupt social order and stand as entrepreneurs for public policies. This inability stems from internal and external constraints. Internally, the institutional and financial fragility makes any idea of autonomy and self-sufficiency to be delusive, but also creates distrust of established political order. At the external level, the authoritarian political context generates serious constraints, especially with regards to the will of some organizations and individual to participate out of formally instituted fields and standards. In addition, the risk of sanctions, together with institutional and organizational difficulties, significantly contributes to discard the issue of children and HIV/AIDS from national priorities, and even among priorities in fighting HIV/AIDS.

References

Bayart, J.-F. (1985). *L'Etat au Cameroun. Références* (2nd ed.). Paris: Presses de Science Po.

Becker, H. (1985). *Outsiders. Etudes de sociologie de la déviance* (3rd ed.). Paris: Métailié.

Bergeron, H., Castel, P., & Nouguez, E. (2011). Un entrepreneur privé de politique publique: la lutte contre l'obésité, entre santé publique et intérêt privé. *Revue Française de Science Politique, 61*(2), 201–229.

Bigombé Logo, P., & Menthong, H.-L. (1996). Crise de légitimité et évidence de la continuité politique. *Politique Africaine, 62*, 15–23.

Bourdieu, P. (2000) *Esquisse d'une théorie de la pratique*. Paris: Editions du Seuil, (Essais).

Cobb, R., & Elder, C. (1972). *Participation in American politics: The dynamics of agenda building*. Baltimore: John Hopkins University Press.

Eboko, F. (2002). La lutte contre le sida au Cameroun: de la verticlaité à la dispersion. In APAD, M.E. Gruénais (Ed.), *Un système de santé en mutation: le cas du Cameroun*, Bulletin de l'APAD, Vol. 21.

Eboko, F., & Kerouedan, D. (1999). *Politiques publiques du sida en Afrique*. Travaux et Documents du CEAN, Bordeaux, CEAN.

Eboko, F., & Mandjem, Y. (2010). ONG et associations de lutte contre le sida au Cameroun. De la subordination vers l'émancipation. In *Accès décentralisé au traitement du VIH/sida: évaluation de l'expérience camerounaise* (pp. 269–285). Sciences sociales et sida. Paris: ANRS.

Eboko, F., Bourdier, F., & Broqua, C. (2011). *Les Suds face au sida. Quand la société civile se mobilise. Objectifs Suds*. Marseille: IRD Editions.

Eisenstadt, S. N. (1980). Cultural orientations, institutional entrepreneurs, and social change: Comparative analysis of tradition civilizations. *American Journal of Sociology, 85*(4), 840–869.

Femba, S. D. (2007). *Analyse factorielle des correspondances multiples et classification automatique: appliction à la construction d'une grille d'éligibilité des OEV au Cameroun. Mémoire de Master*. Yaoundé: Ecole Nationale Supérieure Polytechnique de Yaoundé.

Fligstein, N. (2001). Social skill and the theory of the field. *Sociological Theory, 19*(2), 105–125.

Garraud, P. (1990). Politiques nationales: élaboration de l'agenda. *L'Année Sociologique, 40*, 17–41.

Gillespie, S., Norman, A., Finlay, B. (2005). *Child, vulnerability and HIV/AIDS in Subsaharan Africa: What we know and what can be done*. [http://www.ids.ac.uk/files/dmfile/gillespieovcsynth.pdf. Accessed 25 Oct 2008.

GTC-CNLS. (2008). *Rapport de progrès n 3*. Yaoundé: GTC/CNLS.

GTC-CNLS. (2012). *Estimation des ressources et des dépenses 2010 de lutte contre le VIH, le sida et les IST au Cameroun (REDES/NASA)*. Yaoundé: GTC/CNLS.

GTC-CNLS. (2013). *Rapport annuel sur l'épidémie de sida 2013*. Yaoundé: GTC/CNLS.

Hassenteufel, P. (2010). Les processus de mise sur agenda: sélection et construction des problèmes publics. *Informations Sociales, 1*(157), 50–58.

Hunter, S., & Williamson, J. (2000). *Children on the brink: Executive summary. Updated estimates and recommendation for intervention*. Washington, DC: USAID.

Jobert, B., & Muller, P. (1987). *L'Etat en action*. Paris: PUF.

Kingdon, J. W. (1984). *Agendas, alternatives and public policies*. Boston: Little Brown and Co.

Kojoué, L. (2013). *Enfants et VIH/sida au Cameroun. Construction et implications de l'agenda politique*. Thèse pour le doctorat en science politique. Bordeaux: Université Bordeaux IV/ED SP2/LAM, UMR 5115.

Lagroye, J. (2003). *La politisation*. Paris: Belin.

Lagroye, J. (2006). *Sociologie politique*. Paris: Presses de Science Po.

Moleux, M., Schaetzel, F., & Scotton, C. (2011). Les inégalités sociales de santé: déterminants sociaux et modèles d'action. http://www.ladocumentationfrancaise.fr/var/storage/rapports-publics/114000580/0000.pdf, http://www.ladocumentationfrancaise.fr/var/storage/rapports-publics/114000580/0000.pdf. Accessed 6 June 2011.

Moulin, B. (2004). *Missions d'Etudes sur le Fonctionnement des Instances de Coordination Pays (CCM). Cameroun* (p. 55). Paris: CREDES.

Muller, P. (2000). L'analyse cognitive des politiques publiques: vers une sociologie de l'action publique. *Revue Française de Science Politique, 50*(92), 189–207.

ONUSIDA. (2013). *Rapport mondial: Rapport ONUSIDA sur l'épidémie mondiale de sida 2013*. Genève: ONUSIDA.

Paxton, N. (2012). Political science(s) and HIV: A critical analysis. *Contemporary Politics, 18*(2), 141–155.

Piot, P. (2010). *L'épidémie du sida. Mondialisation des risques, transformations de la santé publique et développement, Leçon inaugurale, Chaire de recherché Savoirs contre pauvreté 2009–2010*. Paris: Collège de France.

Pommerolle, M.-E. (2008). La démobilisation collective au Cameroun: entre régime postautoritaire et militantisme extraverti. *Critique Internationale, 3*(40), 73–94.

Sindjoun, L. (1996). Le champ social camerounais: désordre inventif, mythes simplificateurs et stabilité hégémonique de l'Etat. *Politique Africaine, 62*, 57–67.

Sindjoun, L., & Courade, G. (1996). Introduction au thème. Le Cameroun dans l'entre-deux. *Politique Africaine, 62*, 3–14.

Singhal, A., Howard, S., & Esack, F. (2003). *The children of Africa confront AIDS: From vulnerability to possibility*. Athens: Ohio University Press.

Skinner, D., Tsheko, N., Mtero-Munyati, S., Segwabe, M., & Chibatamoto, P. (2004). *Defining orphaned and vulnerable children, Social Aspects oh HIV/AIDS and Health Research Programme*. Capetown: HSRC.

Stone, D. A. (1989). Causal stories and the formation of policy agendas. *Political Science Quaterly, 104*(2), 281–300.

UNAIDS, UNICEF, & USAID. (2004). *Children on the brink 2004. A joint report of new orphan estimates and a framework for action*. New York: UNICEF.

UNICEF. (2006). *Les générations orphelines et vulnérables d'Afrique. Les enfants affectés par le sida*. New York: UNICEF.

UNICEF. (2013). *Enfants et SIDA: sixième bilan de la situation 2013*. New York: UNICEF.

Williamson, J. (2008). *Children made vulnerable by HIV and AIDS. A look back from where we've come*. Washington, DC: USAID.

Chapter 17
Disclosure as a Positive Resource: The Lived Experiences of HIV-Positive Adolescents in Botswana

Vivian Midtbø and Marguerite Daniel

Contents

17.1 Introduction

In the context of antiretroviral treatment (ART), an increasing number of children infected with HIV are now surviving into adolescence and adulthood. In the early days of the epidemic, before the roll out of ART, children who were born with HIV were not expected to survive into adolescence. The roll out of ART has given this group of children a chance to live, and to live a close-to-normal life (see also Chap. 22 in this volume). This also means that a new generation of patients has emerged,

V. Midtbø (✉) • M. Daniel
Department of Health Promotion and Development, University of Bergen, PO Box 7807, 5020 Bergen, Norway
e-mail: vivian_1979@hotmail.com; marguerite.daniel@uib.no

P. Liamputtong (ed.), *Children and Young People Living with HIV/AIDS*, Cross-Cultural Research in Health, Illness and Well-Being,
DOI 10.1007/978-3-319-29936-5_17

together with issues that were not considered in the early days of the epidemic. Some of these new issues include disclosure; telling children and adolescents about their HIV status, and how to provide treatment and support to this new group of patients, to enable them to live a good quality life.

Botswana has the second highest prevalence rate of HIV in the world, with an estimated infection rate of 340,000, and 23 % of the population between 15 and 49 years old, and 11,000 children between the age of 0–14, being infected (UNAIDS 2013). Most of the adolescents living with HIV in Botswana today were born with it or contracted HIV as infants via breastfeeding. Furthermore, the AIDS epidemic has left many of the children and adolescents orphaned, having to adapt to new family arrangements. A large number of HIV-positive adolescents have for a great part of their life been unaware of their diagnosis, as their parents or caregivers have kept it a secret. This trend continues for children entering adolescence in spite of evidence pointing to the positive effects of disclosing adolescents' HIV status to them (Mellins et al. 2002; Bikaako-Kajura et al. 2006; Vaz et al. 2008). In Botswana, it is not common to speak openly about HIV and AIDS, and many keep their diagnosis a secret in fear of being stigmatized, discriminated and isolated from the rest of the community (Thupayagale-Tshweneagae 2010; see also Chaps. 5 and 6 in this volume).

According to UNAIDS, it was estimated that 49 % of those eligible for ART in Sub-Saharan Africa received treatment in 2010 (WHO/UNAIDS/UNICEF 2010). ART is not a cure, but it can slow down the development of HIV and AIDS for many years (see also Chap. 22 in this volume). Botswana introduced its ART program in 2002, aiming to offer treatment for all HIV-positive citizens (Bussmann et al. 2008), and by 2012, 86 % of those eligible[1] for treatment were receiving ART (UNAIDS 2013). ART is mostly supplied by the Botswana national government, however, international organizations, such as the Baylor International Pediatric AIDS Initiative (BIPAI), are involved in organizing the services around the treatment. In Botswana, these services include facilitating treatment to HIV-positive children and the provision of psychosocial services like Teen Club. Teen Club is a peer support group for HIV-positive adolescents between 13 and 19 years old, it can be found at several different sites in Botswana, and aims to improve the adolescents' clinical and mental health outcomes. In order to become a member of Teen Club, the adolescents have to have received disclosure (Baylor International Pediatric AIDS Initiative 2011).

Existing studies have looked at disclosure of children's and adolescents' HIV status in relation to barriers to disclosure (Kouyoumdjian et al. 2005; Vaz et al. 2008; Hejoaka 2009; Vreeman et al. 2010), positive effects of disclosure (Mellins et al. 2002; Bikaako-Kajura et al. 2006; Vaz et al. 2008), and the disclosure process

[1] A CD4 test is usually used to determine when a person should start ART. It measures the number of T-helper cells, which are an essential part of the immune system. HIV damages and destroys T-helper cells, resulting in a weakened immune system (WHO 2012). WHO recommends starting ART when a person with HIV has a CD4 count lower than 350 (WHO 2009).

in itself (Abadía-Barrero and LaRusso 2006; Lesch et al. 2007). Most of the studies are conducted from the perspective of caregivers (Hejoaka 2009; Vreeman et al. 2010; Vaz et al. 2011) or health care professionals (Gerson et al. 2001; Pfaff 2004; Salter-Goldie et al. 2007). Very few have focused on the adolescents' points of view, especially within Sub-Saharan Africa (Vaz et al. 2008, 2010). The literature mostly focuses on problems and challenges experienced by children and adolescents living with HIV, and to what degree they experience these problems compared to the general population. All of the above are important studies. However, few studies have evaluated HIV-positive adolescents who are thriving, in spite of living with a chronic and much stigmatized disease, and what resources contribute to their well-being. Literature tends to explore the negative aspects of living with HIV while few studies focus on adolescents' perspectives or the resources they draw on to cope, especially in Sub-Saharan Africa. As more HIV-positive children now enter adolescence, these are important gaps to fill in order to gain knowledge about what promotes well-being in this group of adolescents, and to enable them to reach their health potentials.

In this chapter, we explore the attitudes to disclosure of HIV-positive adolescents and their lived experiences before and after disclosure, especially regarding their understanding of their life situation, and accessing positive resources that enables the adolescents to live healthily with HIV.

17.2 Theoretical Framework

This chapter is based on the concept of 'thriving' which denotes growth and development, in spite of – or because of – adversity (Feeney and Collins 2014). According to Ickovics and Park (1998: 238), thriving implies that "challenge can provide the impetus for growth and greater well-being". Carver (1998: 247) defines thriving as a situation where "a person can be better off after adversity than beforehand" and distinguishes it from resilience where a person simply returns to their prior situation after adversity. With resilience, a person may develop a resistance to the adversity or the ability to 'bounce back faster' when adversity hits again, but a person who thrives will be able to function at a higher level. Ryff and Singer (2003) refer to the linked concept of posttraumatic growth where severe suffering is followed by significant beneficial change in both cognitive and emotional spheres. Carver (1998) admits that thriving may be difficult to evaluate but he suggests three features to look for, namely skills and knowledge, confidence, and strengthened personal relationships. Acquired skills and knowledge may help a person to deal with future problems and uncertainty with greater flexibility. Surviving adversity (along with increased skills and knowledge) can lead to greater confidence and sustain the person's efforts to cope. Adversity has social consequences, for example, if a person experiencing adversity receives help, this can develop a sense of security in the relationships involved. Thriving is transformative in the sense that "it is contingent on a fundamental cognitive shift in response to a challenge" (O'Leary 1998: 430).

17.3 The Study

The findings presented in this chapter are based on data collected in Botswana between June and September 2011. This phenomenological study sought to explore the lived experiences of adolescents living with HIV. The study received ethical approval from both the Norwegian Social Sciences Data Services (NSD) and the Regional Committee for Medical and Health Research in Norway as well as from the Ministry of Health in Botswana. Ethical guidelines were rigorously followed and written informed consent (assent for those under 18) was obtained from all the participants; for those under the age of 18, written or oral consent was obtained from their caregivers as well.

Data were collected from two sites, a hospice in one of the poorest suburbs of a city and a village hospital. Participants were purposively recruited with the help of staff at each institution to include adolescents between the ages of 12 and 20, who had received disclosure, and were on ART. In addition, the purpose was to include as participants adolescents who were coping well with their life situation. Adolescents who were in a state of acute illness were, for ethical reasons, not included. Participants (see Table 17.1) in the study included 16 adolescents (10 girls and 6 boys) and 3 staff members.

Individual interviews were conducted with all the staff and all the adolescents at the hospice. Two focus groups were conducted at the village hospital and from participants in the groups, four adolescents were selected for individual interviews. Semi-structured interview guides were used throughout. Staff were asked for their perspectives on the adolescents' experiences of living with HIV, using ART and coping with stigma. Adolescents were asked about resources that helped them to cope, relationships with families and friends, their experiences of and thoughts about disclosure, and how they coped with challenges and stigma. With the exception of one girl, we worked with an interpreter for all interviews with adolescents. All interviews and focus group sessions were recorded, with permission, and later transcribed. The Setswana sections were transcribed by a second assistant (not the interpreter) and translated by a third assistant. The first author participated in several of the group activities on offer to the adolescents. This provided additional insight into the adolescents' environment and their relationships with each other.

Data were analyzed using Attride-Stirling's (2001) thematic network analysis within the framework of the objectives of this chapter. Eighteen basic themes emerged (see Table 17.2 below) which were then grouped into seven organizing themes and further clustered into three global themes. The analysis has helped structure our findings section below.

Table 17.1 Overview of study participants

	Female	Male	Age
Adolescents	10	6	12–20
Staff	2	1	

Table 17.2 Themes emerging from data analysis

Basic themes	Organizing themes	Global themes
Seeking reasons for treatment	Before disclosure things did not make sense	Disclosure enables the adolescents to understand life situation
Feeling of anger and confusion		
Refused to take medications	Problems with adherence before receiving disclosure	
Using medications wrong		
Want to know their status	Adolescents think it is important to know their status	
Thankful to the one who disclosed/ lifesaver		
To know who they are/their identity		
Knows importance of medicines	Disclosure makes adhering to treatment regimen meaningful	Disclosure enables the adolescents to deal with their disease
Knowledge about HIV		
Access to guidance on how to live healthy	Disclosure enables the adolescents to take control over their health	
Know how to take care of themselves		
Advise others to follow treatment regimen		
Friends in Teen club	Participation in Teen Club meetings	Disclosure facilitates access to social support
Share their problems		
Support from others in the same situation through Teen club		
Social confidence	Disclosure contributes to a secure base	
Disclose to a friend		
Resist stigma		

17.4 Disclosure and Understanding of Life Situation

All the participants enrolled in this study had received disclosure. All of them wanted to know their status, and they thought it was important that they knew. Receiving disclosure helped them to understand aspects of their life, which had previously made them confused and angry.

Most of the adolescents remembered the time before disclosure. Many of them reported on aspects of life that were difficult, or confusing, before receiving disclosure, for instance being on a medication regimen without knowing why, and a sense of not knowing what was going on in their life.

17.4.1 Before Disclosure Things Did Not Make Sense

Understanding one's life situation is difficult when information about why things are happening is lacking. Many of the participants reported having to continue taking medications without knowing why. Kasigo,[2] 19, explained that she could not

[2] All names are pseudonyms.

understand this: “Why should I keep on taking the same medicine?” When asking for reasons for the never-ending medication regimes, the most common answer the adolescents received was “to make you feel better”.

> They said for me to get better. They just told me that if I don’t take the pills I will continue getting ill (Kasigo, 19)

Henry, 12, explained the uncertainty before receiving disclosure by telling how he used to find himself at the hospital without knowing what was going on. This feeling of confusion was confirmed by several of the other participants.

17.4.2 Before Receiving Disclosure Many Had Problems with Adherence

Before knowing the reason for the medication regimen, participants found adherence meaningless and difficult. Kasigo, 19, explained:

> Because I was angry with them…why do I keep on taking these pills, then they just told me… It is important to know. Sometimes I just refused to take my pills.

Only once she started to question her medication regimen did Kasigo finally receive disclosure. Problems with adherence prior to receiving disclosure were also confirmed by several others, one of the girls, Kefilwe (19) said: “I used to refuse to drink pills until I was told when I was 16 years old”.

Incidences of wrong use of medications before disclosure were also reported. Lerato, 14, told us that although she was only supposed to take the medications in the morning and in the evening, she also used to take it during the day if she had a headache, because she had been told that the medications would make her feel better. Kefilwe, 19, confirmed this issue: “If we are not addressed, there is a possibility that we can overdose on them”.

Staff confirmed many of the issues that the adolescents reported. Kefentse explained how children and adolescents who had not received disclosure were curious about their medication, as they grew older. Because HIV is talked about on TV and radio, and they also saw the medications on TV, the children were able to make the connection between what they saw and their own medication. When they had not received disclosure, they were left with their suspicions about what their medications were for.

> Most of them will just be taking their medication not knowing this why…But as they grow up they wonde, because they hear about the HIV on TV and radio. (Kefentse, staff)

17.4.3 Adolescents Think It Is Important to Know Their Status

When discussing whether children and adolescents should receive disclosure or not, all the adolescents participating in the study made it clear that they wanted to know their status, and they expressed that it was important for them to know. Thobo, 19, explicitly described how he saw disclosure as a lifesaving event for him.

> It is important to know because I feel like that person who told me...saved my life... Without that person, maybe I would have been dead by now.

If he had not been told, he would not have known how to live with the disease and how to take care of himself. Tebogo, 19, saw disclosure as important in relation to learning to accept his situation: "So that I can accept my status...be comfortable and to accept everything that happens in my life".

Not only disclosure contributed to explain events from the past, it could also lead some of the adolescents to redefine themselves. Thobo, 19, pointed out the importance of not losing hope when he received disclosure:

> I have to do whatever it takes to feel better, to be the Thobo who I saw myself as. I don't have to feel like now is the end of the world for me...my mother died of HIV...so I knew maybe that was the reason why it happened...So I am glad I am alive

Some adolescents also raised the question why they had not been told earlier, suggesting that earlier disclosure could prevent the shock of receiving the truth about their HIV status when they had become teenagers. When the first author suggested that their caregivers might have been worried that the child would be scared or upset, Lerato, 14, stated: "That is why they have to start early".

The adolescents' statements about the importance of disclosure were reflected in the interviews with staff, who also saw disclosure as important. They also thought the adolescents themselves saw it as important to receive disclosure. The staff related disclosure to enabling the adolescents to understand what was going on in their lives:

> They find it important for them to be disclosed to. So they really know what is happening in their life...they are starting to realize who they are, to take care of themselves... (Boitumelo, staff)

17.5 Disclosure as a Positive Resource for Dealing with the Disease

17.5.1 Disclosure Made Adhering to Treatment Regimen Meaningful

Before disclosure, many of the participants had been taking medications and attending check-ups at the hospital without knowing why. Serama, 13, talked about the importance of disclosure in relation to her medication regimen: "Because I was not going to understand why I am taking treatment". The staff also pointed to how non-disclosure affected the adolescents in the way that they did not have a chance to understand the consequences of not following up, or adhering to their treatment: "They should understand how it will affect them if they don't take their medications" (Kefentse, staff). Some participants also remarked that before receiving disclosure, they did not really know the meaning of HIV: "I only heard that there was something like HIV...not really knowing the meaning of it" (Henry, 12).

17.5.2 Disclosure Enabled the Adolescents to Take Control of Their Health

After receiving disclosure, the adolescents were able to access more knowledge and information regarding their status, and how to live safely with HIV. This particularly occurred through treatment services like their regular check-ups at the hospital and Teen Club meetings. Teen Club is a social support group for HIV-positive adolescents aged 13–19 years old, which can be found in several sites throughout Botswana. During the first author's stay in the field, she attended Teen Club meetings in both the city and village. The program combines access to knowledge and information on various themes, with health personnel available to answer questions, and sports and games activities. Themes discussed in the meetings included HIV, treatment, reproductive health, how to prevent transmission of the virus, and how to deal with different challenges related to HIV such as disclosure, stigma and discrimination. These services were a source of guidance on how to live a healthy life. Kasigo, 19, explained how the nurse at the hospital: "Just kept on supporting, just guiding, what to do and what not to do". Disclosure enabled the adolescents to have meaningful conversations with the health personnel during their check-ups, regarding their disease, advice and guidance on how to live with it.

For most participants, because they knew their status they were better able to take care of themselves. One of the girls, Marea, 14, stated that because she knew her status she knew how to take care of herself when she grew up. Kasigo, 19, too expressed that "…we have to grow up knowing our status and how to live, to share our problems with others". The staff emphasized that although receiving an HIV diagnosis could be difficult, it gave the adolescents a chance to take care of themselves and the opportunity to live a healthy life.

> They can feel sad, but after all they know…they know how to look after themselves and handle themselves. (Letsego, staff)

The adolescents' knowledge on aspects of their disease was also evident in their answers when asked what they would advise other adolescents who had just received disclosure.

> If you are positive or negative, just don't practice the MCP, multi concurrent partner, don't do it. (Kasigo, 19)

> I just tell them to drink their medications in time, go to the check-ups regularly, and not to have many partners. (Marea, 14)

The adolescent's statements show that they are aware of how the virus transmits, and from these statements it is also evident how important the medication regimen is to them.

> I can advise him not to give up, take his treatment in a good way, and accept his status. (Katie, 16)

17.6 Disclosure and Access to Social Support

Disclosure brought opportunities that the adolescents would not have benefited from without disclosure. Receiving disclosure gave adolescents access to Teen Club, where they met other adolescents in the same situation. In Teen Club, the adolescents could be open about their status, and they found social support from other adolescents in the same situation. Thobo, 19, explained that "I have a lot of friends here…we are having a good time". Kasigo, 19, too suggested that it was important to seek support from others:

> If she or he has a problem, just share with someone, someone which you think will just help.

Kasigo went on to explain how she met others in the same situation as herself through Teen Club, and how they were open to talk to each other and to share the same problems. The teens were very comfortable in each other's company, and it seemed that they had a strong relationship. When the first author observed them at the club meeting, they seemed to have a lot of fun in each other's company, they were chatting, laughing a lot, dancing together to the music from their mobile phones.

Many of the adolescents participating in this study seemed to be very strong and confident, in spite of living with a very stigmatizing disease, indicating that they somehow had a secure base. Confidence was expressed though active participation in games and discussions, and taking part in organizing activities. During the discussion sessions with staff, the adolescents also showed a great level of knowledge regarding the themes discussed. Teen Club seemed to contribute to building the adolescents' confidence and belief in themselves.

Due to fear of being stigmatized, most of the adolescents reported that they would not disclose their status to anyone outside the family or the treatment system. Serama, 13, expressed: "They will discriminate me from their friends". Thobo, 19, also feared how he would be treated if he disclosed his status to others:

> No I feel like they will abandon me, you know. Sometimes I feel like they really don't know anything about HIV.

The staff problematized how everyone was hiding their status from each other:

> Sometimes they think: "I'm not the same as that child". Maybe they are the same,…they don't know whether they are positive just because they can't get open to each other. They don't know, each and everybody is hiding their status. (Letsego, staff).

However, three of the participants reported to have disclosed their status to one or a few close friends. They did this because they wanted their friends to understand their situation and because it felt better when someone knew.

> I chose to tell, because there was a time when I…came for a check-up every month, and he just wanted to know why…then I told him. (Kasigo, 19)

Instead of having to hide the reason for all the hospital check-ups, Kasigo found it better to tell the truth. Marea, 14, told us that she felt better after disclosing to some of her friends, she wanted them to understand.

Stigmatization of people living with HIV and AIDS remains a challenge in Botswana, and is the main reason why people choose to keep their status a secret. However, many of the participants in our study showed that they were able to cope with disclosing to others, and they somehow managed to turn the knowledge of their status into something positive when dealing with stigma. Many of them seemed to find confidence in knowing their status in the sense that they at least knew how to live their lives with HIV, compared to those who did not know their status. Being part of a support group, such as Teen Club, also seemed to make them more able to resist stigma, knowing that they had friends in the same situation that would support them.

17.7 Discussion

The findings suggest that disclosure is a positive resource, which contributes to the adolescents experiencing more control over their health.

17.7.1 Disclosure Enables the Adolescents to Understand Their Life Situation

There are different patterns of disclosure, from not disclosing anything at all, to partial disclosure, to full disclosure. According to Wiener et al. (2007), partial disclosure is the most common form of disclosure, which means that the child is told something, but not everything about his/her condition. In addition, several studies suggest that a relatively high number of caregivers provide their children with deflecting information about their disease, with evidence from Sub-Saharan Africa, Europe, and Asia (Waugh 2003; Oberdorfer et al. 2006; Vaz et al. 2011). Giving the child deflecting information includes telling the child that he or she has a lung disease, allergy, or explicitly lying to the child by saying that he or she is sick, but does not have HIV (Oberdorfer et al. 2006; Vaz et al. 2011). In our study, many of the participants had received partial disclosure before receiving full disclosure. Before disclosure, they were told that they had to take the medications to stay healthy and to prevent them from getting ill, or to make them feel better. This often caused confusion and they did not understand what was going on in their life in relation to having to take medications every day and go to hospital check-ups when they did not feel ill.

One participant in our study, Kasigo, reported that she sometimes refused to take her medications because she was angry for not knowing why she had to take them.

There were similar findings in a study in Uganda where children who had received only partial disclosure had poor adherence, questioned their medication regimen, took medications at the wrong times or in the wrong dosages (Bikaako-Kajura et al. 2006). Studies from South Africa and the United Kingdom reveal that children frequently ask questions about their disease, and that caregivers still avoid disclosing to the child, giving explanations other than the truth or avoiding the question (Waugh 2003; Kouyoumdjian et al. 2005).

In a case study from South Africa, Pfaff (2004) discusses the dilemma of keeping the HIV status secret from a child. He discusses the concept of beneficence of knowing versus non-maleficence. However, Pfaff also admits that one has to consider the situation and the child's environment and cultural factors. He highlights how western cultural values focus on individual rights, while in an African context one has to consider a more family centered approach. Pfaff (2004) recommends that disclosure should be carefully planned and that one should avoid the child discovering his or her diagnosis accidentally.

Thobo, one participant in our study, showed clearly that he managed to relate previous life experiences to his diagnosis when he eventually received disclosure. His mother died from AIDS when he was around 11 years old. When he received disclosure at the age of 13, he knew he had the disease because his mother also had it. In spite of the experience of losing his mother and being told the truth about his HIV diagnosis, Thobo was glad that he was alive, and felt that the person who told him he had HIV had saved his life. He adhered to his medications and stated that he was strong and able to lead a normal life like everyone else. Thobo's experiences and response can be described as an example of the beneficence of knowing as theorized by Pfaff (2004).

For many of the participants in our study, some aspects of their life, such as the medication regimens and hospital check-ups, were difficult to understand prior to disclosure. Disclosure enabled the adolescents to make sense out of these life events, and also helped them to see them as meaningful and important.

17.7.2 Disclosure Is a Positive Resource That Enables the Adolescents to Deal with Their Disease

The participants in this study found disclosure important in relation to several aspects, but the most frequently mentioned one was that disclosure enabled them to take care of themselves. They related this to the opportunity to learn how to live with their condition by gaining information and knowledge about HIV and the treatment regimen, enabling them to adhere to treatment, to use the medical and support services more actively, and to protect themselves and others from re-infection and infection of the virus (see also Chaps. 5, 6, and 22 in this volume).

It was clear that receiving disclosure was important for all participants. When we were discussing the issue of disclosure, the adolescents had strong opinions on it, and discussed it actively. Studies from both Tanzania and the DRC (Vaz et al. 2008, 2010; Midtbø et al. 2012) report similar findings, where children prefer to know their status. In studies conducted by Vaz and colleagues (2008, 2010) from the DRC, children expressed gratitude that they received disclosure as children and not when they were adults. In spite of negative feelings at the moment of disclosure, they thought it was better to know what they were suffering from. The health care personnel's view in this study was consistent with reports from previous studies, which suggest that health care personnel support disclosure to children and adolescents more often than the children's caregivers (Pfaff 2004; Lesch et al. 2007).

Several participants in our study expressed that if they did not know their status, they would not be able to take care of themselves and learn to live with their condition. They related being able to take care of themselves to knowledge about the virus itself and their treatment regimen. Studies from Uganda and the DRC have found disclosure of HIV status to children and adolescents to be one of the factors that facilitates good adherence to drug regimens (Bikaako-Kajura et al. 2006; Vaz et al. 2008). Studies from Kenya and Thailand also suggest that caregivers, in spite of not disclosing their children's HIV status, still perceive positive outcomes of disclosure such as improved adherence to ART (Oberdorfer et al. 2006; Vreeman et al. 2010). Strong statements like the way Thobo expressed gratitude to the one who told him about his positive HIV status clearly illustrate how important he found disclosure to be. Thobo felt that if he had not been told he might have been dead by now. All the adolescents in our study saw the importance of adhering to their treatment, and medication was among the most important things in their lives (see also Chaps. 4, 5, 6, and 22 in this volume). This coincides with statements from children in the study by Bikaako-Kajura et al. (2006) from Uganda, where children who received disclosure reported that they depended on the drugs, and made sure they did not miss a dose even if it involved hiding somewhere while taking their medicine, because they did not want others to see them take it. With evidence like this pointing to important, potentially lifesaving, effects of disclosure to children and adolescents, and also when considering how important disclosure was to the participants in our study, the continuing low level of disclosure implies that many HIV-positive children and adolescents have their chances of survival undermined.

Disclosure also enabled the participants to use the medical and support services more actively; because they now knew what they were there for, they were no longer going to check-ups without knowing why. They could ask questions and seek advice from the health care personnel when attending their check-ups. Communication with the health care personnel improves after disclosure compared to when the patient does not know the real reason for the consultation (Midtbø et al. 2012). Before disclosure, the patient is not in a position to ask relevant questions about his or her health condition, and it is difficult for the health care personnel to give the patient advice about how to best handle his or her condition. Vaz et al. (2010), in a study in the DRC, confirm this dilemma, reporting that children rarely communicated directly with health care providers about their illness before disclosure. A study from Romania (Ferris et al. 2007) suggests that children and adolescents, in the context of ART, who are informed about their HIV status, might receive closer clinically monitoring, and that the opportunity to discuss their HIV status in light of ART might have an empowering effect on the adolescents. Kouyoumdjian et al. (2005) also argue that children with HIV will not be able to reach their full health potential if they are not able to discuss HIV, including with their families.

Many of the participants showed a very constructive way of dealing with their situation, and they were clear that they would not have been so well off if they were not informed about their HIV status. Even those as young as 12–14, demonstrated a high level of knowledge, for instance detailed knowledge about HIV, the medication, issues concerning reproductive health and how to keep themselves and others safe from transmission. These findings are very similar to those found in a Tanzanian study, where children and adolescents who had received disclosure and were enrolled in a treatment regimen also showed a significant level of knowledge, even referring to their improving CD4 counts (Shirima 2012). Our participants gained a lot of this knowledge through Teen Club and conversations with health care staff. Similarly, the participants from the Tanzanian study accessed knowledge and skills through group activities and seminars arranged as part of their treatment regimen (Shirima 2012). Such important knowledge would have been difficult to access if the adolescents had not received disclosure, enabling them to participate in these groups.

Knowledge is one of the features Carver (1998) identifies as evidence of thriving. Certainly, in the case of the participants in our study, the knowledge that could only be gained after disclosure led to growth and development (Ryff and Singer 2003; Feeney and Collins 2014) as they gained confidence and competence and took control of their health and medication.

17.7.3 Disclosure Facilitates Access to Social Support

The findings from the study did not imply that any of the participants had suffered from receiving disclosure; rather the opposite was the case. One of the most important reasons for supporting disclosure was that with disclosure comes improved access to social support and treatment services, compared to if one has not received disclosure. Social support is identified by several authors as contributing to thriving (Carver 1998; Ryff and Singer 2003; Feeney and Collins 2014). When identifying features of thriving, Carver (1998: 252) uses the term "strengthened personal relationships" which is more than just receiving social support, it implies having meaningful relationships where one is sufficiently secure to share at a deeper level.

The relationship between disclosure and improved access to social support became evident through Teen Club, which can only be accessed by those who have received disclosure. Teen Club was an invaluable resource for the adolescents, both when it came to social support and gaining knowledge about their condition. Members trusted each other, were supportive and cared about each other. This relationship between social support and disclosure has also been discussed by Menon et al. (2007: 349), who argue that "interventions to promote disclosure could facilitate access to emotional and peer support". Kasigo, one participant in our study, mentioned how disclosure was important to her in relation to being able to share problems with others. Her statement shows how it can be strengthening to engage with others who have similar life experiences, which can prevent feelings of loneliness in one's situation and enhance the feeling of belonging (Correll and Park 2005). Teen Club provided the opportunity to meet other adolescents in the same situation, and in a safe environment where they did not worry about being looked down at or discriminated because of their HIV status. The participants expressed that it was good to have a place where they could be completely open. Petersen et al. (2010), in a study from South Africa, suggest that being with others in the same situation is particularly helpful, which is also supported by the findings in this study. The adolescents saw others living healthily with HIV, which helped them to not feel alone in their situation. Also the staff thought Teen Club made a considerable difference in these adolescents' lives, and had a very positive attitude towards the support group. When the club-meetings were held, one of the staff from the adolescents' treatment venue was always present which may have contributed to the adolescents feeling comfortable and safe within their support group.

Teen Club contributed to the participants adhering to their treatment regimens. Being in a group together, sharing the same challenges makes it easier to approach and deal with them, especially because of the feeling of not being alone in their situation. Previous studies have found that being member of a social support group has a positive effect on adhering to medication regimens (Gerson et al. 2001; Steele et al. 2007).

In relation to supportive networks, it was quite evident how Teen Club was a positive resource for the adolescents in our study. For those who have not received disclosure, it is likely that they miss out on important social support by not being able to access Teen Club, or meaningfully make use of other types of social support.

Three of the participants had disclosed their status to a few, or one, good friend that they trusted outside their family and the treatment system. In a setting where fear of discrimination and stigmatization due to HIV is deeply rooted in the society, adolescents who disclose their positive HIV status to someone outside the family or the treatment system are extraordinary. The participants' motivation for disclosing their status to others was that it felt good that their friends knew, and they wanted them to understand. It was also easier to explain why they had to miss school on the days when they had to go to the hospital for check-ups. These findings corroborate findings from studies in the USA and Switzerland (Wiener and Battles 2006; Michaud et al. 2009), where participants experienced that disclosure made the situation easier. Another study from the USA also suggests that greater disclosure is associated with increased social support, social self-competence and decreased problem behavior (Battles and Wiener 2002). By disclosing their status to peers, the adolescents in our study showed that they were empowered and in a position to take their own decisions regarding who to disclose to and where to seek support. This is clearly relating to the features of thriving; this is an example of security in relationships mentioned by Carver (1998).

To disclose their status to friends could also be related to seeking acceptance for who they were, which in turn can also be helpful in creating a feeling of normalcy, to not having to lie and hide aspects of one's life. This finding contradicts findings in a study from Botswana, assessing adolescents' behaviors to prevent stigmatization (Thupayagale-Tshweneagae 2010) where adolescents kept silent to avoid people finding out they had HIV. However, Thupayagale-Tshweneagae's finding is consistent with those adolescents in our study who had not disclosed their status to friends. Similar to the adolescents in Thupayagale-Tshweneage's study, they kept silent to avoid being stigmatized and discriminated against. Keeping ones status secret is common, not only in Botswana, but also elsewhere in Sub-Saharan Africa as well as countries outside of Africa (Wiener and Battles 2006; Michaud et al. 2009; Daniel 2015). One of the challenges in combating the spread of HIV is the remaining stigma that surrounds HIV, which in turn contributes to people's fear to talk about the disease (Duffy 2005; Thupayagale-Tshweneagae 2010). Looking at these resources in a greater perspective, disclosure together with social support groups, such as Teen Club, giving the adolescents confidence to disclose their status to friends, could potentially contribute to the breakdown of the stigma associated with HIV.

In our study, the staff did not recommend that adolescents disclose their status to others, due to the possibility of being stigmatized. However, the adolescents were able to be careful and strategic in the process of whom to disclose to. Although they chose to share their status with some friends, they were still selective and would not tell everyone, due to fear of stigmatization. Literature on adolescents in Sub-Saharan Africa disclosing their status to friends, or someone outside the family, treatment system or school system is rare. However, there is some literature on the theme from the USA, suggesting that adolescents who disclose their status to peers, have a significantly larger increase in their CD4 count compared to those who have not disclosed their status, and that they are able to have a more open and satisfactory relationship with their friends, not having to worry about what will happen if their friends find out about their status (Sherman et al. 2000; Wiener and Battles 2006). On the contrary, public disclosure has also been found to be associated with lower self-competence (Battles and Wiener 2002). However, studies suggest that most adolescents keep their status secret from people outside of the family and the treatment system, like the participating staff in our study also advised (Mellins et al. 2002; Petersen et al. 2010; Daniel 2015). WHO (2011) has recommended the issue of social disclosure, or the benefits of identifying a 'safe' person outside the family, as one that needs further research, as there is not much empirical literature written on the subject.

The adolescents in our study can be described as thriving: they were functioning at a higher level since disclosure (see also Chaps. 5 and 6 in this volume). They demonstrated all aspects mentioned by Carver (1998) as features of thriving. Disclosure led to knowledge which in turn contributed to their confidence and competence in managing their own medication and interacting with the health services. Along with knowledge and confidence these adolescents had significantly strengthened personal relationships making them stronger and better off than they were before they received disclosure. Their response to disclosure had transformed their understanding, competence and social relationships.

Disclosure on its own, without access to knowledge and social support such as Teen Club, might not facilitate the same level of thriving as we found in this group of adolescents. It seems the combination of disclosure and social support gave the adolescents a unique group feeling, a feeling of belonging, which seemed to be some of the key factors in their development of self-esteem and coping with HIV (also important in relation to adherence to treatment). It seems that this type of support also can enhance the process of disclosing own HIV status to others, outside the family, like disclosure to friends.

17.8 Conclusion

Receiving disclosure was an important positive resource for the adolescents who participated in this study, and they especially related this to how disclosure enabled them to take care of themselves in relation to living with HIV. Disclosure enabled them to actively take part in their treatment regimens and many of them showed a high level of knowledge concerning the nature of their disease and how to handle it. Disclosure also helped the adolescents to understand their life situation in the sense that their treatment regimen made sense and they were able to make sense out of previous disease-related experiences. Another very important resource facilitated by disclosure was the opportunity to access social support through support groups such as Teen Club, and seeking support from family and friends. Some of the participants reported seeking support by disclosing their status to friends outside of their family or treatment system.

References

Abadía-Barrero, C. E., & LaRusso, M. D. (2006). The disclosure model versus a developmental illness experience model for children and adolescents living with HIV/AIDS in Sao Paulo, Brazil. *AIDS Patient Care & STDs, 20*(1), 36–43.

Attride-Stirling, J. (2001). Thematic networks: An analytic tool for qualitative research. *Qualitative Research, 1*(3), 385–405.

Battles, H. B., & Wiener, L. (2002). From adolescence through young adulthood: Psychosocial adjustment associated with long-term survival of HIV. *Journal of Adolescent Health, 30*(3), 161–168.

Baylor International Pediatric AIDS Initiative (2011). *Programs for Botswanas HIV-infected adolescents*. Retrieved March 27, 2012, http://bipai.org/Botswana/adolescent-programs.aspx#teenclub.

Bikaako-Kajura, W., Luyirika, E., Purcell, D. W., Downing, J., Kaharuza, F., Mermin, J., et al. (2006). Disclosure of HIV status and adherence to daily drug regimens among HIV-infected children in Uganda. *AIDS and Behavior, 10*, S85–S93.

Bussmann, H., Wester, C. W., Ndwapi, N., Grundmann, N., Gaolathe, T., Puvimanasinghe, J., et al. (2008). Five year outcomes of initial patients treated in Botswana's national antiretroviral treatment program. *AIDS, 22*(17), 2303–2311.

Carver, C. S. (1998). Resilience and thriving: Issues, models, and linkages. *Journal of Social Issues, 54*(2), 245–266.

Correll, J., & Park, B. (2005). A model of the ingroup as a social resource. *Personality and Social Psychology Review, 9*(4), 341–359.

Daniel, M. (2015). Keeping the secret: How HIV positive children in Iringa, Tanzania respond to the perceived need for silence and secrecy. *Journal of Child & Adolescent Mental Health, 26*. doi: 10.2989/17280583.2014.947995.

Duffy, L. (2005). Suffering, shame and silence: The stigma of HIV/AIDS. *Journal of the Association of Nurses in AIDS Care, 16*(1), 13–20.

Feeney, B. C., & Collins, N. L. (2014). A theoretical perspective on the importance of social connections for thriving. In M. Mikulincer & P. R. Shaver (Eds.), *Mechanisms of social connection: From brain to group* (pp. 291–394). Washington, DC: American Psychological Association.

Ferris, M., Burau, K., Schweitzer, A., Mihale, S., Murray, N., Preda, A., et al. (2007). The influence of disclosure of HIV diagnosis on time to disease progression in a cohort of Romanian children and teens. *AIDS Care, 19*(9), 1088–1094.

Gerson, A. C., Joyner, M., Fosarelli, P., Butz, A., Wissow, L., Lee, S., et al. (2001). Disclosure of HIV diagnosis to children: When, where, why, and how. *Journal of Pediatric Health Care, 15*(4), 161–167.

Hejoaka, F. (2009). Care and secrecy: Being a mother of children living with HIV in Burkina Faso. *Social Science & Medicine, 69*(6), 869–876.

Ickovics, J. R., & Park, C. L. (1998). Paradigm shift: Why a focus on health is important. *Journal of Social Issues, 54*(2), 237–244.

Kouyoumdjian, F. G., Meyers, T., & Mtshizana, S. (2005). Barriers to disclosure to children with HIV. *Journal of Tropical Pediatrics, 51*(5), 285–287.

Lesch, A., Swartz, L., Kagee, A., Moodley, K., Kafaar, Z., Myer, L., et al. (2007). Paediatric HIV/AIDS disclosure: Towards a developmental and process-oriented approach. *AIDS Care, 19*(6), 811–816.

Mellins, C. A., Brackis-Cott, E., Dolezal, C., Richards, A., Nicholas, S. W., & Abrams, E. J. (2002). Patterns of HIV status disclosure to perinatally HIV-infected children and subsequent mental health outcomes. *Clinical Child Psychology and Psychiatry, 7*(1), 101–114.

Menon, A., Glazebrook, C., Campain, N., & Ngoma, M. (2007). Mental health and disclosure of HIV status in Zambian adolescents with HIV infection: Implications for peer-support programs. *Journal of Acquired Immune Deficiency Syndromes, 46*(3), 349–354.

Michaud, P.-A., Suris, J.-C., Thomas, L. R., Kahlert, C., Rudin, C., & Cheseaux, J.-J. (2009). To say or not to say: A qualitative study on the disclosure of their condition by human immunodeficiency virus–positive adolescents. *Journal of Adolescent Health, 44*(4), 356–362.

Midtbø, V., Shirima, V., Skovdal, M., & Daniel, M. (2012). How disclosure and antiretroviral therapy help HIV-infected adolescents in sub-Saharan Africa cope with stigma. *African Journal of AIDS Research, 11*(3), 487–497.

O'Leary, V. E. (1998). Strength in the face of adversity: Individual and social thriving. *Journal of Social Issues, 54*(2), 425–446.

Oberdorfer, P., Puthanakit, T., Louthrenoo, O., Charnsil, C., Sirisanthana, V., & Sirisanthana, T. (2006). Disclosure of HIV/AIDS diagnosis to HIV-infected children in Thailand. *Journal of Paediatrics and Child Health, 42*(5), 283–288.

Petersen, I., Bhana, A., Myeza, N., Alicea, S., John, S., Holst, H., et al. (2010). Psychosocial challenges and protective influences for socio-emotional coping of HIV+ adolescents in South Africa: A qualitative investigation. *AIDS Care, 22*(8), 970–978.

Pfaff, C. (2004). Telling a child he is HIV positive. *South African Family Practice, 46*(9), 35–40.

Ryff, C. D., & Singer, B. (2003). Flourishing under fire: Resilience as a prototype of challenged thriving. In C. L. M. Keyes & J. Haidt (Eds.), *Flourishing: Positive psychology and the life well-lived* (pp. 15–36). Washington, DC: American Psychological Association.

Salter-Goldie, R., King, S. M., Smith, M. L., Bitnun, A., Brophy, J., Fernandes-Penney, A., et al. (2007). Disclosing HIV diagnosis to infected children: A health care team's approach. *Vulnerable Children and Youth Studies, 2*(1), 12–16. doi:10.1080/17450120701238235.

Sherman, B. F., Bonanno, G. A., Wiener, L. S., & Battles, H. B. (2000). When children tell their friends they have AIDS: Possible consequences for psychological well-being and disease progression. *Psychosomatic Medicine, 62*(2), 238–247.

Shirima, V. L. (2012). *Thriving despite stigma: A qualitative study of HIV positive children in Dar es Salaam, Tanzania. Salutogenic approach.* Unpublished Master's thesis, University of Bergen, Bergen.

Steele, R. G., Nelson, T. D., & Cole, B. P. (2007). Psychosocial functioning of children with AIDS and HIV infection: Review of the literature from a socioecological framework. *Journal of Developmental & Behavioral Pediatrics, 28*(1), 58–69.

Thupayagale-Tshweneagae, G. (2010). Behaviours used by HIV-positive adolescents to prevent stigmatization in Botswana. *International Nursing Review, 57*(2), 260–264.

UNAIDS. (2013). *Global report: UNAIDS report on the global AIDS epidemic 2013*. Geneva: UNAIDS.

Vaz, L. M. E., Corneli, A., Dulyx, J., Rennie, S., Omba, S., Kitetele, F., et al. (2008). The process of HIV status disclosure to HIV-positive youth in Kinshasa, Democratic Republic of the Congo. *AIDS Care, 20*(7), 842–852.

Vaz, L. M. E., Eng, E., Maman, S., Tshikandu, T., & Behets, F. (2010). Telling children they have HIV: Lessons learned from findings of a qualitative study in sub-Saharan Africa. *AIDS Patient Care and STDs, 24*(4), 247–256.

Vaz, L. M. E., Maman, S., Eng, E., Barbarin, O. A., Tshikandu, T., & Behets, F. (2011). Patterns of disclosure of HIV status to infected children in a Sub-Saharan African setting. *Journal of Developmental & Behavioral Pediatrics, 32*(4), 307–315.

Vreeman, R. C., Nyandiko, W. M., Ayaya, S. O., Walumbe, E. G., Marrero, D. G., & Inui, T. S. (2010). The perceived impact of disclosure of pediatric HIV status on pediatric antiretroviral therapy adherence, child well-being, and social relationships in a resource-limited setting. *AIDS Patient Care and STDs, 24*(10), 639–649.

Waugh, S. (2003). Parental views on disclosure of diagnosis to their HIV-positive children. *AIDS Care, 15*(2), 169–176.

WHO. (2009). *Rapid advice: Antiretroviral therapy for HIV infection in adults and adolescents*. Retrieved November 24, 2011, from http://www.who.int/hiv/pub/arv/advice/en/index.html.

WHO. (2011). *Guideline on HIV disclosure counselling for children up to 12 years of age*. Geneva: World Health Organization. Retrieved April 6, 2016, from www.who.int/entity/hiv/pub/hiv_disclosure/en/

WHO. (2012). *CD4+ T-cell counting technology*. Retrieved April 11, 2012, from http://www.who.int/diagnostics_laboratory/faq/cd4/en/.

WHO/UNAIDS/UNICEF. (2010). *Global HIV/AIDS response: Epidemic update and health sector progress towards universal access*. Retrieved March 26, 2012, from http://www.unaids.org/en/targetsandcommittments/15millionaccessingtreatment/.

Wiener, L., & Battles, H. B. (2006). Untangling the web: A close look at diagnosis disclosure among HIV-infected adolescents. *Journal of Adolescent Health, 38*(3), 307–309.

Wiener, L., Mellins, C. A., Marhefka, S., & Battles, H. B. (2007). Disclosure of an HIV diagnosis to children: History, current research, and future directions. *Journal of Developmental and Behavioral Pediatrics, 28*(2), 155–166.

Chapter 18
The Power of Online Patient Communities for HIV Youth

Gonzalo Bacigalupe, Kathryn Cantrell, and Rachel Chickerella

Contents

18.1 The Power of Online Patient Communities for HIV Youth

Xavier is a 19-year-old Black male with HIV. Living in Memphis, Tennessee, Xavier reports struggling with stigma, racial discrimination, and homophobia. As a result, Xavier shares that he rarely discloses to others the HIV-status or his sexual orientation. Likewise, because of the stigma, he avoids meeting others with HIV in his hometown for fear of inadvertent disclosure. His counselor, aware of these barriers, introduced Xavier to an online community of patients diagnosed with HIV. Being able to share his story candidly, Xavier felt more capable of helping others and providing mentorship to those newly infected with HIV. Xavier continues to keep his status hidden in his hometown, but he has become an

G. Bacigalupe (✉) • K. Cantrell
College of Education and Human Development, University of Massachusetts Boston, 100 Morrissey Blvd., Boston, MA 02125, USA
e-mail: Gonzalo.Bacigalupe@umb.edu; kathryn.cantrell001@umb.edu

R. Chickerella
Trilogy Behavioral Health, 1210 W. Granville Unit 101, Chicago, IL 60660, USA
e-mail: chickerellar@gmail.com

P. Liamputtong (ed.), *Children and Young People Living with HIV/AIDS*, Cross-Cultural Research in Health, Illness and Well-Being,
DOI 10.1007/978-3-319-29936-5_18

HIV patient advocate online. A mentor to youth across the globe, he frequently recalls how being able to help others virtually has infused his life of meaning and has enabled a resilient stance towards the HIV diagnosis.

Currently, young people ages 13–24 account for nearly 26 % of all new HIV infections each year (Centers for Disease Control 2012). While the disease is becoming increasingly manageable with advances in antiretroviral therapy, young people with HIV (YHIV) face the additional challenge of learning how to cope with the disease throughout their lifetime (Kahana et al. 2013). For YHIV, the social stigma attached to the diagnosis remains a central stressor accounting for increased social isolation among the community (Battles and Wiener 2002). This stigma also inhibits soliciting support for health management (Battles and Wiener 2002; Hazra et al. 2010; Cantrell et al. 2013). This has a lasting impact as sub-optimal medical adherence is the leading cause of AIDS progression and eventual death in YHIV (Zanoni and Mayer 2014).

Social network technologies makes access to social and informational support available for those with HIV such as Xavier (Fox and Purcell 2010; Kahana et al. 2013). For YHIV, online patient communities (OPCs) are growing steadily as an option, not limited by geographical restrictions, to seek social and emotional support for coping with the diagnosis and its treatment. The ability to control the level of anonymity and confidentiality in online communities is conducive in providing safety and comfort to a population stifled by stigma. Overcoming geographical barriers, OPCs enable patients to connect with others also coping with the illness (Reeves 2001; Bacigalupe 2011). From a narrative perspective, virtual communication provides individuals with the ability to explore illness stories, personal disclosure, and stigma experiences in an open and anonymous format. Previous literature supports that participation in OPCs increases patient empowerment, which has been shown to enhance adherence in YHIV; thus, participation in OPCs has long-term epidemiological benefits (Barak et al. 2008; Van Uden-Kraan et al. 2009; Bartlett and Coulson 2011; Mo and Coulson 2012; Bacigalupe 2013).

We contend that the social power of OPCs can aid in community support and provide opportunities for story-telling and meaning-making that social stigmatization inhibits. While OPCs afford individuals with opportunities to build social networks that provide support and experience outlets for the patient narrative, the digital divide can often prevent against the utilization or research of OPCs for YHIV. This chapter argues for the social benefit of OPCs while also highlighting the gaps in research and implementation that require greater attention.

18.2 HIV Impact in Youth

Mariana is a fifteen-year-old Latin American adolescent living in Brooklyn with her mother although she has been in and out of the foster care system. Marianna's mother had a significant drug problem, is now on recovery. She disclosed her HIV status to her daughter revealing details that included that she was intravenously infected and that Marianna was born with HIV. Following the disclosure, Marianna is in shock and unsure of what to do next. The only information she had about HIV, she acquired from her peers. Her concept is that HIV is a fatal disease that only spreads to people who do "bad things." She is angry, confused, sad, and feels misunderstood. Marianna decides to follow her mother's example and not tell anyone about the disease, choosing instead to hide her diagnosis.

Developmentally, adolescence can be a stressful time. For YHIV, a chronic illness diagnosis is an additional burden that requires complex management including hospital visits, and adverse side effects of medication (see also Chaps. 4 and 22). Youth's identity formation can impact negatively the strict adherence requirements for viral suppression and disclosing to peers and partners can influence coping and create barriers to safe sexual practices. The number of HIV infections in adolescents and young adults from ages 13–24 ranges between 56,000 and 80,600 in the United States (Zanoni and Mayer 2014). From 2006 to 2009, there was a 21 % increase in HIV incidence among youth aged 13–29 over this time period (Zanoni and Mayer 2014). This rise in new HIV infections is occurring primarily in the young black men-who-have-sex-with-men (MSM) population. From 2006 to 2009, 53 % of HIV/AIDS among MSM were between the ages of 13 and 24 years (Zanoni and Mayer 2014). In 2010, African Americans accounted for 57 % of new HIV infections, while MSM accounted for 72 % of all infections among youths (Zanoni and Mayer 2014). While behavioral transmission is increasing for youth, perinatal transmission is decreasing. Of the approximately 80,000 young people ages 13–24 with HIV, roughly 9,500 of those individuals were infected from birth (Tassiopoulos et al. 2013). Whether infected perinatally or behaviorally, YHIV face social, emotional, and physical challenges to coping positively. In subsequent sections, we expand on the aspects of coping with HIV that can be augmented through virtual formats.

18.2.1 Psychosocial Impact

Stigma is one of the most cited barriers to care for YHIV (Martinez et al. 2012; see Chaps. 2, 3, 4, 6, 9, 12, 14, 15, and 17 in this volume). Despite public health efforts to normalize the diagnosis of HIV, stigma continues to impact coping. Thus, caring for YHIV requires comprehensive medical and psychological care that works to alleviate the stigma experienced in the community. Clinical care should facilitate the validation of stories and relationships silenced by the dominant social discourse (Martinez et al. 2012). For individuals with HIV, active efforts to cope are intimately tied to both physiological and psychosocial functioning (Carver and Vargas 2011). In the context of stigma, coping is the intentional efforts to deal with a threatening or harmful situation (Carver and Vargas 2011). For clinical providers, understanding the complexities of coping with the stigma surrounding HIV is essential in ensuring treatment adherence by YHIV.

Disclosing intimate life events including illness, loss, and family functioning are necessary to establish close relationships. For the YHIV like Mariana, stigma surrounding the illness may limit this ability, adding secrecy to new friendships or romantic relationships (Hogwood et al. 2013). Many YHIV, however, see disclosure as an inevitable experience as some point, particularly as they engage in sexual activity. This inevitability can cause stress as many young people worry about identifying the right timing and methods for disclosure (Cantrell et al. 2013; Hogwood et al. 2013). Following disclosure, however, youth identify the admission as a desirable conversation leading to improved peer relationships, more social support with medication adherence, and decreased stigma (Hogwood et al. 2013). Thus, disclosure plays a large role in dissolving social stigmatization surrounding HIV (see Chap. 17 in this volume).

In addition to stigma and disclosure, mental health conditions are a concern for clinicians and researchers responding to the growing cohort of YHIV. The risk for depression or anxiety is higher for YHIV than the general population (Gadow et al. 2012). For many YHIV, lower levels of social support, higher viral load, disclosure to acquaintances, and identifying as LGBT are significantly correlated with mental health conditions (Lam et al. 2007; see also Chaps. 4, and 12 in this volume). PHIV youth face wide-ranging challenges from developmental disabilities, stigma, and family death to toxic environmental factors including poverty, racism, and violence. Youth may also experience multiple caretaker transitions due to death, illness, or family disruption (Pearlstein et al. 2014). These stressors combined with social stigmatization increase the prevalence of mental health conditions.

The implications on mental health differ between those who are perinatally- and behaviorally-infected with HIV. In a study of youth with perinatal HIV, 70 % met the criteria for a DSM-IV diagnosis. For youth perinatally-infected with HIV, a higher viral load predicts depressive symptoms (Gadow et al. 2012). Likewise, youth with perinatally-infected HIV are more likely to be on psychotropic medication than their peers without HIV (Gadow et al. 2012). Behaviorally-infected youth are more likely to be concerned about stigma, putting them at an increased risk of depression. Furthermore, behaviorally-infected youth are more likely to be male, a sexual minority, and a have a history of substance abuse (MacDonell et al. 2013). Despite these distinctions, it is clear that there is a need in YHIV to address mental health, social stigmatization, and personal disclosure.

18.2.2 Relational Impact

From a systems perspective, the HIV experience for youth impacts the entire family. For youth living with HIV, having a supportive family is integral to well-being and medication adherence. Many families live in fear of disclosure because of stigma. For parents of youth with perinatally-acquired HIV, disclosure means confronting personal responsibility and acknowledging the behaviors that led the parent, as well as the child, to be infected (Vranda and Mothi 2013). As in the case of Mariana, both parent and child internalize the shame, putting the family at an increased risk for mental health concerns (Vranda and Mothi 2013). Likewise, the family that has a child infected with HIV is often a family coping with discrimination, illness, lack of resources, and isolation. Thus, efforts to support each member of the household are necessary for augmenting adjustment and coping (see also Chap. 3 in this volume).

Supportive communities impact the quality of life of YHIV. The quality of HIV-infected patients' personal relationships is associated with how adaptively they manage the diagnosis and may predict their ability to cope (Macapagal et al. 2012). There is a relationship between poor medication adherence for YHIV and depression (Kang et al. 2014). One of the major factors that influences depression in YHIV is social isolation (Kang et al. 2014). A benefit of the group process is the ability for patients to form friendships and acquire an opportunity for interpersonal learning and growth. Youth may achieve greater self-awareness through interacting with a group. YHIV may struggle to make or maintain friendships depending on the severity of their illness, and supportive communities provide a space for that interaction. Therefore, in addition to supporting the family system, it is imperative to provide YHIV with a welcoming community to promote social support.

Another relational aspect of the HIV experience is the clinician-patient relationship. A strong clinician-patient relationship is associated with greater social functioning and quality of life in YHIV (Macapagal et al. 2012). The clinician-patient alliance is crucial for the management of HIV. With the clinician-patient relationship being so central to living with HIV, it is essential for clinicians to focus on alliance within their programming. This consideration in addition to family systems and community support, comprise the relational elements of living with HIV that can be impacted through virtual interventions.

18.2.3 Physical Health Impact

The psycho-social and relational impacts of an HIV diagnosis are extensive. However, the physical health implications of the diagnosis should not be ignored. For many patients, combination antiretroviral therapy has transformed HIV from a progressive, fatal infection to a manageable chronic illness (Hazra et al. 2010). Rather than focusing just on survival and avoidance of opportunistic illnesses, YHIV must now focus on long-term disease management, sexual partner disclosure, vocational aspirations, reproductive health, and transitioning to adult medical care (Hazra et al. 2010). After a lifetime of taking antiretroviral therapy, youth with perinatally-infected HIV experience treatment fatigue and apathy associated with medication burnout (Hazra et al. 2010). Furthermore, transition to the adult medical care model takes time and advance planning, as the pediatric and adult chronic care models are vastly different.

While youth with behaviorally-infected HIV may not experience the same treatment fatigue of those with perinatally-infected HIV, many experience a host of other complications. Youth with behaviorally-infected HIV, particularly the African American MSM population, are still being infected at alarming rates and, due to lack of access, are unable to seek treatment in a timely manner (Zanoni and Mayer

2014). The incidence of new HIV infections in these populations remains disproportionately high compared to the general population (Zanoni and Mayer 2014). Because many YHIV are MSM, they may experience the dual stigmatization of sexual minority status and HIV infection, resulting in increased internalizing stigma, depressive symptoms, and subsequently, increased disease progression (Kemeny 2011; see also Chaps. 11, 12, and 13 in this volume).

Near-perfect (>95 %) adherence is necessary to achieve optimal viral suppression and prevent antiretroviral drug-resistance (Reisner et al. 2009). Unfortunately, for YHIV, lack of medication adherence is high and can result in poor health outcomes (Reisner et al. 2009; see also Chap. 22 in this volume). For youth with medical conditions, some degree of suboptimal adherence is common, especially for those with chronic conditions such as HIV (Zanoni and Mayer 2014). Young adults face more barriers to adherence than younger adolescents, especially as they gain independence in their medication routine (Arnett et al. 2007; Zanoni and Mayer 2014). For many YHIV, medication adherence can be supported by a number of interventions including contingency management, MEMs caps, pillboxes, and caregiver supervision (Reisner et al. 2009). Despite these behavioral efforts, many youth cite that social stigmatization, lack of community, and fear of disclosure inhibit the efforts of behavioral interventions (Gunther et al. 2014).

Emotional, social, and physical barriers to taking medication are consistently difficult to tackle through psychosocial interventions. Because social connectedness promotes medication adherence, interventions aimed at enhancing a sense of community should be encouraged. With the growing format of technology, there are more opportunities than ever before for researchers and clinicians to focus on the social and emotional components of an arduous routine such as antiretroviral treatment. In this section, we have explored the psychosocial, relational, and physical impact of HIV diagnosis in youth. Each of these aspects of an HIV diagnosis can be ameliorated through social support. In subsequent sections, we argue that virtual interventions can provide an ideal format for promoting social support in YHIV.

18.3 What Are Online Patient Communities?

Joshua is a 21-year-old male living with perinatally-infected HIV in a rural community in Kentucky. A student at a local technical college, Joshua lives at home with his family that includes 8 other adoptive children with various health conditions. Joshua has grown up as a quiet support for his parents, often sacrificing peer friendships to stay at home and care for his siblings. With few friends and discomfort in social situations, Joshua utilizes online communities to chat with others. Finding more comfort in written communication over face-to-face interactions, Joshua has a growing network online that provides him with social support. Due to his geographical isolation within a rural community, Joshua has never met in person someone his age who also has an HIV diagnosis. However, within a 3-D virtual environment for youth with HIV, Joshua has dozens of friends who share stories regarding medication, transmission, and disclosure. His avatar—Joshua's virtual identity—is confident and communicative.

A growing number of individuals connect online to seek social support and information for various health conditions. Virtual communities are ideal vehicles for countering isolation due to chronic illness. OPCs vary in structure, participants, and targeted outcomes. They are communities of patients and caregivers seeking support and guidance and where the chronically ill interact virtually. Despite the variability of definitions, their scope and significance is supported by research in multiple disciplines with dozens of unique terms identifying OPCs (Bacigalupe et al. 2014). Each OPC originates a unique culture. Communities take different forms based on participant's needs, the organizations that sponsor the communities, the format (open, closed, and semi-closed) and access. Professionals, for instance, facilitate some communities whereas others are made up solely of patients with similar conditions (Nguyen et al. 2008; Bletsos et al. 2013). Based on the size and participation rates of communities, some may comprise a large network of experts and social support, although others might be limited to a handful of individuals providing emotional support. Differences also occur in facilitation, as some have an assigned facilitator while others are based on peer-to-peer interaction. The presence or lack-thereof of a facilitator impacts the community's culture. Based on the community's mission, the necessity of a facilitator varies. For instance, some communities promoting self-efficacy and disease management might contain an e-health curriculum requiring facilitation whereas communities promoting social support might lack a facilitator. Healthcare providers, researchers, or patients may fill the facilitator(s) role.

In recent years, online support has continued to expand in structure and form. Youth are using social network platforms to connect for psychosocial support and self-management resources. Many young people with chronic illnesses already have social network accounts, making access to certain types of forums easy. Likewise, blogs have been found to be an effective medium to foster conversation and support (Neal and McKenzie 2011). Whatever the format or platform, the essential element to any OPC is the community itself and the bonds created by its members. Its impact on the doctor patient relationship is significant too as OPCs can promote communication between patient and physician (Donnelly et al. 2008; van Uden-Kraan et al. 2008; Bartlett and Coulson 2011; Chorbev et al. 2011). They can lead to greater disease management and self-efficacy (Bender et al. 2011; Rains and Young 2009; Samoocha et al. 2010). Most participants in OPCs report increased disease knowledge, social support, and decreased depressive symptoms (Mo and Coulson 2008; van Uden-Kraan et al. 2008; Idriss et al. 2009; Rains and Young 2009). Communities also significantly impact a patient's coping and quality of life (Samoocha et al. 2010; Bartlett and Coulson 2011). In sum, OPCs can support patients' coping with chronic illness and promote positive health behaviors. Most importantly, though, as in Joshua's story, OPCs provide social support by connecting others from across the globe to offer empathic support, information, and comfort. In subsequent sections, we outline the specific elements of OPCs that allow YHIV to garner social support.

18.4 What Are the Advantages of Connecting Virtually?

Nookie is a 13 year-old Black female with perinatally-acquired HIV. The discussion of diagnosis with her counselor prompts a new awareness of how it will impact her self-identity. Upon meeting with her counselor, Nookie states: "I just feel so gross, like no one would ever love me because I'm nasty." Her peers call HIV "the bug" and the connotation surrounding the diagnosis in school is "nasty." When reconciling these labels, Nookie expresses that these connotations have influenced her own self-esteem as well as the image she has of her mother. The counselor and Nookie discuss the use of anonymous writing through a community of bloggers. Nookie and her counselor set up a blog for Nookie to reflect on the meanings assigned to her diagnosis and garner support from others online. Within this environment, Nookie is able to write about her illness and the connotations of labels with the protection of anonymity.

Technological affordances are defined as the capacities facilitated by the technology and how users adapt the technology to meet the communication needs of the embedded culture (Boyd 2010). Thus, affordances are at the intersection of technology design and how it is adapted to meet user needs. The possible uses that YHIC can make of the technology are particularly significant in bridging social isolation, stigmatization, and lack of understanding (see Chap. 12 in this volume). The present attributes of emerging technology may fulfill the needs for many youth who face the challenge of sharing their story, constructing identity, or making supportive connections free of stigma. While Internet accessibility bridges geography and social isolation, the digital divide hinders accessibility for many populations. This digital divide impacts marginalized populations. The marginalization experienced by YHIV due to stigma is mirrored within the literature on OPCs for YHIV: the research literature is scarce and almost inexistent in this area. While the research is limited, clinical evidence supports the therapeutic benefits of OPC participation. Subsequent sections explore literature chronicling individual online communities for YHIV and their impact on the HIV experience when considering connection, story-telling, and health outcomes.

18.4.1 Connection

People from across the globe can connect and provide emotional support through OPCs (Conole and Dyke 2004), and can be a dynamic vehicle for connection, altruism, and mentorship, just like an in-person support group or a close friend. In a rural community, a young person like Joshua may be the only person with a chronic condition like HIV. Bridging the gap of geographic isolation, OPCs provide individuals with chronic illnesses a way to access others with the same diagnosis despite living far apart.

The range of virtual environments for individuals with chronic health conditions is vast and most of these communities are fully searchable online (Boyle and Cook 2004; Conole and Dyke 2004). Technological interventions, specifically OPCs, have been shown to benefit an individual's need for community (Donath 1998; Bers et al. 2001, 2007; Bers 2009). Mo and Coulson (2013) found that members of an HIV OPC who participated more frequently reported lower levels of perceived loneliness. Because loneliness is one of the most common stressors associated with YHIV, online participation has the potential to reduce feelings of isolation by facilitating online social connection with others also living with HIV (Mo and Coulson 2012, 2013). Similarly, Battles and Wiener (2002) studied the psychosocial effects of STARBRIGHT WORLD, an interactive virtual world for children with life-threatening illness. 32 outpatient caregiver-child dyads participated from across the United States. The mean age of the children who participated was 13.5 years and 78 % were living with HIV, 12.4 % with cancer, 6.3 % with chronic granuloma disease, and 3.2 % with neurofibromatosis. Upon the study's completion, researchers discovered that "SBW appears to provide a sense of connectedness to sick children who may feel otherwise disconnected from their peers" (Battles and Wiener 2002: 62). Particularly impressive was that children who use SBW only four times for 1 h or less over a period of 6–9 months experienced "less loneliness and appeared to their parents to be less withdrawn than they were before they used it" (Battles and Wiener 2002: 62). Simply knowing that there is a community only clicks away seems to provide significant comfort for children who may be isolated.

Researchers have also studied the impact of OPCs for YHIV in promoting patient empowerment. Mo and Coulson (2013) found that participants with higher levels of online participation reported higher levels of optimism and of empowerment as a result of receiving useful information and social support, finding positive meaning, and helping others. In addition to empowerment and social support, researchers have also noted how OPCs provide opportunities for affirmation. Thematic analyses of 5,000 online community postings from individuals with HIV in an OPC reveal that positive emotional support was exchanged more frequently than other forms of communications online. Moreover, three main categories of group interactions including sharing personal experience, expression of gratitude, and offering congratulations; each of which can facilitate positive social support exchanges among group members (Coursaris and Liu 2009).

In sum, participating in a supportive group environment online, YHIV can enhance protective factors against loneliness by developing a community of positive support. For someone newly diagnosed with HIV, others in the group in different stages of their diagnosis may be able to provide the connection needed to aid in the adjustment process. The OPC environment enables youth with chronic conditions to exert empathic behavior, listen, and contain the experiences of their peers. Thus, OPCs work much like an in-person support group, providing community and connection when it may not be easily accessible.

18.4.2 Story-Telling

Social technologies have the potential to open up new forms of dialogue and communication (Boyle and Cook 2004; Conole and Dyke 2004). The vast range of possible modes of communication can allow individuals to find an appropriate niche for sharing information and story telling. Virtual communities also afford YHIV like Nookie with opportunities for constructing a preferred identity. These broad options for communication (including real-time chat, forums, blogs, and micro-blogging) provide youth with the opportunity to re-write and re-author their story in multiple forms, promoting a healthy disclosure process and a coherent illness narrative. Likewise, the permanency of many online platforms allows for individuals to re-read their narratives and provide the opportunity for continuous collaborative editing. Archiving, an affordance of social technology enables a continuous individual and collective telling and sharing of experiences. Considering the importance of identity formation, OPCs offer the possibility of negotiating the level of anonymity and thus YHIV can explore multiple roles, experiment with disclosure, and through written communication, re-author their stories, and to have a community witnessing this process without fearing inadvertent disclosure.

Couched by the ability of participants to negotiate the levels of disclosure, OPCs afford youth the exploration of possible selves and re-construction of identity while others act as witnesses. Because the way individuals narrate their HIV experiences impacts coping in addition to identity formation, narrative efforts to support adjustment are imperative to psychosocial and physiological well being in HIV populations. The stigma surrounding an HIV diagnosis leaves many illness narratives unshared. The narrative exercise in OPCs is especially important for reclaiming a sense of worth in the face of cultural stigmatization and prejudice. Ezzy (2000) found that HIV illness narratives were polyphonic, many narratives had multiple and sometimes contradictory plot lines and stories overlaid one upon another. The inability to share an illness story openly may inhibit the opportunity to fully synthesize an illness experience into a narrative structure. This can have a detrimental impact on an individual's ability to understand and maintain a chronic illness like HIV. The capacity to rescue one's story can be an empowering experience that enables social connection. Bar-Lev (2008) found that stories housed within an OPC of those with HIV called HOPE contained significant dramatization of emotions. Not shared elsewhere, the emotionally charged messages posted on the OPC constitute narratives written primarily with the intent of implicating and involving the audience, giving rise to a discursive empathic community containing a web of interwoven emotional tales of stigma, medication, and conflict (Noy 2004; Bar-Lev 2008). Within an OPC, participants interactively formulate an emotional ethic, as they discuss their problematic relations with the self and others and give voice to non dominant stories (Bar-Lev 2008).

The degree to which a person secures a coherent personal identity can predict risk-taking behaviors in young adulthood. A person insecure in identity is more likely to engage in risk taking behavior. However, identity commitment is compromised when a life stressor such as a chronic illness diagnosis impedes a healthy development (Dumas et al. 2012). Online, participants can negotiate, redefine, and reinvent existing cultural codes to make sense of their illness experience and how it impacts identity formation (Bar-Lev 2008). They try on different hats and test them out within the group, comparing the social norms within the OPC to the ones outside the virtual forum. In an OPC for LGBT youth, the anonymity of the online format allowed for more comfort in exploring identities (DeHaan et al. 2013). The story below highlights how the anonymity of an OPC may afford youth with the ability to have conversations regarding identity.

> I could never do that in person to anyone, even if they identified themselves as gay…I would have isolated myself away from them…I would never have had them in person with anyone ever because these people were not necessarily real in my mind. They were not actual (…) like if they were real people, it would have been a completely different discussion. It wasn't until I met the first couple of guys on the Internet, the first two, that it was like suddenly I was having, like I was verbalizing some of these things, and it was really strange for me (…). On the Internet I have a different personality, almost (DeHaan et al. 2013: 430).

Narrative therapy offers a useful framework to comprehend the power of OPC for the creation of story as a community enterprise. Peterkin and Prettyman (2009) hypothesize that the inability to speak candidly about an illness experience may make narrative therapies more helpful as story-telling is a natural process that has been repressed, silenced. Dean (1995) advocated that narrative therapies in the form of therapeutic writing groups allow members with HIV to celebrate their identity within a context of acceptance and expand their concept of self. Likewise, in their research, Peterkin and Prettyman (2009) suggested that a narrative therapy intervention for individuals with HIV had numerous psychological benefits including newfound clarity surrounding life experiences, new insight into problems, and satisfaction at having created something that will live on as a testimonial. In addition to these benefits in constructing narratives, housing stories online provides opportunities for audiences to see various perspectives of those coping with HIV. For example, Mo and Coulson (2013) found that members of an OPC who participated more frequently were more optimistic about their disease; authors argue that this could result from the ability to read the successful stories posted by other members within the OPC (Van Uden-Kraan et al. 2009). In sum, OPCs provide YHIV opportunities to construct their illness narratives while also reading the narratives of others.

18.4.3 Health Outcomes

YHIV may have never met a peer who is also managing the disease. Imparting information regarding diagnosis and care may be shared through an OPC including information about mental health, physical illness, and day-to-day self-care strategies. Education can be a very important part of what an OPC can offer, especially if the community leader(s) provide evidence-based information. The opportunities are far reaching, as people from different parts of the world may have different medical and psychological practices regarding illness management.

Disclosure rates of those with HIV/AIDs are low (Greeff 2013). Qualitative studies have revealed that youth fear disclosure because of fear of negative responses from others, lack of self-efficacy, a fear that witnesses to the disclosure will tell others, and parental attitudes towards onward disclosure (Evangeli and Foster 2014; see also Chaps. 4, 5, 6, 7, 17, and 20 in this volume). Online anonymity can promote candid story-telling, allowing youth to honestly share the details of their HIV experience uninhibited. Some may be concerned that the anonymity of the online medium simply reinforces lack of disclosure. However, connecting virtually may be the first step in youth gaining the self-esteem and confidence to disclose their status to others in the community.

Disclosure matters not only to the YHIV, but others present in that person's life. In intimate partner relationship, YHIV are faced with the burden of partner disclosure, possibly jeopardizing the relationship. Within the world of OPCs, the ability to construct an illness narrative anonymously provides users a format for rehearsing and exploring the potential outcomes of disclosure. It also provides opportunities for social support surrounding disclosure. Peterson (2009) studied an asynchronous online group, AIDStired, targeted to men and found many examples of social support surrounding disclosure. One participant in Peterson's study (2009: 532), who provided emotional support to a new member of the OPC, remarked:

> Today was the day I divulged my status to Tim. He was extremely supportive even more than I thought he would be. You know that divulging your status is not an easy thing and people have different views on this matter.

OPCs combine social support with health information tailored to the needs of YHIV. In a survey of HIV patients, researchers found that health-related Internet use was associated with HIV disease knowledge, active coping, information-seeking coping, and social support. Therefore, the use of the Internet for health-related information can result in health benefits for HIV patients (Kalichman et al. 2002, 2003, 2005). Therefore, communities that integrate health literacy information with social support can aid in the coping process. YHIV in an OPC alternate between messages of emotional and informational support. Advice messages typically provided suggestions or guidance for coping with the difficulties associated with HIV. One participant in Mo and Coulson's study (2008: page 372) referred to books on how to cope with the disease in those newly diagnosed: "There is a great book called [book title], by [author]. Between that book and the help you get from your friends here, you will be just fine". In this sense, participants within an OPC can gather informational support in conjunction with emotional and social support.

OPCs can also lead patients to increased communication with the medical team (Donnelly et al. 2008; van Uden-Kraan et al. 2008; Bartlett and Coulson 2011; Chorbev et al. 2011; Wentzer and Bygholm 2013). Many patients are uncomfortable communicating some concerns with clinicians, or may not be sure what questions to ask. While some information online may be inaccurate, the ability to independently find evidence can promote patients to ask doctors relevant questions, leading to an increase in understanding of their condition and treatment options (Penson et al. 2002; Barker 2008; Wicks et al. 2010; Griffiths et al. 2012; Ziebland and Wyke 2012). Furthermore, for healthcare professionals, OPCs have the ability to provide insights to the needs of patients and help clinicians deliver a higher standard of care (Collins and Lewis 2013; Heisler 2010). Patients with diabetes, for instance, find that OPCs are more important for receiving support than providers (Schubart et al. 2011). In sum, the quality of health care could be impacted by participation in these communities.

Central to treatment of HIV is the tracking of health indicators. OPCs provide tools for tracking and therefore, have a positive effect on disease management (Glasgow et al. 2012). In one community for young men with HIV, users sought social support for HIV-related questions through asynchronous chat (Peterson 2009). A participant in Peterson's study (2009: 532) wrote:

> I got the results of my initial blood work in today. CD4: 513, Viral load: 76,400. The doctor said I could start meds, but I've decided NOT to do so yet :/ Very distressed over this actually :(

Responses to this statement were supportive and also included peer education regarding starting antiretroviral. One person responded, "Starting meds is a very personal decision that you and only you can make and your doctor should be behind you. He can help you with the thinking process. Your CD4 count is quite good and very close to normal which is anywhere between 600 and 1200…" (Peterson 2009; 532). Other responses, both normalize and educate. Feeling less isolated with the daily struggle of remembering the treatment may help motivate patients to higher treatment adherence. Overall, the OPC can also be a place to record health data and gain insight into health behaviors.

OPCs are also a preventative tool for youth at risk for HIV. Community health workers use online social networks to spread awareness and information regarding prevention or HIV prophylaxis (also known as PREP) (Ybarra and Bull 2007). However, research demonstrates that participation in online formats for discussing prevention requires face-to-face buy-in first. Researchers studying a youth-led, hybrid face-to-face and online social network designed for HIV prevention in homeless youth, found that youth requested in-person connection before meeting online to discuss prevention (Rice et al. 2012). Like any OPC, youths' participation in the design of the community is a requirement. This is not different in the case of HIV prevention, YHIV should participate in the development of OPCs. In a study by Bull et al. (2007), researchers found that youth wanted the online prevention community to house role-model messages regarding HIV/STD risks, condom attitudes, and norms and self-efficacy for negotiation. In this case, the youth desired more than data regarding risks but also methods for negotiating situations of risk with their peers. The prospect of OPCs for prevention is promising and more research is needed. In sum, OPCs also act as a virtual tool for health behaviors such as adherence.

18.5 Recommendations and Future Directions

Brittany is a 21-year-old woman with HIV who is expecting her first child. Wanting to be as proactive as possible about her healthcare while pregnant, Brittany has maintained 100 % adherence to her antiretroviral. However, she is interested in learning more information about ways to prevent passing HIV along to her baby. Brittany decides to join an online forum for HIV positive women expecting children. While online, she meets another young woman who lives in her hometown of Detroit, Michigan. After exchanging health information, the two decide to meet in person to continue their conversation. The result is a friendship built on emotional and informational support. The young women stay in contact throughout their pregnancies, checking in about medical appointments, reminding one another to take medication, and sharing health information online.

OPCs are virtual environments where information, social support, and storytelling, counter the discrimination, marginalization, and stigmatization that YHIV confront. OPCs support the work of clinicians helping these youth. They are a teaching ground for learning about the needs and ways in which youth live with the illness. Most communities are born as a result of the interactions among youth in formal virtual spaces designed for this purpose or through adaptations of other technologies—a Twitter hash tag, a closed group in a popular social network like Facebook, and so on. Geographical distance becomes less of a hurdle for youth to find a social network that fulfils needs arising from the diagnosis and treatment of a stigmatizing chronic illness.

Adolescent and young adult disclosure of participation in OPCs may vary. For clinicians working with YHIV, trust needs to be developed before a patient will open up regarding involvement in a community (Dedding et al. 2011). Often, patients do not report what communities they have joined for fear of their clinician discounting the value of the information and support housed online. These spaces may have become a safe haven for YHIV, a place where they can interact with peers separate from the stresses of day-to-day life. Clinicians, therefore, should inquire on patients' participation, but not necessarily expect a full response. Moreover, clinicians should encourage patients to participate in an OPC. Being open to the possibility will encourage disclosure in the clinical encounter as well as involvement by those who may be unaware of OPC's existence.

A patient-centered approach should include conversations about patients' involvement in social networks. This relationship is not only recommended for strengthening medical adherence, but is core in uncovering potential misconceptions, isolation, the role of stigma, and so on. The encouragement by clinicians for patients to participate in OPC may alleviate and prevent the debilitating impact of mental health conditions. Since YHIV have higher rates of depression, anxiety, and risk taking behaviors, OPCs may be the support YHIV need, as evident in Brittany's case.

Research analyzing the impact of OPCs in YHIV is limited and a multitude of questions are necessary to better understand this emerging medium. The impact of the digital divide as well as the barriers posed by health literacy levels has not been conclusive. The well educated and well off have greater access to the Internet as compared to those in the middle and lower class (Korp 2006). YHIV are likely of a lower SES, thus the reliability and access to digital communication technologies is lower. Even when access is not a barrier, racial and cultural disparities in communities may prevent accessibility (Jean-Jacques et al. 2012). As a result, barriers imposed by social inequity limit those who could benefit the most from participating in OPCs. Bridging the technological divide is, as a result, of primary significance. Providing regular access to the Internet may be cost effective considering the resources required to treat this illness at later stages as well as the potential gains in quality of life for these patients. The health outcome gains as a result of participating in these communities and how they may ensure adequate resources for this community of patients is still a question that requires systematic research. Similarly, we are not confident that simple participation in an OPC, if the access barriers are lifted, will necessarily overcome social determinants of health that are at the core influencing access to and treatment adherence.

Research and clinical evidence, despite its scarcity, suggest that OPCs are beneficial to chronic illness patients. Despite the myth that online information is less reliable, the crowdsourcing of information makes health resources reliable and useful to patients. Clinicians need to be aware of the communities and the kind of information that patients access to allow for a shared analysis to dispel myths and uncover useful sources of information that other patients can benefit from. The online medium, therefore, facilitates a patient centered approach. Healthy disclosure is central in self-care and thus the relevance of OPCs. Another area for future study is the impact of disclosure, anonymity, and trust. The community ability to foster or threaten healthy disclosure is still not well understood although the clinical and anecdotal evidence suggest that the ability to manage the online identity can offer better ways to negotiate the level of disclosure. We assume that the community participation will aid patients to affirm their ability to disclose to supportive family members, peers, and the community at large.

Questions of privacy, in particular the archiving of health information, bring up complex questions for patients online. For patients carrying on a stigmatized illness, the protection of confidentiality while creating a forum for sharing will require continuous attention from patients, clinicians, policy makers, and information technology professionals. Ensuring that information is owned and released according to the patients' needs and preferences is a shared requirement for all patients participating in communities online. However, for YHIV, this dilemma will continue to be a central dimension. Paradoxically, it is collective action that will determine the ways in which the illness stops being stigmatized and the way in which the experience of illness is normalized for those suffering it. It is not the ability to maintain anonymity the most important characteristic of online community participation but the ability of a person to manage their identity according to their needs and preferences. This is a fluid process that highlights the relevance of an empowering narrative. This re-storying may, in turn, promote self-efficacy, better self-care, the recruitment of appropriate help, and empowerment. Building community—online or in real life—is a complex, arduous, and never ending process. Designing a community online is, as a result, not a technical challenge but a relational one.

18.6 Conclusion

OPCs are growing as an option for YHIV needing social, narrative, and health management support. With the affordances of being able to bridge geography, stigma, and health disparities, OPCs connect YHIV to others who can provide community. Other affordances such as being able to control the level of anonymity and confidentiality online allows YHIV to create friendships, narrate their stories, and track their health behaviors in an open and anonymous format. Previous literature supports that participation in OPCs increases patient empowerment, which has been shown to enhance adherence in YHIV; thus, participation in OPCs has long-term epidemiological benefits (Barak et al. 2008; Van Uden-Kraan et al. 2009; Bartlett and Coulson 2011; Mo and Coulson 2012; Bacigalupe 2013). In this chapter, we contend that the social capabilities of OPCs can aid in social support and provide opportunities for story-telling and meaning-making that social stigmatization inhibits in YHIV. While OPCs afford individuals with opportunities to build social networks that provide support and experience outlets for the patient narrative, the digital divide can often prevent against the utilization or research of OPCs for YHIV. Researchers and clinicians should continue to explore the efficacy OPCs for promoting social support, narrative opportunities, and health management in chronic illness populations.

References

Arnett, J. J., Grusec, J., & Hasting, P. (2007). Socialization in emerging adulthood. In J. Grusec & D. Paul (Eds.), *Handbook of socialization: Theory and research* (pp. 208–239). New York: Guilford Press.

Bacigalupe, G. (2011). Is there a role for social technologies in collaborative healthcare? *Families, Systems & Health, 29*(1), 1–14.

Bacigalupe, G. (2013). *Chronic patients and social networking: Research lessons from a virtual community in the basque country.* Paper presented at the 141st APHA annual meeting (November 2–November 6, 2013).

Bacigalupe, G., Cantrell, K., & Chickerella, R. (2014). *Online patient communities emerging clinical and research trends: A systematic review of the research literature.* Paper presented at the American Psychological Association annual convention, Washington DC. August 11, 2014.

Barak, A., Boniel-Nissim, M., & Suler, J. (2008). Fostering empowerment in online support groups. *Computers in Human Behavior, 24*(5), 1867–1883.

Barker, K. K. (2008). Electronic support groups, patient-consumers, and medicalization: The case of contested illness. *Journal of Health and Social Behavior, 49*(1), 20–36.

Bar-Lev, S. (2008). "We are here to give you emotional support": Performing emotions in an online HIV/AIDS support group. *Qualitative Health Research, 18*(4), 509–521.

Bartlett, Y. K., & Coulson, N. S. (2011). An investigation into the empowerment effects of using online support groups and how this affects health professional/patient communication. *Patient Education and Counseling, 83*(1), 113–119.

Battles, H. B., & Wiener, L. S. (2002). From adolescence through young adulthood: Psychosocial adjustment associated with long-term survival of HIV. *Journal of Adolescent Health, 30*(3), 161–168.

Bender, J. L., Radhakrishnan, A., Diorio, C., Englesakis, M., & Jadad, A. R. (2011). Can pain be managed through the Internet? A systematic review of randomized controlled trials. *Pain, 152*(8), 1740–1750. doi:10.1016/j.pain.2011.02.012.

Bers, M. U. (2009). New media for new organs: A virtual community for pediatric post-transplant patients. *Convergence: The International Journal of Research into New Media Technologies, 15*(4), 462–469.

Bers, M. U., Gonzalez-Heydrich, J., Raches, D., & DeMaso, D. R. (2001). Zora: A pilot virtual community in the pediatric dialysis unit. *Studies in Health Technology and Informatics, 1*(1), 800–804.

Bers, M., Chau, C., Satoh, K., & Beals, L. (2007). *Virtual communities of care: Online peer networks with post-organ transplant youth.* In Proceedings of the 8th international conference on computer supported collaborative learning (pp. 78–80). New Brunswick, NJ: International Society of the Learning Sciences.

Bletsos, K., Alexias, G., & Tsekeris, C. (2013). Towards a fourth cosmology of doctor-patient relationship: A reflection on the virtual patient community PatientsLikeMe. *tripleC: Communication, Capitalism & Critique, 11*(1), 136–144.

Boyd, D. (2010). Social networks as networked publics: Affordances, dynamics, and implications. In Z. Papacharissi (Ed.), *Networked self: Identity, community and culture on social network sites* (pp. 39–58). New York: Routledge.

Boyle, T., & Cook, J. (2004). Understanding and using technological affordances: A commentary on Conole and Dyke. *Research in Learning Technology, 12*(3), 295–299.

Bull, S. S., Phibbs, S., Watson, S., & McFarlane, M. (2007). What do young adults expect when they go online? Lessons for development of an STD/HIV and pregnancy prevention website. *Journal of Medical Systems, 31*(2), 149–158.

Cantrell, K., Patel, N., Mandrell, B., & Grissom, S. (2013). Pediatric HIV disclosure: A process-oriented framework. *AIDS Education and Prevention, 25*(4), 302–314.

Carver, C. S., & Vargas, S. (2011). Stress, coping, and health. In H. S. Friedman (Ed.), *The Oxford handbook of health psychology* (pp. 162–188). New York: Oxford University Press.

Centers For Disease Control and Prevention. (2012). *Estimated HIV incidence among adults and adolescents in the United States, 2007–2010.* Basic information about HIV and AIDS.

Chorbev, I., Sotirovska, M., & Mihajlov, D. (2011). Virtual communities for diabetes chronic disease healthcare. *International Journal of Telemedicine and Applications, 11*, 1–8. doi:10.1155/2011/721654.

Collins, S. E., & Lewis, D. M. (2013). Social media made easy: Guiding patients to credible online health information and engagement resources. *Clinical Diabetes, 31*(3), 137–141.

Conole, G., & Dyke, M. (2004). What are the affordances of information and communication technologies? *Association for Learning Technology Journal, 12*(2), 113–124.

Coursaris, C. K., & Liu, M. (2009). An analysis of social support exchanges in online HIV/AIDS self-help groups. *Computers in Human Behavior, 25*(4), 911–918.

Dean, R. G. (1995). Stories of AIDS: The use of narrative as an approach to understanding in an AIDS support group. *Clinical Social Work Journal, 23*(3), 287–304.

Dedding, C., van Doorn, R., Winkler, L., & Reis, R. (2011). How will e-health affect patient participation in the clinic? A review of e-health studies and the current evidence for changes in the relationship between medical professionals and patients. *Social Science & Medicine, 72*(1), 49–53.

DeHaan, S., Kuper, L. E., Magee, J. C., Bigelow, L., & Mustanski, B. S. (2013). The interplay between online and offline explorations of identity, relationships, and sex: A mixed-methods study with LGBT youth. *Journal of Sex Research, 50*(5), 421–434.

Donath, J. S. (1998). Identity and deception in the virtual community. In P. Kollock & M. Smith (Eds.), *Communities in cyberspace* (pp. 29–59). London: Routledge.

Donnelly, L. S., Shaw, R. L., & van den Akker, O. B. (2008). eHealth as a challenge to 'expert' power: A focus group study of Internet use for health information and management. *Journal of the Royal Society of Medicine, 101*(10), 501–506.

Dumas, T. M., Ellis, W. E., & Wolfe, D. A. (2012). Identity development as a buffer of adolescent risk behaviors in the context of peer group pressure and control. *Journal of Adolescence, 35*(4), 917–927.

Ezzy, D. (2000). Illness narratives: Time, hope and HIV. *Social Science & Medicine, 50*(5), 605–617.

Fox, S., & Purcell, K. (2010). *Chronic disease and the Internet*. Washington, DC: Pew Internet & American Life Project.

Gadow, K. D., Angelidou, K., Chernoff, M., Williams, P. L., Heston, J., Hodge, J., & Nachman, S. (2012). Longitudinal study of emerging mental health concerns in youth perinatally infected with HIV and peer comparisons. *Journal of Developmental and Behavioral Pediatrics, 33*(6), 456–468.

Glasgow, R. E., Kurz, D., King, D., Dickman, J. M., Faber, A. J., Halterman, E., Woolley, T., Toobert, D. J., Strycker, L. A., Estabrooks, P. A., & Osuna, D. (2012). Twelve-month outcomes of an Internet-based diabetes self-management support program. *Patient education and counseling, 87*(1), 81–92.

Greeff, M. (2013). Disclosure and stigma: A cultural perspective. In *Stigma, discrimination and living with HIV/AIDS* (pp. 71–95). Springer Netherlands.

Griffiths, F., Cave, J., Boardman, F., Ren, J., Pawlikowska, T., Ball, R., …, & Cohen, A. (2012). Social networks–the future for health care delivery. *Social Science & Medicine, 75*(12), 2233–2241.

Gunther, M., Foisy, M., Houston, S., Guirguis, L., & Hughes, C. (2014). Treatment beliefs, illness perceptions, and non-adherence to antiretroviral therapy in an ethnically diverse patient population. *International Journal of Clinical Pharmacy, 36*(1), 105–111.

Hazra, R., Siberry, G. K., & Mofenson, L. M. (2010). Growing up with HIV: Children, adolescents, and young adults with perinatally acquired HIV infection. *Annual Review of Medicine, 61*, 169–185.

Heisler, M. (2010). Different models to mobilize peer support to improve diabetes self-management and clinical outcomes: Evidence, logistics, evaluation considerations and needs for future research. *Family Practice, 27*(suppl 1), i23–i32.

Hogwood, J., Campbell, T., & Butler, S. (2013). I wish I could tell you but I can't: Adolescents with perinatally acquired HIV and their dilemmas around self-disclosure. *Clinical Child Psychology and Psychiatry, 18*(1), 44–60.

Idriss, S. Z., Kvedar, J. C., & Watson, A. J. (2009). The role of online support communities: Benefits of expanded social networks to patients with psoriasis. *Archives of Dermatology, 145*(1), 46. doi:10.1001/archdermatol.2008.529.

Jean-Jacques, M., Persell, S. D., Thompson, J. A., Hasnain-Wynia, R., & Baker, D. W. (2012). Changes in disparities following the implementation of a health information technology-supported quality improvement initiative. *Journal of General Internal Medicine, 27*(1), 71–77.

Kahana, S. Y., Rohan, J., Allison, S., Frazier, T. W., & Drotar, D. (2013). A meta-analysis of adherence to antiretroviral therapy and virologic responses in HIV-infected children, adolescents, and young adults. *AIDS and Behavior, 17*(1), 41–60.

Kalichman, S. C., Weinhardt, L., Benotsch, E., DiFonzo, K., Luke, W., & Austin, J. (2002). Internet access and Internet use for health information among people living with HIV–AIDS. *Patient Education and Counseling, 46*(2), 109–116.

Kalichman, S. C., Benotsch, E. G., Weinhardt, L., Austin, J., Luke, W., & Cherry, C. (2003). Health-related Internet use, coping, social support, and health indicators in people living with HIV/AIDS: Preliminary results from a community survey. *Health Psychology, 22*(1), 111–116.

Kalichman, S. C., Cain, D., Cherry, C., Pope, H., Eaton, L., & Kalichman, M. O. (2005). Internet use among people living with HIV/AIDS: Coping and health-related correlates. *AIDS Patient Care & STDs, 19*(7), 439–448.

Kang, E., Delzell, D. A., Chhabra, M., & Oberdorfer, P. (2014). Factors associated with high rates of antiretroviral medication adherence among youth living with perinatal HIV in Thailand. *International Journal of STD & AIDS*, 0956462414545524.

Kemeny, M. E. (2011). Psychoneuroimmunology. In H. Freidman (Ed.), *The Oxford handbook of health psychology* (pp. 138–161). New York, NY: Oxford Handbook Online.

Korp, P. (2006). Health on the Internet: Implications for health promotion. *Health Education Research, 21*(1), 78–86.

Lam, P. K., Naar-King, S., & Wright, K. (2007). Social support and disclosure as predictors of mental health in HIV-positive youth. *AIDS Patient Care and STDs, 21*(1), 20–29.

Macapagal, K. R., Ringer, J. M., Woller, S. E., & Lysaker, P. H. (2012). Personal narratives, coping, and quality of life in persons living with HIV. *The Journal of the Association of Nurses in AIDS Care, 23*(4), 361–368.

MacDonell, K., Naar-King, S., Huszti, H., & Belzer, M. (2013). Barriers to medication adherence in behaviorally and perinatally infected youth living with HIV. *AIDS and Behavior, 17*(1), 86–93.

Martinez, J., Harper, G., Carleton, R. A., Hosek, S., Bojan, K., Glum, G., & the Adolescent Medicine Trials Network, J. (2012). The impact of stigma on medication adherence among HIV-positive adolescent and young adult females and the moderating effects of coping and satisfaction with health care. *AIDS Patient Care and STDs, 26*(2), 108–115.

Mo, P. K., & Coulson, N. S. (2008). Exploring the communication of social support within virtual communities: A content analysis of messages posted to an online HIV/AIDS support group. *CyberPsychology & Behavior, 11*(3), 371–374.

Mo, P. K., & Coulson, N. (2012). Developing a model for online support group use, empowering processes and psychosocial outcomes for individuals living with HIV/AIDS. *Psychology & Health, 27*(4), 445–459.

Mo, P., & Coulson, N. (2013). Online support group use and psychological health for individuals living with HIV/AIDS. *Patient Education and Counseling, 93*(3), 426–432.

Neal, D. M., & McKenzie, P. J. (2011). Putting the pieces together: endometriosis blogs, cognitive authority, and collaborative information behavior. *Journal of the Medical Library Association: JMLA, 99*(2), 127.

Nguyen, H. Q., Donesky-Cuenco, D., Wolpin, S., Reinke, L. F., Benditt, J. O., Paul, S. M., & Carrieri-Kohlman, V. (2008). Randomized controlled trial of an Internet-based versus face-to-face dyspnea self-management program for patients with chronic obstructive pulmonary disease: Pilot study. *Journal of Medical Internet Research, 10*(2). Retrieved from http://www.ncbi.nlm.nih.gov/pmc/articles/PMC2483918/.

Noy, C. (2004). Performing identity: Touristic narratives of self-change. *Text and Performance Quarterly, 24*(2), 115–138.

Pearlstein, S. L., Mellins, C. A., Dolezal, C., Elkington, K. S., Santamaria, E. K., Leu, C. S., & Abrams, E. J. (2014). Youth in transition: Life skills among perinatally HIV-infected and HIV-exposed adolescents. *Journal of Pediatric Psychology, 39*(3), 294–305.

Penson, R. T., Benson, R. C., Parles, K., Chabner, B. A., & Lynch, T. J. (2002). Virtual connections: Internet health care. *The Oncologist, 7*(6), 555–568.

Peterkin, A. D., & Prettyman, A. A. (2009). Finding a voice: Revisiting the history of therapeutic writing. *Medical Humanities, 35*(2), 80–88.

Peterson, J. L. (2009). "You have to be positive": Social support processes of an online support group for men living with HIV. *Communication Studies, 60*(5), 526–541.

Rains, S. A., & Young, V. (2009). A meta-analysis of research on formal computer-mediated support groups: Examining group characteristics and health outcomes. *Human Communication Research, 35*(3), 309–336. doi:10.1111/j.1468-2958.2009.01353.x.

Reeves, P. M. (2001). How individuals coping with HIV/AIDS use the Internet. *Health Education Research, 16*(6), 709–719.

Reisner, M. S. L., Mimiaga, M. J., Skeer, M. M., Perkovich, M. B., Johnson, M. C. V., & Safren, S. A. (2009). A review of HIV antiretroviral adherence and intervention studies among HIV–infected youth. *Topics in HIV Medicine, 17*(1), 14–35.

Rice, E., Tulbert, E., Cederbaum, J., Adhikari, A. B., & Milburn, N. G. (2012). Mobilizing homeless youth for HIV prevention: A social network analysis of the acceptability of a face-to-face and online social networking intervention. *Health Education Research, 27*(2), 226–236.

Samoocha, D., Bruinvels, D. J., Elbers, N. A., Anema, J. R., & van der Beek, A. J. (2010). Effectiveness of webbased interventions on patient empowerment: A systematic review and meta-analysis. *Journal of medical Internet research, 12*(2). doi: 10.2196/jmir.1286.

Schubart, J. R., Stuckey, H. L., Ganeshamoorthy, A., & Sciamanna, C. N. (2011). Chronic health conditions and internet behavioral interventions: A review of factors to enhance user engagement. *Computers, Informatics, Nursing, 29*(2), 81–92. doi:10.1097/NCN.0b013e3182155274.

Tassiopoulos, K., Moscicki, A.-B., Mellins, C., Kacanek, D., Malee, K., Allison, S., & Paul, M. (2013). Sexual risk behavior among youth with perinatal HIV infection in the United States: Predictors and implications for intervention development. *Clinical Infectious Diseases, 56*(2), 283–290.

van Uden-Kraan, C. F., Drossaert, C. H., Taal, E., Shaw, B. R., Seydel, E. R., & van de Laar, M. A. (2008). Empowering processes and outcomes of participation in online support groups for patients with breast cancer, arthritis, or fibromyalgia. *Qualitative Health Research, 18*(3), 405–417.

Van Uden-Kraan, C. F., Drossaert, C. H., Taal, E., Seydel, E. R., & van de Laar, M. A. (2009). Participation in online patient support groups endorses patients' empowerment. *Patient Education and Counseling, 74*(1), 61–69.

Vranda, M. N., & Mothi, S. N. (2013). Psychosocial issues of children infected with HIV/AIDS. *Indian Journal of Psychological Medicine, 35*(1), 19–22.

Wentzer, H. S., & Bygholm, A. (2013). Narratives of empowerment and compliance: Studies of communication in online patient support groups. *International Journal of Medical Informatics, 82*(12), e386–e394.

Wicks, P., Massagli, M., Frost, J., Brownstein, C., Okun, S., Vaughan, T., & Heywood, J. (2010). Sharing health data for better outcomes on PatientsLikeMe. *Journal of Medical Internet Research, 12*(2), 1–28.

Ybarra, M. L., & Bull, S. S. (2007). Current trends in Internet-and cell phone-based HIV prevention and intervention programs. *Current HIV/AIDS Reports, 4*(4), 201–207.

Zanoni, B. C., & Mayer, K. H. (2014). The adolescent and young adult HIV cascade of care in the United States: Exaggerated health disparities. *AIDS Patient Care and STDs, 28*(3), 128–135.

Ziebland, S., & Wyke, S. (2012). Health and illness in a connected world: How might sharing experiences on the Internet affect people's health? *Milbank Quarterly, 90*(2), 219–249.

Chapter 19
The Power of Peers: Self-Stigma Impacts, Peer Support and Engagement

Magda Conway

Contents

M. Conway (✉)
The Children's HIV Association for the UK and Ireland,
12 St Thomas Street, Bristol BS1 6JJ, UK
e-mail: magdaconway@blueyonder.co.uk

P. Liamputtong (ed.), *Children and Young People Living with HIV/AIDS*,
Cross-Cultural Research in Health, Illness and Well-Being,
DOI 10.1007/978-3-319-29936-5_19

19.1 Introduction

We can't change the world, unless we change ourselves.
Biggie Small (Rapper) (http://www.searchquotes.com/quotes/author/Biggie_Smalls/)

This chapter explores the self-stigma felt by many people living with HIV and how this impacts on perinatally-infected children and adolescents. I argue that protectionist practice with children and adolescents living with HIV (C&ALHIV), in partnership with family silence, societal attitudes and misinformation, impacts on the individual and nurtures self-stigma.

This chapter offers a historical context to children and HIV and how these still influences current practice, and then explores issues faced by C&ALHIV, looking specifically at unintended stigma and the impact of self-stigma. It then explores psycho-social support provision through two evaluated models that fare based on child-centered/children's rights approaches, demonstrating how effective these can be. Although the examples provided are from the UK, I contend that the issues presented and practice models are relevant to C&ALHIV across the globe.

Parts of this chapter are based on my personal experiences. I have spent 12 years working with C&ALHIV, which includes running therapeutic peer groups and one-to-one support. Over the last 5 years, I have run therapeutic group work at a residential support camp (set out in Sect. 19.4.2), each year working with 100 ALHIV. To that end, elements of what is presented are based on observations, reflection and open conversations with close to 400 ALHIV, rather than research findings.

19.2 How the History of HIV Impacts on Current Practice with C&ALHIV

When considering effective psycho-social and peer work with C&ALHIV, it is import to acknowledge the historical context of children and HIV, how and why practice has developed as it has and how this historical context still influences core elements of practice today. The advent of what is now referred to as the 'HIV epidemic' began in the early 1980s. The initial (and sustained) media coverage prior to HIV being 'discovered' constructed many of the myths surrounding HIV today. In 1982, the medical establishment referred to this unknown illness as GRID (gay-related immune deficiency)[1] and a year later in the USA, it was colloquially known as the "4-H Club" reflecting those who were believed most at risk of acquiring this disease: homosexuals, hookers (or hemophiliacs), heroin addicts and Haitians.[2] HIV was linked with drug use, sex work, perceived 'deviate' sexual activities and

[1] AVERT http://www.avert.org/history-aids-1986.htm

[2] AVERT http://www.avert.org/history-aids-1986.htm

immigrant groups. Even before HIV was named, it was publically linked to groups who faced multiple prejudice and social exclusion.[3]

In 2010, the National AIDS Trust (UK) public knowledge and attitudes poll reported that 33 % of the 2000 people polled would not feel comfortable working with a colleague who was HIV-positive. Other statistics were that 10 % thought people could catch HIV from spitting and 9 % from kissing, showing that although medical science has progressed extraordinarily since the 1980s, attitudes and knowledge are still some way behind this.

Prior to the advent of antiretroviral therapy (ART), the life expectancy of perinatally-infected children was expected, for the majority, to be between 2 and 5 years. It has only recently been shown by Ferrand et al. (2009) that a third of these children actually lived to the means age of 16 without ART. This expectation of imminent death, coupled with negative public perceptions could be seen as one of the drivers in the general practice to not name HIV to the child.

Today, the medical outcomes for C&ALHIV who have access to ART are starkly different, but the scientific progress has not been mirrored in the management of the psycho-social needs of these children. HIV, being 'different' from other medical conditions due to the need to protect children, is still a general practice. Protectionist practice, which stems from a good place, has led to C&ALHIV being excluded from rights, inclusion and engagement agendas that have been successfully developed in other pediatric medical conditions. In 1989, the UN Convention on the Rights of the Child (UNCRC) was produced, affording children numerous rights as autonomous beings, this included Article 12:

> States Parties shall assure to the child who is capable of forming his or her own views the right to express those views freely in all matters affecting the child… (United Nation 2009: 3)

Twenty-five years on from publishing the UNCRC, UNICEF undertakes extensive global work with HIV-positive children. Yet this group, unlike their HIV-negative peers, are not afforded these rights as critical information about themselves – their HIV status – is being withheld from them.

19.3 Issues Facing C&ALHIV

To understand self-stigma and support C&ALHIV, practitioners need to understand the non-health issues faced by this group. In the UK, C&ALHIV are a low prevalence group, and although they are growing up in one of the world's most affluent countries, the majority come from poor socio-economic groups and face some shared social issues to their HIV-positive peers around the world. This section briefly sets out these shared experiences.

[3] AVERT http://www.avert.org/history-aids-1986.htm

19.3.1 HIV in the Family

Being born with HIV presents a different experience to acquiring HIV in adolescence or adulthood. The key differences being that HIV is a family issue and that the child has no other experiences other than a life with HIV. Many C&ALHIV in the UK have faced single or multiple bereavements during childhood, are being brought up by relatives or being looked after by the state. Where the mother is still alive, there can be profound feelings of guilt for passing HIV onto their child and this can manifest itself in being over protective and treating the HIV-positive child 'different' from it's HIV-negative siblings (See also Chap. 3 in this volume).

The impact of an HIV diagnosis on an individuals' mental health has been well documented and is explored in more depth later on. When looking at this cohort of children, the primary carers' mental health and well-being has huge impacts on that child's development and well-being. Where a parent is struggling with mental health related issues, the child often takes on more caring responsibilities within the home. As Evans and Becker's (2009) research into young carers living with HIV highlights, this can lead to high levels of anxiety for the child and this in-turn impacts on their social integration, education, peer relationships, as well as their own health and happiness.

19.3.2 Secrecy

The historical context of HIV and its links to sex/sexual behavior can heavily influence people's attitudes towards HIV. For many parents, an HIV diagnosis is something that they feel ashamed about, keep secret and fear the judgments and negative actions of others. To that end, family HIV is treated with high levels of secrecy and children across the globe live in households and institutions where they are told to keep HIV a secret from siblings, other members of their household, they hide medication and hospital appointments, do not tell school or their peers (see also Chaps. 1, 3, 4, 5, 6, and 17). From the point of a child's diagnosis, there is a strong '*do not tell*' culture that can cause multiple issues for the child as they develop into an adult. A simple example that I have seen multiple times is an ALHIV unable to say 'HIV'. Secrecy in the family – unless this secret is a surprise present or party – can be toxic.

The Adolescent HIV Testing, Counselling And Care produced by the WHO (2014) specifically focuses on the need for ALHIV to communicate with one-another and to their HIV-negative peers. Yet we cannot presume that any perinatally-infected HIV-positive adolescent whose live is based in secrecy and very limited conversations about HIV (if these happen at all) will have the vocabulary to talk about it. As this cohort are now predicted to live through to middle age and beyond, they need the language to talk about HIV when they want to be with friends, family, sexual partners and those providing their health care.

19.3.3 Social Exclusion and Naming a Child's HIV

In the UK, the cohort of C&ALHIV are primarily of African origin due to the high levels of HIV in these countries as a result of the historical links formed during colonialism, rather than common myths of health tourism that sporadically surface in the UK media (National AIDS Trust 2008). Many families spend time in the asylum system, with poor housing, being moved regularly by the state and with little money (Conway 2006). This can cause huge levels of anxiety and instability in a child's life.

In the UK, an adolescent diagnosed with HIV will consent to the test and be central to decisions relating to their treatment and care.[4] A child born with HIV will not be told their diagnosis until either the parent/guardian feels it is the right time, or the health care provider feels they can no longer treat the child without them knowing due to their age and – within the context of the UK – the legal obligations of that professional to gain the child's consent to treatment. Therefore, the perinatally-infected child has a very different health care experience to their horizontally-infected peers.

19.3.4 Sex and Talking to Others About HIV

The above shows the often all-encompassing level of secrecy these children can live with. Yet as they progress into adolescents, where the peer group becomes more significant and where thoughts and feelings about sex, sexuality and relationships become increasingly strong, this group has specific sexual health and relationship needs, which include a thorough understanding of HIV routes of transmission.

ALHIV in the UK have reported that their sexual health education in school is poor, and in the clinic, can be very varied, with many pediatric staff finding this area uncomfortable, having known their patients from a young age. That this group obtaining high quality, non-judgmental sex education from an early age is critical, not only to prevent onward transmission of HIV, but to ensure positive self-perceptions around sex and relationships. I annually run sexual health sessions with ALHIV and often hears remarks like "no-one will love me", or "no-one would want to marry me", which reflects low-levels of self-esteem and in essences means, "no one will want to have sex with me because I have HIV". Early, age appropriate conversations about sex have been shown in the Northern European Nordic countries to positively impact on teenage pregnancy rates. Having these conversations from an early age shows that talking about such things is not a taboo and the child feels empowered not only by the information they have, but also by the trust and confidence developed through open and honest conversations.

[4] British Medical Association (2001) Consent, rights and choices in health care for children and young people. London: BMJ Publishing Group.

Where a child has HIV, they are facing a sexual debut with a highly stigmatized, sexually transmitted disease, which in some countries (including the UK) they can be prosecuted for transmitting. Condom use and the ability to negotiate safer sex (and the sex they want) are essential, and to negotiate safer sex takes a high level of confidence and understanding. These children need this information to support them to make good decisions, but they also need to have had conversations about sex and feel empowered, knowing they are entitled to have sexual desires and sexual relationships.

19.3.5 Adherence

Committing to an ongoing regular medication regime has been a challenge for most adolescents; no matter what health condition they are managing (Taddeo et al. 2008). At best, this is 'adherence fatigue', where they are tired of having to take medication every day (McDonald 2011; see also Chaps. 4, 5, 6, 17, 18, and 22 in this volume). Yet poor adherence can be the outcome of many different factors, some of which relate to the internal struggle the individual is having with a life with HIV, and this will be looked at in more detail when exploring self-stigma.

19.3.6 Transition to Adult Care

There will come a time when each child living with HIV will need to leave pediatric services and transition into adult clinical services, which by their very nature, are different. In general, pediatric medicine is more nurturing and many ALHIV will have known their doctor for many years. Adult HIV services are often based in genitourinary medicine and sexual health services, and some ALHIV find these environments overwhelming or intimidating (see also Chaps. 4, 5, 6, and 20 in this volume).

In some areas of the UK, there are now specialist adolescent clinics to support the process of transition. These create a 'half-way-house', supporting the adolescent to take control over their health and health care decisions, whilst still offering a higher level of support and time than they would receive in adult services. But where this is not available, some ALHIV have struggled and been lost to following up. Once an ALHIV is disengaged with their healthcare provider, it can be challenging to re-engage them until they become ill. A child born with HIV entering adulthood has had a life-time of varied clinical experience, from being the passive patient (not knowing their HIV diagnosis), to having this name and then to being expected to self-care. Many factors influence successful transition, and some of these will begin early in that child's life (Hamblin 2011).

19.4 Stigma

There is a common thread through most of the issues faced by C&ALHIV and this is not, "HIV the manageable chronic condition", but "HIV the stigmatized health condition". This sets HIV apart from other health conditions and what needs to be openly addressed in psycho-social work with this group. For C&ALHIV living in the UK, with access to free healthcare and medication, the most debilitating impact of being born with HIV is the real and perceived stigma they face, how they internalize this and how this then influences their engagement with healthcare, adherence, mental health and their feelings about themselves.

It is important to reflect on what is meant by stigma, as this is a term often used but rarely explained. The Concise Oxford English Dictionary defines it as, "a mark of disgrace associated with a particular circumstance, quality, or person" (Tenth Edition 1999: 1410). In its 2003 fact sheet on stigma and discrimination, UNAIDS defines HIV-related stigma as: "… a 'process of devaluation' of people either living with or associated with HIV and AIDS … Discrimination follows stigma and is the unfair and unjust treatment of an individual based on his or her real or perceived HIV status." (UNAIDS 2003: 1; see also Chap. 1).

HIV-related stigma exists in many forms; the obvious would be societal attitudes that lead to negative behavior towards those living with the virus. This could be seen as 'intentional stigma' and relates to media representations and people whose knowledge is poor and therefore respond in negative ways (see also Chaps. 1, 2, 3, 4, 6, 9, 12, 14, 15, and 18 in this volume).

19.4.1 Unintended Stigma

More significant to the child born with HIV is the unintended stigma they experience and the self-stigma they create from these experiences. Unintended stigma can stem from protectionism – not telling a child they have HIV to protect them from this; not wanting to worry a child or adolescent so not fully and clearly explaining what is happening; not wanting to bring up conversations about HIV fearing it will upset the child; not having a child or adolescent party to decision making about their own health and health care. I have found that at times those supporting a child or adolescent will not talk about HIV because it can lead to difficult conversations, and they feel ill-equipped or not confident in managing these properly, so it is easier to just not start them.

In the UK, it is now a common practice to include children in discussions and decisions about their health care. The British Medical Associations guidance (2001) states that children's health care is enhanced by their involvement in decision-making, whether or not they are competent to make final decisions. This necessarily means having age appropriate conversations with that child about their health condition, empowering them by providing the appropriate information and building a trusting and non-judgmental relationship with them so they can be involved in health care decisions.

Some argue that HIV is ‘different’, and this chapter has shown how HIV does present difficulties for the individual due to the stigma associated with it. Yet by treating HIV differently in medical settings, this is unintentionally feeding into and modelling wider intentional stigma. If we look to history, we can see the practice of not telling a patient their diagnosis due to societal stigma occurred with diseases such as cancer. Daniel K Sokol set out the historical context of this in his 2006 article in the Journal of the Royal Society of Medicine, ‘*How the doctor's nose has shortened over time; a historical overview of the truth-telling debate in the doctor-patient relationship*’. He quotes findings from a 1953 article in the same journal, where 444 doctors in the Philadelphia area completed questionnaires about tell patients about life-limiting health conditions: “Sixty nine per cent of the respondents indicated that they never or usually did not inform the patient of a diagnosis of cancer”. Practice in most of the world has moved on significantly since this time, acknowledging the patients needs and rights.

Many ALHIV have reported anger and frustration of having HIV “kept a secret from them”, that “everyone knew apart from me and it's about”. If we consider the psychological impact this can have on an individual, the lesson the child or adolescent learns here is that HIV is a ‘*bad thing*’ that needs to be kept from people, including the person who has it. In reality, most people do not share their health information or conditions with others, whatever this is. Most people consider this personal, but with all other health conditions, this information is shared with the child living with it, which has been shown to support the child in managing their own health and accepting a life with a long-term health condition. Yet with HIV the historical context and societal responses still influences practice today. In 2011, the World Health Organization changed its guidance on naming HIV to a child, stating:

> Children of school age [from the age of 6] should be told their HIV positive status; younger children should be told their status incrementally to accommodate their cognitive skills and emotional maturity, in preparation for full disclosure. (WHO 2011: 12)

However, there is a growing minority of practitioners who are promoting open and honest conversations with children in health care setting from the point of diagnosis, in an attempt to counter self-stigma and reclaim HIV as a health condition that should be treated as all other health conditions are, rather than something ‘different’.

A child may also face unintended stigma in the home. This can come from parents/guardians who feel unable or unwilling to talk about HIV if household members are not aware of HIV in the family. Most ALHIV will say HIV is not spoken about in the home, and siblings are not officially aware – although limited research, such as those by Miah (2004), which shows that most HIV-affected children find out there is HIV in their family years before being told officially. At its most extreme, I have worked with ALHIV where new partners of their primary carer are not told about the child's HIV and a web of secrecy is woven around medication routines and hospital appointments. Where the home is not a 'safe' environment to be HIV-positive, or not a place where this and the impact of it can be discussed openly, it can create unintended stigma.

19.4.2 Self-Stigma

There has been much produced on the impacts of HIV stigma on prevention, testing and accessing treatment. But the internal impacts of HIV stigma is less well documented, with little reference to the impact of self-stigma on children and adolescents, whose experience of HIV is different from their adult counterparts.

Self-stigma is where the individual internalizes the perceived (and real) stigma of their community/society, believing that they are unacceptable and feeling worthlessness and low self-esteem. A number of audits undertaken by the HIV Young Person Network (HYPNet) have concluded that the impacts of HIV-related stigma on individuals can lead to them not attending appointments, taking medication, emotional distress, feelings of intense isolation, increased psychological issues and at worst, mortality.

External attitudes and behavior impacting on the individuals' internal perceptions are nothing new; we see this in many different areas of people's lives, such as the influence of the media on adolescents' behavior relating to body image. We also know that a child will mirror the behavior of the environment in which he/she grows up. For example, Cancer research UK (2014) states on their website that if a parent smokes, a child is three times more likely to become a smoker in adulthood. We see this correlation between the parent and child's ART adherence, attitudes to HIV, and their ability to talk about it. Where the child's peer group voices negative views on HIV, it is likely that without a strong peer 'counter-argument', the child will believe these to be true and internalize them.

When looking at how to meet the psycho-social needs of C&ALHV, self-stigma is central to understanding how HIV impacts upon the child, and the importance of creating environments where C&ALHIV can explore their experiences and attitudes towards HIV and have these challenged. Self-stigma is a combination of their experiences of having HIV and what they learn from those around them, so what they have learnt from health care providers, the family/home, school and society. Nadine Ferris France (2012) explores this in her research on empowering children and how this relates to HIV self-stigma. She quotes JL Hymas research, 'Do children have rights?':

> …children must be empowered to make their own decisions, with certain parameters. This process is one of "trusting, affirming, and building self esteem in children" (Hymas 1999: 5).

To limit its impact, self-stigma needs to be challenged from the start of a child's life with HIV, and in every area of their lives. The child needs to be empowered with information, support and being included in decision-making to equip them with knowledge and increased self-esteem to manage the possible impacts of stigma on their feelings of self-worth and value.

19.5 Psycho-social Well-Being and Support

In the WHO's 2014 online resource, *Adolescent HIV Testing, Counselling and Care*,[5] defines psycho-social well-being as:

> A person's physical health, mental health, emotional life (feelings, thoughts, beliefs, attitudes) and social life (relationships, attitudes, cultural values and the influences of family, school, peers and community) all affect psycho-social well-being. (Living Positively section)

It goes on to underline the merits of psycho-social support for ALHIV, stating this is 'essential' and that,

> Psycho-social support can help patients as well as their caregivers gain confidence in themselves and their coping skills. (Living Positively section)

In the context of peer support, this is not holding a group where C&ALHIV go bowling, play football or simply 'hang out' – these are youth clubs. Psycho-social support must use therapeutic models and structures, have clear objectives relating to the needs of those attending and openly explore issues relating to living with HIV. It is a facilitated environment where the facilitator has good knowledge on the topic. It provides a non-judgemental space for sharing experiences, thought and feelings safely. It allows facilitators to challenge misinformation and misconceptions and to equip C&ALHIV with knowledge, confidence and skills to be able to manage a life with HIV. It is also a place where C&ALHIV can build their own support network that they will take with them into adult life (see also Chaps. 5, 6, 16, 17, 18, and 20 in this volume).

C&ALHIV will potentially, at different times, face multiple needs not relating to HIV. Maslow's Hierarchy of Need, a theory in psychology proposed by Abraham Maslow in his 1943 paper "A Theory of Human Motivation" (1943) offers a simple template that acknowledges an individual needs for personal security (food and shelter) before they would have the capacity to explore their relationship with a life with HIV.

19.5.1 Understanding Adolescents

When supporting adolescents, it is important to have an understanding of child development and the 'norms' for this time in a child's life. During adolescents, the individual becomes more aware of their place in society and how society views

[5] http://apps.who.int/adolescent/hiv-testingtreatment/page/Psychosocial_well_being

them. Peer relationships become more significant for the individual and the peer group can have an increased influence over behavior and beliefs during this time. The issues adolescents present may be seen as significantly challenging to parent/guardian and practitioners.

The secrecy that HIV demands can mean that ALHIV feel a profound sense of difference and isolation within their perceived HIV-negative peer group (see also Chaps. 6 and 17 in this volume). As Dodds (2011) shows, bringing C&ALHIV together has a profound impact on these feelings of isolation. In the process of trying to alter perceptions and behavior relating to self-stigma and accepting a life with HIV, using peer groups has also been shown to have positive outcomes.

19.5.2 *Example of Psycho-social Peer Support: 'Freedom To Be' (F2B)*

The Children's HIV Association (CHIVA) is a UK-based NGO that developed from a network for professionals offering health care to C&ALHIV, and now offers direct service provision to ALHIV across the UK and Ireland. F2B is central to this and is a therapeutic residential intervention for 100 ALHIV that provides psycho-social support, peer support and youth-friendly information/workshops on issues relating to growing up with HIV. It was developed by a group of experts on ALHIV form health and social care and a group of ALHIV. In the UK, unlike in North American, residential camps are not the norm, although a number of UK NGOs now use this model to bring children who share a medical experience together.

19.5.2.1 Core Values of F2B

What is critical to F2Bs success is the core set of values and ethos behind the model. Although this model is specific to low-prevalence areas, the core values behind the work and activities are also relevant to high prevalence areas. These values are respect, non-judgment, equity and acceptance.

Respecting everyone, not judging them for their behavior or life choices (or those of their parents) and that everyone's opinions and voice are of equal important ensure that marginalized children and young people – whether they are marginalized due to being born with HIV, through parental drug use, social situations or through acquiring HIV through 'risky' behavior – feel accepted and respected.

All staff and volunteers are trained to be active listeners, accepting the ALHIV and not trivializing what they say. The needs of the ALHIV and ensuring they are safe (both physically and emotionally) are central to everyone's practice.

Humor is incredibly important and supports building relationships with those attending and ensures that F2B is a fun place to be. The adolescents are never lied to, all questions are answered and no topics avoided. All staff and volunteers aim to build relationships of trust with one-another and with the adolescents they are supporting.

For any individual that has faced adversity and difficult experiences, being in an environment where they are respected, listened to, encouraged to express himself or herself in a way that psychically and emotionally safe can be extremely powerful. All these values are upheld from management to volunteers, and the ALHIV are encouraged to behave this way with one-another.

19.5.2.2 Structured Support

'Freedom To Be' was named by a 17 year old as this needed to be a place where HIV-positive children were free to properly be themselves, unlike in all other aspects of their lives. It had to be a place where HIV could be talked about openly and without shame or fear.

This has been embraced, with many HIV-positive volunteers openly talking about their experiences of living with HIV and medicine being taken openly at meal times. HIV is mentioned in all correspondence with the child and family prior to F2B, spoken about openly throughout F2B, explored in youth-friendly workshops, and in therapeutic and creative activities. Although at times this can seem a little excessive, over the week the attendees become more and more comfortable talking about HIV and 'my HIV'.

F2B has a core group of experienced paid staff that have worked for years supporting ALHIV, with backgrounds in social work, participation, youth work and psychotherapy. All volunteers must attend training prior to F2B where issues relating to HIV, safeguarding children and behavior management are explored. There is a strong ethos of supporting young adults who where once attendees to become volunteers, but this is undertaken in a supportive way, with mandatory training and professional supervision for all volunteers whilst at F2B.

19.5.2.3 Accessibility

An aim of F2B is that every ALHIV has the opportunity to attend once. To that end, each year at least half of those attending are coming for the first time. There is a policy of 'open access' so ALHIV attend with various physical disabilities, cognitive impairments, behavioral and emotional difficulties and impairments. This inclusion extends to adolescents who have experienced sexual exploitation, acquired HIV in early adolescents and those known to the police. Any child with additional needs is risk assessed to ensure F2B can meet their needs and keep them safe during their stay. Each adolescent is given a specific key worker (who is a volunteer) and where there are additional needs, the ALHIV is paired with someone who has experience or expertise in this field.

19.5.2.4 Therapeutic Activities

As previously stated, psycho-social peer support work has to explore issues relating to a life with HIV. Every year, F2B has a structured program of youth-friendly therapeutic activities. The program starts with a theme, previous themes being: 'Stigma', 'the power to change' and 'facing HIV together' (the themes are chosen by the CHIVA Youth Committee). This theme runs through all the workshops and activities held at camp. There are specific HIV workshops run by experts and cover knowledge and understanding HIV; adherence and its links with self-esteem; talking to others about HIV; understanding stigma and self-stigma. To date, these topics are covered annually in different ways, as they are considered the key issues faced by this group. There are also gender/age specific sexual health sessions run one afternoon which include condom demonstrations and the opportunity to confidentially ask questions about sex.

Example: Captain Straight Talk

This workshop was developed when the program theme at F2B was 'Power To Change' and all workshops had names relating to superheros. When the children are told their HIV diagnosis, they are told not to tell anyone. Yet at some point in their lives, it will be important to share this and they should feel confident and comfortable in making that decision and prepared for varied responses. The difficulty is that, if for a number of years they have kept HIV a secret, the psychological shift they need to make to be in a position to feel comfortable telling can be overwhelming. The purpose of this short workshop was for ALHIV to start to explore all the above and start to move towards a position of choosing not to tell from a positive position, such as "I will choose who to share it with", rather than from a position of fear and enforced secrecy.

Activity 1: Why do we talk to people about things?

Look at the different reasons to talk to others, from passing on information, developing friendships, that it is good to talk to people sometimes.

Activity 2: Why don't HIV-positive people talk to others about HIV?

The group were asked to shout out all the reasons they thought why people did not talk about their HIV, then asked to break these answers into 'outside' (external) and 'inside' (internal). They explored the difference between the reasons, so how sometimes we keep things to ourselves because they are private, whereas other times it is because we are afraid of how others will react. Stigma and self-stigma were specifically explained, and how we cannot control what others think of us, but we can control how we think about ourselves.

Activity 3: Role-play

The participants broke into groups and prepared a short role-play of how 'not to tell' and how 'to tell' someone you are HIV-positive. After each role-play, the group was asked what useful phrases and advice came from that and produce their 'top tips'.

19.5.2.5 Impacts of Psycho-social Peer Support

Often, psycho-social models of support are not thoroughly evaluated and even when they are, it can be difficult to say that an intervention was solely responsible for behavioral changes or impacts on an individual. The pilot of F2B was evaluated by Sigma Research (2010), a leading UK-based HIV academic research organization. The evaluation consisted of three different data collection phases, with attendees invited to voluntarily complete each of three linked questionnaires: phase one before F2B, phase two on the final day before leaving F2B, and phase three, 3 months after F2B.

Phase one findings suggested that those participating described HIV in their lives as overwhelmingly negative. They focused on secrecy, their self-stigmatizing, the difficulties in adhering and their fears of future and how HIV will impact upon that.

> It keeps you from having a full relationship with someone because you have to keep a massive part of you away from them. (16 year old)

Phase two revisited these themes, but also evaluated their experience during their time at F2B. Where it was possible to compare individuals' responses to a similar question from phase one, the majority (71 %) had met most of the information needs they had talked about before F2B. When asked what they had learned about themselves from this experience, most participants talked about their new-found confidence, and that they had learned to talk more openly about HIV. When asked about meeting other ALHIV, the majority (93 %) said this had been incredibly important to them and most of these said they would keep in touch with the people they had met.

> Arguably the most compelling information of all comes from some of the open-ended responses about participants' overarching impressions of camp, and what participants recalled learning there. How to tell people – that helped me tell my boyfriend. (15 year old)
>
> The elements of camp that were of greatest value to those who took part were (in order): making new friends with HIV, taking part in new activities, learning more about HIV and being in a fun and open atmosphere. (Dodds 2011: 5)

Phase three showed that many of the participants now considered they had numerous HIV-positive friends, with 97 % remaining in contact with a number of ALHIV they met at F2B. As Dodds (2011: 5) concludes:

> The overwhelming majority of the responses, even three months on from the event, were full of praise and gratitude for a life-changing, or at the very least, beneficial intervention. (Dodds 2011: 5)

Additionally to evaluating the ALHIV experiences, an anonymous survey of health care providers who had sent patients to F2B was run to see if they had noticed any changes in their patients. The most significant points were that 90 % felt their patient was now more inquisitive about their care; 80 % felt their patient had higher level of self-esteem; 70 % that they were better informed about potentially having conversations with others about their HIV and that 60 % better knowledge around their medication and adherence.

> They both expressed how great it was and the fact that they were able to meet so many young people who may experience the same problems with regards to medicines and disclosure. They were also able to exchange tips and strategies to deal with such issues (Healthcare Professional). (Harris 2010: 5)

19.5.3 Psycho-social Support: Conclusion

Self-stigma is complex, and in perinatally-infected children and adolescents, can develop over a long period of time and for many different reasons. It impacts on that child's core beliefs about HIV and about themselves, but happens in a silent way – silent as it is internalized, and silent as it can be a response to the silence that surrounds HIV in the child's life.

Using a model where the adolescent is central, respected, educated but also required to discuss HIV and have some of their views challenged has been shown to be highly effective. Bringing the peer group together to share their experiences, explore challenges and develop personal support networks that will survive into adulthood, goes someway to 'normalizing' HIV for this group. Peer support on its own can offer much, but where self-stigma runs deep within an individual, this should be part of a care package, linked to health care providers and promoting open and honest practice with this group of children.

19.6 Participation

Having children and adolescents meaningfully involved in their healthcare and personal decision-making can have an extremely positive impact on them. This participation should extend beyond their healthcare and include activities that will effect or impact upon them, such as service delivery and development in both health and social care. Within the context of this chapter, participation is used to mean involving C&ALHIV in having a voice in service development, influence public opinion, and inform policy.

Youth participation has become common best practice in the UK and is about ensuring children and young people are central to the process of indentifying needs, solutions, they are key to decision making and planning and developing work. Only this year, the UK government set up a specific piece of work to engage young people in NHS (National Health Service) developments. CHIVA has been striving to support ALHIV to have a voice in the development and delivery of health care provision, representation with policy-makers and with the public through the media and social networking.

Through this level of involvement and engagement, there is a very real sense of ownership and the experience for the individuals involved can be empowering. At its best, participation is about handing power over to those who the service or project is for and to this end, ensuring that their needs are central to developments and improves their lives.

19.6.1 Example: CHIVA Youth Committee (CYC)

C&ALHIV are a group that have decades of experience of living with HIV, yet their voices and experiences are seldom heard both nationally and internationally. AVERT reports that in 2011 there were 3.3 million perinatally-infected children living with HIV across the world,[6] yet it is still rare to find them as keynote speakers or advocates at international events relating to HIV in childhood and adolescents or as long term survivors.

In 2009, CHIVA began to develop a youth committee, with the aim to have representation of perinatally-infected adolescents and young adults from across the UK to influence medical guidance and practice in the UK. Once ALHIV were engaged, the aims of the CYC extended to having an outward facing voice to share their experiences, influence policy-makers and the public and try to reduce stigma. This work eventually received funding in 2012, and the CYC developed a formal constitution, specific roles, meets four times a year (as well as being involved in many additional activities) and has a Participation Officer to support them. The role of the CYC has and is still developing in response to issues the members locate.

CYC members have been involved in numerous consultations, in an advisory capacity on studies, clinical trials and individual research projects. Members have spoken at a number of events, having a regular slot at CHIVA's two annual conferences for health and social care professionals, running sessions on 'how doctors should communicate with us' or their experiences of sexual health education. They present at other medical meetings, one representative went to UNAIDS 33rd Board Meeting as a speaker, and two attended the International AIDS Conference 2014, speaking at the symposium on pediatric HIV there. They have met with parliamentarians, developed a campaign to educate schools about their pastoral care needs and they run a Twitter campaign to challenge HIV-related stigma, @freedom2spk. One member has also joined the youth board of the Children's Commissions Office for England that focuses on all children living in England. CYC members have given interviews on national and local radio, television and to newspapers. They are actively involved in the planning of F2B each year, running evening activities throughout the week.

The support they are offered extends beyond practicalities. Where they are liaising with the media, CHIVA staff will negotiate confidentiality inline with what the adolescent's wishes are and will accompany them so they feel supported and know that if at any point they decide they are uncomfortable, they will be supported to terminate the interview.

[6] AVERT: http://www.avert.org/worldwide-hiv-aids-statistics.htm

The CYC has a clear mandate to be advocates and are supported to do this through discussion and training. To that end, they will tell their own stories, but will also strive to represent all the experiences of C&ALHIV in the UK. They have control over how much personal information they share, are never pressured into undertaking any activities and are supported to feel empowered and not exploited.

19.6.2 The Impacts for ALHIV Being Involved in Participation Work

Although it is difficult to solely evaluate the impact of participation, as many factors in a person's life will influence how they are feeling and how they respond, two different evaluations have been undertaken to at the very least present some picture of impacts.

The first was an audit of healthcare providers to see if they had noticed any changes in their patients during their time as CYC members. Eight questions were asked, all being very specific to health, well-being and self-esteem changes that the health care provider had witnessed. The most significant impacts reported were 100 % (n=7) reporting positive changes in attitudes towards healthcare and HIV and 86 % (n=6) in general confidence (Carter 2013).

> I am really impressed with the opportunities that being part of the CHIVA youth committee presents. The young people that I know have had the experience of speaking at national conferences and also planning material to be used at the national summer camp, in addition to taking part in publicity campaigns raising the awareness of HIV. (Nurse) (Carter 2013: 5)

Although only seven health care providers participated in this audit, out of a potential 12, the findings do clearly demonstrate the positive impacts on these adolescents from being involved in this initiative. These second was a set of qualitative interviews undertaken by an external evaluator with CYC members to explore the impacts of membership on individual self-esteem and improved ability to cope with the challenges of living with HIV. The interviews attempted to gauge how the young people described the way they feel about themselves, and whether any increase in self-esteem could in any way be attributed to their experiences on the committee. They also explored the adolescent's future aspirations, as an indicator of an improved ability to cope with the challenges of living with HIV.

This report concluded that membership to the CYC and having the opportunity to participate fully and influence change had a very real impact on the self-esteem of these adolescents. Toocaram (2014: 11) also felt CYC members' experienced improved "ability to cope with the challenges of living with HIV". She located the following key areas of increase:

- The acquisition of interpersonal skills around public engagement and teamwork, helping members to confidently voice their opinion and advocate for others.
- A wider arena of social engagement, where CYC members are exposed to different opinions and experiences that develop their maturity.

- Social engagement with distinguished figures, whose willingness to hear the voices of CYC members affords these young people with a sense of self-worth.
- Feeling valued and respected in the role of CYC member.
- Feeling a sense of pride in the work achieved as a CYC member.
- An increased confidence in being able to achieve aspirations.

Toocaram reported that the ability to cope with the challenges of living with HIV, has increased for CYC members through the following ways:

- Being a CYC member has contributed to an improved view of HIV status.
- Working with other positive young people has contributed toward an empowering sense of collective action, and the feeling of control over one's [HIV] status.
- The safe environment of CYC, where all members are 'in the same boat,' allows for trust between members: members can be open and honest about their status, potentially lessening the psychological burden of secrecy and improving their ability to cope.

Toocaram's final conclusion was that the "increases in self-esteem for these young people through CYC membership is significant" (p. 11).

> Being on the youth committee gives me a sense of control of my status and position. Being on the youth committee helped improve my views toward it and my coping on a daily basis.' (ALHIV) (Toocaram 2014: 11)

19.6.3 Participation: Conclusion

Participation in all realms of life is incredibly important both for those participating and for improved outcomes. This chapter has explored how protectionist practice has developed around this group of children and how this, and the fear and reality of the stigma of having HIV, can profoundly impact on individuals sense of self and lead to self-stigmatizing thoughts and decision-making. Providing opportunities for supported and meaningful participation can have positive impacts on any group of people, but for C&ALHIV, with their collective experience of isolation, silence and secrecy, this impact can be profound.

Structured and supportive models of participation with C&ALHIV both have a positive impact on the individuals involved, but also ensure better quality healthcare, a better understanding of their varied experiences and give this group a national voice in policy and practice development and in the media. The support offered to adolescents undertaking such work is critical for its success both for them as individuals and for maximum impact. It is extremely important to let these children speak in an equitable environment and that those who provide services for them or who can influence policy actually listen to what they have to say.

19.7 Conclusion

Once an HIV-positive child or adolescent has access to food, shelter and ART, the biggest issue they will face will be self-stigma. For too long, focus has been on external stigma, how we need to change public perceptions and negative attitudes towards HIV. Yet little thought of how the behavior of those supporting C&ALHIV can quietly build a picture for a child where HIV is something they have to "fight"; how it is not a bad thing, but "we haven't told you about it before and now don't tell anyone"; how it is kept from all realms of the child's life, from their siblings, extended family and school.

Self-stigma can be profoundly debilitating for individuals self-esteem, self-worth and mental well-being. This, in-turn, can impact on their engagement with their health care and their relationship with HIV. Successful engagement of C&ALHIV must be open, honest, supportive and non-judgmental and this includes trust and child-centered and child-led practice. Bringing the peer group together to either explore issues relating to living with HIV or to work together to have their voices heard, has been shown to have hugely positive effects. Building resilience and empowering this group to see that stigma comes from ignorance and lack of knowledge, not that they are someone who is 'disgraced' or 'devalued' due to their medical condition.

C&ALHIV globally have large HIV education, support and sexual health needs, the self-stigma they feel can have an overwhelming impact on their life choices and life expectancy. This group of children faces the adversity of a life managing a long-term health condition, those supporting these children should ensure they are afforded the basic rights under the UN Convention of the Rights of a Child. They need to 'own' their own HIV diagnosis, be party to make decisions about their own healthcare and have their voices heard.

References

British Medical Association. (2001). *Consent, rights and choices in health care for children and young people*. London: BMJ Press.

Carter, A. (2013). *Finding from the survey: The impact of being a member of the CHIVA Youth Committee*. London: The Children's HIV Association.

Conway, M. (2006). *Children, HIV, asylum & immigration*. London: National Children's Bureau.

Dodds, C. (2011). *Freedom to be summer camp: Outcome evaluation*. London: Sigma Research.

Evans, R., & Becker, S. (2009). *Children caring for parents with HIV and AIDS*. Bristol: The Policy Press.

Ferrand, R., Corbett, E., Wood, R., Hargrove, J., Ndhlovu, E., Cowan, F., Gouws, E., & Williams, B. (2009). AIDS among older children and adolescents in Southern Africa: Projecting the time course and magnitude of the epidemic. *AIDS, 23*(15), 2039–2046.

Ferris-France, N. (2012). *HIV and self-stigma core belief sheet*. Dublin: Open Heart House and Trinity College.

Hamblin, E. (2011). *Just normal young people: Supporting young people living with HIV in their transition to adulthood*. London: National Children's Bureau.

Harris, J. (2010). *Health care professionals and parents/carers evaluation: The impact of the CHIVA summer camp reported by the health care providers and parents/carers*. London: The Children's HIV Association.

Hymas, J. I. (1999). Do children have rights? citing Cullen, S., *Empowering children*. Retrieved from www.congcreator.com/ifcw99/cullen2.htm at www.nhsexposed.com/patients/child health/childrights.shtml.

Maslow, A. H. (1943). A theory of human motivation. *Psychological Review, 50*(4), 370–396.

McDonald, S. (2011). *HYPNet adherence audit*. BHIVA 2011.

Miah, J. (Ed.). (2004). *Talking with children, young people and families about chronic illness and living with HIV*. London: National Children's Bureau.

National AIDS Trust. (2008). *The myth of HIV health tourism*. London: NAT.

Taddeo, D., Egedy, M., & Frappier, J.-Y. (2008). Adherence to treatment in adolescents. *Paediatric Child Health, 13*(1), 19–24.

Toocaram, L. (2014). *Impact upon self-esteem of being a member of the CHIVA Youth Committee*. London: The Children's HIV Association.

UNAIDS (2003). *AIDS epidemic update,* December 2003. Retrieved on April, 20, 2016, from http://data.unaids.org/pub/Report/2003/2003_epiupdate_en.pdf.

United Nation (2009). *Convention on the rights of the child*. Retrieved on April, 20, 2016, from http://www2.ohchr.org/english/bodies/crc/docs/AdvanceVersions/CRC-C-GC-12.pdf.

WHO. (2011). *Guideline on HIV disclosure counseling for children up to 12 years of age*. Geneva: World Health Organization.

WHO. (2014). *Adolescent HIV testing, counselling and care: Implementation guidance for health providers and planners*. Geneva: World Health Organization.

Chapter 20
Teens and Transitions: Supporting Youth with HIV to Move Successfully from Pediatric to Adult Healthcare

Corry Azzopardi, Robyn Salter, Stephanie Savage, Jason Brophy, Ari Bitnun, and Stanley Read

Contents

C. Azzopardi (✉)
Division of Pediatric Medicine, The Hospital for Sick Children, 555 University Avenue, Toronto, ON M5G 1X8, Canada
e-mail: corry.azzopardi@sickkids.ca

R. Salter • A. Bitnun • S. Read
Division of Infectious Diseases, The Hospital for Sick Children, 555 University Avenue, Toronto, ON M5G 1X8, Canada
e-mail: robyn.salter@sickkids.ca; ari.bitnun@sickkids.ca; stanley.read@sickkids.ca

S. Savage
The Teresa Group, 124 Merton Street, Suite 104, Toronto, ON M4S 2Z2, Canada
e-mail: SavageS@teresagroup.ca

J. Brophy
Division of Infectious Diseases, Children's Hospital of Eastern Ontario, 401 Smyth Road, Ottawa, ON K1H 8L1, Canada
e-mail: jbrophy@cheo.on.ca

P. Liamputtong (ed.), *Children and Young People Living with HIV/AIDS*, Cross-Cultural Research in Health, Illness and Well-Being,
DOI 10.1007/978-3-319-29936-5_20

20.1 Introduction

Since the advent of human immunodeficiency virus (HIV) more than three decades ago, loss of life from acquired immune deficiency syndrome (AIDS) has been globally devastating. Internationally, an estimated 5.4 million young people (10–24 years) were living with HIV in 2012 due to ineffective or inaccessible prevention programs (UNAIDS 2013). Infants born with perinatally-acquired HIV through the 1980s and into the 1990s were not expected to reach adulthood. Advancements in medical treatment, particularly the introduction of highly active antiretroviral therapy (HAART) in 1997, have led to a remarkable decline in HIV-associated morbidity and mortality (Antiretroviral Therapy Cohort Collaboration 2008). There has been a corresponding shift in the medical community's conceptualization and management of HIV as a chronic condition. While a longer life expectancy for children living with HIV is cause for celebration, it comes in tandem with new and unexpected challenges during transitions to adolescence and adulthood. Healthcare systems are now faced with the difficult task of effectively and sensitively accommodating the first cohort of youth with HIV as they progress from pediatric to adult care (see also Chaps. 5, 6, 18, 19, and 21 in this volume).

HIV infection is one of a host of chronic conditions requiring lifelong medical management and psycho-social care. In western societies, youth tend to transition from the pediatric healthcare system into the adult healthcare system in their late-teen years. There is, however, significant variation in age of transition policies and practices between and within different jurisdictions, ranging from 15 to 25 years (Burke et al. 2008; Gilliam et al. 2011). A recent Canadian study found that the majority of service providers agreed that transitioning should occur after the age of 18, a sentiment that stands in contrast to current models of care in many institutions (Clark et al. 2014). In addition to chronological age, it is important to consider developmental status, particularly for those with cognitive delays, and state of readiness for the transition process. It is generally recommended that transition interventions be continuous, coordinated, culturally appropriate, compassionate, and family-centered (Cervia 2013). While HIV shares some similarities with other chronic illnesses, there are important differences that must be taken into account when devising responsive models of transitional care (Laufer and Scott 2000; Fair et al. 2010; Andiman 2011). HIV-specific social stigma, HIV transmission prevention, and drug resistance consequent to non-adherence, for example, are some of the many unique complexities to consider (Green 1995; Rao et al. 2007; Valenzuela et al. 2011).

Despite growing recognition of the importance of thoughtful and seamless transition through the phases of HIV care, the present state of clinical and empirical knowledge of how best to assist youth as they progress into adulthood is notably limited. Our ill-preparedness is thought to be, at least in part, due to the reality that HIV-infected children were, in the not so distant past, not expected to survive into adulthood (Wiener et al. 2007; Dowshen and D'Angelo 2011; Boudreau and Fisher 2012). This chapter provides an overview of selected literature examining the unique lived experiences and clinical needs of adolescents with HIV and best practice models for transitioning from pediatric to adult healthcare. We draw on our multidisciplinary perspectives and practices in pediatric healthcare to address some of the challenges commonly encountered by patients and families affected by HIV and propose practical strategies for successful transitions.

20.2 Adolescents Living with HIV: Unique Medical and Psycho-Social Challenges

To fully appreciate the complexities of transitioning from pediatric to adult healthcare, it is helpful to gain some understanding of the medical and psycho-social challenges commonly faced by young people living with HIV. Adolescence is a transitional stage of human development between childhood and adulthood wherein a person typically matures physically, emotionally, psychologically, socially, and sexually. During this formative period, aspects of one's social environment, family influences, and peer relations are continuously being integrated into evolving concepts of self and others. The transition to adulthood is marked by gradual independence from caregivers and increasing responsibilities. For teens coping with HIV, ordinary adolescent struggles may be compounded by the unique issues stemming from their medical condition such as stigmatization and marginalization, loss and trauma, family problems, bio-psycho-social concerns, and treatment adherence challenges (see also Chaps. 4, 5, 6, 7, 8, 9, 10, 15, 17, 18, 19, and 21 in this volume).

20.2.1 Social Stigma, Status Disclosure, and Sexual Health

There has been longstanding social stigma associated with HIV and AIDS that continues to have powerful impact on the lives of those affected (Green 1995; Fielden et al. 2006; Rao et al. 2007; Vijayan et al. 2009). Perinatally-infected youth may be subjected to less stigmatization by virtue of their 'innocent' mode of transmission.

Nevertheless, real and perceived fears of being marginalized and ostracized render the decision to disclose one's HIV status to family members, friends, school systems, and others in the community an arduous one requiring serious contemplation of the consequences. Adolescents and their parents may have divergent thoughts on when and with whom to share their diagnosis, potentially creating additional conflict for some families. One study described stigma as underscoring and compounding all other challenges faced by teens living with HIV (Vijayan et al. 2009). Concerns over stigma compel some young people with HIV to conceal their status, thus restricting their access to social support, contributing to further isolation, and exacerbating feelings of shame (Fielden et al. 2006; Fair et al. 2010; Ross et al. 2010; see also Chaps. 4, 5, 6, 7, 9, 15, 17, and 18 in this volume).

Sexual development is a normal, exciting, and sometimes confusing part of puberty. Because HIV can be sexually transmitted, HIV-infected adolescents who are exploring their sexuality encounter additional burdens. Engaging in intimate relationships is further complicated by having to negotiate status disclosure with partners and potentially face rejection (Fielden et al. 2006; Fair and Albright 2012). In many parts of the world, persons knowingly living with HIV are considered ethically and legally responsible to disclose their positive status to sexual partners, and may face criminal prosecution for failing to do so. Pediatric care providers have expressed concerns regarding the pervasive lack of resources to allow provision of appropriate sexual and reproductive healthcare in pediatric settings (Vijayan et al. 2009; see also Chap. 19 in this volume).

20.2.2 Loss, Trauma, and Family Problems

Many youth living with HIV are coping with complex family dynamics and stress. For those who were perinatally-infected, they will have had one or more biological parents, and possibly siblings and extended family members, also living with HIV. Thus, they are likely to struggle with chronic physical and mental illness in the family. The passing of one or both parents ultimately results in single parenthood or being orphaned, and possibly placement with alternate caregivers and unstable living arrangements. These experiences can trigger intense grief reactions, feelings of abandonment, and disruptions in attachment security (see also Chaps. 2, 3, 4, 5, 6, 7, 15, and 16 in this volume).

HIV-infected mothers commonly struggle with self-blame and guilt because the virus was transmitted from them to their child, which can manifest in the form of overprotective parenting (Spiegel and Futterman 2009). Deciding when to disclose a child's HIV status to them can be very difficult for parents, sometimes leading to delayed disclosures and crises of trust (Salter et al. 2007). Family functioning can be further complicated by physical and mental health disorders, conflict, intensified parenting stress and burden, chronic sorrow, stigma, isolation, and fear (Antle et al. 2001). Immigrant and refugee populations face additional marginalization and challenges stemming from the stresses of adapting to a new culture, losses and traumas in their country of origin, social exclusion, inadequate housing, food insecurity, barriers to employment, poverty, and inaccessible healthcare (Mikkonen and Raphael 2010).

20.2.3 Developmental Functioning and Mental Health

Children and adolescents with perinatally-acquired HIV have a higher propensity for neuro-developmental delays and poor academic performance. In their study examining pediatric psycho-developmental functioning, Nozyce et al. (2006) found lower cognitive and developmental scores and more behavioral problems among young people with HIV in comparison to expected norms. While poor school achievement is often attributed to developmental deficits, there may be other contributing factors at play, such as school absenteeism due to medical appointments, adverse effects of medications, anxiety and depression, and altered self-image (Battles and Wiener 2002; Nozyce et al. 2006; DiRisio et al. 2011).

While many adolescents with HIV demonstrate remarkable resilience, the mental health implications of living with HIV infection can be pervasive (see also Chaps. 4, 12, and 18 in this volume). Youth with HIV confront countless psychological, emotional, and social stressors from which most same-aged peers are protected, including issues related to extensive loss and bereavement, insecurity and instability, rejection and isolation, low self-esteem, and sense of not being 'normal' (Fielden et al. 2006). Unsurprisingly, they are more likely to experience psychiatric illness, substance abuse, and other high risk behaviors, all of which may have adverse health effects (Mellins et al. 2006, 2009). Moreover, infected youth are twice as likely to be prescribed psychotropic medications than their uninfected peers (as cited in Boudreau and Fisher 2012).

20.2.4 Treatment Adherence Challenges and Health Implications

Optimal adherence to HAART regimens correlates positively with virologic suppression, increased CD4 count, and reduced mortality (Van Dyke et al. 2002; Lima et al. 2008). Sustained viral suppression, however, requires at least 95 % compliance with prescribed treatment (Paterson et al. 2000). The risk of virologic rebound and drug resistance is substantial when adherence drops (Sethi et al. 2003; Harrigan et al. 2005). With almost half of HIV-infected youth in high-income countries estimated to be less than 75 % adherent (Simoni et al. 2007), compliance with demanding treatment regimens can be particularly challenging for young people, thus exposing them to detrimental health repercussions. Several studies have observed a decline in treatment adherence as children age (Mellins et al. 2006; Williams et al. 2006), suggesting developmental influences as adolescents begin to gain independence from caregivers and assume more responsibility for their healthcare. Because the adverse health effects of poor adherence are not immediate (in contrast to other chronic conditions such as diabetes mellitus), it is difficult for adolescents to truly grasp and foresee the consequences of their poor adherence.

Although findings tend to be discrepant across research studies, some of the many known impediments to HIV therapy adherence among youth include mental health and cognitive impairments, limited social support, stigma, disclosure status, complicated treatment courses, treatment fatigue, forgetfulness, inconsistent routines, schedule disruption, medication side effects, lack of appreciation for the importance of compliance when feeling well, substance use, low caregiver involvement, caregiver dysfunction, poor family relations, and service disparities (Murphy et al. 2003; Vreeman et al. 2008; Reisner et al. 2009; Vijayan et al. 2009; Naar-King et al. 2013; Azzopardi et al. 2014; see also Chaps. 4, 5, 6, 17, 18, 19, and 22 in this volume).

20.3 Transitioning from Pediatric to Adult Healthcare: Advantages, Disadvantages, and Barriers

For pediatric populations living with HIV, the shift to the adult healthcare system is inevitable, for better or for worse. There is a small but growing body of research with HIV-infected youth, their parents or caregivers, and service providers regarding their perspectives of and experiences with healthcare transitions. Transitions usually elicit mixed emotions, from fear and sadness to relief and excitement. Some youth embrace the transition to adult care and welcome the satisfaction of autonomy from caregivers and personal responsibility for medical management (Miles et al. 2004; Bundock et al. 2011; Valenzuela et al. 2011; Fair et al. 2012a, b). According to some transitioned youth, adult care helped them to develop skills for living independently, making healthier choices, having a more positive outlook, and even giving back to their community (Valenzuela et al. 2011). Caregivers have also identified some advantages of transitioning, including relinquishing control and responsibility to their children, preparation for adulthood, and improved healthcare (Fair et al. 2012a, b). Notwithstanding these benefits, there are a number of potential disadvantages associated with the movement to adult-oriented care and barriers to effective transitions, including discrepant service provision, unsupportive environments and ill-preparedness, socio-economic constraints, and deteriorating treatment adherence and adverse health effects.

20.3.1 Confidentiality, Discrimination, and Service Disparities

Recognizing the stigma and shame surrounding HIV infection, there is a concerted effort in many pediatric HIV settings to ensure that services are offered in a private, sensitive, and confidential manner. This entails respecting the informed decisions of patients and families to maintain status nondisclosure, both within and outside of the family. One way in which some pediatric healthcare programs protect confidentiality is by offering interprofessional HIV care along with services for other common health conditions in shared clinic settings. The adult system tends to be more fragmented in their provision of medical and psycho-social care, and less likely to take the appropriate steps to safeguard privacy. In addition, the patient to allied health professional ratio is often much higher in the adult system, which impairs healthcare providers' ability to provide needed support. For some, fears of inadvertent status disclosure results in delayed or difficult transitions (Gilliam et al. 2011; Valenzuela et al. 2011). This is compounded by concerns of discrimination by adult healthcare providers or other patients based on assumptions of viral acquisition through high risk behaviors such as unprotected sexual relations or injection drug use (Miles et al. 2004; Vijayan et al. 2009; Wiener et al. 2011).

Not all adult healthcare providers are trained to work effectively with adolescents. Transition service discrepancies may be particularly evident for lesbian, gay, bisexual, and transgender (LGBT) youth with HIV, who require adult care providers with the specialized knowledge and skills required to competently and sensitively address critical issues related to sexual orientation, gender identity, and reproductive health in the context of HIV infection (Garofalo et al. 2006; Wiener et al. 2011; Cervia 2013).

20.3.2 Rapport, Trust, and Adaptations to New Healthcare Settings

Many children and adolescents with HIV develop strong, trusting relationships with pediatric service providers over time, often never knowing a life without them. Indeed, for some, the healthcare team is considered family and the clinic feels like home. The inevitable transition to adult care marks the end of these relationships and is often experienced as a significant loss, particularly for youth with strong attachments to their pediatric team (Thorne et al. 2002; Miles et al. 2004; Vijayan et al. 2009; Maturo et al. 2011; Fair et al. 2012a, b; Sharma et al. 2014). For bereaved youth in particular, severing connections with pediatric services may trigger familiar feelings of loss, abandonment, anxiety, and insecurity. For children in foster care, the coincidental loss of foster care services at the age of transition (in some jurisdictions) is an additional burden. These losses may hinder the transition process and obstruct rapport with new care providers. In the absence of a trusting relationship, having to retell their stories to unfamiliar staff in clinics oriented to adults can be emotionally daunting, especially for behaviorally-infected youth (Cervia 2007; Valenzuela et al. 2011). Likewise, pediatric service providers themselves often have a hard time letting go, putting faith in youth to attend to their own healthcare, and trusting the expertise of adult facilities (Viner 1999).

While some adolescents prefer adult-oriented medical settings (Bundock et al. 2011), for others, the contrasting physical environments of 'fun' child-centered clinics versus more serious adult-centered clinics can be a difficult adjustment (Fair et al. 2012a, b). For example, some transitioned youth have expressed surprise with adult focused décor and messaging, predominance of gay male patients, and small number of other youth in adult settings (Miles et al. 2004). Pediatric and adult facilities also tend to differ in patient volume, appointment length, integration of medical and psycho-social services, and level of practical support offered. A multidisciplinary approach to healthcare is less common in adult systems, leaving some youth without necessary developmental and mental health care and thus posing a barrier to successful transition (Reiss et al. 2005; Gilliam et al. 2011; Valenzuela et al. 2011; Wiener et al. 2011). Moreover, adult care providers tend to be less family-centered and less inclined to offer the practical support that many adolescents have grown accustomed to in pediatric settings, such as appointment reminders, transportation assistance, and help with medication adherence (Sharma et al. 2014). While 'hand-holding' may discourage independence and autonomy, some transitioning youth, particularly those with developmental limitations, require additional support during this process.

20.3.3 Adolescent Autonomy and Preparedness for Transitioning

As HIV-infected children transition through adolescence and into early adulthood, caregivers and service providers generally become less directly involved in supervising treatment regimens in order to promote independence and readiness for lifelong healthcare management. This process is sometimes hampered by parental reticence to relinquish control, poor communication or tendency to minimize the impact of the disease, premature assumption of self-sufficient care, or discrepancies in roles and responsibilities, resulting in some youth failing to acquire the autonomy, knowledge, and skills required for successful transitions to adult care (Reiss et al. 2005; Vijayan et al. 2009; Naar-King et al. 2013; Clark et al. 2014).

Furthermore, healthcare providers differ in the ways in which they conceptualize and approach transition. While some view transitioning as a gradual and deliberate process requiring education and capacity building, others consider transition an isolated event involving a transfer from one clinic to another (Gilliam et al. 2011), perhaps resulting in disparate levels of support and youth preparedness.

20.3.4 Socio-Economic Well-Being and Access to Healthcare

Access to healthcare and navigating complicated social service bureaucracies can pose significant barriers to successful transitions from pediatric to adult systems (Dowshen and D'Angelo 2011). As a consequence of their challenging social context, infected youth are more likely to experience poverty than those without HIV, and less likely to have health insurance than other age groups with HIV (Cervia 2013). In countries without universal healthcare, lack of medical insurance, against the backdrop of poverty and deprivation of resources, renders some youth with HIV at high risk for being denied access to medical services (UNAIDS 2013). Socio-economically disadvantaged patients tend to have the poorest health outcomes, highlighting the vital influence of the social determinants of health (Mikkonen and Raphael 2010; Liamputtong et al. 2012).

20.3.5 Treatment Non-Adherence and Compromized Health Post-Transition

Studies have shown that some youth experience a decline in treatment adherence and health status following their transfer from pediatric to adult healthcare (Murphy et al. 2003; Gilliam et al. 2011; Wiener et al. 2011), underscoring the importance of preparation and ongoing support. One study, for instance, found that HIV-infected youth who were newly established in an adult clinic demonstrated lower rates of virologic suppression, higher rates of viral rebound, and higher rates of attrition compared to matched adult controls (Ryscavage et al. 2011). Some of the common barriers to optimal treatment adherence, such as depression, substance abuse, or lack of health insurance, may intensify post-transition, leaving young people especially vulnerable to compromised health during this critical period of change. Conversely, another study reported no significant difference in CD4 count between those who remained in pediatric care and those who transitioned to adult care (Wiener et al. 2011).

20.4 Helping Adolescents Transition: Models of Care and Best Practices Approaches

Interventions to facilitate the transition from child- and family-centered to adult-oriented healthcare settings aim to prepare adolescents for increasingly independent care, alleviate fears and anxieties associated with the shift in care, and streamline the transition process to ensure continuity of quality care in a planned and purposeful way. There is wide variation in approaches to youth transition across healthcare settings and limited guidance available on best practices with HIV populations.

Established transition models for comparable chronic illnesses offer a useful template; however, HIV transition interventions must respond to the unique needs of HIV-infected teens and adults. Despite multilevel challenges and potential obstacles, positive transitions from pediatric to adult HIV services can be promoted with personalized care plans that address known barriers and incorporate facilitators.

20.4.1 Strategies for Transitioning and Indicators of Success

Facilitators of successful youth transitions to adult HIV care, according to the perspectives of healthcare providers, include acceptance of the diagnosis, health literacy, family support, effective communication between pediatric and adult providers, and post-transition reminders (Clark et al. 2014). Transition models generally encourage pediatric care providers to engage in conversations about eventual transitioning with patients and families in early adolescence, regardless of whether the physical transition occurs at a predetermined age or based on individual readiness (Paone et al. 2006; Fair et al. 2010; Maturo et al. 2011; Gilliam et al. 2011; Valenzuela et al. 2011; Committee on Pediatric AIDS 2013). Facilitating an introductory meeting between adolescents and adult care providers before the physical transition occurs can also help to reduce anxiety and enhance preparedness. Pediatric social workers can play a pivotal role in easing the transition process (Fair et al. 2012a, b).

Fundamental to successful youth transition is accurate disease-specific knowledge and capacity to assume responsibility for treatment and independent decision-making, as well as an orientation toward future goals, including good health and long-term survival (Cervia 2013). Some healthcare professionals utilize standardized measures or documentation of patient knowledge to monitor readiness for transition (Gilliam et al. 2011). To ensure uninterrupted care, comprehensive, individualized care plans should be developed collaboratively with adolescents, caregivers if appropriate, and multidisciplinary care providers. In addition to a detailed treatment regimen, formal care plans should include concrete, agreed upon goals and timelines, delegation of responsibilities, and strategies for overcoming anticipated obstacles such as those related to the logistical and financial aspects of care or developmental vulnerabilities of the patient. When the time comes, graduation from pediatric care can be celebrated with a ceremonial event or certificate that marks the end of one phase of healthcare and beginning of another.

Policy statements, best practice guidelines, and tools have begun to emerge to assist HIV care providers in promoting successful transitions (e.g., Children's HIV Association 2011; New York State Department of Health AIDS Institute 2011; American Academy of Pediatrics 2013). Nevertheless, there is a paucity of HIV-specific empirical research examining the efficacy of youth transition programs due to a host of conceptual and methodological challenges, including the absence of tracking mechanisms post-transition and poorly or inconsistently operationalized indicators of success. For example, empirical markers of positive transitions range from patient perceptions (e.g., ownership of healthcare), adherence to clinic appointments, adequate medication adherence, and/or maintenance of viral suppression. As such, extant transition literature tends to be limited to program descriptions, care provider perspectives, and patient or caregiver concerns, in the absence of robust empirical data (Freed and Hudson 2006; Fair et al. 2011). There is, however, some evidence to suggest that a personalized transition intervention increases readiness and decreases anxiety for youth with HIV (Wiener et al. 2007).

20.4.2 One Interprofessional Pediatric Healthcare Team's Approach to Transition

We conclude this chapter by sharing some of the insights we have gained through our work with children, adolescents, and families in a pediatric HIV healthcare setting in Toronto, Canada. We draw on our experiences with a growing number of transitioned or transitioning youth to offer key strategies for successful transitions. The HIV Comprehensive Care Program at the Hospital for Sick Children (SickKids, an urban-based, tertiary care, pediatric teaching hospital) was established in 1988 and has since become one of the largest pediatric HIV programs in the country. Our multidisciplinary team comprises healthcare professionals from pediatric medicine, nursing, social work, pharmacy, physiotherapy, psychiatry, and psychology (for educational testing). Of the almost 200 pediatric patients with HIV followed in our clinic to date, 60 (born between 1987 and 1997) have, or are preparing to, transition to adult healthcare. Of the 60 transitioned or transitioning youth, most (92 %) were perinatally-infected. The majority (85 %) are from families who came to Canada as immigrants or refugees, mostly from African or Caribbean countries. Nearly two thirds (62 %) experienced the loss of one or both biological parents, either from death or family disruption, often requiring placement with alternate caregivers. Many are living in poverty, with more than a third (35 %) relying on social assistance or disability pensions.

Our HIV team follows the hospital's general model of transition, *Good2Go* (see http://www.sickkids.ca/good2go), which has been adapted to the specific needs of young people living with HIV in a specialized version of the model, *Positively Good2Go* (see http://www.sickkids.ca/Go-Positive/Graduating-from-SickKids/index.html). The program includes several formal components, including educational materials and a dedicated website, as well as a transition readiness checklist for patients and knowledge assessment checklist for caregivers, both completed at six-month intervals (Bitnun et al. 2012).

The following case study of '*Sara*' illustrates some of the clinical complexities and common challenges faced by patients and families impacted by HIV. We will revisit this case to explore the strategies implemented by our team to facilitate this patient's transition from our pediatric hospital to an adult care facility.

Sara is a 17-year-old female who has been followed by the HIV clinic at SickKids since her diagnosis of perinatally-transmitted HIV infection at two years of age. She and her parents, both HIV-positive, immigrated to Canada from West Africa when Sara was an infant. Sara's younger sibling was born uninfected in Canada. Sara's father died from AIDS-related complications 10 years ago. Sara's mother struggled to support the family financially while also coping with her own deteriorating health. She was actively involved in Sara's healthcare, attending all clinic appointments and supervising her medication adherence. The pediatric HIV team introduced Sara and her mother to the topic of transitioning to adult care in her early-teen years. Sara's mother, with the support of the healthcare team, fostered Sara's independence from a very early age through education and skill building. Following Sara's mother's death when Sara was 13 years of age, she and her sister were placed in the care of relatives. As a result, they were uprooted from their home and had to transfer to a new school. Sara was deeply affected by the loss of her parents, neighborhood, and close friends. She experienced significant difficulty coping, began to withdraw from school and family activities, and expressed fear of being stigmatized by her new peers should her HIV status be disclosed or discovered. While her extended family members were supportive, none had HIV infection and, from Sara's perspective, could not truly understand what she was going through. With the exception of assistance with transportation to and from clinic appointments, Sara has assumed full responsibility for her healthcare. She does, however, rely on appointment reminders from the clinic and sometimes forgets to fill her medication prescriptions.

Many of our patients, like Sara, present with histories of loss and trauma while simultaneously coping with social stigma as peer relationships become increasingly important in their lives. Individual and family strengths-based counseling is offered to promote healthy coping. Most have had a longstanding relationship with the HIV team, which enhances the experience of care and fosters trust. The strength of these long-term relationships and attachments can, however, make it very difficult for some youth to make the move to adult care as they approach the standard age of transition (18–19 years). We, therefore, approach transition as a gradual process of deliberate preparation beginning in early adolescence, assuming developmental capacity for understanding. In place of a structured protocol, customized transition plans are designed for each of our graduating patients based on their individual developmental and emotional needs and strengths. Equipping youth with a solid knowledge and skill base to maintain good health, while instilling confidence for independent care is a fundamental component to our transition model.

Interprofessional collaboration and communication are key to the success of this approach. Given the potential for sexual transmission of HIV, we try to ensure that youth understand 'safer sex' practices, contraceptive choices, and the importance of partner disclosure prior to sexual contact. This information is integrated into discussions about healthy relationships and readiness for sexual activity.

The multidisciplinary team worked closely with Sara to ensure that she fully understood the nature of her health condition and modes of transmission, the purpose and schedule of medications, the importance of strict adherence and potential consequences of non-adherence. They also provided psychoeducation regarding recognition and management of the stigma associated with HIV, status disclosure decision-making, and healthy relationships, including potential sexual partnerships. To promote positive adaptation and the likelihood of success post-transition, the social worker offered ongoing counseling to help Sara work through the grieving process following the loss of her parents, adjust to her new environment, and constructively cope with the many sources of stress impacting her life. In counseling sessions, Sara shared that she wanted to honor the memory of her parents by taking good care of her health so that she can graduate from university and achieve her career goals. Sara's caregivers were included in these discussions at her discretion. To reduce feelings of isolation, the team collaborated with Sara to develop disclosed social support networks. Sara was referred to a therapeutic support group for teens held in the clinic just before medical visits.

Youth with HIV who disclose their HIV status to other infected youth often unearth a world of understanding, shared experiences, and support. Peer support can help to reduce feelings of isolation, shame, and anxiety during the transition process. It can also offer an empathetic outlet for exploring and preparing for discussions of HIV in romantic/sexual relationships. Therapeutic support groups, summer camps, one-to-one facilitated discussions, and online chat groups are some examples of sources for developing disclosed peer support (see Chaps. 6, 15, 18, 19 and 21 in this volume). Our clinic is fortunate to have a formal partnership with a community-based agency for children, youth, and families infected and affected by HIV that offers hospital-based therapeutic support groups for adolescents with HIV until the point of transition to adult care (Shindler and Tangelder 2010). These groups have been shown to foster safety and support, education and learning, normalization, mutual aid, treatment adherence, and transition (Muskat et al., submitted manuscript). Summer camps provide another opportunity for youth to connect in a fun environment where their diagnoses do not take center stage (see Chap. 6). For those who are uncomfortable with group settings, private one-to-one meetings between two or more consenting young people with HIV can be facilitated in the clinic. Online support groups can offer youth with HIV who prefer to remain anonymous a venue for developing meaningful social relations (see Chap. 18). For example, in the province of Ontario, there is an advocacy and capacity building coalition of agencies serving positive youth that is in the process of developing a youth support program, which includes a website with a private chat room (developed by a young person with HIV and monitored by a professional) to promote and support social connections among youth living with HIV (see http://www.thepozzy.org). Many of the bonds formed through disclosed peer support networks continue long after graduation from pediatric care.

Our approach to transition involves collaborating with adolescents and their parents or guardians to identify tangible goals, appropriate timeframes for achieving them, and evaluation plans. This includes discussions of the differences between pediatric and adult healthcare settings, anticipated obstacles, and potential strategies for overcoming them. An important step early in this process is identifying suitable adult healthcare providers based on patient needs and preferences. This may entail inviting adult healthcare providers to the pediatric clinic or facilitating visits to various adult facilities until reaching a goodness-of-fit. For those who are uncomfortable going to an adult facility on their own for the first time, we provide individual or group visits to selected adult facilities accompanied by our clinic social worker or nurse. We also offer an overlapping period of alternating pediatric and adult clinic appointments to ease the transition process.

Some young people also require resource counseling on applying for and maintaining drug insurance and financial support according to their eligibility. This is an essential skill for transitioning youth who may require guidance on how to obtain necessary verification documents, manage confidentiality, and decide with whom and when to disclose their HIV status.

During a multidisciplinary meeting with the clinic social worker, nurse, and physician, Sara expressed feeling nervous yet excited about her impending transition to adult healthcare. The team normalized and validated Sara's mixed emotions. At Sara's request, the social worker accompanied her to an adult facility, introduced her to the new healthcare providers, and supported her through the discussion. Sara was apprehensive but connected well with the team. She was looking forward to less travel time to the new clinic, meeting new people, and reconnecting with friends from the support groups who had recently transitioned to the same clinic. Toward the end of her time with

(continued)

the pediatric team, Sara was invited to work with her social worker to write a transition summary report to share important psycho-social information with her new care providers. Sara demonstrated remarkable resilience and in the end, embraced her transition to adult care. In her first year post-transition, she maintained a close connection to the pediatric team. These visits gradually decreased as Sara became increasingly independent and confident.

It is important to acknowledge and validate the range of feelings that young people and their caregivers commonly experience throughout the transition process. In addition to medical discharge reports, we use individualized psycho-social transition summaries to help young people further develop insight and awareness that will assist them and their new adult healthcare providers with the transition process. Through therapeutic discussions and writing sessions with their social worker, patients are encouraged to document relevant information related to their psycho-social situations, strengths and needs, coping strategies, support networks, disclosure decisions, finances and drug insurance, education and employment plans, and transition plans (refer to the Appendix for a sample template). The transition summary also marks an important milestone as patients graduate from pediatric care. With consent, this report is shared with adult care providers to highlight important issues and promote continuity of care. Maintaining some connection with transitioned youth, while being mindful to encourage independence, can help to reduce anxiety post-transition and facilitate relationships with new healthcare providers. The scope to which this can occur in other settings will be shaped by organizational policies and program mandates.

20.5 Conclusion

The success of medical advances in the treatment of pediatric HIV has been life-saving for children living with this condition. With this success has come new and welcome challenges for youth graduating from pediatric to adult healthcare, therefore calling for further research to explore optimal strategies for effective transitions. Early engagement and individualized transition plans promote the likelihood of successful entry into adult care and maintenance of good health. Collaborative efforts among youth, their families, and pediatric and adult healthcare providers are essential to facilitating coordinated and seamless transitions. Young people living with HIV deserve such efforts and can live long and healthy lives as a result.

Appendix

Individualized Psycho-Social Transition Summary (Sample)

(to be completed by the transitioning youth and social worker)

Name: ____________________

Date of birth: ____________________

Medical record number: ____________________

Transition plan (adult facility and team contact information, if known):

Study and employment information:

Applied for disability status in my post-secondary school?

Family background and living situation:

Relationships, friendships, and social life:

People who know my HIV status:

Income source and drug insurance:

Past and present activities, programs, and agencies:

Important healthcare issues:

Things I do to manage my physical/mental health (treatment adherence, transmission prevention, coping strategies):

People who support me and things they do that are helpful:

Drug/alcohol use, if any:

Concerns/worries:

Other relevant information:

Social work summary of strengths and needs (written to client):

Consent: I have reviewed this information with my social worker, ________________, and agree that she/he can share this summary with my new social worker, ________________, and healthcare providers at ________________.

Signature: ________________ **Date:** ________________

References

American Academy of Pediatrics. (2013). Policy statement: Transitioning HIV-infected youth into adult care. *Pediatrics, 132*, 192–197. Retrieved from http://pediatrics.aappublications.org/content/early/2013/06/19/peds.2013-1073.full.pdf+html.

Andiman, W. A. (2011). Transition from pediatric to adult healthcare services for young adults with chronic illnesses: The special case of human immunodeficiency virus infection. *Journal of Pediatrics, 159*, 714–719.

Antiretroviral Therapy Cohort Collaboration. (2008). Life expectancy of individuals on combination antiretroviral therapy in high income countries: A collaborative analysis of 14 cohort studies. *Lancet, 372*, 293–299.

Antle, B., Wells, L., Salter Goldie, R., DeMatteo, D., & King, S. (2001). Challenges of parenting for families living with HIV/AIDS. *Social Work, 46*, 159–169.

Azzopardi, C., Wade, M., Salter, R., MacDougall, G. M., Shouldice, M., Read, S., & Bitnun, A. (2014). Medical nonadherence in pediatric HIV: Psychosocial risks and intersection with the child protection system for medical neglect. *Child Abuse and Neglect, 38*, 1766–1777.

Battles, H. B., & Wiener, L. S. (2002). From adolescence through young adulthood: Psychosocial adjustment associated with long-term survival of HIV. *Journal of Adolescent Health, 30*, 161–168.

Bitnun, A., Kerrison, C., MacDougall, G., Louch, D., & Read, S. (2012). Transition from pediatric to adult HIV care: Patient perception of transition readiness and healthcare provider assessment of HIV-related knowledge. *Canadian Journal of Infectious Diseases and Medical Microbiology, 23*(Suppl. SA), 6–128.

Boudreau, M. E., & Fisher, C. M. (2012). Providing effective medical and case management services to HIV-infected youth preparing to transition to adult care. *Journal of the Association of Nurses in AIDS Care, 23*, 318–328.

Bundock, H., Fidler, S., Clarke, S., Holmes-Walker, D. J., Farrell, K., McDonald, S., et al. (2011). Crossing the divide: Transition care services for young people with HIV – Their views. *AIDS Patient Care & STDs, 25*, 465–473.

Burke, R. T., Spoerri, M., Price, A., Cardosi, A., & Flanagan, P. (2008). Survey of primary care pediatricians on the transition and transfer of adolescents to adult health. *Clinical Pediatrics, 47*, 347–354.

Cervia, J. S. (2007). Transitioning HIV-infected children to adult care. *Journal of Pediatrics, 150*, e1.

Cervia, J. S. (2013). Easing the transition of HIV-infected adolescents to adult care. *AIDS Patient Care & STDs, 27*, 692–696.

Children's HIV Association. (2011). *CHIVA Guidance on Transition for adolescents living with HIV.* Retrieved from http://www.chiva.org.uk/files/guidelines/transition.pdf.

Clark, M., Samson, L., Rusley, J., Bowes, J., & Brophy, J. (2014). *Adult and pediatric HIV care providers in Canada agree on the importance of developmental readiness in the transition of youth living with HIV from pediatric to adult care*. Poster presented at international AIDS conference 2014. Melbourne, Australia.

Committee on Pediatric AIDS. (2013). Transitioning HIV-infected youth into adult health care. *Pediatrics, 132*, 192–197.

DiRisio, M., Ballantyne, P. J., Read, S. E., & Bendayan, R. (2011). "HIV isn't me…": HIV+ adolescents' experiences in a positive context of support and treatment. *AIDS Care, 23*, 694–699.

Dowshen, N., & D'Angelo, L. (2011). Health care transition for youth living with HIV/AIDS. *Pediatrics, 128*, 762–771.

Fair, C. D., & Albright, J. (2012). "Don't tell him you have HIV unless he's 'the one'": Romantic relationships among adolescents and young adults with perinatal HIV infection. *AIDS Patient Care & STDs, 26*, 746–754.

Fair, C. D., Sullivan, K., & Gatto, A. (2010). Best practices in transitioning youth with HIV: Perspectives of pediatric and adult infectious disease care providers. *Psychology of Health and Medicine, 15*, 515–527.

Fair, C. D., Sullivan, K., & Gatto, A. (2011). Indicators of transition success for youth living with HIV: Perspectives of pediatric and adult infectious disease care providers. *AIDS Care, 23*, 965–970.

Fair, C. D., Albright, J., Lawrence, A., & Gatto, A. (2012a). "The pediatric social worker really shepherds them through the process": Care team members' roles in transitioning adolescents and young adults with HIV to adult care. *Vulnerable Children and Youth Studies, 7*, 338–346.

Fair, C. D., Sullivan, K., Dizney, R., & Stackpole, A. (2012b). "It's like losing a part of my family": Transition expectations of adolescents living with perinatally acquired HIV and their guardians. *AIDS Patient Care & STDs, 26*, 423–429.

Fielden, S. J., Sheckter, L., Chapman, G. E., Alimenti, A., Forbes, J. C., Sheps, S., et al. (2006). Growing up: Perspectives of children, families and service providers regarding the needs of older children with perinatally-acquired HIV. *AIDS Care, 18*, 1050–1053.

Freed, G. L., & Hudson, E. J. (2006). Transitioning children with chronic diseases to adult care: Current knowledge, practices, and directions. *Journal of Pediatrics, 148*, 824–827.

Garofalo, R., Deleon, J., Osmer, E., Doll, M., & Harper, G. W. (2006). Overlooked, misunderstood and at-risk: Exploring the lives and HIV risk of ethnic minority male to female transgender youth. *Journal of Adolescent Health, 38*, 230–236.

Gilliam, P. P., Ellen, J. M., Leonard, L., Kinsman, S., Jevitt, C. M., & Straub, D. M. (2011). Transition of adolescents with HIV to adult care: Characteristics and current practices of the adolescent trials network for HIV/AIDS interventions. *Journal of the Association of Nurses in AIDS Care, 22*, 283–294.

Green, G. (1995). Attitudes towards people with HIV: Are they as stigmatizing as people with HIV perceive them to be? *Social Science and Medicine, 41*, 557–568.

Harrigan, P. R., Hogg, R. S., Dong, W. W. Y., Yip, B., Wynhoven, B., Woodward, J., et al. (2005). Predictors of HIV drug-resistance mutations in a large antiretroviral-naïve cohort initiating triple antiretroviral therapy. *Journal of Infectious Diseases, 191*, 339–347.

Laufer, M., & Scott, G. (2000). Medical management of HIV disease in children. *Pediatric Clinics of North America, 47*, 127–153.

Liamputtong, P., Fanany, R., & Verrinder, G. (Eds.). (2012). *Health, illness and well-being: Perspectives and social determinants*. Melbourne: Oxford University Press.

Lima, V. D., Harrigan, R., Murray, M., Moore, D. M., Wood, E., Hogg, R. S., & Montaner, J. S. G. (2008). Differential impact of adherence on long-term treatment response among naïve HIV-infected individuals. *AIDS, 22*, 2371–2380.

Maturo, D., Powell, A., Major-Wilson, H., Sanchez, K., De Santis, J. P., & Friedman, L. B. (2011). Development of a protocol for transitioning adolescents with HIV infection to adult care. *Journal of Pediatric Health Care, 25*, 16–23.

Mellins, C. A., Brackis-Cott, E., Dolezal, C., & Abrams, E. J. (2006). Psychiatric disorders in youth with perinatally acquired human immunodeficiency virus infection. *Pediatric Infectious Diseases Journal, 25*, 432–437.

Mellins, C. A., Brackis-Cott, E., Leu, C. S., Elkington, K. S., Dolezal, C., Wiznia, A., et al. (2009). Rates and types of psychiatric disorders in perinatally human immunodeficiency virus-infected youth and seroreverters. *Journal of Child Psychology and Psychiatry, 50*, 1131–1138.

Mikkonen, J., & Raphael, D. (2010). *Social determinants of health: The Canadian facts*. Toronto: York University School of Health Policy and Management.

Miles, K., Edwards, S., & Clapson, M. (2004). Transition from paediatric to adult services: Experiences of HIV-positive adolescents. *AIDS Care, 16*, 305–314.

Murphy, D. A., Sarr, M., Durako, S. J., Moscicki, A. B., Wilson, C. M., & Muenz, L. R. (2003). Barriers to HAART adherence among human immunodeficiency virus-infected adolescents. *Archives of Pediatrics and Adolescent Medicine, 157*, 249–255.

Muskat, B., Salter, R., Shindler, S, Porter, M., & Bitnun, A. (Submitted manuscript). *Here you feel like it's not taboo: Evaluation of a hospital-based, community-leader led, group support program for children/youth with HIV*.

Naar-King, S., Montepiedra, G., Garvie, P., Kammerer, B., Malee, K., Sirois, P. A., et al. (2013). Social ecological predictors of longitudinal HIV treatment adherence in youth with perinatally acquired HIV. *Journal of Pediatric Psychology, 38*, 664–674.

New York State Department of Health AIDS Institute. (2011). *Transitioning HIV-infected adolescents into adult care*. Retrieved from http://www.hivguidelines.org/wp-content/uploads/2012/11/transitioning-hiv-infected-adolescents-into-adult-care-11-06-2012.pdf.

Nozyce, M. L., Lee, S. S., Wiznia, A., Nachman, S., Mofenson, L. M., Smith, M. E., et al. (2006). A behavioral and cognitive profile of clinically stable HIV infected children. *Pediatrics, 117*, 763–770.

Paone, M., Wigle, M., & Saewyc, E. (2006). The ONTRAC model for transitional care of adolescents. *Progress in Transplantation, 16*, 291–302.

Paterson, D. L., Swindells, S., Mohr, J., Brester, M., Vergis, E. N., Squier, C., et al. (2000). *Annals of Internal Medicine, 133*, 21–30.

Rao, D., Kekwaletswe, T. C., Hosek, S., Martinez, J., & Rodriguez, F. (2007). Stigma and social barriers to medication adherence with urban youth living with HIV. *AIDS Care, 19*, 28–33.

Reisner, S. L., Mimiaga, M. J., Skeer, M., Perkovich, B., Johnson, C. V., & Safren, S. A. (2009). A review of HIV antiretroviral adherence and intervention studies among HIV-infected youth. *Topics in HIV Medicine, 17*, 14–25.

Reiss, J. G., Gibson, R. W., & Walker, L. R. (2005). Health care transition: Youth, family, and provider perspectives. *Pediatrics, 15*, 112–120.

Ross, A., Camacho-Gonzalez, A., Henderson, S., Abanyie, F., & Chakraborty, R. (2010). The HIV-infected adolescent. *Current Infectious Disease Report, 12*, 63–70.

Ryscavage, P., Anderson, E. J., Sutton, S. H., Reddy, S., & Taiwo, B. (2011). Clinical outcomes of adolescents and young adults in adult HIV care. *Journal of Acquired Immune Deficiency Syndromes, 58*, 193–197.

Salter, R., King, S. M., Smith, M. L., Bitnun, A., Brophy, J., Fernandes-Penney, A., et al. (2007). Disclosing HIV diagnosis to infected children: A health care team's approach. *Vulnerable Children and Youth Studies, 2*, 12–16.

Sethi, A. K., Celentano, D. D., Gange, S. J., Moore, R. D., & Gallant, J. E. (2003). Association between adherence to antiretroviral therapy and human immunodeficiency virus drug resistance. *Clinical Infectious Diseases, 37*, 1112–1118.

Sharma, N., Willen, E., Garcia, A., & Sharma, T. S. (2014). Attitudes toward transitioning in youth with perinatally acquired HIV and their family caregivers. *Journal of the Association of Nurses in AIDS Care, 25*, 168–175.

Shindler, S., & Tangelder, M. (2010). Beneath the mask: A group therapy model supporting children infected and affected by HIV/AIDS. *Social Work with Groups, 33*, 308–322.

Simoni, J. M., Montgomery, A., Martin, E., New, M., Demas, P. A., & Rana, S. (2007). Adherence to antiretroviral therapy for pediatric HIV infection: A qualitative systematic review with recommendations for research and clinical management. *Pediatrics, 119*, 1371–1383.

Spiegel, H. M., & Futterman, D. C. (2009). Adolescents and HIV: Prevention and clinical care. *Current HIV/AIDS Reports, 6*, 100–107.

Thorne, C., Newell, M. L., Botet, F. A., Bohlin, A. B., Ferrazin, A., Giaquinto, C., et al. (2002). Older children and adolescents surviving with vertically acquired HIV infection. *Journal of Acquired Immune Deficiency Syndromes, 29*, 396–401.

UNAIDS. (2013). *Global report: UNAIDS report on the global AIDS epidemic 2013*. Retrieved from http://www.unaids.org/sites/default/files/en/media/unaids/contentassets/documents/epidemiology/2013/gr2013/UNAIDS_Global_Report_2013_en.pdf.

Valenzuela, J. M., Buchanan, C. L., Radcliffe, J., Ambrose, C., Hawkins, L. A., Tanney, M., & Rudy, B. J. (2011). Transition to adult services among behaviorally infected adolescents with HIV: A qualitative study. *Journal of Pediatric Psychology, 36*, 134–140.

Van Dyke, R. B., Lee, S., Johnson, G. M., Wiznia, A., Mohan, K., Stanley, K., et al. (2002). Reported adherence as a determinant of response to highly active antiretroviral therapy in children who have human immunodeficiency virus infection. *Pediatrics, 109*, e61.

Vijayan, T., Benin, A. L., Wagner, K., Romano, S., & Andiman, W. A. (2009). We never thought this would happen: Transitioning care of adolescents with perinatally acquired HIV infection from pediatrics to internal medicine. *AIDS Care, 21*, 1222–1229.

Viner, R. (1999). Transition from paediatric to adult care: Bridging the gaps or passing the buck? *Archives of Disease in Childhood, 81*, 271–275.

Vreeman, R. C., Wiehe, S. E., Pearce, E. C., & Nyandiko, W. M. (2008). A systematic review of pediatric adherence to antiretroviral therapy in low-and middle-income countries. *Pediatric Infectious Disease Journal, 27*, 686–691.

Wiener, L. S., Zobel, M., Battles, H., & Ryder, C. (2007). Transition from a pediatric HIV intramural clinical research program to adolescent and adult community-based care services: Assessing transition readiness. *Social Work in Health Care, 46*, 1–19.

Wiener, L. S., Kohrt, B. A., Battles, H. B., & Pao, M. (2011). The HIV experience: Youth identified barriers for transitioning from pediatric to adult care. *Journal of Pediatric Psychology, 36*, 141–154.

Williams, P. L., Storm, D., Montepiedra, G., Nichols, S., Kammerer, B., Sirois, P. A., et al. (2006). Predictors of adherence to antiretroviral medications in children and adolescents with HIV infection. *Pediatrics, 118*, 1745–1757.

Chapter 21
"I Can Still Be Happy, I Can Still Get My Life Again": Psychological Interventions with Children, Young People and Families Living with HIV in the United Kingdom

Tomás Campbell and Jayne Griffiths

Contents

T. Campbell (✉)
Consultant Clinical Psychologist, WhizzKids United Health Academy, Pietermaritzberg, South Africa
e-mail: tomascampbell@btinternet.com

J. Griffiths
South Essex Partnership University NHS Foundation Trust, Southend University Hospital, Prittlewell Chase, Westcliff-on-Sea, Essex SS0 0RY, UK
e-mail: jayne.griffiths@southend.nhs.uk

P. Liamputtong (ed.), *Children and Young People Living with HIV/AIDS*, Cross-Cultural Research in Health, Illness and Well-Being,
DOI 10.1007/978-3-319-29936-5_21

21.1 Introduction

The last 20 years have seen extensive advances in the detection and treatment of HIV infection. The early years of the epidemic in the United Kingdom (UK) affected gay men in particular. Heterosexuals and children were initially much less affected although there were small numbers of intravenous drug users and haemophiliacs who acquired HIV (Jones 1990). Haemophiliac children also acquired HIV through blood products.

In the 1990s the pattern of those who acquired HIV infection began to change, and from 1995 to 2003, the percentage of Black African people diagnosed with HIV increased from 17 to 54 % (Harker 2010). This change reflected patterns of migration to the UK from former British colonies in Africa, an increase in the numbers of people seeking political asylum from African countries and economic migrants. Most of this population acquired HIV through heterosexual sex: many in their countries of origin but increasingly within the UK. Black African women were disproportionately affected as 21 % of infections in 2009 were amongst this group despite the fact that there are over 100 times more white than black African women in the population as a whole. As a consequence, there was a significant increase in the number of children with HIV (and their uninfected siblings) arriving with, and born to African women in the UK.

The epidemic amongst children, young people and their families in the UK has had particular characteristics that have shaped and defined the range and kinds of psychological interventions provided. Firstly, many people were newly arrived in the UK with similar issues and problems of any immigrant population such as legal issues with regard to immigration status, financial, employment and housing concerns, and language barriers. Concerns about health (especially HIV) were often not a priority. Secondly, many African people (and women disproportionately) had experienced oppression in their country of origin that had been an important factor that led to immigration or seeking asylum in the UK. The oppression had taken many forms including discrimination and political intimidation, torture, internment and rape. High levels of psychological and physical trauma were common which compounded personal responses to HIV infection. Lastly, many sub-Saharan African people came from countries where they already had personal experience of the devastating impact of high prevalence of HIV which, at the time, resulted in certain death (e.g. in 1993 the HIV prevalence amongst pregnant women in Zambia was approximately 30 %) (Campbell and Kelly 1995). Many had experienced HIV-related deaths in their own families and had witnessed at first hand the sense of helplessness and hopelessness that accompanied this disease. Many had also witnessed the accompanying impact of HIV stigma as communities often responded with fear and anger towards those who had HIV/AIDS. A diagnosis of HIV often became the point at which these factors interacted and presented challenges both to those living with HIV and the clinicians caring for people with HIV.

This cohort and their characteristics presented clinicians with many challenges including how to effectively engage troubled and distressed parents, how to work effectively through interpreters, the complexities of cultural understandings of the impact of HIV and its association with psychological distress. Psychologists and psychotherapists became aware that their psychotherapeutic models were heavily influenced by western understandings of the nature of distress and the therapeutic models we had developed to understand, address and alleviate psychological and emotional suffering were not always appropriate to working with diverse clients groups.

In this chapter, we will explore some of the contextual issues that have influenced psychological interventions with this cohort of children, young people and families living with, and affected by HIV. We will describe the ways in which psychological interventions have attempted to engage therapeutically to address some of these issues. We will describe some of the psychological models and therapeutic approaches that have influenced us in our own work and we will present some of the outcomes and evaluations of our interventions. Lastly, we will make suggestions about how interventions might be designed and implemented in the future.

21.2 Epidemiology of HIV Amongst Children and Young People in the UK

Children and young people with HIV disease are now surviving into adolescence and adulthood with a consequent reduction in HIV-related morbidity and mortality (Foster et al. 2009). In 2013, there were 1070 children living with HIV and attending HIV clinics in the UK of whom just over half (52 %) were female, 48 % were born in the UK or Ireland, 80 % were of black African ethnicity, and nearly all (96 %) were known to have been infected through mother-to-child transmission (Summary data: Collaborative HIV Paediatric Study website 2014). HIV prevalence is highest in the most deprived areas in England; this is particularly evident in London, where diagnosed HIV prevalence is as high as 7.0 per 1000 in the most deprived areas and less than 2.4 per 1000 in the least deprived areas (Aghaizu et al. 2013). Fifty percent of children with HIV in the UK were being seen at clinics in London, 39 % in the rest of England, 4 % in Scotland, 1 % in Wales and <1 % in Northern Ireland. This is an aging cohort: in 2012, 37 % were aged 15 years or older (Summary data: Colloborative HIV Paediatric Study website 2014).

In 2012, the prevalence of HIV was approximately 30 times higher for men-who-have sex-with-men (MSM) and black-African men and women in comparison to the general population in England. Individual, societal and structural factors such as sexual behaviors, infections acquired abroad, migration and HIV-related stigma and discrimination contributed to this disparity (Aghaizu et al. 2013).

21.3 The Effects of HIV on Families in the UK

Despite the welcome medication advances in recent years that have made HIV disease a treatable condition HIV remains a chronic disease which may affect several family members simultaneously and, as such, requires a whole family medical and psycho-social focus (Davey et al. 2008). Clinical services that integrate health and social support for both adults and children have been identified as the most effective way of ensuring good clinical and psycho-social outcomes for HIV-positive children (Richter and Sherr 2009) and several family-focused HIV clinics have been established in the UK that provide co-ordinated multi-disciplinary medical, psychological, nursing and social care for all HIV-positive members of the family (Gibb et al. 1997). This has been easier to achieve in London where 50 % of these children live and it has been far more difficult to achieve this in areas of the country where there has not been a population to support such an integrated care approach. However, recent research has indicated that there are often significant gaps in knowledge about various important aspects of the lives of these families particularly with regard to our knowing how many children in the family have been tested, the location of these children and how HIV testing decisions are made (Astill et al. 2012).

Challenges facing HIV-positive parents including medical concerns (e.g. more than one HIV-positive member of the family, side-effects to highly active antiretroviral (HAART) medication); psychological issues (e.g. acceptance of personal HIV status, adherence to medication); legal issues (e.g. immigration/asylum issues, housing, employment) and social difficulties (e.g. language and cultural differences, stigma, disclosure of status to others) (Waugh 2003; Wilkins et al. 2007). Discussion and disclosure of HIV status is a common difficulty and talking about HIV in more general ways also appears to be very difficult (Michaud et al. 2009). The effects of secrecy may also have an impact on family coping; many parents fear their children will be psychologically damaged by the disclosure of their HIV status and may be exposed to HIV-related stigma (Wiener et al. 2007; Murphy 2008). Keeping the diagnosis secret may affect that parental ability to adequately address new challenges in their families' life (e.g. planning for effective transition from of HIV-positive children from pediatric to adult medical care, adolescent sexuality issues, adherence to medication) which require sharing of status and which may require different and/or new coping mechanisms (Wilkins et al. 2007). Overall, these factors may negatively affect caregivers' capacity to provide the best possible care for children (Richter and Sherr 2009; see also Chaps. 3, 4, 5, and 6 in this volume).

HIV-positive young people are an under-researched group with regard to the psycho-social impact of the disease. Foster et al. (2009) point out that little is known about adherence to antiretroviral medications amongst HIV-positive adolescents in the UK. Some studies have pointed to higher rates of emotional and behavioral difficulty in HIV-positive children (Melvin et al. 2007) and younger children have been reported to have more difficulties with psychological adjustment to their status than older children (Sopena et al. 2010). Little too is known about the psychological and emotional impact of parental death (often HIV-related) which is common amongst this group (Melvin et al. 2007; Foster et al. 2009; Campbell et al. 2014). While behavioral and emotional difficulties have been reported to be more common (prevalence of 14 %) in this group than the general population (Melvin et al. 2007), it is not clear the extent to which other factors such as poor parental/family coping, bereavement, immigrant status and parental ill-health play a role.

21.4 The Impact of HIV Stigma

There is increasing acceptance that HIV stigma has complex and mostly negative effects on HIV-positive people (e.g. poorer social support, poorer mental health) (Logie and Gadalla 2009), lower adherence to HAART (Dlamini et al. 2009) and can be a barrier to accessing health care. With regard to young people specifically, Martinez et al. (2012) reported that higher levels of stigma in HIV-positive young women in particular was associated with poorer adherence to antiretroviral medication.

However, the concept of stigma has been very hard to define, there is little concurrence in the literature about how to operationalize the term (Mahajan et al. 2008) and stigma prevention efforts are not a priority or remain unfunded (Piot 2006). Stigma may operate at the level of the individual and also at organizational and societal levels and may be affected by different cultural or national settings and it has been difficult to measure the extent and impact of stigma, both on individuals living with HIV and wider healthcare and societal structures.

Much of the research to date has focused on adults' perceptions of stigma, the impact on mental health and the barriers thrown up by societal stigma to accessing HIV testing, health care and HAART. Interventions in the UK have sought to change negative perceptions of people with HIV through mass media campaigns, education about transmission and enactment of laws to prevent discrimination. However, little is known about the effectiveness of these interventions although recent UK data suggest HIV stigma is stubbornly resistant to change. The National AIDS Trust 2010 Survey (NAT 2011) reported that 64 % of respondents agreed that there is still a lot of stigma in the UK. White people were more likely than those from BME backgrounds to agree that people with HIV deserve as much support and respect as people with cancer (75 % vs. 65 %) and 62 % believed that their employer should tell them if one of their colleagues was HIV-positive.

21.5 HIV Stigma and Young People in the UK

There is little literature on the impact of HIV-related stigma and young people but the context in which young HIV-positive people are developing and maturing is one in which HIV stigma is a reality and is expressed in many ways. Disappointingly,

HIV stigma in the UK may be highest in the very communities from which most young HIV-positive people themselves come as most young people with HIV in the UK are of African origin (National AIDS Trust 2011). In contrast with adults with HIV who acquired the infection via sex, transfusion or drug use young people who acquired HIV perinatally have lived with HIV all their lives. They may not have not always have known about their diagnosis, and, as the young person matures, the unfolding and often unwelcome realization of the complexity of both the disease and societal attitudes toward HIV becomes a lived reality (Campbell et al. 2010a, b; see also Chaps. 5, 6, 18, and 19 in this volume).

Swendeman et al. (2006) discuss the notion of stigma as a layered experience. This idea refers to HIV being particularly prevalent in certain groups or associated with sexual behaviors or drug using behaviors all of which are already stigmatized. In this way, HIV stigma also becomes attached to other "traits or behaviours that are undesirable" (Swendeman et al. 2006: 502) and may layer the experience of stigma. As such, the interaction of personal characteristics which may already have stigma attached to them (e.g. young age, female gender, Black ethnic origin, African ancestry) and HIV disease provides a context in which the importance of the individual factors become blurred and stigma is experienced at many levels (See also Chaps. 1, 2, 3, 4, 6, 14, 15, 17, 18, 19, 20, and 21 regarding stigma and young people in this volume).

More recently within the published literature, a distinction has been made between perceived stigma (the extent to which a stigmatized person fears or anticipates discrimination) and enacted stigma (actual experiences of discrimination) which allows an exploration of more subtle aspects of HIV stigma and the ways in which they are separate but interconnected. Some of these issues were explored in an American study of HIV-positive young people (Swendeman et al. 2006). The study examined experiences of perceived and enacted stigma in two US sites; 89 % of participants reported perceived stigma and 64 % enacted stigma with 31 % within the previous 3 months. Males reported less perceived stigma than females and females tended to have higher levels of anxiety and depression. In a small study of 21 young people aged 12–21 years Campbell et al. (2014) explored experiences of stigma using an adapted version of the stigma scale devised by Swendeman et al. (2006). In the study, females reported more experiences of enacted stigma than males. The most common experience of stigma was hearing AIDS jokes (39 % of females vs. 12.5 % males) followed by loss of a friend because of HIV status (31 % vs.12.5 %). Females also reported experiences of being shut out by family members and having to move house because of their HIV status (16 % vs. 0 %).

Generally, 34 % of participants reported they had felt socially rejected by their HIV status and 31 % that they had felt shame. Only a small percentage had felt that people avoided them socially because of their HIV status. More females than males had felt socially rejected (43 % vs. 20 % – but roughly equal numbers had felt ashamed about their status (31 % vs. 29 %).

There were clear gender differences with regard to disclosure of the young person's status in their family. More females than males reported that family members knew their status and females had a higher number of friends than males who were aware of their status. Males were more likely to have friends who were completely unaware of their status. Compared with the American data on stigma in young people it seems that UK youth appear less stigmatized than American young people. However, there are many cultural and contextual differences between the UK and the USA and these differences may be reflected in the data shown here. There were marked gender differences in the experiences of enacted stigma with females reporting more experiences than males. Males felt less stigmatized than females on all measures but roughly equal percentages had felt ashamed of their status. Males had fewer family members and friends who were aware of their status and perhaps this may account to some extent for the higher rate of enacted experiences among females: if no-one knows your status they cannot discriminate against you.

It is interesting to speculate why there were fewer people and friends who knew males' status. This may reflect the different ways in which males and females organize their friendship groups and the emphasis that females may place on sharing intimate or confidential information. While this strategy may be effective in seeking support it also makes females more vulnerable to perceived or enacted stigma if the friendship breaks down. On the other hand, males did not seem to disclose their status at all. This may be because the effect of HIV stigma has already been very effective at keeping them silent or it may be that discussion of feelings and swapping personal information is not part of the culture of these young males. Perhaps it is an interaction of both factors and more research is required to understand this phenomenon more clearly.

Kim et al. (2014), in a systematic review and meta-analysis of published studies regarding adherence patterns to antiretroviral therapy for adolescents and young adults living with HIV, reported that there are wide variations in patterns worldwide. Adherence was reported to be highest in Africa and Asia and lowest in Europe and North America. The authors proposed several possible explanations to explain the differences: firstly, young HIV-positive people in Europe and North America were more likely to be from an already marginalized community (Black African or Hispanic) and the interaction of HIV status and membership of a marginalized group increased vulnerability to non-adherence. Secondly, African and Asian HIV-positive young people were more likely to become pregnant in their second decade of life and may have an increased motivation to be adherent in order to prevent vertical transmission. Lastly, there may have been fewer cultural and social differences between young HIV-positive people in Africa and Asia and the adult population in the same setting, especially when they are a bit older (16–24 years). They were more likely to have already worked and may have had children of their own compared with the adolescent population in Europe and South America where there are bigger social and socio-economic differences between adults and adolescents. While this meta-analysis did not control for the effect of stigma this study suggests that membership of a marginalized group is associated with poorer adherence and the mediating factor may the effects of stigma.

There is little published literature about anti-stigma interventions for young people. Kidd et al. (2003) developed an intervention for use in anti-stigma training in African countries. While the interventions were not specifically targeted at young people the toolkit aimed to support HIV trainers to work together to confront HIV stigma, promote more care and support for people living with PLHIV and to defend their rights. Campbell and Griffiths (2013) described a model for delivering an anti-stigma group workshop for UK based young HIV-positive people in which there were three components: firstly, an explanatory model of what is stigma, what are the effects and why are people stigmatized was developed. Secondly, participants were invited to consider which groups of people have been historically stigmatized and the possible reasons why. Lastly, participants worked together to identify the domains of their lives in which they had personally experienced stigma and developed self-statements to counter the effects of stigma.

The intervention was based on two psychological models. Strategies based on cognitive-behavioral theory were utilized to give participants an explanatory structure within which to understand what stigma is and the cognitive, emotional and behavioral responses to it. CBT informed the development of strategies to new self-statements to counter the negative effects of stigma. Participants took part in an exercise called “a letter from future self”. This technique derives from narrative therapy and encouraged participants to consider how they might use the tools they have learnt in a practical way in the coming year. Participants were invited to consider their personal goals and elaborate the process by which these might be achieved and to congratulate themselves (in advance) for their success.

We evaluated the impact of this intervention by recording participants’ responses to three questions about their experiences (Campbell et al. 2011a). Responses indicated that the young people expressed optimism for their ability to cope with stigma related challenges and emphasized seeking help from family members and health professionals. They also emphasized the benefits of taking HAART and of maintaining good self-esteem as counters to negative events. The results presented a picture in which they felt confident to face HIV- -related challenges. However, as we knew these young people well and were knowledgeable about the ways in which they and their families coped with HIV, we considered that the responses were unrealistic about the effectiveness of their responses. These results emphasized to us that developing effective responses to stigma was a long-term goal and required regular intervention.

21.6 Supporting HIV-Positive Parents

There has been a welcome recent focus on strategies to strengthen families’ capacity to respond most effectively to the challenge of HIV. Advocates for a family-focused approach point to a number of reasons for this perspective. Firstly, HIV infections frequently occur within the family context via sexual relationships, pregnancy, delivery and breastfeeding. Secondly, the family is the unit in which most HIV-positive children are raised and the one best placed to meet their needs – both developmentally and medically. Lastly, all members of the family (both positive and negative) are affected by the social consequences of HIV, including stigmatization, social exclusion and discrimination (Leeper et al. 2010).

Perinatally-infected HIV-positive young people are developing into adulthood and are now having children of their own and we are seeing a new generation of people and families in which there is HIV. Growing numbers of young people also acquire HIV sexually and this is particularly true in Africa (Christofides et al. 2014). To date, there is little research on how young people who were perinatally-infected are who are now parents themselves are coping with the effects of HIV on their lives and this is an obvious area for further research (but see also Chaps. 5, 6, 10, and 19 in this volume for research that involved perinatally-infected young people). However, Elgalib et al. (2010) noted there is significant overlap between the social, demographic and behavioral determinants of teenage pregnancy and the characteristics of adolescents living with HIV. Psycho-social stressors may increase vulnerability to teenage pregnancy for young women through such factors of increased substance misuse, sexual risk taking and inadequate family and social support.

In their study of 58 HIV-positive young women in London, Elgalib et al. (2010) noted that all but one teenage reported that they were unaware of the infection at the time of pregnancy. Most were diagnosed antenatally. It is impossible to know how many had acquired the infection vertically but it is unlikely they all acquired it sexually. Many had significant and complex psycho-social problems that may have contributed to vulnerability to pregnancy. About half (44 %) lived alone and had poor social support and financial difficulties (62 %). Other issues included housing problems (58 %), a history of domestic violence (10 %) and a history of sexual abuse (45 %).

The availability of HAART has transformed the management of HIV disease in pregnancy and many of these young parents can look forward to delivering HIV-negative infants. However, complexities remain and the issues of parental adherence to HAART, disclosure of status to sexual partners, family members and perhaps children may place a strain on their ability to cope.

Clinical services that integrate health and social support for both adults and children have been identified as the most effective way of ensuring good clinical and psycho-social outcomes for HIV-positive children (Richter and Sherr 2009) and several family-focused HIV clinics have been established in the UK that provide co-ordinated multi-disciplinary medical, psychological, nursing and social care for all HIV-positive members of the family (Gibb et al. 1997).

Family-focused care can be difficult to define as there is no generally accepted definition of what constitutes a 'family', what appropriate treatment and care should be and how should it be delivered. Family-focused approaches have tended to focus on mothers and children for many reasons: they are easier to access as a population via child health and immunization clinics, mothers' gender and social roles emphasize that child care and rearing is a female responsibility and fathers have historically been very absent from child-focused health settings compounding the difficulty of delivering health interventions. There is a growing awareness that males and fathers should be more involved and that new strategies need to be developed and implemented to achieve this aim (Hosegood and Madhavan 2010).

Nonetheless, a review of this area suggested that a family-focused approach is effective for recruiting HIV-positive women into treatment and consequently reduces mother to child transmission, supports adherence and improves pediatric adherence to antiretroviral medication (Leeper et al. 2010). Models of care that support effective family functioning have been demonstrated to be effective in supporting good outcomes for children including better psycho-social functioning in children (Nostlinger et al. 2006) and have been demonstrated to assist parents in making decisions about disclosure of HIV status, planning for childrens' long term adjustment to HIV (Rotherham-Borus et al. 2001), and the development of long term coping skills to cope with HIV infection (Nyandiya-Bundy et al. 2009). There is some evidence that providing group based interventions for parents aimed at strengthening skills regarding issues such as disclosure can be effective (Nyandiya-Bundy et al. 2009). Supportive group interventions utilizing cognitive-behavioral theory and psycho-education have also been demonstrated to be effective in enhancing mood and coping behaviors and reducing negative affect (Chesney et al. 2003). However, family-focused programs have been less successful in recruiting males and fathers into treatment and care and programs and have reported mixed success regarding supporting disclosure of HIV status between females and their male partners. Finally, studies have also shown that HIV-positive adults in care did not consistently and routinely refer their children to the same treatment center or program where they themselves were receiving treatment (Leeper et al. 2010).

We developed a parenting course within our own clinical context to address some of these issues (Campbell et al. 2011b). The course grew out of a single workshop run in collaboration with a voluntary sector organization in which we had focused on some of the challenges faced by HIV-positive African parents raising their children in a UK cultural context. Over subsequent years, this collaboration grew between National Health Service (NHS) clinical psychologists and a voluntary sector organization and the course developed into a 6-weekly intervention run during the school summer holidays.

The intervention was informed by social action theory (Gore-Felton et al. 2005) which proposes that coping behaviors are located within three psychological domains: responses to internal affective states that influence the self-regulation process, the self-regulation capabilities of the individual and the external environmental context. Within this model, interventions are aimed at increasing coping skills, improving communication skills between parents, children, other family members and new sexual partners, and psycho-education about child and adolescent development. Enhancing parental confidence and skills in relation to coping with HIV was a focus for each session, including topics such as: exploring fears of and approaches to the disclosure of parental HIV status and of HIV-positive childrens' status; promoting ongoing conversations about HIV within the family rather than a 'one-off' disclosure conversation; enhancing children's resilience in the face of HIV-related stigma; dealing with parental fears of adolescence within the context of HIV. While each workshop was designed to be a stand-alone event, participants were encouraged to attend the whole course in order to gain maximum benefit. In practical

Box 21.1: Questionnaire

Demographic information:

Name
Gender
Contact details
Relationship status
Length of time in the UK
Immigration status
Number of children: HIV+ and HIV-
Ages of children
Location of children (whether in UK or elsewhere)
Disclosure of parental HIV status to children?
Disclosure to child(ren) of their HIV status?

Participant self-evaluation of confidence/coping in the following domains:

Disclosure of parental HIV status to children
Disclosure of child's positive status to the child
Ability to communicate about sexual matters
Global assessment of family coping
Knowledge of UK educational and social services systems

terms, we provided crèche facilities and lunch and provided travel expenses in order to facilitate attendance.

Underpinning the intervention was a commitment to the active participation of participants in the design and delivery of the intervention. Previous cohorts were invited to co-design the content and structure of the course and to co-deliver workshops. This grounded the intervention in the lived experience of HIV-affected parents, and acted as form of ongoing intervention for previous participants.

In relation to intervention evaluation, participants completed a specifically designed pre and post questionnaire focused on self-evaluation of coping in different domains (see Box 21.1).

We evaluated the effectiveness of this intervention (Campbell et al. 2011b). The results indicated that by the end of the intervention participants reported an increase in confidence or knowledge with regard to most of the questionnaire items compared with baseline scores these changes were not statistically significant. These data also suggested that post-intervention participants were more confident talking to their children about their own HIV status, and their children's HIV status (for those who had HIV-positive children). Parents also reported feeling more confident talking to HIV-negative children about HIV.

However, despite expressing more confidence with HIV-related discussion, there was also a drop in confidence to help their families cope with HIV and participants agreed more strongly at evaluation than at baseline that it was more difficult to raise children in London than in Africa. Whilst neither of these responses were statistically significant, they may suggest that raising emotionally sensitive issues may lead to a reduced sense of coping in the short term as parents become more aware of the complexities they face. Being exposed to new ideas about coping strategies may have led to a re-evaluation of previous coping styles. For many parents, this was the first time they had explored such issues and their previous coping styles had developed in a context of secrecy and fear and without exposure to a range of other strategies. Indeed, most participants had never talked about such issues with other parents.

Despite the course was heavily advertised as being relevant to fathers and mothers, most participants were female which may indicate that childrearing is considered to be a female rather than a male concern. Certainly, during the course the lack of male participants was commented on by the females who considered that it reflected widely held stereotypical views about gender roles. Interestingly, and despite encouragement, none of the male partners of the female participants attended the course with them. If family focused coping with HIV is influenced by gender roles then males (i.e. fathers) are at a potential disadvantage because they may not attend interventions focused at increasing coping capacity.

Disclosure of status is an issue that most people with HIV struggle and this cohort was no exception. Most participants' children were HIV-negative and the issue that participants faced most commonly was disclosure of parental status to these children. The data suggests that participants' confidence regarding this issue had increased at the end of the course. Confidence with regard to disclosure of HIV-positive childrens' status had also increased.

Parents sometimes do not know the HIV status of their children. This is not uncommon amongst African parents who live in the UK (Eisenhut et al. 2008) and particularly for children who live in Africa. Parents may decide not to have their children tested because of a perceived lack of effective medical interventions for HIV infection in the country in which the child(ren) lives and the fear of the possible negative impact on the carers of the child.

Parents may fear that their child will be treated badly and/or discriminated against if they have a positive diagnosis. A child's HIV-positive diagnosis also opens the question of where the child acquired HIV and parents fear that this will result in an unwanted disclosure of mother's HIV status (if the child acquired HIV in utero). They may fear that this will have profound negative effects on family and community relationships. The fact that these children remain untested may also be an indication of how complex are the emotional and social aspects of testing and disclosure.

21.7 Supporting Young People

21.7.1 Supporting Transition Between Services

As the UK cohort of adolescents living with HIV ages, HIV services have increasingly been facing the challenge of developing mechanisms to facilitate young people in making the transition from pediatric or family services to adult-centered care. Transition is defined as the "purposeful, planned movement of adolescents and young adults with chronic physical and medical conditions from child-centred to adult-oriented health care systems" (Blum et al. 1993: 570).

This stage of movement between services is traditionally a time where young patients become lost to follow up. Young people can be unprepared for the increased self-management of out-patient appointments; they are unfamiliar with the stricter structure and protocol of adult services; puberty has begun and young people are exploring identity and sexuality and may not want to think about medical issues; services and families may be unprepared to allow the young person to grow up, or conversely, expect them to behave as 'adults' in relation to their care.

In our context, we consulted a group of HIV-positive young people about their experiences of and preferences for transition as a part of developing a local transition clinic for HIV-positive adolescents, and in order to maximize engagement and minimize loss to follow up (Campbell et al. 2010a, b). We undertook a focus group with 20 adolescents (12 female, 8 male; age range 12–19 years; all Black African ethnic origin and all vertically infected) at different points in the transition process. Questions focused on: preferred ways of managing the medical, social and psychological transition from pediatric to adolescent services; physical/practical aspects of transition clinics; views on how to maximize clinic attendance rates. The session was transcribed verbatim and data were compared and analyzed for inter-rater reliability, commonly recurring themes and subjected to a thematic analysis.

The overarching theme was the importance of the quality of therapeutic relationship clinic staff developed with young people, with all participants identified this as key in both exiting from pediatric services and entering more adult focused services. A key theme in relation to managing transition was viewing transition as a process rather than an event, with attention paid to the process of 'saying goodbye' to trusted pediatric staff in a planned way over time (e.g. acknowledgement of the sadness of saying goodbye by both young person and staff; transitioning in small groups rather than as individuals). Key themes in relation to engaging young people included: the importance of practical factors (e.g. modernizing communication methods, clinic spaces as young-person friendly); mixed views over the use of rewards and incentives (e.g. monetary rewards for attendance and/or adherence); the importance of a 'good beginning' with new clinic staff and of staff actively working to build positive relationships (e.g. friendly receptionists, doctors asking questions about all aspects of a young person's life rather than focusing on HIV and adherence only); a desire to be supported to take more responsibility for managing their health condition in a staged manner (e.g. involving parents in consultations initially).

The data suggested that young people had clear views about their preferences about the transition to adult services and for transition clinics themselves, with a particular emphasis on the importance of the quality of relationship with individual clinic staff. It is important that attention and planning be paid to the relational and emotional aspects of transition, in particular the loss of valued relationships with pediatric staff and the anxiety of developing new relationships in more adult services. Individual transition plans developed in collaboration with young people are an important way of supporting young people in this process and responding to their request to have a more active role in managing transition. Young people identified the importance of family remaining involved and clinic staff who may be more familiar with working with adults may need to be supported to develop competencies around working with adolescents generally, and skills around working with parents/carers whilst working to foster independence. Clinics may need to consider adapting communication methods and clinic spaces to become more developmentally appropriate rather than replicating adult-focused approaches (see also Chaps. 5, 6, 19, and 20 in this volume about transitional care and young people with HIV/AIDS).

21.7.2 Transition Through Adolescence into Adulthood: Supporting Well-Being

Transition not only involves ensuring that young people are prepared for new clinical settings but also equipping them for all aspects of adolescent and adult life in the context of their diagnosis. Studies conducted in other countries have noted that psycho-social support and preparation for such challenges for HIV-positive young people is rare (Bitsindou et al. 2007; Lesch et al. 2007) and have highlighted the need for equipping adolescents with the necessary psychological and emotional skills to enable them to cope in the long term with a highly stigmatized illness (Bitsindou et al. 2007). An important component of this process is equipping young people with skills to take responsibility for their own health, psychological and emotional needs.

We developed a program called the 'Looking Forward Day' (LfD) as a way of engaging with young people and giving them the opportunity to discuss their diagnosis, medication and any related difficulties with other HIV-positive young people and professionals. Because of the sexual nature of HIV transmission, it also creates the opportunity to give the young people essential information about sex and sexual health and skills with regard to negotiation around sexual relationships.

LfDs are held four times a year during school holidays and are co-facilitated by clinical psychologists and clinical nurse specialists, with the input of a variety of multidisciplinary professionals, such as HIV physicians, pharmacists and sexual health workers. Emphasis is placed on giving parents as much information about the events in advance as possible and also the opportunity to explore any fears or concerns about the content. Potential participants are also told that lunch at a popular local restaurant is included as is a £10 gift voucher. A clinical setting was considered inappropriate and a local church hall with good transport links was selected as the venue.

In terms of program content, each LFd differs in focus, but information about HIV and what it is, what it does and how people acquire it is always included. Other themes which we address include:

(a) Medication: how it works, how to take it and how their families manage adherence to medication.
(b) Their disclosure: how the young people were disclosed to about their diagnosis, how they have faced this ways of adjusting to/coming to terms with this.
(c) Family management of HIV: how HIV is talked about within their families, to whom they can talk about their diagnosis, and how they relate to their siblings who may either be HIV-positive or -negative.
(d) Romantic and sexual relationships: disclosure and negotiation skills around sex as well as protection and prevention of onward transmission; working to depathologize narratives around sex and HIV and ensure that the importance of sex and pleasure is recognized; addressing fears about fertility and reproduction.
(e) Managing disclosure within friendship/platonic relationships.
(f) Communication with health professionals: increasing confidence and behavioral skills to communicate more clearly and remain in contact with services.

An overarching Narrative Therapy approach underpins the LfDsIn terms of program content. Narrative Therapy sees problems as occurring when the dominant narratives people have available about themselves are pathologizing and unhelpful, and where as a result people begin to elaborate problem-saturated descriptions of themselves. We felt that this strengths-based approach which attempts to make more visible the relationship between these dominant narratives and power in society was particularly relevant to young people living with a highly stigmatized health condition. A focus has been to work alongside young people in resisting the effects and influences of problem stories and deficit descriptions which can surround the label of 'HIV'.

We have also used psychodrama approaches to exploring emotions, enhancing and practicing (and re-practicing) skills. Psychodrama, developed by Moreno (cited in Fox 1987) employs guided dramatic action to enact problems in a creative way rather than remain at the level of 'talk'. By recreating real-life situations or problems, and acting them out in the present, the young people have an opportunity to evaluate their behavior, practice new roles safely and to develop and rehearse new skills. The 'director' supports the group to explore newer solutions to old problems, and the whole group is actively involved.

The process of addressing HIV in a safe and engaging manner is essential. Young people may not have talked about HIV in any detail beforehand and/or had negative experiences of doing so. Our philosophy has been one of adopting a 'playful approach to serious problems' (Epston et al. 1997) and to constantly update and modify how issues are covered in order to facilitate ongoing attendance and engagement.

We evaluated the effectiveness of the intervention by use of a specifically designed self-report questionnaire (Campbell et al. 2010b). The data suggested that the events were effective in answering questions about HIV that the young people were not able to ask elsewhere. Most questionnaire responses indicated that after attending a LFP day the young people felt more optimistic for the future, were able to talk to a family member about coming to the event and what had been discussed and had increased comfort talking to a HIV specialist doctor or nurse and taking their anti-HIV medication. There was a wider range of responses to questions about personal emotional responses to their HIV status. This may indicate that coming to terms with their HIV status is more problematic than acquiring behavioral skills to better manage their disease. However, as we do not have a baseline that measured HIV related emotional distress it is difficult to interpret this data.

21.7.3 Supporting Adherence

Adolescence in general, and the time of transition from child to adult services, are both associated with poorer adherence, both for HIV and for other long term health conditions in childhood (see also Chaps. 4, 5, 6, 17, 18, 19, 20, and 22 in this volume). Evidence suggests that 25 % of children have failed first line therapy and that one in eight children have triple class failure within 4 years of starting ART, with poor adherence as the most common factor (Foster et al. 2014). A recent audit of HIV deaths following transfer to adult care in the UK demonstrated that established poor adherence in pediatrics persisting into adult care resulted in 9 of 11 deaths reported, with the remaining two deaths due to suicide (Fish et al. 2014). This study emphasized the complex medical and psycho-social issues faced by these young people and reported high levels of mental health problems, unstable home circumstances and prevalent drug and alcohol use. As such, the mental health needs of young people need to be a priority in identifying needs and supporting access to child and adolescent mental health services (see also Chaps. 4, 9, 12, 18, and 20 in this volume).

A mapping exercise of our adolescent clinic cohort showed that 45 % had adherence problems, that young people often lived in one-parent families with high levels of parental depression, and where almost a quarter had had contact with social services (Campbell et al. 2014). As such, it is important to intervene early at the parent and family level as a preventative measure. This includes maximizing stability within the home environment by ensuring that parents have good access to legal, social and mental health support where applicable. It includes supporting parents with their own complicated relationship to HIV and adherence as a way of increasing their ability to manage their children's health and medication adherence. This has included enhancing parental ability to communicate about HIV with their children so that they are more equipped when adolescence arrives, and facilitating a 'good' disclosure to children of their HIV diagnosis in a gradual, staged manner.

At the adolescent level, facilitating increased autonomy and involvement in consultations with their medical team is important, as is an increased understanding of their health condition and responsibility for medication taking. Accessible communication using text-message reminders and email has also been an important service change to ensure that we maximize opportunities to communicate rather than create barriers for adolescents.

There is evidence that motivational interviewing (MI) approaches are useful when working with young people around HAART adherence. MI was developed in the 1980s as a counseling strategy to promote behavior change in alcohol and substance abuse patients and has been utilized for many other types of health behavior interventions, such as smoking cessation (Colby et al. 2005), diabetes self-management (West et al. 2007), and medication adherence (Ogedegbe et al. 2008). Hill and Kavookjian (2012) conducted a review of the literature to identify studies analyzing the effect of a MI intervention on HAART adherence. Three of the five RCT studies examined showed a significant increase in adherence rates, two studies reported a significant decrease in viral load, and one study showed an increase in CD4 cell count as a result of the intervention.

A more recent and innovative approach to ART adherence in the UK is one of financial incentives. Financial incentives have been used with different client groups in the UK, and there has been evidence for improved health outcomes in drug abstinence (Lussier et al. 2006), completion of tuberculosis therapy (Volmink and Garner 2000) and smoking cessation during pregnancy (Bauld and Coleman 2009). In the UK, Foster et al. (2014) have reported on a pilot project using financial incentives combined with motivational interviewing with a small number of young people with established poor adherence and advanced disease. Eleven eligible young people (16–25 years, non-adherent, CD4 count <200) received motivational interviewing and financial incentives for a 1 year period (dependent on having a reduction in viral load or maintaining an undetectable viral load and up to a maximum of £200). Outcome data showed that nine achieved a viral load of under 50, five sustained an undetectable viral load. The project showed considerable gains a year after the cessation of incentives with six maintaining a viral load of <50. They suggest that novel approaches such as this can work to reverse poor patterns of adherence established since childhood, and that achieving improved virological and immunological outcomes is possible with minimal expenditure. Whilst this intervention was with a limited number of young people, it shows promising results and underlines the importance of addressing psychological barriers in addition to taking health economics into account via financial incentives.

Within this complicated context, a multi-disciplinary and multi-factorial approach is key. Early identification of families in which there are adherence difficulties allows the team to discuss and develop a strategy to support adherence. Active follow-up of young people and families who do not attend appointments is crucial. Identification of parental issues (poor mental health, financial worries, domestic violence) that may contribute to non-adherence may be helpful. Likewise, early identification of adolescents and young people who are struggling with adherence allows different strategies to be tried out such as motivational interviewing approaches regarding medication and negotiating with them keeping in contact with services at times of reduced adherence.

Another key approach has also been to educate the multidisciplinary team on adolescence and adherence in relation to normalizing a change in adherence in previously-concordant children. In our experience, multi-disciplinary team members can often find this sudden change challenging and perplexing, which can lead to a sense of being de-skilled and feelings of anger toward the young person. This can lead to conversations which young people experience as 'lecturing' and unhelpful, and which can unwittingly serve to reinforce their reduced adherence. Expecting and being prepared for a change in adherence can support professionals to have more helpful conversations with young people.

21.8 Conclusion

Many of HIV-positive children acquired HIV vertically but an increasing number acquired the infection as the result of sexual activity and this is particularly true of young females. These young people are now in late adolescence and this data shows the scale of the challenge of effectively managing the medical, psychological and social consequences of the infection in young people.

In this chapter, we have emphasized that, as HIV is a family issue for many young people, this context cannot be ignored as there are many potential factors that affect the psychological capacity to manage this life-long condition. Parental coping factors are very important not least that they model ways of managing the disease to children and young people. It seems reasonable to conclude that children and young people who are exposed to poor parental coping will find it harder to develop effective HIV coping strategies themselves. Parental ill-health (both mental and physical), loss and bereavement and the broad impact of stigma all effect the development of effective ways of coping for young people. Effective anti-stigma interventions are needed to equip young people with the tools to counter the negative and damaging effects of stigma. However, there is little evidence that such interventions are being implemented especially in high prevalence areas. Such interventions need to be written into national and international guidelines for the effective management of the disease.

Although HAART is more widely available than ever there is still inconsistent global coverage and especially in areas of highest need (see also Chap. 22). However, availability of effective medication is useless unless it is taken consistently. Until there is a cure for HIV, PHIV are likely to have to take medication on a daily basis for the rest of their lives. For young people, this often seems overwhelming and there is good evidence that adherence in this group is fraught with difficulty. However, it seems that clinicians have unrealistic expectations about the likelihood that young people will be adherent consistently during adolescence and young adulthood especially. We contend that adherence difficulties are almost to be expected and that clinicians could plan for periods of inconsistent or non-adherence in advance. Discussions with young PHIV might reveal reasons for non-adherence and this maybe the opportunity to approach this issue with creativity. This may transform what is usually a highly stressful situation for everyone (the young person, their family, the clinicians) into one that demonstrates an understanding of the complexity of this issue for them and moves the conversation from blame and failure to what can be achieved (e.g. treatment interruption for a certain period of time, changing the regimen to the easiest one possible, incentivizing adherence).

Preparation for other life events including pregnancy and parenthood, employment and disclosure of status to new sexual partners is necessary to ensure that young PHIV have the skills and strategies to effectively manage these ubiquitous life events. PHIV have exactly the same desires to be in loving and stable relationships and to be financially prosperous as other young people and it is crucial that we actively attend to the 'whole adolescent' with all of their wishes and goals, and not just to medication adherence and sexual behavior.

Effective psychological interventions to address HIV issues in young people (disclosure, adherence, coping) should take into account the family and systemic factors that contribute to the development of their coping strategies. As we are now in the fourth decade of the disease, we need to ensure that young people are equipped as well as possible with psychological and emotional tools to manage this infection in the long term. However, it is unlikely that one off interventions will be effective in facilitating the development of effective coping strategies. If psychological interventions are to be of maximum efficacy, they need to be interwoven into the provision of medical and social care for young people and their families. There is no doubt that this is a challenge. Health care teams delivering HIV care in the developed world have disproportionate access to such resources and young people in resource poor settings (which is where the bulk of young PHIV live) are much less likely to be able to access sophisticated psychological interventions. However, much of the work that needs to be undertaken does not require sophisticated technology or highly trained staff. It could be argued that what is necessary is a paradigm shift for those who provide the medical care. Being aware of the likely issues that arise at different points of the life span and what are effective interventions to address the common issues that are underpinned by stigma are likely to be successful. We contend that it is through a stance of curiosity about the ways in which HIV is managed in the lives of both individuals and their families that allows for different and transforming conversations to occur.

References

Aghaizu, A., Brown, A. E., Nardone, A., Gill, O. N., & Delpech, V. C. (2013). *HIV in the United Kingdom 2013 report: Data to end 2012*. London: Public Health England.

Astill, N., Anderson, P., Winter, A., Nandwani, R., & MacConnachie, A. (2012). Improvement is needed in the documentation and HIV testing of children of HIV-positive women. *International Journal of STD & AIDS, 23*(1), 55–56.

Bauld, L., & Coleman, T. (2009). *The effectiveness of smoking cessation interventions during pregnancy: A briefing paper*. London: National Institute for Health and Clinical Excellence.

Bitsindou, P., Nzounza, P., Diafouka, M., Sibillle, B., Tran-Minh, T., Mouala, C., Adam, G., Mooney, M., & Mattei, J-F. (2007). *Need for dialogue in talking to children and adolescents living with HIV*. AIDS impact conference (Abstract no. 155), Marseille, France, 1–4 July.

Blum, R., Garell, D., & Hodgman, C. (1993). Transition from child-centred to adult health-care systems for adolescents with chronic conditions: A position paper of the Society for Adolescent Medicine. *Journal of Adolescent Health, 14*, 570–576.

Campbell, T., & Griffiths, J. (2013). *HIV stigma: The mental health elephant in the room. How to implement and develop effective anti-stigma interventions for people with HIV*. 13th AIDS impact conference, Barcelona, Spain, Sept 29–Oct 4.

Campbell, T., & Kelly, M. (1995). Women and AIDS in Zambia: A review of the psychosocial factors implicated in the transmission of HIV. *AIDS Care, 7*(3), 365–373.

Campbell, T., Beer, H., & Wilkins, R. (2010a). *Experiences of and preferences for transition in a group of HIV+ young people*. Unpublished data.

Campbell, T., Beer, H., & Wilkins, R. (2010b). The looking forward day: An evaluation of group work with HIV+ young people in London. *Clinical Psychology Forum, 205*, 26–30.

Campbell, T., Griffiths, J., & Wilkins, R. (2011a). Outcomes of the looking forward day anti-stigma workshop. Unpublished data.

Campbell, T., Griffiths, J., Beer, H., Tungana, J., Bostock, V., & Parrett, N. (2011b). A group approach to facilitate family-focused coping with HIV+ African parents in London. *Clinical Psychology Forum, 220*, 31–36.

Campbell, T., Griffiths, J., Beer, H., Legemah, P., & Saine, M. (2014). HIV+ children and their families in the UK: Results from a family-clinic based 'look-back' exercise in London. *Perspectives in Public Health, 134*(1), 31–37.

Chesney, M. A., Chambers, D. B., Taylor, J. M., Johnson, L. M., & Folkman, S. (2003). Coping effectiveness training for men living with HIV: Results from a randomized clinical trial testing a group-based intervention. *Psychosomatic Medicine, 65*(6), 1038–1046.

Christofides, N. J., Jewkes, R. K., Dunkle, K. L., Nduna, M., Shai, N. J., & Sterk, C. (2014). Early adolescent pregnancy increases risk of incident HIV infection in the Eastern Cape, South Africa: A longitudinal study. *Journal of the International AIDS Society, 17*, 18585. http://www.jiasociety.org/index.php/jias/article/view/18585.

Colby, S. M., Monti, P. M., O'Leary Tevyaw, T., Barnett, N. P., Spirito, A., Rohsenow, D. J., Riggs, S., & Lewander, W. (2005). Brief motivational intervention for adolescent smokers in medical settings. *Addictive Behaviors, 30*(5), 865–874.

Davey, M. P., Duncan, T. M., Foster, J., & Milton, K. (2008). Keeping the family in focus at an HIV/AIDS pediatric clinic. *Families, Systems & Health, 26*(3), 350–355.

Dlamini, P. S., Wantland, D., Makoae, L. N., Chirwa, M., Kohi, T. W., Greeff, M., & Holzemer, W. L. (2009). HIV stigma and missed medications in HIV-positive people in five African countries. *AIDS Patient Care & STDS, 23*(5), 377–387.

Eisenhut, M., Sharma, V., Kawsar, M., & Balachandran, T. (2008). Knowledge of their children's HIV status in HIV positive mothers attending a genitourinary medicine clinic in the UK. *HIV Medicine, 9*, 257–259.

Elgalib, A., Hegazi, A., Samarawickrama, A., Roedling, S., Tariq, S., Draeger, E., Hemelaar, J., Rathnayaka, T., Azwa, A., Hawkins, D., Edwards, S., Perez, K., Russell, J., Wood, C., Poulton, M., Shah, R., Noble, H., Rodgers, M., Taylor, G. P., Anderson, J., & de Ruiter, A. (2010). Pregnancy in HIV-infected teenagers in London. *HIV Medicine, 12*, 118–123.

Epston, D., Freeman, J., & Lobovits, D. (1997). *Playful approaches to serious problems: Narrative therapy with children and their families*. Chicago: WW Norton & Company.

Fish, R., Judd, A., Jungmann, E., O'Leary, C., & Foster, C. (2014). Mortality in perinatally HIV-infected young people in England following transition to adult care: An HIV Young Persons Network (HYPNet) audit. *HIV Medicine, 15*(26), 239–244.

Foster, C., Tookey, P., Tudor-Williams, G., Dunn, D., Shingadia, D., & Butler, K. (2009). Young people in the United Kingdom and Ireland with perinatally acquired HIV: The pediatric legacy for adult services. *AIDS Patient Care & STDs., 23*(3), 159–166.

Foster, C., McDonald, S., Frize, G., Ayers, S., & Fidler, S. (2014). "Payment by results"—financial incentives and motivational interviewing, adherence interventions in young adults with perinatally acquired HIV-1 infection: A pilot program. *AIDS Patient Care & STDs, 28*(1), 28–32.

Fox, J. (1987). *The essential Moreno*. New York: Springer.

Gibb, D. M., Masters, J., Shingadia, D., Trickett, S., Klein, N., & Duggan, C. (1997). A family clinic—optimising care for HIV infected children and their families. *Archives of Disease in Childhood, 77*, 478–482.

Gore-Felton, C., Rotheram-Borus, M. J., Weinhardt, L. S., Kelly, J. A., Lightfoot, M., & Kirschenbaum, S. B. (2005). The healthy living project: An individually tailored, multidimensional intervention for HIV-infected persons. *AIDS Education and Prevention, 17*(Suppl. A), 21–39.

Harker, R. (2010). *HIV and AIDS statistics, SN/SG/2210*. London: House of Commons Library.

Hill, S., & Kavookjian, J. (2012). Motivational interviewing as a behavioral intervention to increase HAART adherence in patients who are HIV+: A systematic review of the literature. *AIDS Care, 24*(5), 583–592.

Hosegood, V., & Madhavan, S. (2010). Data availability on men's involvement in families in sub-Saharan Africa to inform family-centred programmes for children affected by HIV and AIDS. *Journal of the International AIDS Society, 13*(Suppl. 2), S5. doi:10.1186/1758-2652-13-S2-S5.

Jones, P. (1990). HIV infection and haemophilia. *Archives of Disease in Childhood, 65*, 364–368.

Kidd, R., Clay, S., & Chiiya, C. (2003). *Understanding and challenging HIV stigma: Toolkit for action*. Washington, DC: International Center for Research on Women.

Kim, S.-H., Gerver, S. M., Fidler, S., & Ward, H. (2014). Adherence to antiretroviral therapy in adolescents living with HIV: Systematic review and meta-analysis. *AIDS, 28*(13), 1945–1956.

Leeper, S. C., Montague, B. T., Friedman, J. F., & Flanigan, T. P. (2010). Lessons learned from family-centred models of treatment for children living with HIV: Current approaches and future directions. *Journal of the International AIDS Society, 13*(Suppl. 2), S3. doi:10.1186/1758-2652-13-S2-S3.

Lesch, A., Swartz, L., Kagee, A., Moodley, K., Kafaar, Z., Myer, L., & Cotton, M. (2007). Paediatric HIV/AIDS disclosure: Towards a developmental and process-oriented approach. *AIDS Care, 19*(6), 811–816.

Logie, C., & Gadalla, T. M. (2009). Meta-analysis of health and demographic correlates of stigma toward people living with HIV. *AIDS Care, 21*(6), 742–753.

Lussier, J. P., Heil, S. H., Mongeon, J. A., Badger, G. J., & Higgins, S. T. (2006). A meta-analysis of voucher-based reinforcement therapy for substance use disorders. *Addiction, 101*, 192–203.

Mahajan, A. P., Sayles, J. N., Patel, V. A., Remien, R. H., Ortiz, D., Szekeres, G., & Coates, T. J. (2008). Stigma in the HIV/AIDS epidemic: A review of the literature and recommendations for the way forward. *AIDS, 22*(Suppl. 2), S67–S79.

Martinez, J., Harper, G., Carleton, R. A., Hosek, S., Bojan, K., Glum, G., & Ellen, J. (2012). The impact of stigma on medication adherence among HIV-positive adolescent and young adult females and the moderating effects of coping and satisfaction with health care. *AIDS Patient Care & STDS, 26*(2), 108–115.

Melvin, D., Krechevsky, D., Divac, A., Tacconelli, E., Miah, J., & Waugh, S. (2007). Parental reports of emotional and behavioural difficulties on the SDQ for school-age children with vertically acquired HIV infection living in London. *Psychology, Health & Medicine, 12*(1), 40–47.

Michaud, P.-A., Suris, J.-C., Thomas, L. R., Kahlert, C., Rudin, C., & Cheseaux, J.-J. (2009). To say or not to say: A qualitative study on the disclosure of their condition by human immunodeficiency virus–Positive adolescents. *Journal of Adolescent Health, 4*, 356–362. doi:10.1016/j.jadohealth.2008.08.004.

Murphy, D. A. (2008). HIV-positive mothers' disclosure of their serostatus to their young children: A review. *Clinical Child Psychology and Psychiatry, 13*, 105–122.

National AIDS Trust. (2011). *HIV: Public knowledge and attitudes, 2010*. London: National AIDS Trust.

Nostlinger, C., Bartoli, G., & Gordillo, V. (2006). Children and adolescents living with HIV positive parents: Emotional and behavioural problems. *Vulnerable Children and Youth Studies, 1*(1), 29–43.

Nyandiya-Bundy, S., Gatsi, R., Machokoto, S., Beta, N., Montaño, D., & Kasprzyk, D. (2009). *TALC TO PIP: The adaptation of TALC for Zimbabwe*. AIDS impact conference, Gaborone, Botswana, September 22–25.

Ogedegbe, G., Schoenthaler, A., Richardson, T., Lewis, L., Belue, R., Espinosa, E., Spencer, J., Allegrante, J. P., & Charlson, M. E. (2008). An RCT of the effect of motivational interviewing on medication adherence in hypertensive African Americans: Rationale and design. *Contemporary Clinical Trials, 28*(2), 169–181.

Piot, T. (2006). AIDS: From crisis management to sustained strategic response. *The Lancet, 368*(9534), 526–530.

Richter, L., & Sherr, L. (2009). Strengthening families: A key recommendation of the Joint Learning Initiative on Children and AIDS (JLICA). *AIDS Care, 21*(1), 1–2.

Rotheram-Borus, M. J., Lee, M. B., Murphy, D. A., Futterman, D., Duan, N., & Birnbaum, J. (2001). The teens linked to care consortium efficacy of a preventive interventions for youths living with HIV. *American Journal of Public Health, 91*, 400–405.

Sopena, S., Evangeli, M., Dodge, J., & Melvin, D. (2010). Coping and psychological adjustments in adolescents with vertically acquired HIV. *AIDS Care, 22*(10), 1252–1258.

Summary data: Colloborative HIV Paediatric Study website (2014). Available at; http://www.chipscohort.ac.uk/summary_data.asp.

Swendeman, D., Rotherham–Borus, M. J., Comulada, S., Weiss, R., & Ramos, M. E. (2006). Predictors of HIV-related stigma among young people living with HIV. *Health Psychology, 25*(4), 501–509.

Volmink, J., & Garner, P. (2000). Interventions for promoting adherence to tuberculosis management. *Cochrane Database of Systematic Reviews*. doi:10.1002/14651858.CD000010. John Wiley and Sons Ltd.

Waugh, S. (2003). Parental views on disclosure of diagnosis to their HIV-positive children. *AIDS Care, 15*, 169–176. doi:10.1080/0954012031000068317.

Weiner, L., Zobel, M., Battles, H., & Ryder, C. (2007). Transition from a pediatric HIV intramural clinical research program to adolescent and adult community-based care services. *Social Work in Health Care, 46*(1), 1–19.

West, D. S., DiLillo, V., Bursac, Z., Gore, S. A., & Greene, P. G. (2007). Motivational interviewing improves weight loss in women with type 2 diabetes. *Diabetes Care, 30*(5), 1081–1087.

Wilkins, R., Campbell, T., & Beer, H. (2007). Preparing HIV- positive young people for the challenges of adult life: A group work approach. *AIDS & Hepatitis Digest, 119*, 1–3.

Chapter 22
Lay Definitions of Antiretroviral Treatment: Unpacking the Paradoxes and Dilemmas of Therapeutic Efficacy in Rural Tanzania

Mangi J. Ezekiel

Contents

22.1 HIV, AIDS and the Changing Landscape of Risk and Vulnerability

Since AIDS cases were first detected in Tanzania in 1983, the epidemic has spread throughout the country, affecting both rural and urban areas. The predominant mode (78 %) of transmission remains to be heterosexual (NACP 2005). For quite some time, the rate of infection depicted geographical variability with higher prevalence mainly reported in urban areas compared to rural locations (Mnyika et al. 1996; NACP 2005). Nevertheless, as the epidemic evolves, some rural areas have reported significant increases in HIV prevalence in recent years (Mwaluko et al. 2003; Mshana et al. 2006; Mmbaga et al. 2007). Recent statistics show that the overall HIV prevalence among age group 15–49 in the country is estimated to have dropped from 7 to 6 % between 2001 and 2007 respectively (UNAIDS 2008). However, the age group

M.J. Ezekiel (✉)
School of Public Health and Social Sciences, Muhimbili University of Health and Allied Sciences, P O Box 65015, United Nations Road, Dar es Salaam, Tanzania
e-mail: e_mangi@yahoo.com; mezekiel@muhas.ac.tz

P. Liamputtong (ed.), *Children and Young People Living with HIV/AIDS*, Cross-Cultural Research in Health, Illness and Well-Being,
DOI 10.1007/978-3-319-29936-5_22

20–49 years has continued to comprise the largest proportion of HIV infected individuals, with peaks in the age group 25–34 for both sexes (NACP 2005). In the recent past, Kilimanjaro region, to these findings emanate, was one of the most affected regions in the country. Recent studies report that HIV prevalence in the region is increasing (Kapiga et al. 2006; Mmbaga et al. 2006). In some parts of the region, the prevalence of HIV-1 infection was 10.3 % in women and 7 % in their long-term male partners (Kapiga et al. 2006). Young people in particular continued to be among the most at risk population in Tanzania (Ministry of Health 2004). Evidence from the current study setting shows that although HIV prevalence among people aged 15–24 years has been stable in recent years, HIV prevalence and sexual risk practices in the general population have been increasing (Mmbaga et al. 2006, 2007). Despite significant increase in knowledge of HIV/AIDS, 85 % of people are unaware of their HIV status, and for those who are aware are faced with the dilemma of managing status disclosure (Ministry of Health 2007). This suggests that tackling HIV/AIDS requires interventions addressing wider societal constraining HIV management. HIV is a biological entity that is responsive to medical interventions. However, the epidemic has continued to expand, largely due to the failure to tackle societal conditions that increase HIV risk and vulnerability (UNAIDS 2008).

As the HIV pandemic has been evolving, so have the conceptions and perceptions of risk. In the early years after AIDS was detected in Tanzania, there was a general understanding that HIV/AIDS was confined to specific groups in society, such as long distance truck drivers, sex workers and people of certain geographical localities. Some rural residents have also considered AIDS as a problem of urban areas. However, this long held understanding about HIV risk groups are changing as the pandemic is affecting many parts of Tanzania including rural areas such as Kahe (Mmbaga et al. 2006). Similarly, previous evidence has shown that in some rural areas AIDS changed from a "less known disease to a disease of both outsiders (such as people living in urban areas, well-educated, involved in business) and local people" (Haram 1999: 191). As antiretroviral therapy (ART) is currently spreading to rural parts of Tanzania, people are confronting a new reality that may affect existing understanding of HIV/AIDS and the benefits and risks that come with increasing availability of treatment. Increased availability may be seen as beneficial to public health but also be associated with increased probability for some people to engage in risk sexual behaviors. The benefits and potential risks of ART must be understood in the wider context of both individual and societal wide factors that affect the ability of individuals to avoid or manage risk of HIV infection.

22.2 Risk in the Context of Antiretroviral Treatment: Conceptual and Theoretical Approaches

Risk as a concept is a subject of a variety of definitions. Sjoberg (1998: 751) argues that "the word risk is ambiguous and carries contents both of probability and consequence". The concept of risk has sometimes been defined in relation to vulnerability. Thus, taking a probabilistic perspective, the UNAIDS (2008: 65) defines HIV risk and vulnerability as:

> The probability or likelihood that a person may become infected with HIV. Certain behaviors create, increase, and perpetuate risk. Examples include unprotected sex with a partner whose HIV status is unknown, multiple sexual partnerships involving unprotected sex, and injecting drug use with contaminated needles and syringes. Vulnerability results from a range of factors outside the control of the individual that reduce the ability of individuals and communities to avoid HIV risk. These factors may include: (1) lack of knowledge and skills required to protect oneself and others; (2) factors pertaining to the quality and coverage of services (e.g. inaccessibility of service due to distance, cost or other factors); and (3) societal factors such as human rights violations, or social and cultural norms. These norms can include practices, beliefs and laws that stigmatize and disempower certain populations, limiting their ability to access or use HIV prevention, treatment, care, and support services and commodities. These factors, alone or in combination, may create or exacerbate individual and collective vulnerability to HIV.

There have also been attempts to differentiate between the perceived and actual risk. Actual risk includes those behaviors or practices that increase the probability of being infected with HIV such as unprotected sex and multiple sexual partners. Perceived risk is the subjective judgment or evaluation of the likelihood of being infected with HIV. Perceived risk involves processes of self-appraisal of a person's likelihood to become infected. Leventhal and colleagues (1999) suggest that perceptions of risk are related to motivation to act and to action. They also point out that increasing the match between perceived risk (beliefs) and actual risk (reality) will encourage individuals to initiate and maintain preventive and treatment behaviors.

In everyday usage, the concept of risk in Kiswahili usually translates into (or is synonymous to) "danger" (*hatari*). Hence, it has become common in both people's social interactions and official communications to use the concept of danger (to mean risk) in various messages and slogans in communicating about HIV and AIDS. Most messages tended to invoke a sense of danger (such as of imminent death due to HIV/AIDS related illnesses) when someone became HIV infected (see also Chaps. 9 and 11 in this volume). The notion that being infected with HIV/AIDS signals imminent death has been in existence since AIDS was first detected in Tanzania in the 1980s. This may explain the accusations and blame leveled against some HIV-positive persons allegedly deliberately spreading HIV. Thus, the concept of risk involves the belief that once you have sexual intercourse with infected person (whether deliberately or by chance), you are putting oneself 'at risk' (*kwenye hatari*) of HIV infection. It is worth noting that when research participants spoke about risk of spreading HIV with reference to PLHIV, they often attributed the risk to perceived neglect of protective sexual practices among persons receiving antiretroviral treatment. In other words, the positive health outcomes of ART come with some perceived unintended negative consequences considered potentially risky in the community. This chapter borrows UNAIDS' conceptions of risk and vulnerability in order to understand the social and cultural context of ART. It attempts to situate ART as an intervention that shapes social cultural definitions of medicines and influences explanations about risk and vulnerability to HIV. In that sense, pharmaco-therapeutic properties of ART find expression in peoples' lives and social interactions.

22.3 Social and Cultural Approaches to Risk

The fact that antiretroviral drugs are meant to deal with (individual) human health suggests that the risks and benefits of this medical intervention need to be understood in a particular social context (see also Izugbara and Wekesa 2011; Liamputtong et al. 2015). According to Douglas (1992), risk perception is not governed by personality traits, needs, or preferences but it is socially and/or culturally constructed phenomenon. Thus, one may argue that the labels attached to ART and the blame attached to (HIV-positive) persons accused of spreading HIV may be described as socially constructed and shaped by a particular cultural outlook about possible dangerous outcomes of specific undesirable conditions to the prevailing social order (Douglas and Wildavsky 1982). Cultural theory aims at explaining how people perceive and act upon the world around them. The core argument in my study is the competing perspectives about the benefits and potential dangers/risks of antiretroviral treatment in the study community. According to cultural theory of risk, whenever there are potential dangers in the community, there must be some explanations or "someone to be held accountable/responsible for the occurrence" (Tulloch and Lupton 2003: 3). In this context, the fear or perceived danger of being infected with HIV appears to be blamed on the existence of ART and the risk sexual behaviors involving persons receiving ART. Furthermore, cultural theory of risk acknowledges the variations in how members of community attach blame for imminent-potential risks. The theory acknowledges the cultural differences in the distribution of blame and the gap between lay and expert opinion about risk. Douglas (1992: 11–13) has also suggested that "the public does not see risks in the same way as experts". Similarly, Renn (2010) argues that managing risk takes various forms at individual and institutional levels. He points out that in responding to risk, risk perceptions of lay people will usually tend to over regulate (as it is the case with suggestions to pass legislation, physical isolation of persons accused of transmitting HIV and avoiding visiting risky places/villages), while ignoring expert advice. In attempts to manage risk, members of a community may employ a wide range of exclusionary measures to isolate bodies/persons blamed for producing risk in order to reduce harm to individuals and the community at large. Using an imagery of "skin and envelope", Douglas (1992: 115) describes how community attempts to control risk and protect individuals (bodies) from risk may pose intellectual and practical dilemmas:

> The idea of the body includes a weak immunity conferred by the double envelope, the body's own skin, and the community's skin…within a community a person can be safe, so long as entry to the body and to the community is controlled. The most appropriate action to take in the face of an epidemic is consolidation of the community, exclusion of outsiders, and repression of deviants. The first duty is to call home the wanderers who have gone abroad or whose work takes them to dangerous places abroad. Then the categories at risk have to be identified, and isolated. All of this organizing effort is supported by blaming procedures: the population at risk is divided into those needing care and protection and those needing forcible detention. Intellectual dilemmas which arise in the process are not easy to solve honestly.

Renn (2010) identifies three characteristics that underline definition of risk: ambiguity, uncertainty and complexity. Following Renn's characterization, it is fair to say that what is perceived as potential risk associated with increased availability of ART among my participants, could be a result (unintended consequences) of the complexity, uncertainty and ambiguity introduced by this relatively new medical intervention for managing HIV. In other words, ART is evaluated based on established expectations/functions of medication (drug effect) and in relation to a set of behaviors (real and perceived intention to deliberately spread the disease) of PLHIV considered by some research participants as sexually 'deviant' and dangerous to others. Furthermore, the ambiguities arise from the fact that scientific information about ART is not available, limited or misrepresented in official health messages and from peers. The idea that ART might lead to unprotected sex echoes ideas of risk society and risk reflexivity where attempts to control risk (through introduction of technologies) may produce new problems and effects which are not always known and controlled (Beck 1992; Giddens 1998).

Beck (1992) applies the notion of risk society in which risk is narrowed to the responses to technical and environmental risks resulting from unforeseen consequences of industrialization. Beck's definition of risk is "synonymous to hazard and danger" (cited in Tulloch and Lupton 2003: 2). An explanation of risk as resulting from environmental hazards of industrial age is considered insufficient to explain other complex issues of emotional or socio-cultural nature (Tulloch and Lupton 2003). Thus, the cultural approach is adopted as a framework for understanding culturally constructed/given ways to respond to threats of the boundaries of a group, organization or society and its definitions of reality and ways to maintain social order.

Cultural approach is used in qualitative studies as a heuristic in order to analyze the different approaches to risk in organizations and sub groups (Zinn 2006) – as it may be the case with different definitions of ART and risk perception among groups of young people in different villages in Kahe ward. Thus, the cultural approach is powerful and influential in its core concept to link risk perception and responses to processes of identity formation/construction and group formation by the distinction between self and other distinction (Zinn 2006).

The social and cultural approaches to risk also include the perspective offered by Anthony Giddens (1991). Giddens argues that risk is only negotiable in a late modern world in which people have diverse choices. Risk perceptions are linked to self-identity, which becomes reflexively organized through the creation of narratives. The range of possibilities facing individuals both provides them with choice but also creates anxiety and self-doubt and results in an increased awareness of risk. Giddens' formulation can have implications in how risk is perceived at the level of social relations particularly with regard to exposure to modern medical technologies such as ART. It may affect local discourse/narratives about the relative exposure to risks among members of community: for instance among those who self-identify to be not at risk and those thought to be at heightened risk/danger due to increased exposure to modern (as conceptually opposed to traditional) lifestyles or modern technologies.

Although cultural theory is useful in explaining risk, it has been subject to criticism. It has been criticized for its inherent ambiguities and complexities in the diversity of conceptualizations of risk and its powerful embrace of functionalism. Because of being overly functionalist, it fails to recognize the role of agency/power of individuals to pursue their own ends in social relations and variations in individual perception of risk (Boholm 1996). Tulloch and Lupton (2003) criticize the cultural theory for its oversimplification of far more complex dynamic processes of how risk is dealt with and experienced. Despite its weaknesses, the cultural approach to risk recognizes the powerful role of culture-based values and the insight they can provide in the understanding of risk perception. In the context of my study, the cultural theory is strong in its "emphasis on the link between biomedical technologies and fundamental questions about the social and political meaning of technologies and their broader societal implications" (Dake 1992: 23).

In line with Dake's argument (1992), it is important to examine implications of ART in the broader social and cultural context where availability of medication is mediated by structural factors that may shape individual vulnerability. Availability of ART may be constrained by government policies, socio-economic conditions, historical factors, geographical realities and social and cultural arrangements within social groups and communities. Although access to ART has expanded significantly in recent years, many people (particularly in rural areas of Tanzania) have difficulties accessing HIV treatment and care services (Mshana et al. 2006; Stoeckle et al. 2006; Hardon et al. 2007). This is in spite of evidence indicating that HIV/AIDS is gradually becoming a generalized epidemic in many parts of the country including rural areas (Mwaluko et al. 2003; Kapiga et al. 2006; Mmbaga et al. 2008). Because of the patterns of modern social life, risks have become more difficult to calculate and control, crossing national and socioeconomic boundaries (Tulloch and Lupton 2003). Tulloch and Lupton (2003) further argue that risks have broken down previous social and geographic boundaries evident in modern societies. In Kilimanjaro region (where my study was conducted), there is evidence indicating how population dynamics (movement and mobility) caused shifts in disease dynamics. Such shifts were particularly evident in local narratives about HIV and the local manifestations of the HIV/AIDS epidemic (see for example Setel 1999: 53–54). It is worth noting that before and after the introduction of ART, mobility is a subject that has continued to attract considerable attention in explaining risk and HIV spread in Tanzania (Weiss 1996; Setel 1999; Ezekiel et al. 2008; Mmbaga et al. 2008). It is documented that the introduction of ART has often increased concern about the potential for increased HIV related risk sexual behaviors both among infected and uninfected populations (Bateganya et al. 2005; Rice et al. 2006; UNAIDS 2006). ART has emerged as a new medical intervention that appears to affect discourse about persons living with HIV and the policy measures adopted to control the epidemic. Recent evidence shows that people living with HIV have been blamed for engaging in unprotected sex, deliberate spread of disease and sometimes been legally prosecuted (Cameron et al. 2008; Roura et al. 2008).

In the face of increasing awareness about HIV/AIDS and the introduction of ART, there is growing uncertainties about the appropriate responses to risk and the effectiveness of social/institutional mechanisms available to manage the spread of HIV/AIDS. There is an emerging debate about the public health implications of using legal sanctions to prevent and control the spread of the epidemic (UNAIDS 2006; Cameron et al. 2008). Some of the measures to control HIV suggest that HIV-infected individuals deviate from social expectations (self-control of sexual desires). With regard to the implications of HIV treatment for sexual practice, some policy-makers have argued for interventions that focus on the detection, treatment and behavior management of individuals with HIV (Janssen et al. 2001). As will be shown later, my study supports previous assertions that no single institution can prevent risk and that responsibility and blame are usually leveled against individuals thought to be responsible for producing the risks (Tulloch and Lupton 2003).

22.4 The Social and Cultural Life of Antiretroviral Treatment

Social and cultural aspects of ART relate to how different people (individuals, communities or social groups) explain treatment and how beliefs and practices about ART relate to wider definitions about health and disease (see also Izugbara and Wekesa 2011; Liamputtong et al. 2015). Most medicines are defined in terms of how they affect the human body (Helman 1990; Persson 2004). However, the effects of any medication on individuals and society are not solely a function of its pharmacological properties. For instance, Van der Geest and Hardon (2006) suggest that the social and cultural effects of pharmaceuticals need to be taken into account because a number of non-medical effects deeply influence the medical outcomes of medicine use. Effects of medicines are determined by a set of beliefs about the physiological significance, structure and function of the body. It has also been observed that the "effectiveness of medicines is often explained through the body because it is a site of both physical and social reality" (Whyte et al. 2002: 13). Furthermore, the human body is a medium through which information about health and people's behavior is communicated (Helman 1990).

In the context of HIV/AIDS, the body has become an important theme in understanding the social context and management of HIV epidemic. This is because the body is an implicit theme in construction of knowledge about pain, suffering, sickness, disability and death (Williams and Bendelow 1998) which are also central aspects in understanding HIV/AIDS and ART. It has been suggested that there is an "apparent link between therapeutic efficacy of drugs and its effect in modifying bodies" (Whyte et al. 2002: 14). Therefore, in order to understand the social and cultural context of ART, it is useful to take into account both the pharmacological and societal wide processes affecting medicines in a community and the effects of medication on human bodies. Thus, although medicines are usually ingested by individuals, their effects are usually beyond the individuals. A number of elements are taken into consideration including the "attributes of a drug itself, a person/patient receiving treatment, person prescribing/dispensing the drugs and the physical setting in which the drug is prescribed or administered (Helman 2007: 196).

Medicines are also a means of meeting social expectations within family, work place and community; as part of a cultural view of what is acceptable behavior. Social acceptance of drugs is an important part of making them a normal part of life and can lessen stigma attached to disease to which the drug is related (Helman 1990). Normalization of drugs is illustrated by lay beliefs about what is or is not a drug. The extent to which a new form of treatment is integrated into the healing system depends on social values that support its normalization. Normalization is "partly learned from doctors who in turn may be influenced by colleagues and the extensive advertising of the pharmaceutical industry, in newspapers, magazines and television programs" (Helman 2007: 203). It is important to note here that the existence of different sources of information about treatment also opens up the possibilities of multiple perspectives in understanding ART. The introduction of ART presents one of the recent technological interventions that have altered lay understanding about management of HIV/AIDS. ART may be examined and understood in different ways. One way of looking at ART is to consider it as constituting a moral and political enterprise concerned with regulation, surveillance and control of bodies through the medical regimen (Foucault 1990). From an instrumentalist perspective, antiretroviral treatment may also be conceived as a tool to empower individuals (on treatment) to reassert control over subjective experiences of social life (Williams and Bendelow 1998). In other words, the meaning of ART resides both in the objective and subjective realities of human existence. In order to understand ART as a social-cultural entity, it is also important to examine the "motives of individuals, practitioners and members of therapy management groups" (Nichter and Vuckovic 1994: 1510). There is a need to investigate how the different social actors "use discourse for metamedical purposes, that is, for purposes beyond the achievement of physical cure… and also to uncover how the use of medicines to mask symptoms and modify behavior establishes new criteria by which health, illness and acceptable behavior are evaluated" (Nichter and Vuckovic 1994: 1510–1511).

Through different social processes such as stratification, labeling and policies affecting access to health services, medicines may contribute to formation of discourses that have implications on identities of individual living with HIV and HIV risk. For instance, research has shown that persons with HIV are said to be "positioned by their HIV sero-identities in cultural systems of reflective hierarchy and blaming" (Davis 2007: 1006). Furthermore, ART roll out, through intended and unintended consequences, may produce social hierarchy, dominance and control. Policy decisions and clinical rules and criteria may impose restrictions (such as eligibility criteria for starting treatment or through conscious policy and legislative action) on access to treatment. For instance, the decisions to begin ART roll out in tertiary hospitals in Tanzania may have denied treatment opportunities for persons (unable to reach tertiary hospitals) who meet clinical eligibility criteria for enrollment into treatment programs. The aforementioned factors eventually highlight the ways in which a purely biomedical technology is transformed through social processes and contexts. Social and cultural dimensions of ART may also be understood through institutions, discourses, and practices of persons on ART. For instance, research involving persons on HIV treatment suggests an emerging debate about the relevance of terminology such as 'AIDS' following the introduction of more effective HIV treatment (Greene and Ward 2002). This underscores the fact that medicines are usually evaluated based on how they perform a core clinical function, namely, healing (Helman 1990). Cultural labels attached to medicines convey information about how to manage a particular illness (Kleinman 1980) and are often useful tools employed in understanding the social and biomedical aspects of treatment in different communities and social groups. Medicines are cultural entities with particular histories and investments (Persson 2004). They are not only products of human culture but also producers of culture as they carry ideas about self and body, illness, health and responsibility (Van der Geest et al. 1996; Cohen et al. 2001). Therefore, when introducing new forms of disease intervention, it is crucial to examine how the new treatment is evaluated within the existing social and cultural frameworks of health, disease and illness. Taking stock of local discourse and perceptions about ART could form the basis for understanding individual and community wide responses to and preparedness for ART scale up.

22.5 Targeting Young People

As previously indicated, many young people continue to be vulnerable to HIV infection and are affected by HIV/AIDS in different ways (Ministry of Health 2004). However, they are often ignored in sexual and reproductive health and related interventions for different reasons. Poverty, migration, civil unrest, stigma and discrimination are among factors that marginalize young people, increase their vulnerability to infection and reduce their access to services (Van den Bergh 2008; WHO 2008; see also Chaps. 3, 4, 6, 9, 12, 14, 15, 17, 18, 19, 20, and 21 in this volume). Addressing HIV prevention in this group is vital considering the changing risk dynamics in the times of AIDS particularly with availability of new treatment for HIV. The combined hazards of vulnerability and poor access are often most acute among young people. The WHO (2003) suggests that in order to increase access and uptake of integrated HIV services, active entry points are needed to reach out to marginalized populations that do not seek treatment on their own. In recognition of young people's vulnerability to HIV/AIDS, the United Nations General Assembly Special Session (UNGASS) on HIV/AIDS outlined a number of goals and targets focusing on young people aged 15–24. The goals and targets endorsed during the UNGASS on HIV/AIDS not only focus on decreasing HIV prevalence among young people but also on providing access to information, skills and services as well as decreasing vulnerability (WHO 2003).

Reaching out to key marginalized populations at risk of HIV may contribute to increasing awareness and social acceptability of ART. ART roll out programs may benefit by understanding and addressing young people's beliefs, attitudes, perceptions and potential implications of ART on sexual risk behaviors and overall HIV prevention efforts. However, it has been pointed out that studies on ART beliefs and attitudes among young people in sub-Saharan Africa are limited (Cohen et al. 2009). A majority of studies about ART have addressed access to treatment, stigma, treatment adherence and changes in risk sexual behaviors among persons on ART. One study conducted among HIV-infected adults indicated overoptimistic attitudes towards ART through association of ARVs to cure of HIV (Nachega et al. 2005). Furthermore, some studies conducted among persons on treatment reveal that access to treatment promotes safer sex (Bateganya et al. 2005; Bunnell et al. 2006). These studies attest to the neglect and marginalization of this key population group in the context of increased availability of ART. A population-based survey in Kisumu (Cohen et al. 2009) revealed that with increased availability of ART, young people represent not only one of the highest risk groups for HIV acquisition and transmission, but also are the group most likely to become HIV infected during the period in which ART became available. It has been emphasized that understanding of antiretroviral treatment, the side effects of treatment, and belief in treatment efficacy is an important part in assessing individual readiness to start treatment (Gebrekristos et al. 2005). Recent studies in Tanzania revealed that ART-related beliefs and attitudes are hinged primarily on the level of education and knowledge about ART, concerns about stigma and status disclosure (Roura et al. 2008; Zou et al. 2009). Little is understood about the role that ART can play in shaping local discourse about risk and its potential implications on perceptions and existing mechanisms to manage risk among young people.

There are good epidemiological and clinical reasons to study how ART related discourses, beliefs and perceptions relate to the potential sexual risk behaviors among young people as they interact with other members of community. Apart from their social and biological vulnerability to HIV, young people are thought of as a dynamic population in a constantly changing epidemic and as such may experience or exhibit changes in risk behaviors with appropriate and timely interventions (Klepp et al. 2008; Lema et al. 2008). Given their limited access to sexual and reproductive health services and information coupled with their social and biological vulnerability to HIV infection (Jejeebhoy et al. 2005; Luke 2005; Nkosana and Rosenthal 2007; Klepp et al. 2008), targeting young people with appropriate ART-related education addressing treatment beliefs, attitudes and risk reduction is vital (Cohen et al. 2009). Young people have also been shown to employ different strategies to avoid engaging in risk sexual relationships (Nkosana and Rosenthal 2007). Previous evidence of risk sexual behaviors and potential spread of HIV among HIV-infected persons further justifies efforts to better understand ART in the current study (Crepaz et al. 2004; Nachega et al. 2005; Rice et al. 2006). Clearly, an examination of social and cultural discourses around ART and the perceived consequences of treatment on risks and HIV transmission dynamics in Tanzania are timely and warranted. Highlighting the importance of targeting young people in the context of HIV/AIDS prevention, Klepp and colleagues (2008: 7–11) observe that:

> Despite being at the center of HIV epidemic, in terms of transmission, vulnerability and impact, the vast majority of young people and adolescents encounter significant barriers in maintaining their sexual and reproductive health including lack of access to services, information designed to equip them with skills and services for prevention, treatment and care.

A study conducted in Canada (Veinot et al. 2006) showed that many young people on ART were often confused and skeptical about the treatment. While those not on treatments did not believe in antiretroviral treatment, those on treatment did not understand why they were taking medications (see also Chaps. 4, 5, 6, 17, 18, 19, 20, and 21 in this volume). In other contexts, women and young people are among the groups poorly informed about HIV testing and treatment services compared to adult males (IPASC and EQUINET 2009). What Veinot and colleagues concluded in their study may be useful in the context of the current study; that the availability of social programs to provide treatment access does not guarantee that youth will be aware of them. Thus, there is a need for youth-specific outreach programs for young people (Veinot et al. 2006).

While there have been a number of studies investigating ART in relation to sexual behaviors changes, risk taking, treatment access and adherence particularly among individuals on treatment, the study on which this chapter is based explores how the introduction of ART affects local discourses and shapes perceptions about and responses to HIV risk. The study is a further attempt to recognize universal treatment as a key part of HIV prevention for young people especially, in order to support them to stay HIV-negative and mitigate the potential impact of increased availability of ART on HIV transmission dynamics in a rural area.

22.6 Antiretroviral Treatment, the Body and Local Discourse on Healing

Evidence from my study with young people revealed that individuals hold mixed views and responses about the therapeutic value of ART. Participants tended to view treatments and cures differently and thus the discourses on ART were centered around the capacity of medicines to perform both (to treat and cure) functions. Young people used different terminologies to describe ART. Local Swahili terms identified by young people had a combination of the dominant lay, biomedical and official discourses about ART. All terms acknowledged the role of ART in enduring survival while emphasizing different aspects of health and individual well-being. The study shows that local discourses contained some remnants of the previous official or dominant discourses and at the same time embracing new ones. While some terms emanated from official/public discourse (such as life prolonging drugs), others appeared to come from participants' own local experiences (such as fattening injections, pigs' medication). Use of ART was understood as primarily intended to make persons on treatment recover (sometimes temporarily) from illness, become fat and look healthy. ART appeared to be at odds with a socially established body of knowledge about physical symptoms of HIV/AIDS. Assessment of physical symptoms was considered an important determinant of HIV status, participants' interactions with HIV-positive people and consequent sexual decisions. Consequently, healthy appearances among ART users were thought to compromise locally relevant ways of avoiding HIV infection. Structural inequities in access, limited information on therapeutic efficacy, difficulties with status disclosure and limited access to counseling and testing services appear to inform conceptions about and socio-medical implications of antiretroviral therapy.

22.7 Deliberate/Intentional Transmission of HIV

Building upon findings from young people, this chapter also explored sexual and social behaviors that constitute deliberate spread of HIV. It draws on the connection between antiretroviral use and potential risks of spread of HIV. A number of sexual behaviors were perceived to potentially constitute deliberate transmission of HIV/AIDS. Desire for sexual reproduction among HIV-positive persons, marriage and remarriage, intentional misuse of HIV preventive technologies such as condoms and transactional sex were mentioned. Findings also indicate that people on ART face the dilemma between reducing risk of spreading HIV and a desire to maintain socially acceptable sexual and reproductive lives. Although many participants reportedly remained sexually abstinent, they also revealed that some people on treatment from within and beyond study area were believed or suspected to be engaging in sexual activities/practices that were considered to represent a potential for deliberate spread of HIV. The findings also showed that most participants supported the establishment of some form of legal or other mechanisms to control intentional spread of HIV/AIDS. However, some participants were concerned about the practical applicability of legal sanctions to control sexual behaviors. In Tanzania, there is a law that defines various offences and remedies for persons and institutions proven to intentionally spread HIV. Although few participants were aware of this law, they appeared optimistic that if effectively enforced it could be useful in the prevention and control of the spread of HIV/AIDS.

22.8 Discussion

Results of my study indicate that the availability of ART may affect how people experience and define medicines and perceive risk. Pharmacological properties of ART appear to have introduced a paradigm shift in locally shared understanding of therapeutic effects of medicines. Since HIV/AIDS is known to have no cure, the effects of ART introduced a new reality in the social meaning of medicines. ART underscores the central role of the body as a determinant of social definitions about health and illness. Limited access to ART influences how people define antiretroviral medication as a symbol of rural neglect and inequity in health services. ART is described to be a privilege of urban residents and few people in rural areas also considered to be at most risk. However, despite maintaining boundaries of access to treatment, interactions between people of this rural setting and adjacent urban areas appears to have broken boundaries of HIV risk. Risk of HIV is understood to be a function of social practices across time and space and not entirely a property of specific groups of people. While ART is not intended to cure HIV/AIDS, its availability may have both intended and unintended consequences on risk sexual behaviors among HIV-infected individuals and affected members of community. Despite restoring health and improving well-being, ART is thought to have the potential to influence harmful sexual practices such as deliberate spread of the disease. Overall, the findings highlight the increasing tendency towards institutional mechanisms as a strategy to control risk sexual behaviors and prevent spread of HIV and AIDS.

Medicines are reported to take on different meanings as they move across different actors, social groups and cultures (Whyte et al. 2002; Persson 2004; Van der Geest and Hardon 2006). Antiretroviral treatment has also been described and understood based on its pharmacological properties and its restorative capacity (Persson 2004; Roura et al. 2008). Community views of ART have also been reported to attach the significance of treatment to changes in bodily appearance and the potential sexual consequences of restored health (Craddock 2000; Cockroft et al. 2007). The social and cultural discourses around HIV/AIDS are largely influenced by holistic definitions of disease and its implications on social lives. Widespread use of metaphor and local terms to explain antiretroviral medication and its implications on illness is not a new phenomenon. It reflects the widespread use of metaphors to represent HIV and AIDS as it is evident in previous studies (Simon 2002; Stillwaggon 2003; Helman 2007; Liamputtong et al. 2015). Nevertheless, the availability of ART in the current study setting appeared to have introduced a new paradigm in the existing discourses about HIV and AIDS and the meaning and effects of medical treatment. Treatment perspectives tended to blend local socio-cultural realities while borrowing existing and previous biomedical and official discourse about management of AIDS. Generally, the treatment paradigms relate to the notion that not all drugs can or must cure a specific disease it is purported to treat. Furthermore, descriptions of ART reveal that the dominant understanding of HIV/AIDS as a 'death sentence' appears to be shifting. The shift is more pronounced in descriptions of the (disappearance of) bodily manifestations and signs of HIV and resumption of (normal) social roles among persons on ART. Individuals on ART also reported a remarkable shift in particular with regard to the positive evaluation of self-perceived health status experienced after starting treatment. Previous evidence has shown that the changes in meaning and attitudes toward ART were usually associated with positive outcomes of therapy (Schrimshaw et al. 2005; Atuyambe et al. 2008). This is in contrast to the findings from my study, which indicate both positive and negative feelings about ART among study participants.

My study also shows that persons on ART and other members of community do not necessarily hold similar views and attitudes towards ART. The shifting paradigms of antiretroviral treatment are also evident in the paradoxes and dilemmas facing both HIV-infected and affected members in the study setting. While ART is viewed as a way to manage illness and resume normal social roles, it may also become a potential source of stigma, blame and prosecution for harmful sexual conducts. Similar evidence has indicated that apart from helping reduce stigma,

ART may also contribute to emergence of new forms of stigma particularly (Roura et al. 2008; UNAIDS 2008). This underlines the need to manage unintended consequences of ART at all stages of implementation of treatment roll out.

Depiction of some ART users as transmitters of HIV may consequently affect community perspectives about care and support of HIV-infected persons. Local terms and discourses about therapeutic effects of ART may result into a loss of legitimate claims to sick role among persons on ART. Consequently, others in their families, community and neighborhoods may see persons on treatment as responsible for how they present themselves and manifest signs of their illness (Nettleton 2006). What appears to be an important feature in the social definition of ART is how the changes in signs and symptoms of illness (following ART) are 'sexually constructed' among most of the study participants thus affecting how persons on treatment were perceived to present their illness. My study supports the view that individuals have "varied resources available to them to resist or rework the cultural meanings of illness" (Kleinman 1998: 26). This reinforces the view found among many participants in my study and a previous study suggesting that patients receiving treatment who are feeling well may be more prone to engage in unprotected sex (Crepaz et al. 2004). Thus, while the availability of ART was generally sexually constructed and viewed with skepticism among young people in general, it was considered to be a lifesaving intervention among persons on treatment and some young people. Similar findings indicate that people's beliefs about ART may promote unprotected sex and that these beliefs may be amenable to change through prevention messages (Crepaz et al. 2004; Schrimshaw et al. 2005).

Since my study only explored experiences and opinions about deliberate spread of HIV among ART users, it may be useful (in future studies) to explore the causal linkage between ART use and risk sexual practices by conducting a comparative study among persons on ART and those who are not on ART. Recent evidence from population based studies shows that people in the same community may hold different beliefs and attitudes about ART and that ART-related risk compensation was associated with an increased HIV sero-prevalence among young people (Rice et al. 2006; Cohen et al. 2009). My study reveals that while local discourses about ART may serve as a tool for communicating about effects of treatment on illness, they also reveal the level of awareness and knowledge about ART among young people. Recent evidence documented that low treatment literacy not only affects stigma but also been shown to influence attitude and decisions to start ARV if infected (Roura et al. 2008; Zou et al. 2009). It might be important to explore further the existing and potential sources of ART information in the community to understand how they may support on-going treatment programs. Besides limited knowledge, fear of stigma may also make people unwilling to seek ART at the nearest hospital for fear of status disclosure even when treatment was available (Adeneye et al. 2006; Cockroft et al. 2007). Similar feelings about status disclosure expressed by young people in my study underscore the need to include ART messages in HIV interventions targeting young people and persons on ART in order to impart correct information about ART, voluntary status and stigma in the context of increased availability of ART. This is because evidence suggests that removing perceived structural barriers to access alone may not be enough unless supported by measures to address stigma and discrimination against persons living with HIV (Mshana et al. 2006; Roura et al. 2009a). There is evidence showing that misinformation and irrational fears of contagion that trigger some stigmatizing behaviors during pre-ART era may persist in spite of increased availability of ART (Lekas et al. 2006). Mechanisms proposed to control spread of HIV reported in the current study may also potentially evoke fear and result into discrimination particularly among people perceived or suspected to be purposefully spreading the disease.

The different meanings invested in ART further suggest that it is vital to adopt culturally and group specific messages in public health information. This is because different people may hold different views about HIV and the available treatment/healing alternatives. For instance, while most participants in this study viewed HIV from a biomedical perspective (a strange disease with strange medications that does not cure), they also tended to employ both biomedical and popular socio-cultural terminology and beliefs to describe the effects of ART. This appears to be in sharp contrast to the existence of the belief reported among some religious groups that HIV was a regular virus capable of being cured through prayer (Dilger 2007; Zou et al. 2009). It is interesting to note that despite beliefs in prayer, a resort to modern medicine is often the alternative option when prayer appears to be insufficient to address HIV (Zou et al. 2009). Thus, different conceptualizations of HIV/AIDS among different social groups may inform the definition and perceived social efficacy of antiretroviral treatment and health seeking behaviors.

An important entry point to treatment seeking is the availability and functioning of HIV testing services. It has been observed that public awareness and approval of routine HIV testing supports uptake of ART provided through government health facilities (Cockroft et al. 2007). Similarly, the general approval and positive value/meaning attributed to ART among individuals taking antiretroviral medication in the study area may reflect the nature of efforts to sustain treatment regardless of the long distances traveled to access medication at the regional hospital. This underscores the need for public health systems to lay emphasis on early detection and timely care of HIV-positive persons while taking into account the different perspectives about HIV etiology and health care seeking alternatives available in the community.

Descriptions and responses about the availability and the clinical outcomes (both visible and invisible) of antiretroviral treatment appear to have affected dominant notions about the HIV-positive bodies and led to formation of a new identity of individuals living with HIV. As has been previously observed, ART provides evidence of capacity of medicines for restoring bodily normality and multiple transformations (Persson 2004; Liamputtong et al. 2015). My findings suggest that because of ART, the discourse around HIV and AIDS might be undergoing a major shift and transformation. During the early days of epidemic, descriptions, metaphors and images of a HIV-positive body mainly consisted of individuals depicted (as weak, wasted) with signs of advanced HIV disease and opportunistic infections (Lucas et al. 1994; Stillwaggon 2003; Kalipeni et al. 2004; Helman 2007). Such images (a bed-ridden, weak, wasted and sickly body) dominated the public discourse about persons suspected to be HIV infected for quite some time, and actually appeared to form the basis on which participants in my study evaluated therapeutic effects of ART. While these notions appear to persist among participants in my study, their descriptions of effects of ART on the body highlight a shift in physical identity of HIV-positive person. It has also been observed that new identities related to ART may contribute to the formation of new forms of stigma if not accompanied by interventions to promote social acceptability of ART at community level (UNAIDS 2006; Roura et al. 2008). Borrowing Goffman's (1963) conception of stigma, Kleinman (1998) recognizes shifts that usually occur in the (physical) bodily attributes; he describes the attributes as "visible stigmata of the pathology" that society defines as stigmatizing among persons suffering chronic illness (pp. 158–159). Physical attributes associated with clinical outcomes of ART may produce various implications in different contexts and people. It appears that ART is embodied and reflexive. It is reflexive because it involves social definitions emanating from peoples interaction. On the one hand, from the perspectives of persons around the HIV-positive individuals, ART may be explained by concerns about sexual risk of HIV transmission. On the other hand, ART may be a source of optimism brought about by improved health conditions and functional capacity of the body. The aforementioned circumstances highlight ideas about limits and opportunities of what (else) a healthy body can do (Fox and Ward 2008). Thus, despite limited accessibility and mixed feelings about potential public health implications of ART, there is strong rationale for the need to build on positive perceptions of ART (Adeneye et al. 2006). This further underscores the need for HIV prevention and control interventions to adopt dynamic and holistic approaches to inform the public about benefits of ART and avoid targeting specific individuals or groups for blame of spreading HIV.

One of the most talked about impact of ART is the fact that it has transformed HIV/AIDS from a death sentence to a manageable chronic illness (Detels et al. 1998; Kalipeni et al. 2004; UNAIDS 2006; Cohen et al. 2007; WHO 2008). In light of above reality, it seems that the disease which would once have killed the patient can now be managed through treatment enabling infected people to stay well and survive longer than thought before. Consequently, this produces circumstances in which individuals, their families and entire communities need to adjust and accommodate this new reality. Furthermore, this transition suggests that while persons on ART become subjected to the life long requirements and control of medication, there is increasing role for members of affected community and health systems in supporting individuals living with HIV. This may explain the shared hopes, concerns and dilemmas that were collectively shared among young people, persons on ART and health workers.

Overall, my findings suggest that the meanings attached to ART may change or adjust among different social actors in the community. As I have shown, while the antiretroviral medications are ascribed different names and value with regard to their effects in the body, there is also an inherent shift in the understanding and definitions of persons receiving ART. Depending on context and circumstances, persons on ART may be variously labeled as patients, persons looking healthy and HIV-negative, sick people, victims, as well as transmitters of HIV. At the core of the shifting paradigms of medicines is the therapeutic efficacy and symbolic value of ART in the lived experiences of my participants. Findings underscore the need to address beliefs (both positive and negative) about the performative effects of ART and potential short-term and long-term consequences of treatment in the management and control of HIV spread. Meanings attached to ART may play an important role in the actual and potential course of action people will take when faced with an episode of HIV and related illnesses. My findings suggest that the meanings and beliefs about therapeutic effects of ART are shaped by a combination of historical, socio-cultural, economic, epidemiologic and geographical realities of the study setting and how these are related to the organization of health and illness both within and beyond the study setting.

22.9 Conclusion

Local understanding and responses to antiretroviral treatment is shaped by forces generated from within and beyond the borders of the study area. Despite the availability of ART as a new intervention, HIV/AIDS continues to be a folk illness identifiable/described in relation to local discourses about bodily health, geographical and gendered power inequalities and other structural constraints to access to healthcare. Local discourses suggest that the body provides the means through which people use lay methods to assess health status and devise ways to avoid or control HIV infection. Due to the fact that ART is a relatively recent development, there is limited understanding about its clinical significance and possible implications. Limited understanding of therapeutic efficacy of ART leads to misconceptions about the clinical functions, purpose and limitations of ART in the management of HIV/AIDS. Of particular importance is the possible impact of ART scale up on risk sexual behaviors. Limited access to ART in the study area appears to have reinforced existing notions of structural imbalances and rural neglect in access to HIV-related care in particular, and other health services in general. Consequently, geographical variations in access to ART may influence local understandings about relative risk of HIV and AIDS among people in different locations. In one way, the introduction of ART has uncovered perceived successes and weaknesses in the health systems with regard to ART roll out. On the other hand, ART calls for the strengthening of health system capacity to deliver quality treatment, care and support services and explore ways to collaborate effectively with other actors particularly non-governmental organizations, the private sector, individuals receiving treatment, schools and other community organizations. Stigma and discrimination still provide a great challenge to successful implementation of ART programs. Although ART is hailed as an opportunity for people living with HIV to manage illness and move on with their lives, it still poses great challenges in addressing stigma and managing risk sexual behavior both among ART users and affected local communities. A major challenge is encouraging voluntary testing and status disclosure among sexual partners as an entry point to treatment. It is fair to hypothesize that increasing accessibility to ART may contribute to a more open social dialogue about status disclosure in the community and families. It is also important to work with especially vulnerable young people (e.g. both in school and out-of-school) through peer networks and integrate ART within youth friendly health services.

In conclusion, antiretroviral treatment has the potential to produce both positive and negative consequences to public health. ART cannot be divorced from the socio-economic, cultural, political, geographic realities that constrain medical care in different settings. One of the key messages in this work is the need to understand the complex interplay between structural realities and human agency in the quest to understand the social and cultural context of ART. My study underscores how government/policy actions and pharmacological properties of ART may have consequences on the formation of meanings about disease and illness, local perception of risk and discourses around medical treatment. While ensuring universal access to treatment may be a key priority, there is an urgent need to address a set of social, cultural and behavioral issues in order to make HIV treatment part of wider interventions to manage risk and prevent further spread of HIV.

References

Adeneye, A. K., Adewole, T. A., Musa, A. Z., Onwujekwe, D., Odunukwe, N. N., Araoyinbo, I. D., Gbajabiamila, T. A., Ezeobi, P. M., & Idigbe, E. O. (2006). Limitations to access and use of antiretroviral therapy (ART) among HIV positive persons in Lagos, Nigeria. *World Health and Population, 8*(2), 46–56.

Atuyambe, L., Neema, S., Otolok-Tanga, E., Wamuyu-Maina, G., Kasasa, S., & Wabwire-Mangen, F. (2008). The effects of enhanced access to antiretroviral therapy: A qualitative study of community perceptions in Kampala city, Uganda. *African Health Sciences, 8*(1), 13–19.

Bateganya, M., Colfax, G., Schafer, L. A., Kityo, C., Mugynyi, P., Serwadda, D., Mayanja, H., & Bangsberg, D. (2005). Antiretroviral therapy and sexual behavior: A comparative study between antiretroviral-naïve and experienced patients at an urban HIV/AIDS care and research centre in Kampala, Uganda. *AIDS Patient Care and STDs, 19*, 760–768.

Beck, U. (1992). *Risk society: Towards a new modernity*. New Delhi: Sage.

Boholm, A. (1996). Risk perception and social anthropology: Critique of cultural theory. *Ethnos, 61*(1–2), 64–84.

Bunnell, R., Ekwaru, J. P., Solberg, P., Wamai, N., Bikaako-Kajura, W., Were, W., Coutinho, A., Liechty, C., Madraa, E., Rutherford, G., & Mermin, J. (2006). Changes in sexual behaviour and risk of HIV transmission after antiretroviral therapy and prevention interventions in rural Uganda. *AIDS, 20*, 85–92.

Cameron, E., Burris, S., & Clayton, M. (2008). HIV is a virus, not a crime: Ten reasons against criminal statutes and criminal prosecutions. *Journal of the International AIDS Society, 11*(7), 1–7.

Cockcroft, A., Andersson, N., Milne, D., Mokoena, T., & Masisi, M. (2007). Community views about routine HIV testing and antiretroviral treatment in Botswana: Signs of progress from a cross sectional study. *BMC International Health and Human Rights, 7*(5), 1–11.

Cohen, D., McCubbin, M., Collin, J., & Perodeau, G. (2001). Medications as social phenomena. *Health: An Interdisciplinary Journal for the Social Study of Health, Illness and Medicine, 5*(4), 441–469.

Cohen, M. S., Gay, C., Angela, D. M., Kashuba, D. M., Pharm, D., Blower, S., & Paxton, L. (2007). Narrative review: Antiretroviral therapy to prevent the sexual transmission of HIV-1. *Annals of Internal Medicine, 146*(8), 591–601.

Cohen, C. R., Montadon, M., Carrico, A. W., Shiboski, S., Bostrom, A., Obure, A., Kwena, Z., Bailey, R. C., Nguti, R., & Bukusi, E. A. (2009). Association of attitudes and beliefs towards antiretroviral therapy with HIV-seroprevalence in the general population of Kisumu, Kenya. *PLoS ONE, 4*(3), e4573. doi:10.1371/journal.pone.0004573.

Craddock, S. (2000). Disease, social identity, and risk: Rethinking the geography of AIDS. *Transactions of the Institute of British Geographers, 25*(2), 153–168.

Crepaz, N., Hart, T. A., & Marks, G. (2004). Highly active antiretroviral therapy and sexual risk behavior: A meta-analytic review. *JAMA, 292*, 224–236.

Dake, K. (1992). 'Myths of nature': Culture and the social construction of risk. *The Journal of Social Issues, 48*(4), 21–37.

Davis, M. (2007). Identity, expertise and HIV risk in a case study of reflexive medical technologies. *Sociology, 41*(6), 1003–1019.

Detels, R. M. A., McFarlane, G., Kingsley, L. A., Margolick, J. B., Giorgi, J., Shrager, L. K., & Phair, J. P. (1998). Effectiveness of potent antiretroviral therapy on time to AIDS and death in men with known HIV infection duration. Multicenter AIDS cohort study investigators. *JAMA, 280*(17), 1497–1503.

Dilger, H. (2007). Healing the wounds of modernity: Salvation, community and care in a neo-Pentecostal church in Dar es Salaam, Tanzania. *Journal of Religion in Africa, 37*, 59–83.

Douglas, M. (1992). *Risk and blame: Essays in cultural theory*. London: Routledge.

Douglas, M., & Wildavsky, A. (1982). *Risk and culture: An essay on the selection of technical and environmental dangers*. Berkeley: University of California Press.

Ezekiel, M. J., Talle, A., Juma, J. M., Mnyika, K. S., & Klepp, K.-I. (2008). Attitudes and perceived impact of antiretroviral drug therapy on risk sexual behaviour among young people in Kahe, Moshi rural district, Tanzania. *Tanzania Journal of Health Research, 10*(4), 203–212.

Foucault, M. (1990). *The history of sexuality* (Vol. 1, Trans. Hurley). Harmondsworth: Penguin

Fox, N. J., & Ward, K. J. (2008). What are health identities and how may we study them? *Sociology of Health and Illness, 30*(7), 1007–1021.

Gebrekristos, H. T., Mlisana, K. P., & Karim, Q. A. (2005). Patients' readiness to start highly active antiretroviral treatment for HIV. *British Medical Journal, 331*, 772–775.

Giddens, A. (1991). *Modernity and self-identity*. Cambridge: Polity.

Giddens, A. (1998). Risk society: The context of British politics. In J. Franklin (Ed.), *The politics of risk society* (pp. 23–34). Cambridge: Polity.

Goffman, E. (1963). *Stigma: Notes on the management of spoiled identity*. New York: Simon & Schuster.

Greene, R., & Ward, D. (2002). *'Let's call it HIV infection, not AIDS'*. Poster presented at the 4th international AIDS conference, Barcelona, 7–14 July.

Haram, L. (1999). *'Women out of sight': Modern women in gendered worlds. The case of Meru women of northern Tanzania*. Unpublished PhD thesis, University of Bergen, Norway.

Hardon, A. P., Akurut, D., Comoro, C., Ekezie, C., Irunde, H. F., Gerrits, T., Kglatwane, J., Kinsman, J., Kwasa, R., Maridadi, J., Moroka, T. M., Moyo, S., Nakiyemba, A., Nsimba, S., Ogenyi, R., Oyabba, T., Temu, F., & Laing, R. (2007). Hunger, waiting time and transport costs: Time to confront challenges to ART adherence in Africa. *AIDS Care, 19*(5), 658–665.

Helman, C. G. (1990). *Culture, health and illness* (2nd ed.). Oxford: Butterworth-Heinemann Ltd.

Helman, C. G. (2007). *Culture, heaath and illness* (5th ed.). London: Hodder Arnold.

IPASC & EQUINET. (2009). *Acceptability and accessibility of HIV testing and treatment services in Bembeyi, Bunia, North Eastern Democratic Republic of Congo*. Available at www.equinetafrica.org. Accessed 1 June 2009.

Izugbara, C. O., & Wekesa, E. (2011). Beliefs and practices about antiretroviral medication: A study of poor urban Kenyans living with HIV/AIDS. *Sociology of Health & Illness, 33*, 869–883.

Janssen, R. S., Holtgrave, D. R., Valdiserri, R. O., Sherperd, M., Gayle, H. D., & De Cock, K. M. (2001). The serostatus approach to fighting the HIV epidemic: Prevention strategies for infected individuals. *American Journal of Public Health, 91*(7), 1019–1024.
Jejeebhoy, S. J., Shah, I., & Thapa, S. (2005). *Sex without consent: Young people in developing countries*. London: Zed Books.
Kalipeni, E., Craddock, S., Oppong, J., & Gosh, J. (Eds.). (2004). *HIV and AIDS in Africa: Beyond epidemiology*. Malden: Blackwell.
Kapiga, S. H., Sam, N. E., Mlay, J., Aboud, S., Ballard, R. C., Shao, J. F., & Larsen, U. (2006). The epidemiology of HIV-1 infection in northern Tanzania: Results from a community based study. *AIDS Care, 18*(4), 379–387.
Kleinman, A. (1980). *Patients and healers in the context of culture*. Berkeley: University of California Press.
Kleinman, A. (1998). *The illness narratives: Suffering, healing and the human condition*. New York: Basic Books.
Klepp, K.-I., Fisher, A., & Kaaya, S. F. (Eds.). (2008). *Promoting adolescent sexual and reproductive health in East and Southern Africa*. Cape Town: HRSC Press.
Lekas, H., Siegel, K., & Schrimshaw, E. (2006). Continuities and discontinuities in the experiences of felt and enacted stigma among women with HIV/AIDS. *Qualitative Health Research, 16*(9), 1165–1190.
Lema, L. A., Katapa, R. S., & Musa, A. S. (2008). Knowledge on HIV/AIDS and sexual behaviour among youths in Kibaha District, Tanzania. *Tanzania Journal of Health Research, 10*(2), 79–83.
Leventhal, H., Kelly, K., & Leventhal, E. A. (1999). Population risk, actual risk, perceived risk and cancer control: A discussion. *Journal of the National Cancer Institute Monographs, 25*, 81–85.
Liamputtong, P., Haritavorn, N., & Kiatying-Angsulee, N. (2015). Local discourses on antiretrovirals and the lived experiences of women living with HIV/AIDS in Thailand. *Qualitative Health Research, 25*, 253–263.
Lucas, S. B., De Cock, K. M., Hounnou, A., Peacock, C., Diomande, M., Hondé, M., Beaumel, A., Kestens, L., & Kadio, A. (1994). Contribution of tuberculosis to slim disease in Africa. *British Medical Journal, 308*(6943), 1531–1533.
Luke, N. (2005). Investigating exchange in sexual relationships in sub Saharan Africa using survey data. In S. J. Jejeebhoy, I. Shah, & S. Thapa (Eds.), *Sex without consent: Young people in developing countries* (pp. 105–124). London: Zed Books.
Mmbaga, E. J., Hussein, A., Leyna, G. H., Klouman, E., Masenga, E., Sam, N., Mnyika, K. S., & Klepp, K.-I. (2006). Incidence of HIV-1 infection and changes in prevalence of reproductive tract infections and sexual risk behaviours: A population based longitudinal study in rural Tanzania. *African Journal of AIDS Research, 5*(3), 281–288.
Mmbaga, E. J., Hussein, A., Leyna, G. H., Mnyika, K. S., Sam, N., & Klepp, K.-I. (2007). Prevalence and risk factors for HIV-1 infection in rural Kilimanjaro region of Tanzania. Implications for prevention and treatment. *BMC Public Health, 7*, 58. doi:10.1186/1471-2458-7-58. Available at http://www.biomedcentral.com/1471-2458/7/58.
Mmbaga, E. J., Hussein, A., Leyna, G. H., Mnyika, K. S., Sam, N., & Klepp, K.-I. (2008). The role of in-migrants in the increasing rural HIV-1 prevalence pandemic: Results from a village population survey in Kilimanjaro region of Tanzania. *International Journal of Infectious Diseases, 12*(5), 519–525.
Mnyika, K. S., Klepp, K.-I., Kvåle, G., & Ole-King'ori, N. (1996). Risk factors for HIV-1 infection among women in the Arusha region of Tanzania. *Journal of Acquired Immune Deficiency Syndrome and Human Retrovirology, 11*(5), 484–491.
Mshana, G. H., Wamoyi, J., Busza, J., Zaba, B., Changalucha, J., Kaluvya, S., & Urassa, M. (2006). Barriers to accessing antiretroviral therapy in Kisesa Tanzania: A qualitative study of early rural referrals to the national programme. *AIDS Patient Care and STDs, 20*, 649–657.

Mwaluko, G., Urassa, M., Isingo, R., Zaba, B., & Boerma, J. T. (2003). Trends in HIV and sexual behaviour in a longitudinal study in a rural population in Tanzania, 1994–2000. *AIDS, 17*, 2645–2651.

Nachega, J. B., Lehman, D. A., Hlatshwayo, D., Mothopeng, R., Chaisson, R. E., & Karstaedt, A. S. (2005). HIV/AIDS and antiretroviral treatment knowledge, attitudes, beliefs and practices in HIV-infected adults in Soweto, South Africa. *Journal of Acquired Immune Deficiency Syndrome, 38*(2), 196–201.

National AIDS Control Programme (NACP). (2005). HIV/AIDS/STI surveillance report No.19. December 2004. Dar es salaam: Epidemiology Unit, NACP. Ministry of Health, Tanzania Mainland, Issued September 2005.

Nettleton, S. (2006). 'I just want permission to be ill': Towards a sociology of medically unexplained symptoms. *Social Science & Medicine, 62*, 1167–1178.

Nichter, M., & Vuckovic, N. (1994). Agenda for an anthropology of pharmaceutical practice. *Social Science & Medicine, 39*(1), 1509–1525.

Nkosana, J., & Rosenthal, D. (2007). Saying no to intergenerational sex: The experience of schoolgirls in Botswana. *Vulnerable Children and Youth Studies, 2*(1), 1–11.

Persson, A. (2004). Incorporating *pharmakon*: HIV, medicine and body shape change. *Body and Society, 10*(4), 45–67.

Renn, O. (2010). *Precautionary principle: Risk, uncertainty and rational action*. Available at www.allchemeseminars.org. Accessed 25 Jan 2010.

Rice, E., Batterham, P., & Rotheram-Borus, M. J. (2006). Unprotected sex among youth living with HIV before and after the advent of highly active antiretroviral therapy. *Perspectives on Sexual and Reproductive Health, 38*(3), 162–167.

Roura, M., Urassa, M., Busza, J., Mbata, D., Wringe, A., & Zaba, B. (2008). Scaling up HIV stigma? The effects of antiretroviral roll-out on stigma and HIV testing. Early evidence from rural Tanzania. *SexuallyTransmitted Infections, 85*, 308–312.

Roura, M., Busza, J., Wringe, A., Mbata, D., Urassa, M., & Zaba, B. (2009). Barriers to sustaining antiretroviral treatment in Kisesa, Tanzania: A follow-up study to understand attrition from the antiretroviral programme. *AIDS Patient Care and STDs, 23*(3), 203–210.

Schrimshaw, E. W., Siegel, K., & Lekas, H. (2005). Changes in attitudes toward antiretroviral medication: A comparison of women living with HIV/AIDS in the pre-HAART and HAART eras. *AIDS and Behaviour, 9*(3), 267–279.

Setel, P. W. (1999). *A plague of paradoxes: AIDS, culture and demography in northern Tanzania*. Chicago: The University of Chicago Press.

Simon, V. (2002). *Local culture: Risk or resource in times of AIDS? A case study of Mbulu in northern Tanzania*. Unpublished Master of Philosophy thesis, University of Bergen, Norway.

Sjoberg, L. (1998). Why do people demand risk reduction? In S. Lydersen, G. K. Hansen, & H. A. Sandtorv (Eds.), *ESREL-98: Safety and reliability* (pp. 751–758). Trondheim: A.A. Balkema.

Stillwaggon, E. (2003). Racial metaphors: Interpreting sex and AIDS in Africa. *Development and Change, 34*(5), 809–832.

Stoeckle, M., Mchomvu, R., Hatz, C., Battegay, M., Aris, E. A., Mshinda, H., & Tanner, M. (2006). Moving up from 3 by 5. *The Lancet Infectious Diseases, 6*(8), 460–461.

Tanzania Ministry of Health. (2004, December). *National AIDS control programme*. HIV/AIDS/STI surveillance report no.19. Dar es Salaam.

Tanzania Ministry of Health. (2007). *Guidelines for HIV testing and counselling in clinical settings*. Dar es salaam: Ministry of Health.

Tulloch, J., & Lupton, D. (2003). *Risk and everyday life*. London: Sage.

UNAIDS. (2006). *Treatment education: A critical component of efforts to ensure universal access to prevention, treatment and care*. Geneva: UNAIDS.

UNAIDS. (2008). *Reports on the global AIDS epidemic*. Available at www.unaids.org/pub/globalreport/. Accessed 13 Apr 2009.

Van den Bergh, G. (2008). To risk or not to risk? Is it a question? Sexual debut, poverty and vulnerability in the times of AIDS: A case from Kigoma, Tanzania. In K.-I. Klepp, A. Fisher, & S. F.

Kaaya (Eds.), *Promoting adolescent sexual and reproductive health in East and Southern Africa* (pp. 162–182). Cape Town: HRSC Press.

Van der Geest, S., & Hardon, A. (2006). Social and cultural efficacies of medicines: complications for antiretroviral therapy. *Journal of Ethnobiology and Ethnomedicine*, *2*, 48. doi:10.1186/1746-4269-2-48. Available at http://www.ethnobiomed.com/content/2/1/48.

Van der Geest, S., Whyte, S. R., & Hardon, A. (1996). The anthropology of pharmaceuticals: A biographical approach. *Annual Review of Anthropology, 25*(1), 153–178.

Veinot, T. C., Flicker, S. E., Skinner, H. A., McClelland, A., & Saulnier, P. (2006). "Supposed to make you better but it doesn't really": HIV-positive youths' perceptions of HIV treatment. *Journal of Adolescent Health, 38*(3), 261–267.

Weiss, B. (1996). *The making and unmaking of the Haya lived world: Consumption, commoditization and everyday practice*. Durham: Duke University Press.

WHO. (2008). *Towards universal access: Scaling up priority HIV/AIDS interventions in the health sector*. Geneva: WHO.

WHO/UNAIDS. (2003). *Treating 3 million by 2005: Making it happen: The WHO strategy*. Geneva: WHO.

Whyte, S., Van der Geest, S., & Hardon, A. (2002). *Social lives of medicines*. Cambridge: Cambridge University Press.

William, S. J., & Bendelow, G. (1998). *The lived body: Sociological themes, embodied issues*. London: Routledge.

Zinn, J. O. (2006). Recent developments in the sociology of risk and uncertainty. *Historical Social Research, 31*(2), 275–286.

Zou, J., Yamanaka, Y., Muze, J., Watt, M., Ostermann, J., & Thielman N. (2009). Religion and HIV in Tanzania: Influence of religious beliefs on HIV stigma, disclosure, and treatment attitudes. *BMC Public Health, 9*, 75. doi:10.1186/1471-2458-9-75. Available at http://www.biomedcentral.com/1472-2458/9/75.

Part IV
Children, Young People & Research

Chapter 23
Ethical Considerations of Conducting Research among Children and Young People Affected by HIV: A View from an Ethics Review Board

Katie D. Schenk and Saumya RamaRao

Contents

23.1 Introduction

The contents of this book rely on primary data collected among children and young people whose lives have been severely impacted by the effects of HIV and AIDS. Beyond direct measures of HIV prevalence, indirect effects of HIV documented in this book include diverse indicators of social welfare (e.g. increased vulnerability to dropping out of school, elevated exposure to stigma), psychosocial well-being, anthropometry, and school attendance as reflected in data collected from children and members of their household.

K.D. Schenk (✉)
Department of Global and Community Health, George Mason University,
4400 University Drive, Fairfax, VA 22030, USA
e-mail: kschenk@gmu.edu

S. RamaRao
Senior Associate, Population Council, 1 Dag Hammarskjold Plaza,
New York, NY 10017, USA
e-mail: sramarao@popcouncil.org

P. Liamputtong (ed.), *Children and Young People Living with HIV/AIDS*,
Cross-Cultural Research in Health, Illness and Well-Being,
DOI 10.1007/978-3-319-29936-5_23

Children and young people affected by HIV are already vulnerable to a range of detrimental outcomes spanning the physical, social and emotional domains (as indicated by chapters within this volume). However, a further vulnerability is their susceptibility to participation in research without a comprehensive understanding of the risks and benefits thereof. Data collectors seeking information for research purposes are in a powerful position to take advantage of these young research participants due to their limited ability to refuse research investigators. Sadly, without careful planning and delicacy, even the most well-intentioned of research plans may turn out to be bluntly naïve or ill-informed. Even as we endeavor to *do no harm* among the individuals and communities to whom we aim to bring quality of life improvements, researchers frequently face ethical dilemmas reflecting the precarious nature of family circumstances, especially in vulnerable HIV-affected communities (Schenk and Williamson 2005).

As public health researchers, we aim to gather data to inform the development of interventions (e.g., healthcare, education, nutrition) aimed at addressing the needs of children affected by HIV. In order to design, implement and subsequently refine a service that will effect genuine welfare enhancement, we must take special care and precautions to protect the children and families we serve. We must recognize that children have a lower level of access to knowledge, resources and power than adults, elevating their vulnerability to potential exploitation and abuse during the process of data collection, and we must respond by designing additional precautions above and beyond those required for data collection among adult[1] populations.

Every country has a mechanism by which research activities are required to achieve ethical approval, typically from an Ethical Review Committee based at a University or within a government agency. In the United States, any human subjects research conducted by a US-based institution or using US Government funds must gain approval from a federally-mandated Institutional Review Board (IRB) ("Federal policy for the protection of human subjects. Final rule," 1991). As members of one such Institutional Review Board, reviewing up to 60 new protocols for biomedical and behavioral research every year, we have noted the emergence of common themes in the feedback provided to researchers submitting protocols on HIV- and AIDS-related work for review, which we aim to share in this chapter.

We begin with a historical overview to provide a theoretical framework for this discussion. We explore some of the recurrent themes with which we – as members of an ethical review board – have observed researchers grappling when proposing new studies among children affected by HIV. We will provide examples of common pitfalls and share some of the constructive feedback given to researchers before granting ethical approval. We conclude by providing practical guidance to researchers working in this important area of enquiry, aimed at smoothing the path towards the ethical conduct of research.

[1] Similar precautions also apply when working with vulnerable and stigmatized adult populations, such as sex workers or men who have sex with men – but the power imbalance is especially pronounced when working among children.

23.2 Theoretical and Historical Context

23.2.1 Legal Requirements

Responsible conduct of research is required to protect research participants from harm; including certification of investigators in ethical conduct of research, appropriate training of research staff, and systems in place to minimize risk to study participants. Research activities cannot progress without approval from an independent ethical review board (also known as an Ethics Committee or Institutional Review Board, and including community representatives) that has thoroughly reviewed all research plans (protocols).

The conduct of researchers working among human subjects is governed by multiple (and often overlapping) legal and ethical requirements. National regulations may require additional permissions from local scientific institutions. A research protocol may therefore undergo multiple reviews within the country from which funding originates, the institution/s managing and implementing the research, and the country in which research is taking place, before researchers may be granted permission to proceed with their study. Professionals working with children are also subject to professional codes governing their behavior within their discipline, e.g. codes of conduct of the Society of Psychologists. In addition to the professional expertise provided by these mechanisms, use of a Community Advisory Board is also recommended as a formal method for inviting local and civil society inputs.

23.2.2 Belmont Report and Beyond

The central resource guiding the operations of review boards in the USA is the Belmont Report (National Commission for the Proptection of Human Subjects of Biomedical and Behavioral Research 1978). While this document has been subject to various critiques[2] since its publication nearly 40 years ago, its principles remain influential. In this chapter, we examine the conduct of research studies among children affected by HIV by exploring how to address the three fundamental ethical principles of the Belmont Report:

- respect
- beneficence
- justice

[2] Some researchers have alleged that the principles of the Belmont Report, designed with biomedical research studies in mind, do not adequately address the circumstances of public health research, where research goals extend from the individual to the population level. Several alternatives have been proposed for frameworks of public health ethics [e.g. (Soskolne 1991; Kass 2001; Callahan and Jennings 2002; Bernheim 2003; Baum et al. 2007).

We use the practical applications suggested by the Belmont Report to highlight commonly recurring themes with which researchers working among children affected by HIV often struggle, including attention to the informed consent process, employing age-appropriate methodologies, avoiding stigma, and research recruitment design.

23.3 Recurrent Themes

23.3.1 Informed Consent

The principle of *respect for persons* requires that all individuals participating in research must be treated as autonomous agents who can decide for themselves if, when and under what conditions they wish to participate (National Commission for the Protection of Human Subjects of Biomedical and Behavioral Research 1978). Prospective research participants must have as much time and information as they need to decide whether or not they wish to participate in research. The researcher must provide key information (e.g., describing exactly what procedures are involved in participation; explaining that the participant may refuse to participate in any part of the study or decide to withdraw completely at any time; providing full contact details for researchers) in accessible and comprehensible language appropriate to the age, education and developmental stage of the invited participant. After learning about the study, invited participants must be able to make an independent decision about whether or not to voluntarily enroll, without any pressure.

The Belmont Report further emphasizes that those with diminished autonomy are entitled to additional protections. Special arrangements for protection are required when a person's understanding is limited due to age or developmental disabilities. The first line of protection for children is the requirement of seeking consent from their parent or legal guardian to approach the child. Without such agreement, the researcher may not approach the child to seek participation in research.

Once the responsible adult has agreed to the child's participation in research, the child themself should have the opportunity to express views and make choices, assured of the protection of the informed consent process. The active verbal agreement of the child (assent) should be sought in a manner that is appropriate to their understanding.

Children's capacity to make and understand decisions develops as they grow up, depending on the extent and quality of their lived experiences – including opportunities for formal and informal education, and learning from previous decision-making opportunities With less education and life experience upon which to draw to comprehend the nature of the research and to assess the risks and benefits of participation, children are less equipped than adults to make an independent determination as to whether or not they wish to participate in a research study.

Thus, when conducting research among children affected by HIV, researchers must take great care to design informed consent procedures that are appropriate to the comprehension and decision-making abilities of their potential participants, taking into account their age, developmental stage, culture, and education/literacy. Consultation and review with local staff and community members is vital to the acceptability of the informed consent process, ideally through the mechanism of a community advisory board, and meeting all relevant requirements of permission for initial contact with the family through a gatekeeper (community leader, school, healthcare facility) representing the setting in which research is taking place.

Conducting research among children affected by HIV, it is not unusual to come across settings in which there is doubt regarding the effective or legal guardian who can represent a child's best interests (e.g. a child living on the street who is not in contact with their family, a child who is heading a household of younger siblings following the death of their parents, a child caregiver for a parent who is chronically ill), or whether the guardian's interests adequately reflect the interests of the child (e.g. a child at risk of abuse within the home). When parents are dead, sick or absent (and in the absence of a formally appointed legal guardian) it may be difficult to determine who is the appropriate or effective guardian from whom to seek consent. Researchers must make a careful determination to select the most appropriate adult (if any) who will adequately represent the best interests of the child; adults with a vested interest not be aligned with those of the child should be avoided (e.g. obtaining consent from a child's employer when reporting on workplace conditions). Among families in high HIV prevalence settings, researchers frequently encounter a diversity of individual, family and household living configurations. Researchers must make sure that informed consent protocols are explicitly designed to recognize a variety of residential circumstances, including children who are: living in a household where a parent is chronically ill; in the temporary or informal care of someone who is not their legal guardian; in a child-headed household; on the street; in a residential group care setting.

As a last resort, when seeking consent from the child's parent or guardian is difficult or even antithetical to the purposes of the research, we propose two alternative responses:

Emancipated minors

In circumstances in which a child is already taking adult responsibilities and making adult decisions (e.g. marriage, leading a household of siblings, raising a child of their own, living alone on the street) and where permitted by law, it may be determined appropriate to treat the child as an **emancipated minor**. An emancipated minor is deemed competent to make their own decision regarding research participation, using a specially designed informed consent form without recourse to an adult guardian. However, although such children can often be considered emancipated under the law, they may – ironically – be most in need of guidance and ultimately much more vulnerable than children with stable homes and accessible guardians; so careful oversight is crucial.

Child advocates

In situations in which there is any doubt about the protection provided by a guardian, researchers may appoint an **independent child advocate** to represent the best interests of a child who may not legally provide consent alone and to make sure that adequate protection is provided. The advocate is responsible for providing informed consent and for upholding protection from harm throughout the activity. The advocate must be familiar with the child's circumstances and be independent of any other interests, including the research. For example, when working with a child in institutional care, permission from the Director represents the interests of the institution, while consent from an independent advocate represents the interests of an individual child. Depending on the nature of the research, a child advocate may act on behalf of an individual child or may represent the interests of a broader group of children within a single activity. However, researchers and advocates must be alert to any possibility of coercion that may easily occur when working among children in a closed group setting such as a residential care home. An advocate may also act to represent the interests of a child whose parent is sick or unavailable, but if the parent later becomes able to provide informed consent, their decision must be sought and respected.

In either of these cases, procedures should be determined in consultation with community representatives and continually reviewed to ensure that they are consistent with local culture, law and practice, ideally under the supervision of a community review board to make sure that the consent thus sought is sufficiently robust to be genuinely protective of the child's participation. For example, when an adult gives consent to their child's participation in research in a culture in which age is revered, expectations of child obedience to the adult require further examination of the power dynamics at play when seeking child assent. The input of a community review board is often helpful in finding a way to ensure that the child has a true opportunity to comprehend expectations, then decide whether to accept or refuse participation.

23.3.2 Age Limits and Age-Appropriate Methodologies

Conducting research in international settings invokes multiple obligations to abide by the legal standards of the countries from which funding is obtained, the country of the research institution, and the country in which fieldwork is taking place. When we talk about children, we mean someone who is a minor in the eyes of the law, not an adult. For the process of informed consent, local definitions must be used – in particular when defining who is a child. For the purposes of this chapter, we follow the definition of a child as a person below the age of 18 years old (United Nations General Assembly 1989).

Once processes of parent/guardian consent and child assent for participation in research have been completed, research input from participating children may be sought in a manner appropriate to age and developmental stage. In order to identify children's needs and design relevant programs addressing them, researchers seeking child participation in public health intervention studies may be trying to elicit appropriate input regarding tailoring intervention content (e.g. educational assistance, psychosocial support, HIV prevention and treatment programs, food and nutritional services), format (e.g., frequency of contact, type of contact) or delivery modes (e.g., outreach, health center-based, youth center-based). While some see it as intuitive that child-friendly services should be designed to appeal to children, e.g. using appropriately sized furniture and fixtures, the next step is to apply that same logic to making research procedures age-appropriate too.

In order to justify that the involvement of children in the research process researchers must show that their participation is indeed necessary to produce salient findings that willinform decision-making for program development. Research cannot be a speculative endeavor – researchers must verify that child participation in research is actively required in order to help programs meet child and community needs.

Exposing a child to the inherent risks of research is considered a negative possibility, which must be balanced against any positive benefits yet to be generated (whether at the level of an individual child, their family, their community, or more generalized). The principle of beneficence as expressed in the Belmont Report requires that, above all, researchers do no harm – encompassing physical, mental and social dimensions. Doing everything possible to anticipate and avert any potential negative consequences among every research participant, their families and communities is crucial. If researchers are unable to put appropriate safeguards into place, the research activity may not proceed. Monitoring adherence to research requirements must continue as an ongoing process throughout the duration of the study.

In order to tailor research methods to be appropriate to children's age, culture and developmental stage, we emphasize the importance of establishing community consultations regarding research objectives and procedures, especially on the modes and content of research participation to which children will be exposed. An important step is to develop a plan for segmentation of research activities by the age of participants, recognizing the need to make sure that it is not just the *topics* covered but also the *modes* of eliciting information that should be designed in a sensitive manner.

Young children should be excluded from gathering detailed information on potentially traumatic topics that may cause emotional distress, such as discussing a recent bereavement. They may be asked questions about their knowledge of health matters in an agee-approriate manner; however, it is unethical to subject young research participants to the trauma of directly asking intrusive questions addressing sensitive personal traumatic experiences (e.g. sex, abuse) in a research setting.

Segmentation should divide the proposed research participants by age, restricting research activities within each group to those considered strictly age-relevant according to community input. For example, the youngest of research participants might be excluded from survey questions considered more appropriate for older participants, due to their potentially complex or intrusive wording. For example, a survey tool for use among young research participants might come in three distinct versions: for children aged 12–14 years old, children aged 15–17 years old, and youth aged 18–24 years old. The younger groups would be guided towards successively shorter tools recognizing their more limited attention span and shielding them from questions addressing thematically complex or sexually explicit questions. Depending on community input, the older group may no longer require consent procedures to first approach a parent or guardian.

Research methods used among younger research participants should employ methods tending towards more creative approaches, designed by skilled staff experienced in working with children of the appropriate age and cultural setting. Approaches including artistic and dramatic exercises have been used to great effect, e.g. artistic representations of families, dramatic re-enactments of recent events. Researchers are encouraged to explore innovative new methods of research and data capture, employing all the possibilities of new media to make the research process interactive, empowering and inclusive. For example, researchers have provided young research participants with cameras and encouraged them to use their own autonomy regarding what and how to record their own story (Cook and Hess 2007), researchers in Guatemala have asked children to map their community as seen though their own eyes using GPS trackers to locate safe spots and community boundaries (Del Valle 2013). (see chapters in part three of this volume for the use of creative approaches in research with children and young people).

As children grow up and their intellectual capacities develop, they become increasingly able to respond to more searching questions, first as asked through qualitative methods (in-depth interviews), and subsequently through more traditional quantitative methods (surveys). The use of inappropriate methods calls into question the quality of the data collected, as young children may be unable to provide valid and/or reliable responses. In order to elicit genuinely useful information in the most sensitive manner possible, it remains crucial to refrain from asking the wide range of intrusive questions that adults could be asked.

Conducting research into HIV, researchers often aim to ask adults questions about sensitive topics, including their age of sexual debut, experiences of sexual violence, or use of condoms at last sex. Based upon our experiences as members of an ethical review board, we suggest that such questions should in general be avoided. They may asked with appropriate supervision *if and only if* they pertain directly to the respondent being interviewed and will directly contribute to answering the research question. Questionnaire design must include filter questions in which the participant has the opportunity to skip out of questions inappropriate for children's age and stage (e.g. based upon knowledge of sex; experiences of sexual activity). Another way to approach data collection on sensitive topics is to explore whether of these data could be obtained from adults reporting retrospectively on past events. Although retrospective reporting runs the problem of memory lapse, it is nevertheless preferred in order to protect children from any negative repercussions of asking them sensitive or age-inappropriate questions.

23.3.3 Stigma

When conducting research among children and families affected by HIV, researchers must be vigilant to avoid the harmful effects of stigma that could result from inadvertently revealing the HIV-positive status of any individual. Singling out selected individuals or households from a community or classroom for special attention through the research study can have the unintended negative effect of marking them as different and exposing them to harm. Researchers must make every effort to protect children and their families from the inadvertent consequences of stigma associated with the research.

Before commencing research, researchers should hold a community sensitization meeting to consult with local community leaders and members, and seek their input into the design of the proposed activity. Such a meeting provides a good opportunity to clarify the purpose and limits of research activities (including why certain households have been selected to participate), to gain community input into recruitment methods, and for community review of research tools. Community review provides the opportunity to understand how communities recognize vulnerability and how to work with children considered vulnerable without introducing or reinforcing stigma. For example, it may be unacceptable to distinguish between children who are vulnerable due to HIV/AIDS and those whose vulnerability is due to other causes.

Researchers must also be sensitive to the language they use to describe the children with whom they are working. The use of epidemiologically accurate terms to describe core target groups (e.g. "vertically-infected", "HIV orphan") is often inappropriate when working with real people and communities. Local community groups, children, and program staff should be consulted to determine the preferred terminology for local use. Instead of using jargon and labels that may stigmatize, researchers must work with local children and adults to find ways to describe the factual characteristics of the groups and situations they are trying to address, such as children who are disabled, or children who have been forced into sex work.

Participation in research may add to children's vulnerability. Although the stigma surrounding HIV/AIDS has reduced in recent years, there remain concerns due to which maintaining anonymity or at least confidentiality become critical in research. For example, if children are seen to be participating in a study known to be about HIV transmission, they and their families run the risk of being viewed differently within their communities, even if the children themselves are unaware about HIV, sex and sexuality, and transmission issues.

Researchers testing low-cost ways to maintain anonymity and confidentiality during data collection promote options including avoiding the recording of names and addresses, using self-administered questionnaire tools through audio devices (e.g. ACASI), administering multiple versions of questionnaires so that individual participant responses are concealed from neighboring research participants; and employing community-wide census survey methods rather than singling out specific populations for survey attention.

23.3.4 Research Design

Considering issues of research design is justified as an ethical issue because exposing research participants to the risks of research through a poorly designed study incapable of producing relevant results cannot be justified. Worse still, a poorly designed study might lead to erroneous or misleading results, on which basis inappropriate policy and programmatic responses may be formulated. Careful consideration of research design provides additional opportunities to provide protections to children participating in a research study, including considering participant recruitment methods, and the decision of whether or not to use a control group.

Research recruitment / participation

We have learntfrom the principles of the Belmont Report that recruitment must be equitable, in accordance with the principle of justice. When working among children affected by HIV, these concerns are especially heighted, as we must ensure that the risks and benefits of the research are distributed fairly across the research participants, some of whom may be especially vulnerable. In determining who will be invited to participate in research, researchers must select participants equitably in relation to research aims, without bias due to participants' vulnerability (e.g. ease of access to information services, economic circumstances), and must make sure that all participants and their communities will eventually have access to research results. Research design must reflect the power dynamics of children and communities to make sure that all social realities are represented.

If the research pertains to a specific venue in which children congregate, data collection at these specific locations is justified (e.g. using school registers as a starting point for sampling participants in a study of school attainment). However, choosing such venues due to convenience of recruitment when they are not strictly relevant to the research goal is inappropriate and must be avoided (e.g. recruiting participants exclusively from a pediatric ward for a research study regarding the general provision of healthcare).

Control groups

Research studies exploring the operations of interventions to prevent or mitigate effects of HIV among children (e.g. offering youth HIV education; providing HIV counselling and testing services; delivering nutritional, psychosocial or educational support) may include a treatment arm and a control arm[3] receiving the existing local standard of care rather than the new, experimental intervention. While this approach clearly adds rigor, precision and enhanced data quality to research findings, creating a control group deprived of an intervention may be unjustified for some research questions (e.g. feasibility, formative research) where simpler research designs (such as pre- and post-intervention comparisons) might suffice.

[3] Or comparison arm, for quasi-experimental research.

When working among children, it is especially important to consider the implications of creating a control or comparison group, due to the heightened power imbalance between children and researchers. Children enrolling in a research study may lack the scientific judgment to understand the reasoning behind the existence of a control group, and may have unrealistic expectations for their participation.

One response utilized by HIV researchers is to take advantage of the natural dynamics of intervention roll-out to create a "natural" comparison group to which the intervention is scheduled for delivery at a later date. Service providers introducing a new program typically start in one region, gradually expanding and fine-tuning services as they scale up and learn from experience. Under these circumstances it may be possible to explore the circumstances of a pilot community receiving the early intervention and draw a comparison to a community in a location without access to the initial phase. The comparison group would subsequently gain access to the expanded and hopefully improved services when later offered in their location, thus addressing ethical concerns of withholding the intervention. For example, researchers in Rwanda evaluating the wellbeing of vulnerable youth before and after a mentoring intervention collected data from four districts, including two districts in which households were receiving the pilot intervention during the study period. They were compared to two districts in which households were receiving the local standard of care during the study, but slated for subsequent roll-out of intervention services after the conclusion of the research (Brown et al. 2009).

23.4 Conclusion: Moving Forward

Conducting research among children and young people affected by HIV is a politically and emotionally sensitive minefield in which many ethical issues are heightened. In our dual roles as researchers conducting our own studies and also as members of an ethical review board, we have designed and reviewed multiple protocols and provided input on the design and conduct of international behavioral research studies among children and families affected by HIV in a wide variety of settings. We have learnt about the field challenges of adhering to ethical principles while conducting research, and how they might be addressed.

We acknowledge that this is daunting work. Meeting standards of ethical rigor in research when working among such vulnerable people is a demanding but necessary task. As public health researchers aiming to improve quality of life for the families we serve, we are all responsible for minimizing risk and enhancing benefits to the participants of our research. There can be no higher goal than improving the wellbeing of the children and families that we serve, and we must leave no stone unturned to achieve that goal.

We gain encouragement from the recognition that the context in which we work is changing for the better. Researchers (including individuals and institutions) are increasingly mindful of the need for applying ethical standards in research. Funders and stakeholders (including government agencies and civil society groups) are increasingly cognizant of the process and implications of seeking ethical approvals for the conduct of research. Even journal publishers are increasingly requiring certification of ethical approvals before findings can be published. International institutions are increasingly establishing their own ethical review boards to provide locally and culturally relevant mechanisms for research review. Review boards all over the world are working together to establish harmonization and coordination between multiple review options. We want to make sure that the standards set for research are genuinely meeting expectations about how research should be conducted, at all levels.

In summary, in this chapter we have highlighted ways in which to enhance the ethical conduct of research among children and families affected by HIV, based upon our own experiences of implementation and oversight. We have shown that the ethical demands of our research spur us on to achieve higher levels of research rigor and ethical correctness, without sacrificing data quality. Despite concerns to the contrary, it is feasible to conduct ethically sound and high quality research among children and families affected by HIV, and to do it right. We affirm that the value of these lessons reaches far beyond our field of HIV research: we aim to promote these approaches to researchers in other fields working among vulnerable children and families, including malaria and child survival.

References

Baum, N. M., Gollust, S. E., Goold, S. D., & Jacobson, P. D. (2007). Looking ahead: Addressing ethical challenges in public health practice. *The Journal of Law, Medicine & Ethics: A Journal of the American Society of Law, Medicine & Ethics, 35*(4), 657–667. 513.

Bernheim, R. G. (2003). Public health ethics: The voices of practitioners. *The Journal of Law, Medicine & Ethics, 31*(S4), 104–109.

Brown, L., Thurman, T. R., Rice, J., Boris, N. W., Ntaganira, J., Nyirazinyoye, L., … Snider, L. (2009). Impact of a mentoring program on psychosocial wellbeing of youth in Rwanda: Results of a quasi-experimental study. *Vulnerable Children and Youth Studies, 4*(4), 288–299.

Callahan, D., & Jennings, B. (2002). Ethics and public health: Forging a strong relationship. *American Journal of Public Health, 92*(2), 169–176.

Cook, T., & Hess, E. (2007). What the camera sees and from whose perspective fun: Methodologies for engaging children in enlightening adults. *Childhood, 14*(1), 29–45.

Del Valle, A. (2013). *Addressing violence against girls and adolescents through participatory mapping*. UNFPA Webinar Series for the Adolescent Girls Initiative. Population Council.

Kass, N. E. (2001). An ethics framework for public health. *American Journal of Public Health, 91*(11), 1776–1782.

National Commission for the Protection of Human Subjects of Biomedical and Behavioral Research. (1978). *The Belmont report: Ethical principles and guidelines for the protection of human subjects of research*. Bethesda: ERIC Clearinghouse.

Schenk, K. D., & Williamson, J. (2005). *Ethical approaches to gathering information from children and adolescents in international settings: Guidelines and resources*. Washington, DC: USAID, Population Council, Family Health International.

Soskolne, C. L. (1991). Ethical decision-making in epidemiology: The case study approach. *Journal of Clinical Epidemiology, 44*(Supplement 1), 125–130.

United Nations General Assembly. (1989). *Convention on the Rights rights of the child*. New York: United Nations.

United States Department of Health and Human Services. (1991). Federal policy for the protection of human subjects. Final rule. *Federal Register, 56*(117), 28003–28018.

Chapter 24
Can Pictures Influence Policy? Ugandan Children Share Stories Utilizing Photovoice

Bonnie Fournier and Olenka Bilash

Contents

B. Fournier (✉)
Faculty of Nursing, University of Alberta, Edmonton, AB, Canada
e-mail: bonnie.fournier@ualberta.ca

O. Bilash
Department of Secondary Education, University of Alberta, Edmonton, AB, Canada
e-mail: olenka.bilash@ualberta.ca

P. Liamputtong (ed.), *Children and Young People Living with HIV/AIDS*,
Cross-Cultural Research in Health, Illness and Well-Being,
DOI 10.1007/978-3-319-29936-5_24

24.1 Introduction

Photovoice is a method that brings into focus the everyday experiences of individuals whose voices are often forgotten, silenced or not heard (Foster-Fishman et al. 2005). Photovoice was first developed by Caroline Wang and Mary Ann Burris in 1994 and previously termed 'photo novella' to describe their work with rural Chinese women. However, in their seminal article in 1997, they changed the name to Photovoice. They explained, "photo novella, foto novella, and photonovel have also been commonly used to describe a process of using photographs or pictures to tell a story or to teach language or literacy" (p. 369). Wang and Burris felt that there was significant difference between the goals of photo novella and Photovoice and since 1997 have honored this distinction by using only the term Photovoice. They identify three theoretical roots and outline three goals for this research approach, which we describe later.

In a Photovoice project, cameras are provided to individuals, and they are asked to document specific areas of their daily lives in alignment with the focus of the project. Once photographs are taken, they are shared in critical group discussions between participants and researchers, thus providing opportunities for participants to reflect on aspects of their lives and communities, including strengths and areas of greatest concern. Photovoice goes beyond facilitating discussions, to a stage of fermenting action through which change can occur at the individual, community and policy levels. Advocating for social equity through influencing policy is a key aspect of Photovoice and sets it apart from other photo methods (see Wang 1999, 2000, 2003, 2006; Wang and Burris 1994, 1997; Wang et al. 1998, 2004; Wang and Redwood-Jones 2001; Wang and Pies 2004 for further discussions of Photovoice). Photovoice projects culminate with an exhibition in a public space where collaboratively chosen photographs and stories are showcased. The Photovoice exhibitions are intended to reach multiple audiences, including individuals with similar concerns and problems (Erdner and Magnusson 2011), decision makers, policy influencers, and media. Photovoice is not only a method that provides insights into individual lives; it is also one that helps participants and researchers express their vision to policymakers with the purpose of social change, meaning "any alteration in the cultural, structural, population, or ecological characteristics of a social system" (Social Change 2015: 286). The camera and Photovoice process are well suited for use with all ages, including children, offer insight to all involved and can enhance children and young peoples' understanding of their experiences and create new relationships and collaborations in the process of self-discovery (Clark-Ibanez 2004).

In this chapter, we elaborate on the theoretical links of Photovoice, discuss the role children play in political advocacy, share a Photovoice study conducted with Ugandan children who are HIV sero-positive and live in a group home, and identify limitations in reaching the broad and intended audience. In discovering why the project fell short of advocacy, we argue that the responsibility of agency for action cannot lie solely with Photovoice participants, in this case children, but must also be taken up by researchers who thus must become better informed about how to influence policy.

There is a growing body of research that includes children in the research process and demonstrates that one of the many outcomes of this process is that children become health advocates and change agents in their families and communities. However, in the current study, the children were limited in their ability to be change agents due to HIV stigma (see also Chaps. 1, 2, 3, 9, and 14 in this volume). As researchers wanting to improve the health of individuals and communities we found this outcome disconcerting. It forced us to re-visit the study and the Photovoice method to understand how we could improve on Photovoice as a tool to create change. This reflection lead to a realization of our own limitations in understanding the policymaking process. Consequently, we began to seek out strategies that could improve our ability to make change and ultimately improve the health of children living with HIV illness. We turned to political science theories to inform us and thus suggest a revision to the Photovoice method to include two more steps in the process: building knowledge and capacity for policy change and becoming immersed in the local context before conducting a Photovoice study.

24.2 Theoretical Links

The Photovoice method was conceived from the wedding of three theoretical frameworks: empowerment education for critical consciousness, feminist theory, and documentary photography (Wang and Burris 1994). Freire's concept of empowerment education for critical consciousness aims to mobilize individuals into becoming change agents in their community. Developing a critical consciousness occurs through critical group dialogue to foster understanding and action (Freire 1973). Freire (2000) described three levels of increasing consciousness resulting from ongoing dialogue within a community, and states that the highest level of consciousness is reached when community members begin to recognize how their own beliefs and behaviors shape their reality. Freire (2000), while working with various groups, would listen for particularly emotionally charged dialogue, and then translate this into a series of drawings to generate further discussion. Dialogue in this process acts as a means for fostering a critical consciousness about social reality, and an understanding based on knowledge of how people and issues are historically and politically situated (Shor and Freire 1987). Freire's (2000) drawings coupled with further discussions encouraged a co-creation of knowledge with the goal of engaging community members in their own learning and creating a plan of action (Carlson et al. 2006).

Feminist theory has also informed the development of Photovoice as its roots acknowledge that people have expert knowledge of their own lives (Wang and Burris 1994). Feminist theory is based on the notion of equality and the right of individuals to take action toward improving their social, political and economic conditions (Castleden and Garvin 2008). At the root of feminism is the belief that women and other marginalized groups of people must be active agents in any activity concerning their well being, and that these activities must be collaborative and respectful of their experiences (Linton 1990; Liamputtong 2007). Feminist theory also challenges the status quo, prioritizing the needs of marginalized women and establishing plans for action (Linton 1990). As a methodology, women or marginalized groups generate knowledge on their own terms, which can be an empowering experience (Kramarae and Spender 1992; Liamputtong 2007).

Finally, Photovoice has drawn upon elements of documentary photography. The term documentary photography refers to the process of documenting aspects of social life by the photographer. According to Kuo (2007), documentary photography is at once as emotional and compassionate as it is radical and political. Documentary photography has been described as "photographic images that are used to draw attention to social issues; however the images are typically taken from the photographer's outsider viewpoint" (Strack et al. 2004: 49). When documentary photography is combined with participant-defined images rather than photographer-defined images there is a shift in attempting to represent the person as an object (Freidenberg 1998) to participants themselves representing their own reality (Wang et al. 1996). Representing their own reality means in many ways that individuals are able to control the production of knowledge and meaning about themselves and their lives, hence becoming empowered to transform their social reality by becoming change agents.

In weaving these three theoretical threads, Wang and Burris (1997) have generated three goals of Photovoice: to enable people to: (1) Record and reflect their personal and community strengths and concerns; (2) Promote critical dialogue and knowledge about personal and community issues through group discussions of photographs; and (3) Promote social change by communicating issues of both concern and pride to policy makers and society at large.

24.3 Photovoice with Children and Young People

Engaging children and young people as active participants in the research process is gaining momentum in public health research and community based work (Checkoway et al. 1995; Cheatham and Shen 2003; London et al. 2003; Hung 2014). Photovoice as an arts-based method uncovers multiple ways of knowing and subjective realities (Leavy 2009). Harper (2000) echoes this view and states that "the power of the photo lies in its ability to unlock the subjectivity of those who see the image differently from the researcher" (p. 729). It is through imagination that we are able to unlock our subjectivities. The process of creating images and telling stories is an art form and when we engage children in imaginative experiences new things happen – "the boundaries of their experiences expand" (Ehrenworth 2003: 43). Greene (1995) advocates the use of the arts for bringing about new ways of seeing.

A photograph can make visible the experiences of young people whose voices might otherwise be absent from socio-political discussions that affect them (Wang and Burris 1997) as they have little access to decision makers in their daily lives. Utilizing methods such as photography in a participatory way can be a suitable method for children because it involves performing a task, is a fun activity, and as such can help children feel more comfortable. It is also a valuable method for representing children's unique ways of knowing the world. Utilizing Photovoice as a medium to engage children and young people to understand their community issues has been widely published (Wang and Burris 1994; Darbyshire et al. 2005; Wang 2006; Purcell 2007; Rudkin and Davis 2007; Castonguay and Jutras 2009; Fournier et al. 2014a). Participating in a Photovoice project can enhance children and young peoples' process of self-discovery (Clark-Ibanez 2004) and has the ability to transform and heal children and young people.

Greene (1995) argues that the arts provide a language that opens the imagination to possibilities or what she terms 'passion for possibility'. She believes that "imagination and the transformations it makes possible are what defamiliarize the familiar taken-for-granted and allow us to see in a different light" (p. 2). Seen from this view, imagination can be brought to bear on social issues. Such social imagination encourages thinking about the kind of world we would like to live in or what Freire (1994) called 'a lovelier world'. For children and young people, imagining in this way explores boundaries that go beyond their experiences "to awaken, to disclose the ordinarily unseen, unheard, and unexpected" (Greene 1995: 25). Children's imaginative abilities must be cultivated and sensory systems refined to explore visions of possibility beyond their experiences (Eisner 2003). Taking photographs, telling stories and exploring meaning facilitates the activation of their imagination. Eisner (2003: xii) writes: "The most complex or subtle forms of thinking take place when [children] have an opportunity either to work meaningfully on the creation of images . . . or to scrutinize them appreciatively". Complex thinking is needed for critical dialogue among a group of children in a Photovoice project. Thinking about the world we want to live in and discussing through dialogue with others encourages action or social change. By documenting their lives using Photovoice participants have the potential to transform not only themselves but society as well.

In the next section, we share the voices of Ugandan children who are HIV seropositive living in a group home, revealing their many strengths and hardships. Additionally, the children's voices also provide context to the limitations of reaching decision and policy makers within the current study.

24.4 A Case Study: Ugandan Children Living with HIV and Orphaned

The purpose of this study was to explore the experiences of orphaned, HIV seropositive children who live in a group home in semi-urban western Uganda utilizing Photovoice. Children's perspectives are central (Pritchard Kennedy 2012) to understanding the local meanings of psychological, emotional and social well-being, and coping strategies to inform effective supports and interventions. This is important as the AIDS pandemic is having a profound impact on the health of children in Uganda. It is occurring directly through child HIV infection, and indirectly through effects on families, communities and the social and economic functioning of the country (Barnett and Whiteside 2002; Bridge et al. 2006a, b).

24.4.1 Uganda

In Uganda, there is a growing number of orphans (children below the age of 18 and with either a mother or father who has died), with estimates of around 2.5 million of Uganda's 17 million children under the age of 18 (Government of Uganda [GoU] 2010). Of those 2.5 million, 48 % were orphaned due to AIDS (GoU). HIV sero-positive AIDS orphans have a double burden. Not only have they experienced multiple losses but they also have a life-threatening illness. It is unusual for an orphaned child to live in a group home in sub-Saharan Africa, as this is often a last resort option and usually signifies a crisis situation where no one is able to care for the child (The United Nations Children's Fund [UNICEF] 2006).

It is estimated that the HIV prevalence in Uganda is 7.2 %, with 1.5 million children and adults living with HIV (UNAIDS 2012) and 0.7 % among children (GoU 2010). Over 190,000 are children aged 14 years and under (UNAIDS 2012). It is also reported that 18 % of the new HIV infections in Uganda occur through mother-to-child-transmission (GoU). Although there have been progress and increased access and funding for HIV, treatment demand remains greater than the availability of antiretroviral therapy (ART). In 2011, only 313,000 Ugandans who are living with HIV infection and require ART have access to treatment (World Health Organization [WHO] 2013). The number of Ugandan children accessing ART has increased tenfold in the past few years; however, the need still remains extremely high (WHO 2011). Currently, only a fifth of Ugandan children who need treatment are receiving it (GoU). Stigma is reported to be one of the main reasons (GoU); however, the cost of transportation to medical facilities is also a barrier. The limited availability of antiretrovirals (ARVs) has been an ongoing issue. However, since 2010 Uganda has begun to produce its own generic drugs (WHO 2011) with the hope of reducing both the cost and the possibility of running out of the drugs as well as increasing geographic access. However, the ARV rollout in Uganda has faced many challenges due to shortages in healthcare finance, infrastructure, and human resources.

24.4.2 The Study

An exploratory qualitative design was used for the study and as such an open, flexible, and inductive approach was essential. Participant recruitment occurred in June 2010 and data were collected during a 1-month period. The target population included male and female children 12–18 years of age (N = 13, female = 5, male = 8) who were orphaned, HIV-positive, and lived in a home run by a local non-governmental organization (NGO) in Western Uganda. The NGO was chosen based on an established relationship with a University and a NGO in Canada. All the meetings took place at the group home. The home provides basic life needs and psychosocial support for 30 children who are HIV sero-positive and orphaned. Participants spoke their native language, Rutooro, fluently; however they are not able to read it well. Therefore, all the focus group discussions with children were conducted in Rutooro while all written materials for the research team were provided in English. Focus group discussions and Photovoice were the primary data collection methods. For an in-depth discussion of the challenges and solutions that arose due to the multilingual and cross-cultural setting see Fournier et al. (2014b).

According to the Uganda partner NGO that supports the children in this study, the children have been repeatedly told in their home villages that they have "slim" disease (HIV/AIDS) and will soon die. When they go to the health clinic for treatment, they discuss with each other which friend has died since the last visit. The findings from the current study demonstrated that the children face many hardships, especially related to stigma and discrimination at school and in their community (Fournier et al. 2014a). However, they also told stories about how the group home supported key protective factors in their everyday lives and promoted their well-being, and encouraged resilience for coping with challenges such as stigma (Fournier et al. 2014a).

Data collection included a total of eight meetings with the children. Following Photovoice protocol, meetings were divided into five steps: training sessions, devising themes, taking pictures, discussing photos, and planning the display. The children told stories about their lives using the photographs as a focal point, thus improving our understanding of individual and community needs and assets.

Data analysis occurred on three levels. The first was with the participants utilizing the acronym SHOWeD[1] as the framework for telling stories and exploring root causes with some modifications as the research assistants remained flexible to allow the children to discuss what was important to them. The second level was carried out using matrix methodology techniques described by Miles and Huberman (1994) for analyzing the transcripts, as well as a personal journal kept by the field researcher (A. Bridge) along with field notes. A third level of data analysis occurred when A. Bridge and Fournier returned to Uganda to share the emerging themes with the

[1] SHOWeD stands for- What did you **S**ee while you were taking this/these photograph(s)? What is **H**appening in this photograph? How does this relate to **O**ur life? **W**hy does this problem or strength exist do you think? What can be **D**one about this issue?

research assistants, the director and staff of the NGO, two senior public health and health research practitioners in the area, and Konde-Lule, a professor in the Department of Public Health at Makerere University, who was also part of the research team. In separate meetings, the themes were confirmed by agreement and some re-analyzed based on the feedback from all team members.

24.5 Photovoice Outcomes: Improved Understanding of Individual and Community

24.5.1 Needs and Assets

During the focus group discussions the children came together to share their photographs. In this process an understanding emerged of the protective factors and hardships they faced in their daily lives. As a result of the children telling stories about their lives using the photographs in group dialogue, we gained an improved understanding not only of their needs and assets but also of those of their community (group home). Reported here are the children's voices about the strengths and needs they see in themselves and their community.

24.5.1.1 Nature as a Resource

The children took many pictures of the natural environment and described the value of nature, the natural world as "created by God", and how essential these resources are for life and survival. One child described his photo of vegetation by saying:

> These papyrus … act as a home for aquatic animals and we get fish from here, dig it and grow food and sometimes we get herbal medicines in case you have stomach upsets" (see Fig. 24.1).

He summarized the presentation of his photo saying:

> They help us a lot in building houses, making fences… there's a lot of money you can get [from] the papyrus, make mats and sell them to get money.

24.5.1.2 Hopes and Dreams

Almost all of the children's photos and discussions depicted their hopes and dreams. When discussing their photos they described their desire to be successful, contributing members of society. One child described how they "have to work hard to achieve something". Other children described their career aspirations. "I want to become a counsellor. I have gone through many problems and I know some people can learn

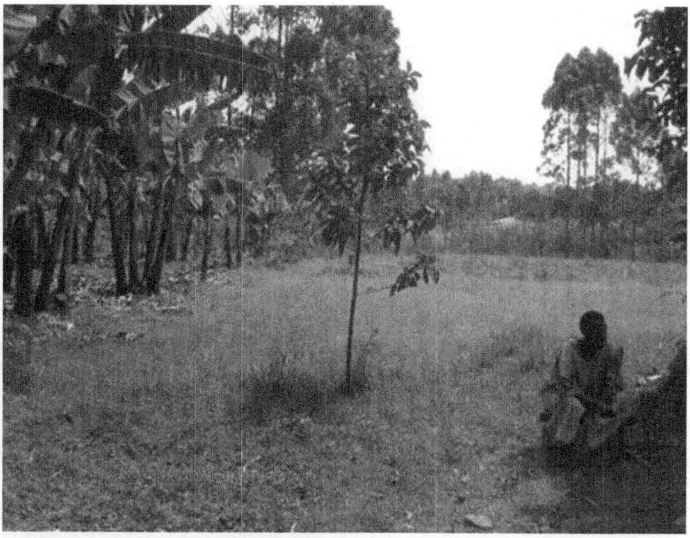

Fig. 24.1 Papyrus tree

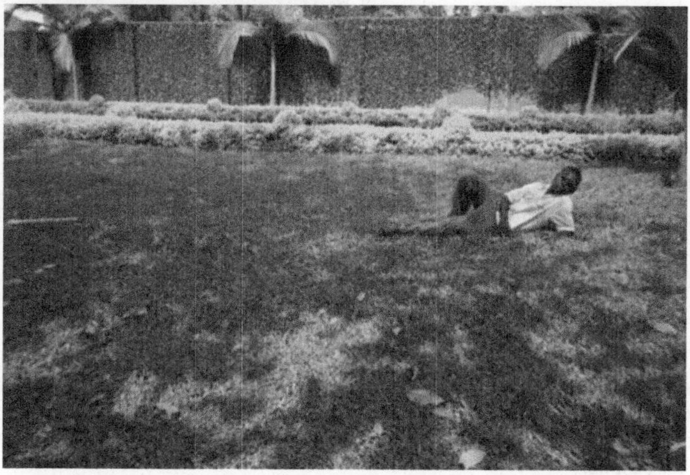

Fig. 24.2 Dreaming on the grass: after getting money, I will build a house

from me." Another stated: "I want to become a doctor and treat patients." Others dreamed of being self-sufficient (see Fig. 24.2): "After getting money, I will build a house. Then start my own business. I want to be self-employed. I will be the happiest person in the world."

Hope flows abundantly through the children's stories, most clearly expressed in the words of one child who declared: "if I take my drugs well and study hard, I know I will get all I need."

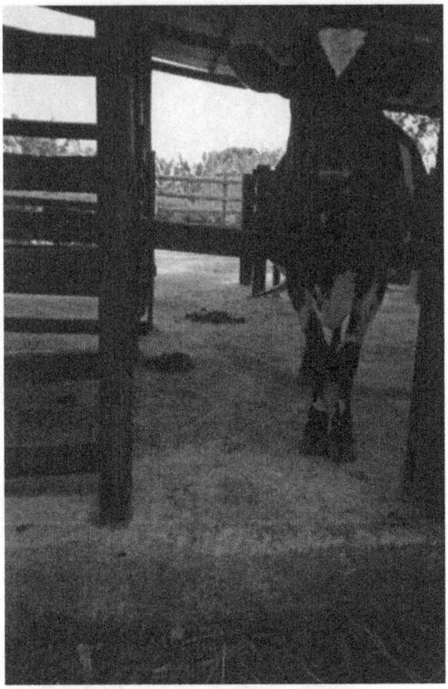

Fig. 24.3 Photo of a cow

24.5.1.3 Material Resources

The children frequently expressed appreciation for the basic life needs and material resources provided at the group home, as described by one child in his photo (see Fig. 24.3): "The cow [at the group home] helps us in giving us a source of milk at the home for drinking, it is why I took this photo to mean that I love the cow and the one who bought it."

Another child spoke of the group home:

> I want to talk about the house [group home]. It has helped so much, it has saved many people's lives… giving them school fees, food, drinks, they can play… it knows all the problems they have, it has helped so much… it even has a water heater, that helps warming water for bathing.

The children were acutely aware of the fact that the material resources at the group home were in stark contrast to the conditions under which they had previously lived:

> Most of us are orphans, if some had stayed in their villages, some would have been beaten to death because you can be tempted to steal because you cannot find food.

24.5.1.4 Social Support

In addition to material resources, the children's photos and discussions highlighted the importance of friends and social support in their lives, particularly at the group home: "Why I took this photo is that there is love between us children and staff [of the group home]." An older child described his relationship with the younger children at the home by saying:

> I love these little children [at the home] so I gathered them and I took a photo together with them ... I want them to always be happy ... I had my aunt ... she loved me so much, would always carry me. That reminds me that I should try to do to the little children what my aunt did to me.

About friendship, one child said:

> If you don't have friends you walk as if you are not walking.

24.5.2 *Hardships*

Although the majority of children's photos and discussions were related to positive aspects of their lives, children also discussed hardships that cause suffering or privation. They described experiences of stigma and discrimination, struggles to cope with their emotions related to stigma, as well as traumatic situations in their communities. It was clear that these hardships impact their psychological, emotional and social well-being. We highlight some examples of the hardships they described from their photos.

24.5.2.1 Stigma and Discrimination

The various forms of stigma children face in the broader community and their impact was a recurring theme. Children spoke about overhearing people in the community talk about others with HIV and AIDS. They also described their experiences being personally singled out as having HIV and AIDS. One child stated:

> The thing that hurts me most is when people point at me, that I am suffering from HIV and AIDS... it hurts me so much. People should stop talking about that.

The "talking about that" referred to people who would not only point fingers but also whisper to one another about the child having HIV and AIDS. One child described overhearing someone in the community saying "that one is finished with his/her AIDS", and then went on to say:

> If you hear that, even if they are not talking about you, you can even collapse and die ... HIV and AIDS came, but people should stop pointing to the infected people.

Compounding this issue of pointing fingers at HIV positive individuals, the group home had also become victim of finger pointing and was labelled an "AIDS home" by community members.

The distress caused by stigma was also shared by the children:

> I hate discrimination and this makes you feel worthless. Another thing is that they should stop pointing fingers to people with HIV and AIDS.

Another child expressed that "most HIV victims are desperate and when you annoy them they can commit suicide or do anything bad which endangers their lives." These statements describe how they feared for their fellow children at the home, and worried about the impact of stigma on themselves, their friends, and other children they care about.

In addition to HIV- and AIDS- related stigma, children discussed other derogatory labels used in the community and by the local government such as "unsanitary", "a thief", "uneducated" or "poor" and their desire to prevent succumbing to this social-status. For example, one child described why a latrine was so important:

> This toilet helps us dispose of our feces … some homes which don't have a specific place to put their feces are dirty homes. The local council … those responsible for health … used to arrest people in the villages who didn't have latrines. Some children would start making fun of those children whose parents were arrested for not having latrines. When I build [my own home], the first thing to do is have a latrine.

A female child described the social stigma of being unsanitary by saying:

> You can leave your house dirty and disorganized, shabby with plates near the toilet door, then on your way to work you get an accident and they take you to hospital. But going back to your home to look for blankets and other equipment to use at the hospital, they find a house in a mess. You can be embarrassed.

For some children there was a stigma connected to being labelled a thief, as one child stated about his photo of a pig:

> [Without a pig] you can suffer a lot. You can even die of hunger or go ahead to steal people's food and everyone will be pointing at you that you are a thief.

24.5.2.2 Psychological, Emotional and Social Challenges

Children described various psychological, emotional and social challenges. Experiencing anger was mentioned frequently, and was related to being abused, bullied in school, and wrongly accused of a crime, as well as witnessing other children suffering. The children expressed feelings of distress related to remembering their past and present losses (such as the loss of parents), being abused by extended family members and coping with the fears and challenges related to living with HIV. One child said:

> I get really angry when someone insults me by abusing me [and saying] that I should bury my mother. Yet she died a long time ago and I buried her.

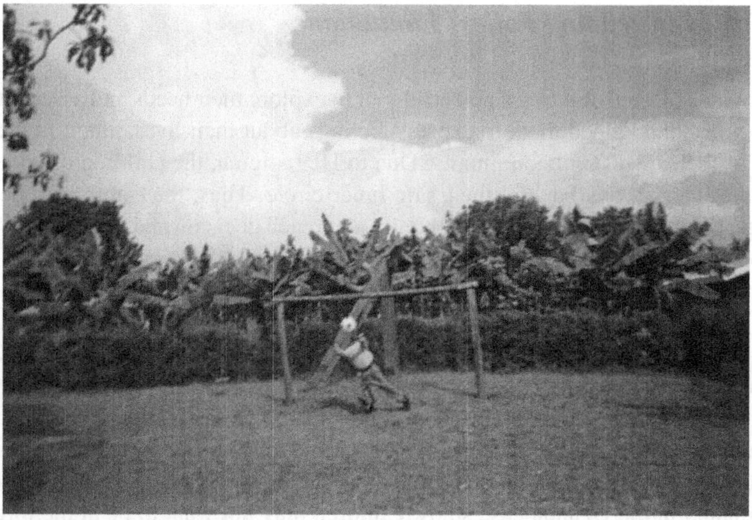

Fig. 24.4 Photo of playing football

Another described coping with fears of death by saying: "Friends can help you in many things. This helps you not to be alone and stop thinking of many things like that you are going to die." And another child discussed not wanting to feel sad and how they positively cope by saying:

> I don't like being sad all the time. So I love playing football. It helps me not to get lost in thoughts". (see Fig. 24.4)

24.5.3 Findings Summary

Putting cameras in the hands of children and young people highlight the often unheard voices of children who are orphaned and living with HIV. In our study, Photovoice offered valuable insights into the children's lives such as how the group was stigmatized, how the children were bullied by other school children, and how the community at large viewed these children. Despite discovering these insights the hope of the research team was that the children would take action, and consequently that social and policy change would occur. Since this did not happen, we were forced to re-visit the study and the methodology. In sharing the shortcomings of the study, our goal is to extend and improve on Photovoice in the areas of policy advocacy. Our hope is that other researchers can be mindful of Photovoice's limitations and take up additional strategies to improve on its effectiveness in reaching policy influencers.

24.5.4 Influencing Policy: Limitations

Photovoice offered children a powerful tool to explore their needs and assets. It gave them voice and helped them to express feelings about their lives, albeit in the confines of their own small community. Due to HIV stigma, the children did not wish to share their stories beyond their safe inner circle. Thus, their ability to become change agents in their broader community and reach decision and policy makers did not occur.

Transforming society requires change agents and the research community is increasingly recognizing children as health agents of change in their communities and households (Smyth et al. 2011; Onyango-Ouma et al. 2005; Kamo et al. 2008) and by NGOs (Rogers 2014). However, understanding the complexity of their involvement needs further attention. An understanding of the socio-political context is needed to assess the appropriateness of advancing children as change agents in a Photovoice study. Further, much caution is needed when HIV stigma plays a role as illuminated in the Uganda case study. Children may not want to be at the forefront of HIV policy or take social action when they feel stigmatized and are perceived or risk being perceived as "immoral" or "not worth anyone's time" "as death is knocking on their door" (Fournier et al. 2014a). Building capacity for advocacy to address stigma in their communities could be a possible next step for a Photovoice project.

Sharing photographs with decision and policy makers or having a public presentation is an important "action" step in the Photovoice method (Wang 1999; Wang and Burris 1997) and is a place to communicate the need for change to the community. However, at this stage of the research process in the Uganda case study, the children were not open to inviting family, school, church, or other community members to their photo display. They only wanted the other children from the group home and the staff to participate. To be true to the Photovoice method the research team tried to communicate the importance of inviting the broader community to the photo display, but to be ethical it remained flexible and honored the children's desire.

The issue of stigma had surfaced earlier in the project, but not understood deeply by the research team (Fournier et al. 2014a), namely when the team suggested going to the school to conduct the focus group sessions, the children said that they did not want to draw more attention to themselves and feared harassment and teasing. It was only later during the dissemination phase of the study that the gravity of this stigma registered with the team, particularly when Bridge and Fournier returned to Uganda and learned that the community had labeled the group home as a home for HIV-positive children and the children living there felt the stigma each day they left the home to walk to school (Fournier et al. 2014a). Despite the fact that the children's life experiences, especially regarding stigma, impact their life in such negative ways, the team decided that in the spirit of collaborative practice and fostering trust it was necessary to follow the children's wishes. As a result, the presentation to policy influencers, the final step in the Photovoice method, did not take place.

Instead, policy recommendations were made to the Director of the NGO to further enhance the care of the children in the group home. Although all recommendations were positively received by the Director, a challenge arose when one of the recommendations bumped up against internal politics in the group home. The children were receiving group counseling sessions of 2–3 h each once a week and as the team heard the stories from the children it was thought that psycho-social individual counseling could also be beneficial. The team took the suggestions to the Director, who at first supported the idea, but later turned it down. Many months later, while still working in the region and building increased contextual knowledge, the research team discovered that the dissonance was related to social status and internal politics.

The lesson learned from this experience was that there are often hidden social, cultural, and political influences that tie the hands of the people who try to keep the best interest of the children as a priority. Applying political science theory to this scenario, as will be seen in the next section, could have helped to understand how windows of opportunity can open to allow change to take place. Fortuitously, almost a year later such a window opened - the political situation had dissipated and individual counseling was instituted at the group home.

24.6 Political Science Theories

Co-creating new knowledge through critical discussions of photographs and translating this new knowledge into action steps through advocacy and public fora have been promoted as a method to support policy change in Photovoice studies (Haque and Eng 2011). For children and young people who are HIV sero-positive, finding ways for their concerns and assets to influence the policy environment to achieve social equity is complex given the many factors that influence their lives. Conceptualizing children as agents of change in their community, as in the work of Freire (1970) on empowerment education, places the burden or the capacity to act squarely on the shoulders of the children themselves. Training children in advocacy work could prepare them to think more about policy solutions and to build their skills in using stories, photographs and written words to influence others, including policy makers. However, children who are living with HIV illness, may not want to engage in such work, as was demonstrated in the Ugandan study discussed earlier, because of the negative attention and risk of additional bullying it might bring them. Thus, researchers must also be equipped with knowledge and skills to influence the policy environment. Understanding political science theories can shed light on the process of policy change and applying them in practice can facilitate creating sustained change to improve the health of individuals and communities. Models of policy-making are thought to be necessary to avoid scattered, imprecise, and ineffective change attempts (Steckler and Dawson 1982). Building the voice of the unheard and often neglected through developing a critical consciousness can go hand in hand with creating a social environment in which decision and policy makers are more likely to listen and take action (Campbell 2014). In this section, we present two limitations within the Photovoice method and recommend three ways to improve Photovoice by applying concepts from political science theories.

24.6.1 Issue/Limitation #1

As stated earlier, one of the goals of Photovoice is to bring an issue to the attention of decision and policy makers through public fora and displays of the photographs. In social science research making findings accessible- moving research into action - is referred to as knowledge translation (KT). Typical KT strategies include presentations, reports, and published summaries. Such passive, unilateral and hierarchical approaches have led to some push back among knowledge users who claim that they do not lead to sustainable change (Henderson et al. 2013). In their place more collaborative approaches, or integrated models of KT (iKT) have emerged to improve the relevance of research to knowledge users (Henderson et al. 2014), thus enhancing its impact on the policymaking process and facilitating sustainable system level change.

24.6.2 Recommendation #1

By including individuals affected by the issue under investigation, Photovoice is a participatory approach to research. In contrast, iKT focuses on integrating the end users of the knowledge being created. This integration can take the form of creating a community advisory committee (CAC) in which decision and policy makers are more closely involved in defining, conducting and implementing the research. A CAC is usually composed of representatives from various community partners, along with individuals whose lives may be affected by the issue under study and community leaders, decision or policy makers. A CAC may also be referred to as a "steering committee" to signify both the advisory as well as the decision-making capacities of the group. The Ugandan study did not have a CAC but may have benefited greatly from the advice of such a group especially regarding the finding of HIV stigma and its consequences. The advocacy potential of Photovoice can be enhanced by integrating both participants and CAC members. However, it must be noted that iKT/CAC alone may not necessarily be enough to influence the policy environment.

24.6.3 Issue/Limitation #2

There is little guidance in the Photovoice literature for those interested in employing Photovoice to achieve policy outcomes through policy approaches. Although many Photovoice studies have been conducted, few appear to discuss the role or method of influencing or changing policy. Photovoice studies tend not to articulate what policy approaches were used nor subsequent policy outcomes. This could be related to the complex nature of policymaking and inadequate knowledge and capacity of researchers to influence the policy environment. Influencing policy in many Photovoice studies is often reported as inviting decision and policy makers to a presentation, relying on linear models of policymaking that assume the existence of a continuum from research to policy change (Bernier and Clavier 2011). As a result, there is an assumption that good data, often in the form of statistics, will produce policy change (Tarantola 2007), which is the rational and logical view of policy making. Freudenberg and Tsui (2014) extend this further to say that policy change at any level does not always come about from providing strong scientific evidence, mobilizing a number of communities, or convincing a few decision makers, but rather results from taking multiple actions in many domains (Freudenberg and Tsui 2014). Minkler, Rubin and Wallerstein (2012) believe it is a combination of "stories and statistics" (p. 12) that facilitate policy change. In the HIV/AIDS context, political will, the level of civil society contribution and the level of stigma and discrimination are often cited as factors influencing policy making and outcomes.

24.6.4 Recommendation #2

Demystifying the policy making process (Minkler et al. 2012) can help researchers engage in policy thinking and facilitate action beyond typical KT or iKT strategies to influence the policy environment. This can be done through understanding and applying concepts from the policymaking process. Here, we offer a sampling of concepts from political science theory that may be helpful for Photovoice researchers to employ. By no means exhaustive, the following list of concepts can help demystify the policy making process: problem identification and issue framing, agenda setting, windows of opportunity, and coalition building. While these concepts are being reported individually, they not only often overlap but are most effective when they work in tandem.

24.6.4.1 Problem Identification and Issue Framing

Not all issues are viewed as problems in the eyes of decision and policy makers. Therefore, any issue under focus in a Photovoice study must be or become perceived as a problem in order to influence policy or reach policy makers. This is often referred to as problem identification in the policy making process. In the early stages and years of HIV activism when thousands of people were dying each day around the world, framing HIV issues as problems was not so difficult. Today, however, the number of deaths has been reduced and new competing issues have arisen. The current HIV/AIDS activist is now challenged to figure out how to engage in the 'mundane' aspects of HIV interventions such as monitoring drug stocks of ARTs (Colvin 2014). Colvin explains how the Treatment Action Campaign (TAC) and Médecins Sans Frontières have come together in South Africa to find ways to "mobilize allies, elicit moral outrage, pursue political and legal strategies, and generate a public narrative or frame for this new struggle" (p.67).

Researchers and practitioners using Photovoice can also benefit from understanding "contentious politics" or the ability of "outsiders" to upset the political context (Tarrow 2005). Social movements such as the civil disobedience campaign in South Africa, can disrupt the political context. Defined as "collective challenges, based on common purposes and social solidarities in sustained collective interaction with elites, opponents and authorities" (Tarrow 1994: 20), social movements can only upset the political context when a problem has been framed such that it is palatable to the public or is the most culturally relevant or appropriate. Capturing the attention of decision and policy makers to promote policy change and facilitate momentum with the general public to accept a solution and pressure for system wide change depends on how well an issue is framed.

24.6.4.2 Agenda Setting

In Photovoice projects, more emphasis needs to be placed on the dynamic interaction between individuals and the social – political context. Why do some issues make the agenda of policy makers while others do not? Understanding 'why' could provide insight to Photovoice researchers and help them plan for particular policy approaches required to bring about social and policy change. Understanding how to get issues on the agenda is referred to as agenda setting in the policy making process, which also includes preventing the issue from falling off the agenda.

Social movements can put the problem on the agendas of governments and multinational corporations such as happened with the campaign of universal access to AIDS treatment. The market transformation of anti-retroviral medications from "high price, low volume to universal access" in high-income countries is an example of change that occurred through the campaign of universal access to AIDS treatment (Kapstein and Busby 2013: 1). Activists found an opportunity or an opening in the fluid nature of the Trade-Related Aspects of Intellectual Property Rights (TRIPS) and were able to create controversy in the global arena, especially regarding the patent protection regime of TRIPS. South Africa in their legal challenge to the TRIPS regime used the media to campaign for lower drug costs highlighting that drugs were being denied to those that needed them in the name of profit (Kapstein and Busby 2013). Activists were able to shape the TRIPS debate and began providing information and advice to low income governments in the global South (Kapstein and Busby 2013). Media advocacy, specifically the tactic of attacking corporate reputations by naming and shaming, was particularly helpful for agenda setting (King and Pearce 2010). Media advocacy was also helpful in the TAC in South Africa (Heywood 2009). With the goal of remedying the inequitable access to health care for underserved people with HIV and AIDS, TAC was able to reframe the notion of equitable access to health care in moral, political, and legal terms as a right guaranteed under the South African constitution and thus point out a human rights violation (Grebe 2011). Not only is this a successful example of framing an issue, it also shows how framing an issue can help it land on the policy agenda, thus setting the agenda for policymaking.

24.6.4.3 Windows of Opportunity

The analytic Multiple Streams Framework (MSF) created by Kingdon (1984) and developed further by Zahariadis (2003, 2007) intends to answer how and why issues appear on the policy agenda (Boezeman et al. 2010). MSF contends that the policy process involves the movement of three independent and constantly flowing streams—problems, policy, and politics—each competing for the attention of decision makers. The moment these three policy-related streams intersect or act together a policy window opens and presents an opportunity to push through policy solutions (Kingdon 1995). A window may open when three things occur simultaneously: a problem has been clearly framed as requiring a solution or different policy; a variety of solutions are available; and some external and unforeseen event shifts public opinion, mood or political climate (Kingdon 1984). Changes in all three streams are needed before windows of opportunity emerge. A wide range of strategies must be employed in order to identify, create, anticipate and sustain a window of opportunity. Policy entrepreneurs (PE's) have been recognized as drivers of the policy agenda and being able to couple the problem, policy and politics streams and open policy windows (Kingdon 1984). PE's seize the opportunity to initiate action during this critical period of coupling because windows may not be open for long. Once a window is closed, the three streams separate, signaling that interest in the issue has dissipated, and the opportunity for action closes until the next window opens. In a Photovoice project, participants in the study could take on the role of a PE with some training. As well, members of a CAC working along side young people who have been trained in advocacy can also act as PEs or change agents.

Participating as change agents helps young people to assume roles that move them beyond being learners to researchers and educators of other youth and adults (Christens and Dolan 2011). This shift in the roles of youth also can promote positive outcomes such as leadership, community involvement, decision-making, psychological well-being, and even academic engagement (Kirshner and Ginwwright 2012). Given the impact of HIV stigma, young people may not want to become PE's. However, positive acknowledgement for such leadership work could help to change public attitude. Alternatively, partnerships with community stakeholders could also fill the role of a PE. Learning how to frame an issue is a key skill for PEs

(Zahariadis 2007) and is a skill that can be taught to young people. Framing facilitates coupling of the streams by enabling PEs to influence decision makers' perceptions of problems and solutions. Zahariadis (2003) explains that framing "may require PEs to become "sellers" where information is framed to highlight certain aspects and to hide others" (p. 91). Framing is a powerful force in shaping agendas (Haider-Markel 2001). Research teams utilizing Photovoice need to have members who can analyze the policy environment and country context in order to identify, anticipate and prepare for windows of opportunity.

24.6.4.4 Coalition Building

The Advocacy Coalition Framework (ACF) developed by Sabatier and Jenkins-Smith (1993, 1999) views policy change as a function of the beliefs of coalitions or policy actors. ACF views the policy process as a competition between coalitions of actors who advocate beliefs about policy problems and solutions. ACF focuses on strengthening policy issues and expanding policy windows of opportunity by emphasizing the alignment of groups or individuals with the same core beliefs, thus coordinating and leveraging their power to achieve shared goals. Belief systems include opinions on values, priorities, perspectives, and assumptions about a policy issue. ACF identifies beliefs as the causal driver for political behavior and acknowledges that in the complex process of policymaking coalitions must specialize in order to be influential (Sabatier and Jenkins-Smith 1993). Coalitions comprise a diverse set of groups and individuals (researchers, journalists, interest group leaders, agency officials, target groups, and so on) who might diverge on non-core beliefs or primary goals. Photovoice researchers can benefit from knowledge of local coalitions.

This framework also emphasizes the importance of the education of change agents and the sharing of scientific/technical information across sectors to influence the political stream. TAC from South Africa is an example of a coalition that joined forces with other allies to use public action campaigns to assert policy beliefs that were then translated into public policies. Advocacy coalitions like the TAC-led coalition in South Africa can bring about the right expertise and political alignment to exploit and trigger windows of opportunity (Brecher et al. 2010). Coalition building can produce large turnouts for campaign activities.

Establishing partnerships with diverse stakeholders who hold similar beliefs about the issue under focus in a Photovoice project early on in the project development can help to build momentum for social and policy change and challenge power held by NGO's and government institutions. Additionally, when policy options have been decided in a Photovoice study finding allies to further the cause increases participation and engagement in the work. Sustaining these partnerships after the project is over is a key consideration when initiating a Photovoice study.

Translating Photovoice findings into policy options can encourage policy related action and help to identify the most appropriate partners with similar beliefs. Influencing the policy environment can take years and working within coalitions to make change can be a slow process. However, if windows of opportunities present themselves, change can happen rather quickly as was seen with the global TRIPS regime. Coalitions can also engage in assessing a community's readiness for policy change by administering the Policy Readiness Toolkit (Nykiforuk et al. 2011). The tool is a self-administered questionnaire that encourages the adoption of healthy public policy within communities or organizations. As well, the tool outlines a number of strategies to encourage healthy policy change.

24.6.5 *Recommendation #3*

Understanding the local policy context and process in the community where the Photovoice project will take place is an important first step to the research endeavor. Spending time in the community where participants inhabit and taking on a more ethnographic inquiry before conducting a Photovoice study would provide a solid background of the socio-cultural-political context. Minkler et al. (2012) have developed a Community-Based Participatory Research framework that can help guide researchers and practitioners in engaging participants and community members in policy development and advocacy.

In summary, researchers and practitioners wanting to use Photovoice must be prepared to engage in efforts to influence the policy environment. Establishing relationships, building trust and mutual respect with decision makers and other allies are essential in the success of any policymaking endeavor and we would argue in any Photovoice study.

24.7 Concluding Thoughts

Photovoice is a powerful tool that gives voice to the often unheard or silenced and attaches meaning to the images that provide insights into the lives of those who take them. As an arts-based method, it engaged the children in a creative way to express themselves and share their experiences with trusted others. While theoretically Photovoice can be a powerful tool for influencing policy, as Wang et al. (1996) demonstrate in their Photovoice project in the Yunnan province of China, applying Photovoice to have a positive effect on children and young people's lives requires a greater understanding of the socio-political context, particularly of how HIV stigma can limit children's ability to be change agents and thus create challenges to the intended outcome of social and policy change. Political science theories can provide some guidance on how to affect change more broadly. Understanding how to frame a problem, push the problem or solution onto the agenda of decision and policy makers, create and optimize windows of opportunity, and join forces with allies to help shape the political arena are key strategies and skills for researchers who use

Photovoice, especially if they aim to influence policy and improve the health and well-being of individuals and communities.

References

Barnett, T., & Whiteside, A. (2002). *AIDS in the twenty-first century: Disease and globalization.* New York: Palgrave Macmillan.

Bernier, N. F., & Clavier, C. (2011). Public health policy research: Making the case for a political science approach. *Health Promotion International, 26*(1), 109–116.

Boezeman, D., Leroy, P., Maas, R., & Kruitwagen, S. (2010). The (limited) political influence of EE: A case study on Dutch environmental policies. *Ecological Economics, 69*(9), 1756–1764.

Brecher, C., Brazill, C., Weitzman, B. C., & Silver, D. (2010). Understanding the political context of "new" policy issues: The use of the advocacy coalition framework in the case of expanded after-school programs. *Journal of Public Administration Research and Theory, 20*(2), 335–355.

Bridge, A., Kipp, W., Jhangri, G. S., Laing, L., & Konde-Lule, J. (2006a). Nutritional status of young children in AIDS-affected households and controls in Uganda. *American Journal of Tropical Medicine & Hygiene, 74*(5), 926–931.

Bridge, A., Kipp, W., Raine, K., & Konde-Lule, J. (2006b). Nutritional status and food consumption patterns of young children living in Western Uganda. *East African Medical Journal, 83*(11), 363–370.

Campbell, C. (2014). Community mobilisation in the 21st century: Updating our theory of social change? *Journal of Health Psychology, 19*(1), 46–59.

Carlson, E. D., Engebretson, J., & Chamberlain, R. M. (2006). Photovoice as a social process of critical consciousness. *Qualitative Health Research, 16*, 836–852.

Castleden, H., & Garvin, T. (2008). Modifying photovoice for community-based participatory indigenous research. *Social Science & Medicine, 66*(6), 1393–1405.

Castonguay, G., & Jutras, S. (2009). Children's appreciation of outdoor places in a poor neighbourhood. *Journal of Environmental Psychology, 29*, 101–109.

Cheatham, A., & Shen, E. (2003). Community based participatory research with Cambodian girls in Long Beach, California: A Case Study. In M. Minkler & N. Wallerstein (Eds.), *Community-based participatory research for health* (pp. 121–134). San Francisco: Wiley.

Checkoway, B., Finn, J., & Pothukuchi, K. (1995). Young people as community resources: New forms of participation. In P. Adams & K. Nelson (Eds.), *Reinventing human services: Community- and family-centered practice* (pp. 189–202). New York: Aldine de Gruyter.

Christens, B. D., & Dolan, T. (2011). Interweaving youth development, community development, and social change through youth organizing. *Youth & Society, 43*, 528–548.

Clark-Ibanez, M. (2004). Framing the social world with photo elicitation interviews. *American Behavioral Scientist, 47*(12), 1507–1527.

Colvin, C. J. (2014). Evidence and AIDS activism: HIV scale-up and the contemporary politics of knowledge in global public health. *Global Public Health, 9*(1–2), 57–72.

Darbyshire, P., MacDougal, C., & Schiller, W. (2005). Multiple methods in qualitative research with children: More insight or just more? *Qualitative Research, 5*(4), 417–436.

Ehrenworth, M. (2003). Literacy and the aesthetic experience: Engaging children with the visual arts in the teaching of writing. *Language Arts, 81*(1), 43–51.

Eisner, E. (2003). The arts and the create on of mind. *Language Arts, 80*(5), 340–344.

Erdner, A., & Magnusson, A. (2011). Photography as a method of data collection: Helping people with long-term mental illness to convey their life world. *Perspectives in Psychiatric Care, 47*(3), 145–150.

Foster-Fishman, P., Nowell, B., Deacon, Z., Nievar, M. A., & McCann, P. (2005). Using methods that matter: The impact of reflection, dialogue, and voice. *American Journal of Community Psychology, 36*(3–4), 275–291.

Fournier, B., Bridge, A., Pritchard Kennedy, A., Alibhai, A., & Konde-Lule, J. (2014a). Hear our voices: A photovoice project with children who are orphaned and living with HIV in a Ugandan group home. *Children and Youth Services Review, 45*, 55–63.

Fournier, B., Bridge, A., Mill, J., Alibhai, A., Kennedy, A. P., & Konde-Lule, J. (2014b). Turning the camera back: A photovoice project with Ugandan children who are orphaned and living with HIV. *Sage Open, 4*(2), 2158244014530997.

Freidenberg, J. (1998). The social construction and reconstruction of the other: Fieldwork in El Barrio. *Anthropological Quarterly, 71*(4), 169–185.

Freire, P. (1973). *Education for critical consciousness*. New York: Continuum.

Freire, P. (1994). *Pedagogy of hope*. New York: Continuum.

Freire, P. (2000/1970). *Pedagogy of the oppressed*. New York: Continuum.

Freudenberg, N., & Tsui, E. (2014). Evidence, power, and policy change in community-based participatory research. *American Journal of Public Health, 104*(1), 11–14.

Government of Uganda. (2010, March). *UNGASS country progress report: Uganda*. Retrieved from: http://www.unaids.org/en/ CountryResponses/Countries/uganda.asp.

Grebe, E. (2011). The treatment action campaign's struggle for AIDS treatment in South Africa: Coalition-building through networks. *Journal of South African Studies, 37*, 849–868.

Greene, M. (1995). *Releasing the imagination: Essays on education, the arts, and social change*. San Francisco: Jossey-Bass Publishers.

Haider-Markel, D. P. (2001). Implementing controversial policy: Results from a national survey of law enforcement department activity on hate crime. *Justice Research and Policy, 3*(1), 29–61.

Haque, N., & Eng, B. (2011). Tackling inequity through a Photovoice project on the social determinants of health: Translating photovoice evidence to community action. *Global Health Promotion, 18*(1), 16–19.

Harper, D. (2000). Reimagining visual methods: Galileo to Neuromancer. In N. K. Denzin & Y. S. Lincoln (Eds.), *Handbook of qualitative research* (2nd ed., pp. 717–732). Beverly Hills: Sage.

Henderson, J., Brownlie, E., Rosenkranz, S., Chaim, G., & Beitchman, J. (2013). Integrated knowledge translation and grant development: Addressing the research practice gap through stakeholder-informed research. *Journal of the Canadian Academy of Child and Adolescent Psychiatry, 22*(4), 268.

Henderson, J., Sword, W., Niccols, A., & Dobbins, M. (2014). Implementing stakeholder-informed research in the substance abuse treatment sector: Strategies used by Connections, a Canadian knowledge translation and exchange project. *Substance Abuse Treatment, Prevention, and Policy, 9*(1), 1–5.

Heywood, M. (2009). South Africa's treatment action campaign: Combining law and social mobilization to realize the right to health. *Journal of Human Rights Practice, 1*, 14–36.

Hung, Y. (2014). East New York farms: Youth participation in community development and urban agriculture. *Children, Youth and Environments, 14*(1), 56–85.

Kamo, N., Carlson, M., Brennan, R. T., & Earls, F. (2008). Young citizens as health agents: Use of drama in promoting community efficacy for HIV/AIDS. *American Journal of Public Health, 98*, 201–204.

Kapstein, E. B., & Busby, J. W. (2013). *AIDS drugs for all: Social movements and market transformations*. Cambridge: Cambridge University Press.

King, B. G., & Pearce, N. A. (2010). The contentiousness of markets: Politics, social movements, and institutional change in markets. *Annual Review of Sociology, 36*, 249–267.

Kingdon, J. W. (1984). *Agendas, alternatives and public policies*. Boston: Little, Brown.

Kingdon, J. W. (1995). *Agendas, alternatives and public policies* (2nd ed.). New York: Harper Collins.

Kirshner, B., & Ginwright, S. (2012). Youth organizing as a developmental context for African American and Latino adolescents. *Child Development Perspectives, 6*(3), 288–294.

Kramarae, C., & Spender, D. (Eds.). (1992). *The knowledge explosion: Generations of feminist scholarship*. New York: Teachers College Press.

Kuo, L. H. (2007). Politicising documentary photography: Ren Jian and Guan Xiao Rong in late 1980s Taiwan. *Javnost-The Public, 14*(3), 49–64.

Leavy, P. (2009). *Method meets art: Arts-based research practice*. New York: Guilford Press.

Liamputtong, P. (2007). *Researching the vulnerable: A guide to sensitive research methods*. London: Sage.

Linton, R. (1990). Toward a feminist research method. In A. Jaggar & S. Bordo (Eds.), *Gender/body/knowledge: Feminist reconstructions of being and knowing* (pp. 273–292). New Brunswick: Rutgers University Press.

London, J. K., Zimmerman, K., & Erbstein, N. (2003). Youth-led research and evaluation: Tools for youth, organizational, and community development. *New Directions for Evaluation, 98*, 33–45.

Miles, M. B., & Huberman, A. M. (1994). *Qualitative data analysis: An expanded sourcebook* (3rd ed.). Thousand Oaks: Sage.

Minkler, M., Rubin, V., & Wallerstein, N. (2012). *Community-based participatory research: A strategy for building healthy communities and promoting health through policy change*. PolicyLink. Retrieved from http://www.policylink.org/atf/cf/%7B97C6D565-BB43-406D-A6D5-ECA3BBF35AF0%7D/CBPR.pdf.

Nykiforuk, C. I. J., Nieuwendyk, L. M., Atkey, K. M., Raine, K., Reed, S., & Kyle, K. (2011). *Policy readiness tool: Understanding a municipality's readiness for policy change and strategies for taking action*. Edmonton: School of Public Health, University of Alberta.

Onyango-Ouma, W., Aagaard-Hansen, J., & Jensen, B. B. (2005). The potential of schoolchildren as health change agents in rural western Kenya. *Social Science & Medicine, 61*, 1711–1722.

Pritchard Kennedy, A. (2012). Systematic ethnography of school age children with bleeding disorders and other chronic illnesses exploring children's perceptions of their partnership roles in family-centred care of their chronic illness. *Child Care Health Development, 38*(6), 863–869.

Purcell, R. (2007). Images for change: Community development, community arts, and photography. *Community Development Journal, 44*(1), 111–122.

Rogers, P. (2014). *Theory of change, methodological briefs: Impact evaluation* (Vol. 2). Florence: UNICEF Office of Research.

Rudkin, J. K., & Davis, A. (2007). Photography as a tool for understanding youth connections to their neighborhood. *Children, Youth and Environments, 17*(4), 107–123.

Sabatier, P. A., & Jenkins-Smith, H. C. (Eds.). (1993). *Policy change and learning. An advocacy coalition approach*. Boulder: Westview Press.

Sabatier, P. A., & Jenkins-Smith, H. C. (1999). The advocacy coalition framework: An assessment. In P. A. Sabatier (Ed.), *Theories of the policy process* (pp. 117–166). Boulder: Westview Press.

Shor, I., & Freire, P. (1987). What is the "dialogical method" of teaching? *Journal of Education, 169*(3), 11–31.

Smyth, C., Cass, B., & Hill, T. (2011). Children and young people as active agents in caregiving: Agency and constraint. *Children and Youth Services Review, 33*, 509–514.

Social change. (2015). In J. Scott & G. Marshall (Eds.), *A dictionary of sociology* (3rd Rev. Ed.). Retrieved from Oxford Reference Online Premium database.

Steckler, A., & Dawson, L. (1982). The role of health education in public policy development. *Health Education Quarterly, 9*, 275–292.

Strack, R. W., Magill, C., & McDonagh, K. (2004). Engaging youth through photovoice. *Health Promotion Practice, 5*(1), 49–58.

Tarantola, D. (2007). Of public health, policy, politics, and trees. *American Journal of Public Health, 97*, 19–33.

Tarrow, S. (1994). *Power in movement: Social movements, collective action and politics*. Cambridge: Cambridge University Press.

Tarrow, S. (2005). The dualities of transnational contention: "Two activist solitudes" or a new world altogether? *Mobilization: An International Quarterly, 10*(1), 53–72.

The United Nations Children's Fund [UNICEF]. (2006). *Africa's orphaned and vulnerable generations: Children affect by AIDS*. Zurich: Author.

UNAIDS. (2012). *Uganda: HIV and AIDS estimates 2012*. Retrieved from http://www.unaids.org/en/regionscountries/countries/uganda/.

Wang, C. C. (1999). Photovoice: A participatory action research strategy applied to women's health. *Journal of Women's Health, 8*(2), 185–19.

Wang, C. C. (Ed.). (2000). *Strength to be: Community visions and voices*. Ann Arbor: University of Michigan.

Wang, C. C. (2003). Using photovoice as a participatory assessment and issue selection tool: A case study with the homeless in Ann Arbor. In M. Minkler & N. Wallerstein (Eds.), *Community-based participatory research for health* (pp. 179–196). San Francisco: Jossey-Bass.

Wang, C. (2006). Youth participation in photovoice as a strategy for community change. *Journal of Community Practice, 14*(1), 147–161.

Wang, C., & Burris, M. A. (1994). Empowerment through photo novella: Portraits of participation. *Health Education & Behavior, 21*(2), 171–186.

Wang, C., & Burris, M. A. (1997). Photovoice: Concept, methodology, and use for participatory needs assessment. *Health Education & Behavior, 24*(3), 369–387.

Wang, C. C., & Pies, C. A. (2004). Family, maternal, and child health through photovoice. *Maternal and Child Health Journal, 8*(2), 95–102.

Wang, C. C., & Redwood-Jones, Y. A. (2001). Photovoice ethics: Perspectives from Flint photovoice. *Health Education & Behavior, 28*(5), 560–572.

Wang, C., Burris, M. A., & Ping, X. Y. (1996). Chinese village women as visual anthropologists: A participatory approach to reaching policymakers. *Social Science & Medicine, 42*(10), 1391–1400.

Wang, C. C., Yi, W. K., Tao, Z. W., & Carovano, K. (1998). Photovoice as a participatory health promotion strategy. *Health Promotion International, 13*(1), 75–86.

Wang, C. C., Morrel-Samuels, S., Hutchison, P., Bell, L., & Pestronk, R. M. (2004). Flint photovoice: Community-building among youth, adults, and policy makers. *American Journal of Public Health, 94*(6), 911–913.

World Health Organization. (2013). *Global update on HIV treatment 2013: Results, impact and opportunities*. Retrieved from http://apps.who.int/iris/handle/10665/85327.

World Health Organization/Joint United Nations Programme on HIV/AIDS/The United Nations Children's Fund. (2011). *Global HIV/AIDS response: Epidemic update and health sector progress towards universal access* (Progress report 2011). Zurich: Author.

Zahariadis, N. (2003). *Ambiguity and choice in public policy: Political decision making in modern democracies*. Washington, DC: Georgetown University Press.

Zahariadis, N. (2007). The multiple streams framework: Structure, limitations, prospects. In P. A. Sabatier (Ed.), *Theories of the policy process* (2nd ed., pp. 65–92). Boulder: Westview Press.

Index

P. Liamputtong (ed.), *Children and Young People Living with HIV/AIDS*,
Cross-Cultural Research in Health, Illness and Well-Being,
DOI 10.1007/978-3-319-29936-5

The manufacturer's authorised representative in the EU is Springer Nature Customer Service Centre GmbH, Europaplatz 3, 69115 Heidelberg, Germany. If you have any concerns regarding our products, please contact ProductSafety@springernature.com

Printed and bound by CPI Group (UK) Ltd, Croydon, CR0 4YY
30/09/2026
02225570-0017